Handbook of Experimental Pharmacology

Volume 99

Pharmacology of Peptic Ulcer Disease

Contributors

S.B. Benjamin, G.M.A. Börsch, S.H. Caldwell, E.L. Cattau
M.J. Collen, J. Doppman, D.E. Fleischer, J.D. Gardner
D.Y. Graham, A. Guglietta, D. Hollander, C.W. Howden
R.H. Hunt, R.T. Jensen, D.A. Johnson, J.H. Lewis, P.N. Maton
R.W. McCallum, L.S. Miller, R.V. Nardi, I.Parikh
J.W. Rademaker, A.M. Rosen, G. Sachs, A. Tarnawski
J. Van Dam, B. Wallmark, M.M. Wolfe, P.N. Yakshe

Editors

Martin J. Collen and Stanley B. Benjamin

Springer-Verlag
Berlin Heidelberg New York London Paris
Tokyo Hong Kong Barcelona Budapest

Martin J. Collen, M.D., F.A.C.P.
Professor of Medicine
Chairman of Research
Division of Gastroenterology
Loma Linda University School of Medicine
Loma Linda, CA 92354, USA

Stanley B. Benjamin, M.D., F.A.C.P.
Professor of Medicine and Chief,
Division of Gastroenterology
Georgetown University Hospital
Washington, DC 20007, USA

With 69 Figures

Library of Congress Cataloging-in-Publication Data. Pharmacology of peptic ulcer disease/contributors S.B. Benjamin ... [et al.] editors, Martin J. Collen and Stanley B. Benjamin. p. cm. – (Handbook of experimental pharmacology; v. 99) Includes bibliographical references.
ISBN-13: 978-3-642-75860-7 e-ISBN-13: 978-3-642-75858-4
DOI: 10.1007/ 978-3-642-75858-4
1. Peptic ulcer – Chemotherapy. 2. Peptic ulcer – Pathophysiology. I. Benjamin, Stanley B., 1948– . II. Collen, Martin J., 1943– . III. Series. [DNLM: 1. Peptic Ulcer. 2. Peptic Ulcer – drug therapy. W1 HA51L v. 99 / WI 350 P5365] QP905.H3 vol. 99 [RC821] 615′.1 s – dc20 [616.3′43061] DNLM/DLC for Library of Congress 91-4647 CIP

Softcover reprint of the hardcover 1st edition 1991

Typesetting: Best-set Typesetter Ltd., Hong Kong
27/3130-543210 – Printed on acid-free paper

List of Contributors

BENJAMIN, S.B., Division of Gastroenterology, Georgetown University Hospital, 3800 Reservoir Road NW, Washington, DC 20007, USA

BÖRSCH, G.M.A., Department of Medicine, Elisabeth-Hospital, Academic Teaching Hospital of the University of Essen Medical School, Moltkestraße 61, D-4300 Essen

CALDWELL, S.H., VAMC, Salem, Bldg. 4, Room 215 (111 G), 1970 Boulevard, Salem, VA 24153, USA

CATTAU, E.L., 6025 Walnut Grove Road, Suite 401, Memphis, TN 38119, USA

COLLEN, M.J., Division of Gastroenterology, Loma Linda University Medical Center and Jerry L. Pettis Memorial Veterans Hospital, 11201 Benton Street, Loma Linda, CA 92357, USA

DOPPMAN, J., Digestive Diseases Branch, National Institute of Diabetes and Digestive and Kidney Disease, National Institutes of Health, Bldg. 10, Rm. 9C-103, Bethesda, MD 20892, USA

FLEISCHER, D.E., Division of Gastroenterology, Room 2118, Georgetown University Hospital Medical Center, 3800 Reservoir Road NW, Washington, DC 20007-2197, USA

GARDNER, J.D., Digestive Diseases Branch, National Institute of Diabetes and Digestive and Kidney Disease, National Institutes of Health, Bldg. 10, Rm. 9C-103, Bethesda, MD 20892, USA

GRAHAM, D.Y., Department of Medicine, Gastroenterology Section, Baylor College of Medicine, and Department of Medicine, Digestive Disease Section, VA Administration Medical Center, 2002 Holcombe Blvd. (111D), Houston, TX 77030, USA

GUGLIETTA, A., Parke-Davis, Pharmaceutical Research Division, Warner-Lambert Company, 2800 Plymouth Road, Ann Arbor, MI 48105-2430, USA

HOLLANDER, D., Division of Gastroenterology, Department of Medicine, University of California, Medical Sciences Building, Room. I, C340, Irvine, CA 92717, USA

Howden, C.W., Division of Digestive Diseases and Nutrition, University of South Carolina School of Medicine, 2, Richland Medical Park, Suite 506, Columbia, SC 29203, USA

Hunt, R.H., Division of Gastroenteroloy, Department of Medicine, McMaster University, 1200 Main Street West, Hamilton, Ontario, L8N 3Z5, Canada

Jensen, R.T., Digestive Diseases Branch, National Institute of Diabetes and Digestive and Kidney Disease, National Institutes of Health, Bldg. 10, Rm. 9C-103, Bethesda, MD 20892, USA

Johnson, D.A., Digestive and Liver Disease Specialists Ltd., 844 Kempsville Road, Suite 106, Norfolk, VA 23502, USA

Lewis, J.H., Division of Gastroenterology, Room 2118, George-town University Hospital, 3800 Reservoir Road NW, Washington, DC 20007-2197, USA

Maton, P.N., Digestive Diseases Branch, National Institutes of Health, Bldg. 10, Rm. 9C-103, Bethesda, MD 20892, USA. Present address: The Oklahoma Foundation for Digestive Research, 711 Stanton Young Blvd., Suite 501, Oklahoma City, OK 73104, USA

McCallum, R.W., Department of Internal Medicine, Division of Gastroenterology, University of Virginia Medical School, Box 145, Charlottesville, VA 22908, USA

Miller, L.S., Digestive Diseases Branch, National Institute of Diabetes and Digestive and Kidney Disease, National Institutes of Health, Bldg. 10, Rm. 9C-103, Bethesda, MD 20892, USA

Nardi, R.V., Parke-Davis, Pharmaceutical Research Division, Warner-Lambert Company, 2800 Plymouth Road, Ann Arbor, MI 48105-2430, USA

Parikh, I., Cato Research Ltd., 4364 S. Alston Ave., Durham NC 27713, USA

Rademaker, J.W., Division of Gastroenterology, Department of Medicine, McMaster University, 1200 Main Street West, Hamilton, Ontario, L8N 3Z5 Canada

Rosen, A.M., Division of Gastroenterology, Room 2118, Georgetown University Hospital Medical Center, 3800 Reservoir Road NW, Washington, DC 20007-2197. Present address: Rockford Gastroenterology Center, 401 Roxbury Road, Rockford, IL 61107–5078, USA

Sachs, G., Veterans Administration Medical Center, West Los Angeles, Bldg. 115, Rm. 203, Wilshire & Sawtelle Bldvds., Los Angeles, CA 90073, USA

TARNAWSKI, A., Veterans Administration Medical Center, Long Beach III G, 5901 E. Seventh Street, Long Beach, CA 90822, USA

VAN DAM, J., Gastroenterology Division, Brigham and Women's Hospital, 75 Francis Street, Boston, MA 02115, USA

WALLMARK, B., Department of Biology, Gastrointestinal Research, AB Hässle, S-43183 Mōlndahl, Sweden

WOLFE, M.M., Gastroenterology Division, Brigham and Women's Hospital, 75 Francis Street, Boston, MA 02115, USA

YAKSHE, P.N., Division of Gastroenterology, Hepatology and nutrition, University of Minnesota, Department of Medicine, G.I. Division, Room 14-124 PWB, 516 Delaware Street S.E., Minneapolis, MN 55455, USA

Preface

Peptic ulcer disease manifested by symptoms and/or mucosal disease is a common problem worldwide. Although there was a great amount of research and clinical interest prior to the 1970s, with the development of the H_2 receptor antagonists and the more frequent utilization of upper gastrointestinal endoscopy there has been a rapid increase in our understanding of most aspects of the pathogenesis, diagnosis, and therapy of peptic ulcer disease. Furthermore, with the development of effective antisecretory and cytoprotective medication, research and clinical interests have shifted from the topic of "effective therapy" to the topics of "refractory disease" and "recurrent disease." Idiopathic gastric acid hypersecretion, epidermal growth factor, and *Helicobacter pylori* have emerged as topics of interest. And, with the recent development of video endoscopy and quantitative computer analysis, there is now an extremely objective means of diagnosis which allows precise documentation of peptic ulcer disease. Nevertheless, there is still no uniform agreement on all aspects of this field. In this book we have endeavored to cover in detail most aspects of the pathophysiology, diagnosis, and therapy of peptic ulcer disease. Our goal was to identify what is most pertinent by inviting contributions from individuals with documented expertise and research experience in special areas pertaining to this field. Because of the diligence and enthusiasm of the many authors who prepared the chapters for the book, the final result is a thorough review of the scientific literature; however, each author has also been allowed to state his own opinions and concepts. The editors are pleased to offer the reader this publication, which we hope will provide a timely update on a number of important issues pertaining to peptic ulcer disease.

MARTIN J. COLLEN
STANLEY B. BENJAMIN

Contents

CHAPTER 2

Epidermal Growth Factor

CHAPTER 3

Gastrin and Other Peptide Hormones

CHAPTER 4

The Role of Essential Fatty Acids in Gastric and Duodenal Protection and Ulcer Therapy

CHAPTER 8

Hypothesis of Peptic Ulcer: A Modern Classification of a Multifactorial Disease

CHAPTER 9

Nonulcer Dyspepsia

CHAPTER 10

The Natural History of Duodenal Ulcer Disease:
Has It Been Altered by Drug Therapy?

CHAPTER 12

Idiopathic Gastric Acid Hypersecretion

CHAPTER 13

Zollinger-Ellison Syndrome:
Advances in Diagnosis and Management

CHAPTER 1

Pharmacology of the Parietal Cell

G. SACHS, P.N. MATON, and B. WALLMARK

A. Introduction

It is well accepted that the level of acid secretion and hence the pH of contents of the lumen of esophagus, stomach, and duodenum and the pH of gastric wall plays a major role in the pathogenesis of ulcer disease. Therefore much effort has been devoted to exploring mechanisms of acid secretion and of resistance to acid in order to be able to treat ulcer disease. In this review, we briefly discuss the cellular biology of gastric acid secretion and relate this to the use of pharmacological agents in the treatment of ulcer disease.

B. Anatomy of Gastric Mucosa

The gastric mucosa is a single-layer infolded epithelium composed of several different cell types (ITO 1987). The surface of the mucosa is composed of surface epithelial cells, columnar in shape, possessing dense mucous granules. Infolding of the epithelium into gastric glands occurs, with the formation of mucous neck cells and then the stem cells of the gastric mucosal epithelium. Deeper within the glands, the two major cell types are the chief cells, which secrete pepsinogen, and the parietal cells, which secrete acid and intrinsic factor (Fig. 1, upper left).

The chief cell is an exocrine cell containing pepsinogen granules, which fuse with the apical membrane upon stimulation of zymogen secretion. The pepsinogen is activated in acid solutions of $pH < 3$, and peptic digestion contributes to acid related damage. Elevation of pH not only prevents the formation of active protease but also inactivates preexisting pepsin.

The parietal cell secretes HCl. It is located in the middle third of the gastric glands of the fundic mucosa. There are about 10^9 parietal cells in the human stomach. The parietal cell appears to be an end cell incapable of further division. The life span of the parietal cell in rat is about 90 days (HUNT and HUNT 1962) and presumably is about the same in man.

The parietal cell is conical, with the apical portion pointed into the lumen of the gastric gland. The base of the cell protrudes from the gland, giving the cell its name, peripheral or parietal. It has a diameter of about 15–20 μm. The content of mitochondria is very high, accounting for about 34% of cell volume. In addition to the numerous mitochondria, the cytoplasm has a

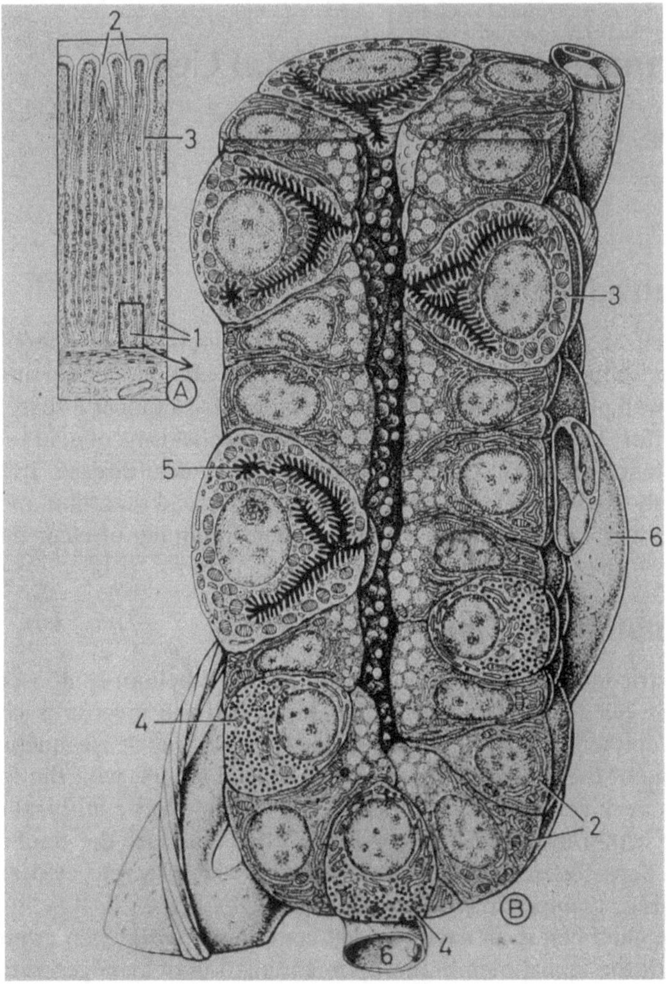

Fig. 1. *Upper left, A*: A cross-section of mouse gastric mucosa, showing surface epithelial cells (*2*), the neck region (*3*), and deeper in the tissue, gastric glands (*1*). *Right portion, B*: Diagram of a mammalian gastric gland showing blood supply (*6*), mature and immature peptic cells (*2,4*), parietal cells (*3*), and secretory canaliculus of the parietal cell (*5*). (Drawing courtesy of Dr. H.F. Helander)

unique structure, the secretory canaliculus, which is an infolding of the apical plasma membrane. In a cell that has not been stimulated to secrete acid, the secretory canaliculus bears a few stubby microvilli and the cytoplasm has a large number of smooth surfaced vesicles or tubules. With stimulation the tubulovesicles decrease in number, and the surface of the secretory canaliculus is expanded by the formation of long microvilli. Morphometric analysis has shown that the loss of tubulovesicular area is compensated for by an increase in canalicular area and vice versa (HELANDER and HIRSCHOWITZ

1974). A diagram of a gastric gland is shown in Fig. 1 and electron micrographs of a resting and a secreting parietal cell are shown in Fig. 2.

Both the tubulovesicles and the stimulated secretory canaliculus show a fuzzy coat which binds a variety of lectins, demonstrating the presence of carbohydrate on the extracellular face (OKAMOTO et al. 1989; HALL et al. 1990). The microvilli of the stimulated cell possess microfilaments in characteristic form, and staining for F- and G-actin using phalloidin derivatives has produced direct evidence for a cytoskeletal rearrangement upon stimulation (WOLOSIN et al. 1983). Quite recently an 80-kd protein has been shown to be involved in rearrangement of the tubulovesicles to secretory canaliculi (URUSHIDANI et al. 1987).

Staining of the parietal cell with antibodies against the gastric H^+,K^+-ATPase showed that in the resting cell the enzyme was present in the tubulovesicles of the cytoplasm, and in the stimulated state, in the microvilli of the secretory canaliculus (Fig. 2) (SMOLKA et al. 1983). The morphological change and relocation of the pump between these two membrane compartments suggest that there is a fusion-retrieval mechanism involved in activation and deactivation of acid secretion by this cell. In fact, expansion of the secretory canaliculus due to insertion of pump containing tubulovesicles appears essential for observable acid secretion by the gastric mucosa.

C. Secretion by the Stomach

I. General

The function of the stomach is to prepare ingested food for digestion by the small intestine. However, the digestive capacity of the lower gut is such that achlorhydria does not appear to have a measurable effect on efficiency of absorption of dietary materials. In man, acid as part of this preparation process was perhaps necessary prior to the cooking of meat since primitive man was probably a scavenger. Modern man appears to survive well with no acid in the stomach. There has been a perception, however, that anacidity can result in overgrowth of gastric flora, with production of nitrosamines, or perhaps infections due to ingested bacteria not killed owing to the elevation of pH. Retention of this property suggests significant function. Indeed, there is some evidence that achlorhydria can increase susceptibility to various infectious agents (HOWDEN and HUNT 1987).

In terms of agents used to treat ulcer disease, neither the H_2 blockers nor the H^+,K^+-ATPase inhibitors produce 24-h achlorhydria. Achlorhydria is found in pernicious anemia, but there appears of little consequence in terms of bacterial overgrowth and consequent nitrosamine production.

The secretory capacity of the stomach is large, producing as much as 1.5 liters of fluid per day. The majority of fluid flow is due to function of the oxyntic glands of fundic mucosa.

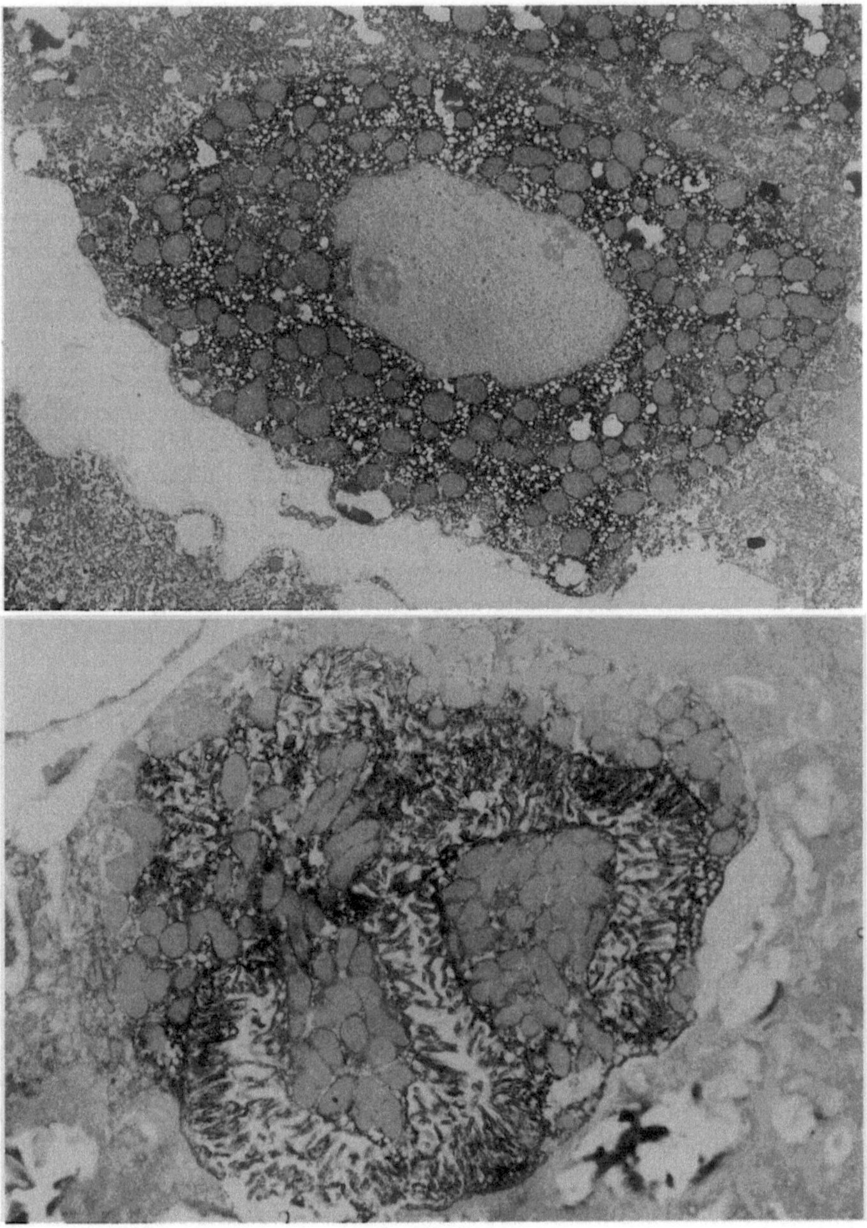

a

b

Fig. 2. **a** A resting parietal cell stained with a monoclonal antibody against the H^+,K^+-ATPase, showing large numbers of mitochondria, and the ATPase present in the smooth surfaced tubulovesicles. **b** A stimulated parietal cell also stained with a monoclonal antibody against the H^+,K^+-ATPase, showing the disappearance of tubulovesicles and relocation of the pump to the villi of the expanded secretory canaliculus

The composition of secreted fluid is essentially isotonic, and it contains about 140 mM HCl, 15 mM K, 5 mM Na, and organic anions. The secretion as measured in the lumen of the stomach is the result of function (secretion, absorption) of the total cell population of the gastric epithelium, namely peptic cells, oxyntic (parietal) cells, mucous neck cells, and surface epithelial cells.

II. Secretion and Absorption by Surface Epithelial Cells

The surface cells of the stomach are thought to have the capacity to secrete HCO_3^-, in part by anion exchange, in part by secondary active transport (FLEMSTROM 1987). The HCO_3^- secretory rate has been estimated to be about 10% of the maximal acid secretory rate. In addition the surface cells are able to reabsorb Na^+ through Na^+ channels that can be blocked by amiloride. The activity of the surface cell layer will therefore modify the primary secretion produced by the gastric glands. Na^+ is reabsorbed by the surface cells along with Cl^-. Anion exchange removes Cl^- and adds HCO_3^-, and the HCO_3^- will react with H^+ to form CO_2 and water. Thus secretion of HCO_3^- by anion exchange results in a decrease in the primary acidity of secretion, as does transport of HCO_3^- by secondary active secretion through HCO_3^- channels.

HCO_3^- secretion by the surface epithelial cells of the gastric mucosa has been considered to be an important part of the gastric barrier (SILEN 1987), the ability of the gastric epithelium to resist acid damage. The gastric barrier includes all properties that endow the gastric mucosal epithelium with resistance to a highly acidic luminal environment.

D. Gastric Barrier

The gastric epithelium forms a continuous layer separating the acidic lumen from the submucosa. There are at least four major cell types: the surface cells, mucous neck cells, parietal cells, and peptic cells. There are likewise several components of the gastric barrier.

Secretion of mucus by the surface and the mucous neck cells has often been invoked as generating a structure giving acid resistance to the gastric epithelium. It has been claimed that a pH gradient is measurable across this mucous layer (ALLEN and GARNER 1980). However, detailed calculations have shown that with HCO_3^- secretion by the surface cells at about 10% of acid secretion, at a bulk pH of less than 3 no pH gradient would exist across the mucous layer (ENGEL et al. 1984). At best, the mucus could serve as an extension of an unstirred layer of higher pH at a relatively low luminal acidity (when the pH exceeds 3). The function of mucus is more likely to be mechanical rather than physical. An experiment illustrating this compared the pH sensitivity of amiloride-sensitive Na uptake in tissue with and without a mucous barrier (stomach and frog skin). The Na uptake titrated with the same apparent pKa in both tissues (MACHEN and PARADISO 1987).

The surface membrane of the gastric cells must constitute a relatively proton-impermeable barrier. It has been shown, using peptic cells in culture, that these cells resist a pH of 2, but not one below that (SANDERS et al. 1985). This would imply that there is a paucity of proton transporting pathways in the surface membrane of this cell type. In the case of the parietal cell, a back leak of H^+ would be compensated for by the activity of the proton pump, the H^+,K^+-ATPase. In the case of surface cells, their apical membranes must also contain few if any proton pathways, given the low pH to which these membranes are exposed. Earlier work had suggested that artificial lipid bilayers are relatively permeable to protons (GUTKNECHT 1984). In the case of the gastric mucosa, with such high hydrogen ion concentrations, it must be that even the lipid bilayer has a low permeability. More recent work on artificial lipid membranes has shown that the high permeability was due to contamination with either weak bases or free fatty acids, either of which would lead to overestimates of proton permeability (GUTKNECHT 1988). Considering these more recent data, it appears more likely that native bilayers have a low proton permeability, comparable to that for other cations, and probably that specialized proteins are used by nature to endow proton (or hydroxyl) permeability to membranes. Presumably such proteins are absent in the apical membranes of gastric cells.

It has been shown in amphibia that tight junctions exist between surface cells, between oxyntic cells, and between mucous neck cells (ITO 1987). A leaky tight junction would allow access of hydrogen ion to the basal lateral surface of the cells, and these membranes, as discussed below, contain several proteins that can transport hydrogen ions. The tight junctions must therefore be relatively proton impermeable. A loss of this property would inevitably result in acidification of the basal lateral environment of the cells, with consequent damage to the cells when the pH regulatory mechanisms of the epithelial cells are overwhelmed. Figure 3a shows the structure, on freeze-fracture, of a tight junction between oxyntic cells of *Necturus* gastric mucosa. This junction shows frequent strands, suggesting that it is a relatively tight, tight junction.

Figure 3b shows La^{3+} infiltration of the same tight junctional region. La^{3+} is present between the cells in the lateral space but does not penetrate the tight junctional region. Electrophysiological and morphological data in this species have shown that the tight junction between surface epithelial cells is also very tight (DEMAREST and MACHEN 1985). Figure 4a shows a model whereby progressive damage to tight junctions results in increased H^+ back leak, which will eventually overwhelm the pH regulatory mechanisms of the cells.

Secretion of HCO_3^- by the surface or parietal cells, apart from partially neutralizing gastric content, also reflects the pH regulatory mechanisms possessed by these cells. For HCO_3^- secretion to occur, intracellular bicarbonate must be raised above the electrochemical equilibrium for this anion across the apical membrane of the cell. There are three known pH regulatory

a
b

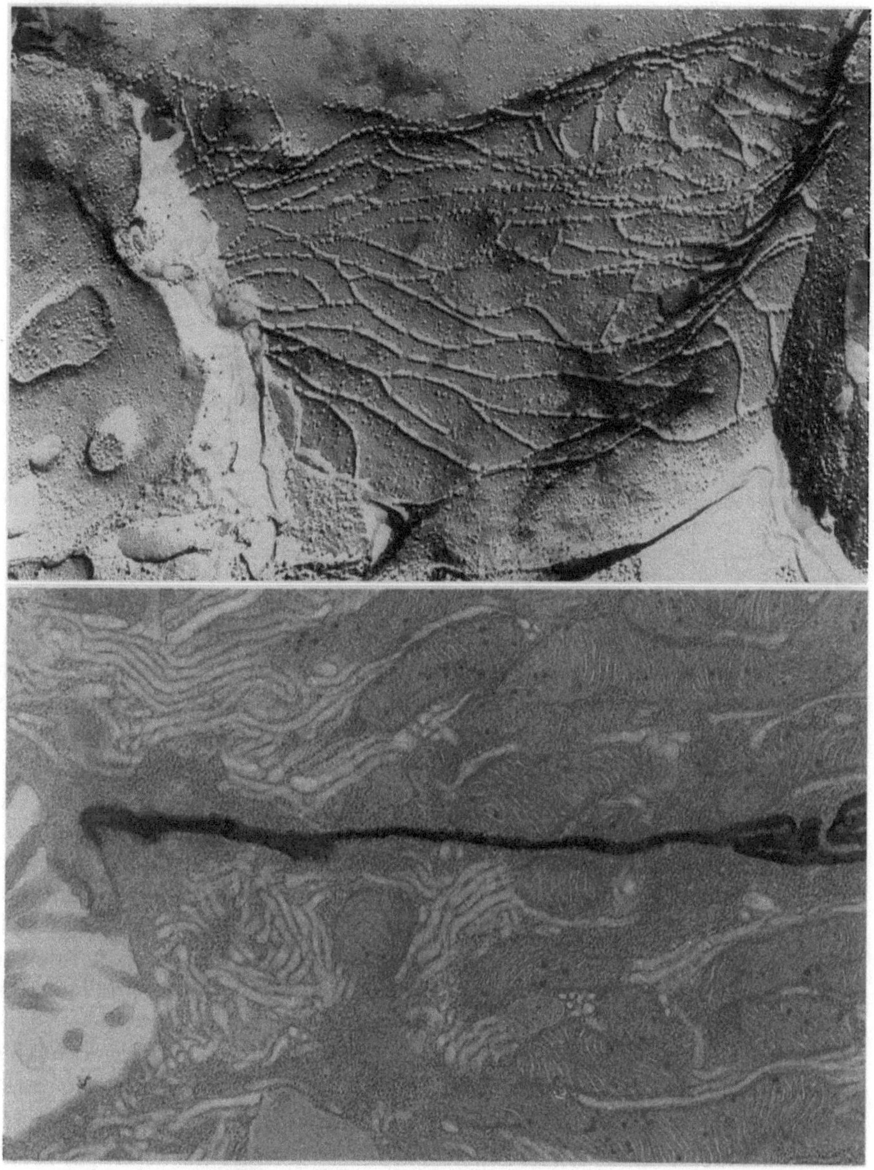

Fig. 3. **a** A tight junction between two oxyntic cells of a *Necturus* gastric gland, showing a large number of strands. The average length of these junctions is 0.556 $\pm$ 0.058 um. The number of interfaces was 30. In the case of surface cells, the dimensions and interfaces are roughly one-half those of the oxyntic cell tight junction. **b** La^{3+} infiltration of a *Necturus* gastric mucosa, showing the presence of La^{3+} in the lateral space and its absence in the tight junction region. With this method, the length of the tight junction region is ascertained as 0.510 $\pm$ 0.059 μm (n = 30). Again, for surface cells the length is about one-half that of oxyntic cells. (Micrographs courtesy of D. Anderson)

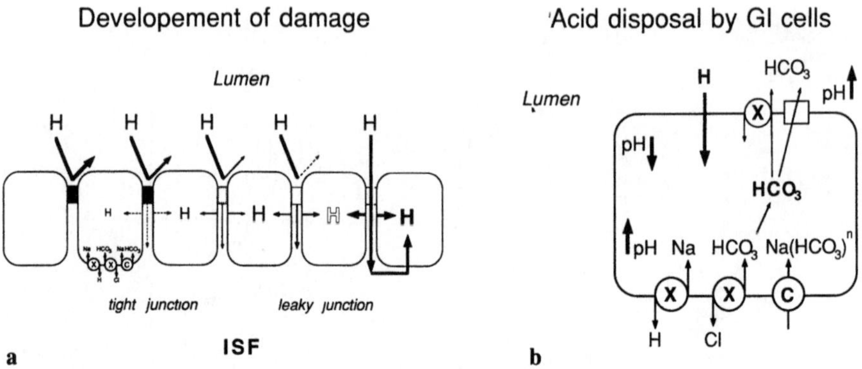

Fig. 4. a A model of gastric epithelial cells separated by tight junctions. Progressive damage to tight junctions results in back leak of H^+, and entry of H^+ into the cells from the basal lateral, not apical surface. Various pH regulatory mechanisms are present in the cells. *ISF*, interstitial fluid. **b** pH_i regulatory mechanisms known to be present in gastric cells. These include cation exchange, anion exchange, and $Na(HCO_3)^n$ cotransport on the basal lateral surface, and anion exchange and bicarbonate conductance on the apical surface

pathways in parietal cells and presumably also in surface cells, although in the latter case they would be regulated differently. The major pathway is Cl^-/HCO_3^- exchange (MUALLEM et al. 1985, 1988; PARADISO et al. 1987), which appears to be rather inactive below pH 7.1. Cell acidification would result in lowered HCO_3^-. With an active anion exchanger, inward HCO_3^- flux coupled to outward Cl^- flux would elevate pH_i. A second exchanger, Na^+/H^+ exchange (MUALLEM et al. 1985, 1988), has been shown to be present and to be activated by histamine in rabbit parietal cells, allowing elevation of pH_i by about 0.2pH units. Another transporter that could both increase pH_i and also serve to power HCO_3^- secretion is the $Na(HCO_3)^n$ cotransporter (CURCI et al. 1987), provided n was 2 or less. In kidney (KONDO and FROMTER 1987) this cotransporter has a stoichiometry of 3 HCO_3^- ions to 1 Na^+ ion, and hence has a net charge of 2. Since cell potential is positive exterior, this carrier would always serve to export HCO_3^- in the kidney, at realistic intracellular $[Na]_i$. In gastric parietal cells, and presumably on the basal lateral surface of surface cells, it appears that the stoichiometry is less, perhaps 2 HCO_3^- for 1 Na^+, with only one negative charge being transported per cycle. This would allow for HCO_3^- entry, depending on the anion and Na^+ gradients and cell potential. Extrusion of HCO_3^- across the apical membrane via conductive pathways or by Cl^-/HCO_3^- exchange would be coupled to the activity of the $Na(HCO_3)_2$ transporter to allow secondary active HCO_3^- secretion. It appears that the cotransporter is inhibited by secretagogues, presumably for maintenance of tight coupling between HCO_3^- production by the pump and Cl^- entry for HCl secretion (CURCI et al. 1987; TOWNSLEY and MACHEN 1990). Finally, a vacuolar ATP-driven proton pump on the basal lateral surface would also serve to export H^+ and alkalinize the cell. However, this has not been demonstrated in the stomach. These pathways are illustrated in Fig. 4b. They are present at different levels in the various cells of the gastric epithelium, and presumably are regulated differently in the different cell types, either by second messengers or by changes in pH_i.

E. Agents Thought to Affect Gastric Barrier Function

In this section, three classes of compound are discussed, sucrose aluminium sulfate (sucralfate, Karafate), prostaglandins, and bismuth compounds.

I. Sucralfate

Sucralfate has been shown to be of benefit in ulcer disease, but its mechanism is unknown (MAY 1989). Various hypotheses to account for its action, such as stimulation of prostaglandin biosynthesis, have not proven correct. Perhaps the best explanation to date is that it binds to the surface of the ulcer crater, thereby aiding the healing process. A similar explanation was put forward for the benefits of a compound no longer in use, carbenoxolone (glycyrrhetinic acid, found in liquorice). Measurements of the action of this latter compound showed that it did indeed change the passive permeability of the tight junction in the antrum, arguing perhaps for a mechanism of action of these compounds on tight junction properties (BAJAJ et al. 1977).

II. Prostaglandins

In ulcer disease, use is made of derivatives of prostaglandins of the E_2 type designed to be more slowly metabolized than the natural product. It is thought that they have at least two actions (WHITTLE and VANE 1987). One is inhibition of histamine stimulated acid secretion, by binding to an inhibitory protein for adenylate cyclase (CHEN et al. 1988). Elsewhere in the gastrointestinal tract, they appear to activate adenylate cyclase and thus stimulate fluid secretion, producing the side-effect of diarrhea. In general, data showing benefit in ulcer healing (EULER et al. 1989) can be interpreted as mainly due to the antisecretory activity, and it is not possible to achieve the potency of other types of receptor antagonist without increasing side-effects. A second action in the stomach has been called "cytoprotective" (WHITTLE and VANE 1987). The precise meaning of this general term is not clear. Experimentally it has been shown that pretreatment with prostaglandins reduces hemorrhage in rat gastric mucosae when rats are treated in vivo with ethanol, alkali, or hot water. It is possible that prostaglandins regulate the various pH_i regulatory mechanisms discussed above, which may help explain some of their cytoprotective action. The contribution of the cytoprotective actions of prostaglandins to treatment of peptic ulcer disease in man is not definite.

A specific therapeutic mechanism of action that has been proposed for ulceration caused by nonsteroidal anti-inflammatory drugs (NSAIDs) is based on NSAID inhibition of cycloxygenase, the system which is responsible for the biosynthesis of prostaglandins from arachidonic acid. It is therefore possible that prostaglandins might be useful in prophylaxis of NSAID induced ulcers (FUKUI et al. 1988). Several types of prostaglandins are manufactured by gut epithelium, and prostaglandins outside the E_2 class may also be beneficial in reducing NSAID induced gastric damage.

III. Bismuth Compounds

Bismuth compounds have been in use for decades in dyspepsia. However, until recently there was no evidence for any specialized action of these chemicals. The discovery of the association of *Helicobacter pylori* (previously named *Campylobacter pylori*) with duodenal ulcer, ulcer recurrence, and gastritis (CHENG et al. 1989), and an action of bismuth compounds in inhibiting the growth of this organism, has sparked renewed interest in bismuth compounds (ARMSTRONG et al. 1987). It does appear that part of their action is due to a decrease in the population of this organism. *Helicobacter* produces large quantities of urease, and therefore NH_4^+. This cation can enter the cells as NH_3, resulting in cell alkalinization and perhaps damage, or *Helicobacter* could produce a toxin damaging to the cells themselves. In either case, disruption of the gastric barrier could result. In the case of helicobacter itself NH_3 production by urease and NH_4 export would allow the organism, to survive is an acid environment.

It does seem that therapy which reduces *Helicobacter* accelerates ulcer healing and reduces ulcer recurrence. The aim of this type of therapy is to eradicate the organism and bismuth compounds have been shown to be able to do this, as have combinations of antibiotics or antibiotics coupled with bismuth. Eradication appears necessary to provide healing data comparable to those of H_2 antagonists.

F. Ion Transport by the Parietal Cell

I. Apical Surface

The parietal cell has several ion transport pathways in its apical surface (canalicular surface) related to Cl^- dependent fluid transport and to secretion of HCl.

There is a secondary active secretion of Cl^-, by a Cl^- entry mechanism uphill across the basal lateral surface, and Cl^- exit via a channel or conductance in the apical membrane. This process accounts for much of the current across the gastric mucosa and also accounts for the transtissue potential oriented lumen negative (HOGBEN 1955).

In terms of mechanism the Cl^- secretion is generally similar to that by other epithelia. This is usually modeled as uphill transport of Cl^- across the basal lateral surface by direct or indirect coupling of Cl^- movement to inward Na^+ entry. The driving force for Cl^- entry is therefore maintained by turnover of the Na^+,K^+-ATPase, which maintains low intracellular Na^+. Electrogenic Cl^- secretion across the apical surface is downhill via a channel or conductance since the transapical potential is positive, exterior (DEMAREST et al. 1990).

The apical surface in the stimulated state also contains a KCl pathway (WOLOSIN and FORTE 1984), to provide K^+ to the H^+,K^+-ATPase and Cl^- for HCl secretion. It is not known whether the KCl pathway is due to coupling between two channels or to a single coupled protein complex. The gastric proton pump, the H^+,K^+-ATPase, is present in the canalicular and apical surface of the stimulated parietal cell (Fig. 5).

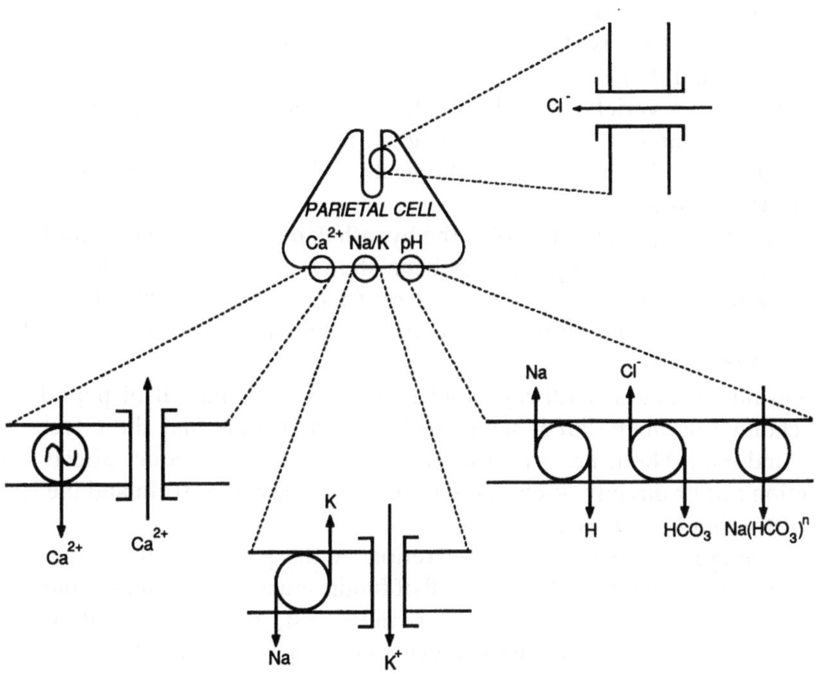

Fig. 5. Composite diagram of the known ion pathways in the parietal cell. Above is the exploded view of the apical surface, below the exploded views of the basal lateral surface. The apical surface contains a Cl^- channel, to allow for transtissue potential even in the absence of secretion. The basal lateral membrane contains the Ca^{2+} pump that is stimulated by calmodulin and a variety of receptor operated Ca channels (*left-hand side*). The Na^+ pump is coupled to K^+ channels and pH regulation as well as Cl^- supply to the apical surface is handled by the Na/H exchanger, the anion (Cl/HCO_3) exchanger, and sodium bicarbonate cotransport

II. Basal Lateral Surface

The known pathway for Cl^- entry basal laterally is the Cl^-/HCO_3^- exchanger, similar in mechanism to the anion exchanger of red cells. Cloning and sequencing of the gastric anion exchanger has shown that it has a large N-terminal extension distinguishing it from the red cell anion exchanger (SHULL, personal communication). There is also Na^+/H^+ exchange and $NaHCO_3$ cotransport. The former appears to be stimulated with secretion (MUALLEM et al. 1988), the latter inhibited (CURCI et al. 1987; TOWNSLEY and MACHEN 1990). In addition to these passive pathways there is the Na^+,K^+-ATPase and a Ca^{2+}-ATPase (MUALLEM et al. 1985) as well as Ca^{2+} entry pathways involved in cholinergic stimulation of the parietal cell (Fig. 5).

III. Stimulation of Acid Secretion

In the absence of stimulus, acid secretory rate is low in man, but not negligible. Food is the major stimulus for acid secretion and has considerable buffering capacity. Nighttime secretion occurs in the absence of luminal buffering and hence is the time when gastric pH is generally at its lowest (FIMMEL et al. 1985).

There are a variety of pathways for regulation of acid secretion, some of which are subject to pharmacological intervention. The pathways for stimulation can be classified anatomically. Thus there are cephalic and peripheral pathways.

The cephalic pathways involve the hypothalamus and vagal outflow to the stomach. A variety of peptides has been shown to affect acid secretion and other gastric functions when injected centrally, but it is difficult to know specifically which peptides play a role in central regulation of gastric secretion (TACHE 1988).

Peripheral neural pathways appear to be a combination of peptidergic and cholinergic fibers but it seems to be the consensus that the effects are often indirect. There are various cells whose secreted product affects acid secretion rather directly, such as the G cell of the gastric antrum and the ECL cell of the fundic mucosa.

The major stimulant of acid secretion by the parietal cell is histamine, (probably) released from the ECL cell of fundic mucosa. Histamine binds to a receptor, the H_2 receptor on the parietal cell, generating both cAMP increases and a transient increase in cytosolic $[Ca]_i$ (CHEW and BROWN 1986). Release of histamine from the ECL cell is due to activation of muscarinic and/or gastrin receptors (BERGQVIST and OBRINK 1979). Histamine release plays a major role in activation of parietal cell acid secretion, but in the dog, for example, atropine is able to block all forms of stimuli, suggesting that muscarinic receptors also have an important role (WALSH 1987). The parietal cell itself has an M3 muscarinic receptor rather than an M_1 receptor; it is blocked by atropine but only weakly by pirenzepine, a selective M_1 antagonist

(PFEIFFER et al. 1988). Activation of this M3 receptor results in both enhanced Ca^{2+} entry and Ca^{2+} release from intracellular stores (MUALLEM and SACHS 1985; NEGULESCU and MACHEN 1988). There is also a gastrin receptor on the parietal cell, which gives a transient elevation of $[Ca]_i$, but the source of this Ca^{2+} is obscure (MUALLEM and SACHS 1985). Only histamine increases intracellular cAMP, accounting for its dominance in the stimulation of parietal cell acid secretion. In all in vitro models tested, cAMP is able to elicit a full secretory response.

The action of gastrin, apart from histamine release, is also trophic for the fundic mucosa (JOHNSON 1987), and whether the Ca^{2+} signal seen for gastrin in parietal cells relates to a secretory receptor or a residual trophic receptor on this non-dividing has not been established.

The complicated interactions between the three known primary stimuli of parietal cell acid secretion make correlation of some of the in vivo pharmacological data with in vitro models somewhat difficult. The scheme shown in Fig. 6 is a personal working model rationalizing a variety of findings in the intact animal. Figure 6b illustrates the cellular events of stimulation.

There is as yet fragmentary knowledge of the targets for the second messengers of the parietal cell. As in other cells, presumably these are proteins phosphorylated by cAMP dependent kinase, or by calmodulin kinase or C kinase.

IV. Mechanism of Parietal Cell Stimulation

Activation of HCl secretion by the parietal cell involves activation of the gastric proton pump, the H^+,K^+-ATPase. This occurs in at least two stages, one involving a relocation of the pump from a cytoplasmic to plasma membrane site, the other a change in transport properties of the pump associated membrane to allow K^+ access to the extracellular surface of the acid pump.

The change in location of the ATPase from cytoplasmic tubulovesicles to the microvilli of the secretory canaliculus has been demonstrated by both morphometric and immunological methods (HELANDER and HIRSCHOWITZ 1974; SMOLKA et al. 1983). It would seem that this change in cellular location of the pump is essential for acid secretion into the lumen of the gastric gland.

It has been shown that the properties of the ion transport pathways associated with the H^+,K^+-ATPase change dramatically. When present in the tubulovesicles of resting cells, the ATPase is inactive because of an absence of K^+ on its extracellular face. K^+ on this face of the enzyme is required to stimulate ATP turnover by the enzyme which catalyzes an exchange of cytosolic H^+ for luminal K^+ (SACHS et al. 1976; WOLOSIN 1985). The membrane of the tubulovesicles has low or no KCl permeability. In the stimulated membrane of the secretory canaliculus, there is adequate KCl permeability to allow pump turnover (WOLOSIN 1985). Thus part of the stimulation is due to activation of KCl pathways in the membrane. The net

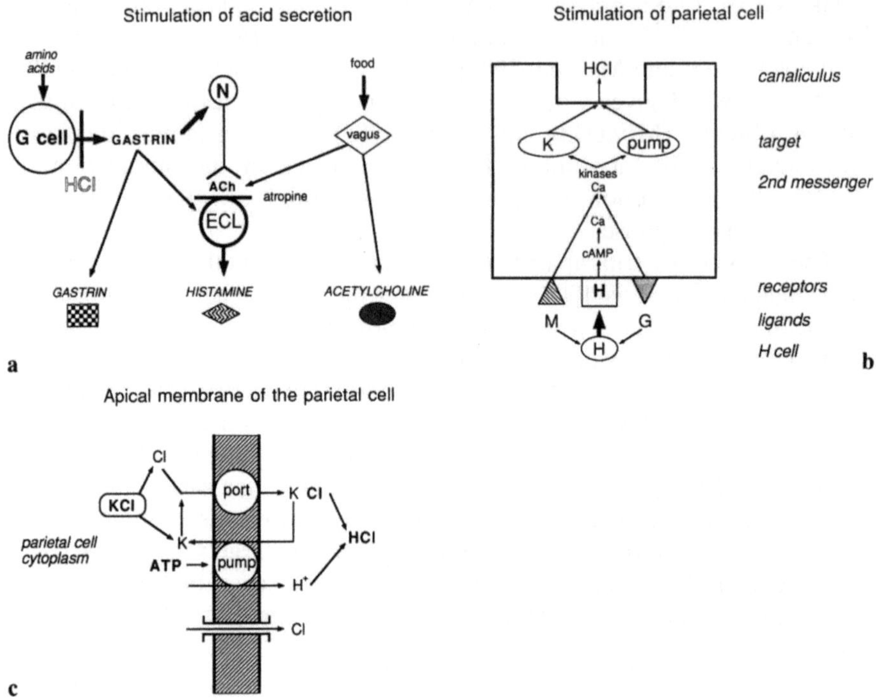

Fig. 6. a Stimulation pathways of the parietal cell, involving neural pathways, paracrine pathways, and receptors on the parietal cell. **b** Intracellular messengers in the parietal cell showing that histamine stimulates both cAMP and Ca, whereas acetylcholine and gastrin stimulate only Ca. The effect of change of second messenger levels is to allow pump insertion into the apical or canalicular membrane and to activate a KCl pathway. **c** Diagram of the pathways known to be present in the stimulated membrane of the parietal cell. The H^+,K^+-ATPase exchanges H for K. K is supplied by a KCl cotransport (or coupled conductance) pathway. In parallel there is a Cl conductance, which may or may not be part of the KCl pathway

effect of this activation of a KCl pathway is to allow KCl efflux from the cytosol of the parietal cell and K^+ reuptake by the pump in exchange for protons, resulting in net HCl secretion (see also Figs. 5, 6c).

G. Receptor Antagonists

As a class, receptor antagonists prevent or reverse stimulation of parietal cell acid secretion (MÅRDH et al. 1988). Histamine appears to play a central role in the receptor hierarchy of the parietal cell; therefore the histamine antagonists are the most effective suppressants of acid secretion. On the other hand, as discussed above, cholinergic mediation of histamine release as well as direct cholinergic activation of parietal cell secretion occurs; hence muscarinic antagonists are also able to reduce acid secretion (Chan and Soll 1988). Inhibition of gastrin receptors or histamine release would also be effective in suppression of acid secretion, but only one rather weak antagonist of gastrin action, proglumide, has been described. Unpublished work has shown that certain types of mast cell stabilizers are able to prevent gastrin stimulation of acid secretion by rabbit gastric glands and of histamine release (A. Kirk et al., unpublished observations).

I. Muscarinic Antagonists

Pharmacological and cloning methods have resulted in the description of five subclasses of muscarinic receptor. These receptors are widely distributed in the body and therefore it is difficult to get a highly selective gastric action of muscarinic antagonists. Selective antagonists show that two types of muscarinic receptor are involved in stimulation of gastric acid secretion. The first appears to be nonparietal cell related, probably a preganglionic M_1 receptor, and therefore selectively blocked by compounds such as pirenzepine or telenzepine (Chan and Soll 1988). On the parietal cell membrane, the receptor appears to be of the M3 subtype, and blocked by selective M3 antagonists (Wilkes et al. 1991). The M3 type of antagonist may have more side-effects (e.g., mydriasis and inhibition of salivary secretion) than the M_1 class, but it should be remembered that none of the known antagonists are entirely selective for one type of receptor. Clinical data using pirenzepine have shown efficacy in duodenal ulcer, but an efficacy inferior to that of H_2 receptor antagonists, as well as significant muscarinic side-effects.

II. H_2 Antagonists

The major change in treatment of peptic ulcer disease occurred with the synthesis of selective H_2 antagonists by Black et al. in 1972. The third generation of these, following on burimamide and metiamide, was cimetidine (Tagamet). It has now been used successfully in several million patients with a variety of peptic ulcer diseases. It appears that the H_2 receptor is found in relatively few tissues – uterus, atrium, and the parietal cell – thus reducing the likelihood of any significant nonspecific drug related effects. As discussed above, the action of the H_2 receptor in the parietal cell appears to be elevation of cAMP and a transient elevation of $[Ca]_i$. The release of histamine is also a crucial action of both cholinergic and gastrinergic stimulation of acid secretion, and therefore H_2 blockade is effective against all three major stimuli of acid secretion under normal circumstances. There have been several reviews on H_2 antagonists, and therefore this section will be brief. Currently at least four H_2 antagonists are available for clinical use: cimetidine (Tagamet), ranitidine (Zantac), famotidine (Pepcid), and nizatidine. They vary somewhat in potency but little in terms of efficacy, and they are all relatively short acting reversible inhibitors. This short plasma half-life or reversible binding is one factor that appears to limit their usefulness in acid related diseases that require more significant inhibition of acid secretion. However, inhibitors are being tested that either show only partial reversibility or have longer plasma half-lives. Such inhibitors should extend the usefulness of H_2 blockade in peptic ulcer disease.

H. Mechanism of Gastric Proton Pump

The molecular mechanism of any biological pump is poorly understood. However, certain generalizations can be made. The scalar energy released by the breakdown of ATP by the catalytic center (cytosolic domain) of the α subunit in the case of this class of pumps is translated into a vectorial displacement of H ion binding sites so that ions are forced through the membrane spanning sector towards the extracellular face of the enzyme. This translation must involve movement of portions of the protein, so that a barrier is raised on the *cis* side of the ion binding site, as the affinity of the site for the ion decreases. This prevents back leak of the ion. A forward barrier must also be lowered to allow escape of the ion from the pump. These transitions of sites and barriers are reversed for the countertransport of K^+.

I. Transport by ATPase

The overall transport properties of this enzyme have been elucidated in the last decade or so. The H^+,K^+-ATPase is a member of the family of transporting ATPases which form a covalent phosphoenzyme during their reaction cycle. Other members of this family in mammalian cells are the Ca^{2+} pumps and the Na^+ pump, which are ubiquitous. In its reaction cycle, the H^+,K^+-ATPase undergoes conformational changes as a function of binding the divalent Mg^{2+} cation, phosphorylation from ATP, and binding of the transported ions, protons or hydronium ions, from the cytosolic surface and K^+ from the extracytosolic surface. The definition of the two major conformations, E_1 and E_2, is based on the orientation of the ion binding sites. In the E_1 conformation, the ion binding sites face the cytosol, whereas in the E_2 conformation they face the extracellular surface. As the ion binding sites alter orientation, there is also a marked change in affinity for the bound ions.

Hydrogen ions are bound at neutral pH from the cytosolic face and released at pH 1, implying a greater than millionfold change in affinity of the transport site as it changes from cellular to extracellular orientation. K^+ is bound on the extracellular face with a K_m (app) of about 0.5 mM and released into the cytosolic solution at a hundredfold greater concentration (SCHACKMANN et al. 1977).

Although physiologically the gastric H^+,K^+-ATPase exchanges H^+ for K^+, it is also able to transport Na^+ in the forward direction (POLVANI et al.

1989) and $Tl^+ > K^+ > Rb^+ > NH_4^+ > Cs^+$ (SACHS et al. 1978) in the reverse direction, as well as Na^+ and Li^+ very poorly back into the cell. Since Na^+ can act as an H^+ surrogate, it seems that the proton is handled by pathways also able to accommodate the small alkali cations, which are much larger than the proton. This makes it likely that the larger hydronium ion, H_3O^+, rather than naked proton is pumped by the enzyme in the forward direction. The larger cations are transported in the reverse direction; therefore one distinction between the structure of the sites in the E_1 or E_2 conformation is the size of ion that can be accommodated. In the E_1 form the ion binding site accommodates the small cations well, and the larger ones poorly. The converse is true for the E_2 form of the enzyme.

II. Reaction Cycle

A simplified catalytic scheme is illustrated in Fig. 7a. The enzyme, in the presence of MgATP, binds a proton and is phosphorylated to form the E_1-P complex. This converts to the E_2-P form of the enzyme, which can now release hydronium to the extracellular solution and bind K^+ from the extracellular solution. With binding of K^+, the enzyme dephosphorylates and converts to first the $E_2 \cdot K$ and then the $E_1 \cdot K$ form, which loses K^+ into the cytosolic solution upon binding ATP (WALLMARK et al. 1980; STEWART et al. 1981).

Figure 7b is a representation of the transport events associated with the simplified catalytic cycle discussed above. The ion binding region of the pump is shown as changing position with respect to the membrane. The pump is represented as having a large cytosolic domain and a membrane spanning domain (the extracellular domain is not shown). The ion binding site contains a histidine and accepts $H^+(H_2O)$ from the cytosol. Since Na^+ can also be transported, the site is considerably larger than necessary just for proton binding, so it is modeled as large enough to allow water entry as well as the hydrogen ion. At this time the pump is phosphorylated (E_1-$P \cdot H^+ \cdot H_2O$) and the binding site changes conformation, so that the affinity for H^+ decreases and a barrier is formed that prevents reflux of H^+ back into the cell [E_1-$P(H_3O^+)$]. In this state, the proton is occluded in the binding site. Part of this change involves removal of the histidine from the site, lowering the proton binding affinity and allowing the symmetric cation, H_3O^+, to form. A second conformational change allows escape of the ion into the extracellular solution (from E_2-$P \cdot H_3O^+$), followed by binding of K^+ from the extracellular solution (E_2-$P \cdot K^+$). Binding of the hydronium ion to the carbonyl groups in the E_2 conformation of the binding site allows pumping of hydrogen ions into a solution of low pH, without postulating a large shift in the pK_a of carboxyl groups. This could be achieved by closeness of arginine or lysine groups, but these are absent in the predicted membrane spanning sequences of the enzyme. Basically, once the "hydronium" binding site is formed, this cation can be handled just like Na^+ is handled by the Na^+,K^+-ATPase. The enzyme

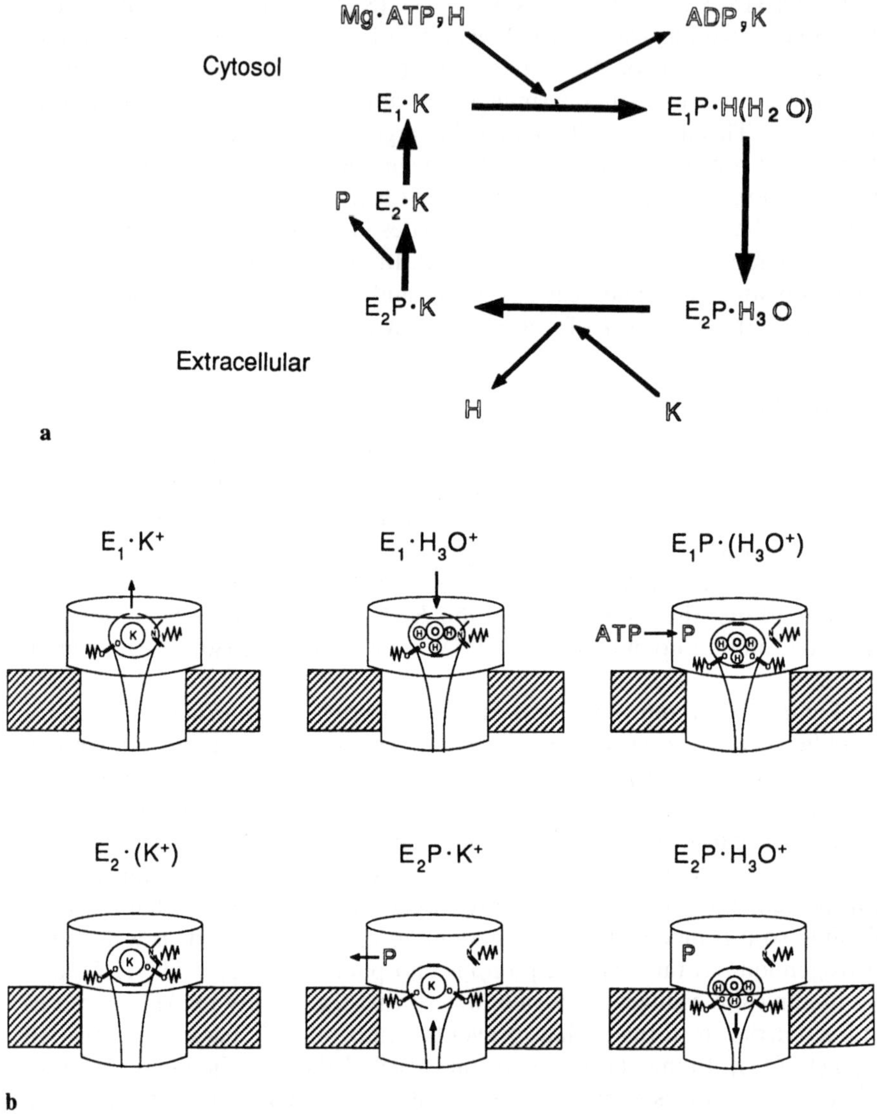

Fig. 7. a A simplified catalytic scheme of the reaction cycle of gastric H^+,K^+-ATPase. The enzyme exists in two major conformations, E_1, with the ion binding site facing the cytosol, and E_2, with the ion binding site facing the extracellular face. With binding of the proton, in the presence of Mg, the E_1-P form of enzyme is formed. This converts to the E_2-P·H_3O^+ form. Proton is released and K^+ binds to the E_2-P form, i.e., from the extracellular face, resulting in enzyme dephosphorylation to the E_2·K form, which then converts to E_1·K. Binding of ATP results in displacement of K^+ and the cycle reinitiates. **b** A graphic representation of the pump cycle. The overall structure of the enzyme is shown as having a large cytosolic domain and a narrower membrane spanning domain. The ion binding site in the E_1 conformation is closer to the cytosolic domain and can bind a proton to a histidine in the site. The site is large enough also to accommodate Na^+, but at a lower affinity and lower catalytic efficiency. Thus water is

then dephosphorylates and a barrier prevents release of K^+ back into the extracellular space $[E_2 \cdot (K^+)]$. The ion site then converts to the cytosolically facing, conformation, $E_1 \cdot K^+$, allowing release of K^+ back into the cytosol. ATP binding accelerates the loss of K^+ from the enzyme.

In the model illustrated the ion binding site is shown as moving with respect to the plane of the membrane, a piston type model. It is equally possible that the sidedness and affinity of the sites change due to twisting and untwisting of protein helices, a peristaltic model. Both models are illustrative of a chemomechanical pump.

As shown in both the catalytic cycle and the graphic model, the initial binding is that of a proton, presumably to histidine. The site is large enough, however, to accommodate water. In the E_2 form of the site, the histidine is not present and the released cation, bound to carbonyl oxygens, is the hydronium ion H_3O^+. This allows a large change in affinity without invoking highly abnormal pKa values for the amino acids in the E_2 form of the site, and represents a site large enough to accommodate cations such as K^+.

III. Structure of Gastric H^+,K^+-ATPase

The pump membrane appears to consist of at least two types of protein. One is responsible for the binding and breakdown of ATP. The second type is heavily glycosylated and may be another subunit of the ATPase. The larger, catalytic, subunit has been sequenced by cDNA methods (Shull and Lingrel 1986; Maeda et al. 1988). In hog, it is composed of 1033 amino acids. Hydropathy plots suggest possibly ten to twelve membrane spanning sectors (about 160–240 amino acids), a large cytosolic domain, and a minor extracellular domain. This, the catalytic subunit, is the subunit that is phosphorylated by ATP and is considered responsible for the transport reactions of the enzyme. This is the α subunit of the H^+,K^+-ATPase. Associated with this subunit is a heavily glycosylated β subunit, composed of 291 amino acids in the rabbit (Reuben et al. 1990). This subunit was discovered by treating gastric vesicles from hog by a N-glycanase and showing the appearance of a 35 kdalton peptide on SDS gels (Okamoto et al. 1989;

---

shown as being able to be accommodated in the E1 configuration. Following phosphorylation, a barrier is raised to prevent backflux of protons, and the histidine is removed from the site as it moves deeper into the membrane, allowing a large decrease in affinity for protons, and now indeed hydronium occupies the site made up of carbonyl liganding groups. The barrier on the extracellular surface is now lowered and hydronium can escape into the extracellular solution. K^+ is then bound, the enzyme dephosphorylates, and the site changes conformation with a barrier being raised to prevent K^+ backflux into the extracellular solution. The cytosolic barrier now decays, allowing movement of K^+ back into the cell. This step is accelerated by the binding of ATP and then proton rebinds, reinitiating the cycle

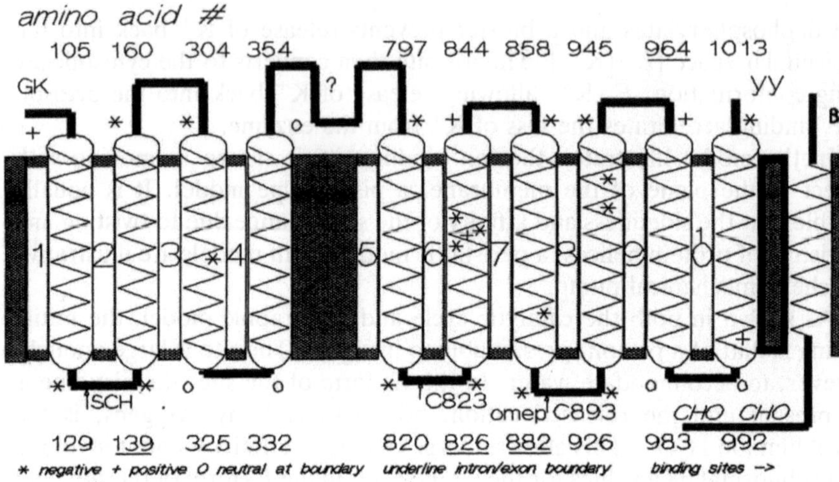

Fig. 8. Diagram of the structure of the H^+,K^+-ATPase. The enzyme is shown as being composed of two subunits. The catalytic subunit is larger in terms of protein and is shown as threading in and out of the membrane ten times. There is some glycosylation of this subunit. The second or β subunit is shown as passing across the membrane only once, but its large extracellular domain is heavily glycosylated and is associated closely with the catalytic or α subunit. Other membrane spanning sequences are possible between H4 and H5 (?). The region binding SCH 28080 and the sites of omeprazole labeling are shown (*SCH, omep*). Amino acid numbers are based on aDNA sequence.

HALL et al. 1990). Digestion of this band with protease V8 resulted in the production of peptides which were similar in sequence to the β subunit of the Na^+,K^+-ATPase (HALL et al. 1990). This allowed cloning of the β subunit from a rabbit gastric library (REUBEN et al. 1990) and a rat gastric library (SHULL 1990). The amino acid sequence of this subunit suggests the presence of a small cytosolic domain, only a single membrane spanning domain with most of the protein in the extracellular domain. There are six cysteines in this region, presumably in disulfide linkage since they do not react with acid activated omeprazole. The rate of biosynthesis of both subunits in the parietal cell appears to be equivalent based on rougly equal levels of mRNA (REUBEN et al. 1990).

A diagram of the postulated structural arrangement of the cytosolic sectors, membrane spanning domains, and the extracytosolic face of the enzyme is given in Fig. 8, with arrows indicating identified sites of interaction with known inhibitors of this ATPase as discussed below.

J. Inhibitors of H^+,K^+-ATPase

An alternative to receptor antagonists as a method for controlling acid secretion is inhibition of the H^+,K^+-ATPase. Although this enzyme shows a considerable degree of homology to the Na^+,K^+-ATPase, 40% of the sequence is different. In particular, the N terminal region and membrane spanning sequences towards the C terminal end show considerable deviation. Further, the putative β subunit is also not identical to the β subunit of the sodium pump. It seems also that the enzyme is confined to the parietal cell. Evidence for other locations of the pump is partial. For example, there is immune cross-reactivity with a protein in the ciliary body nonpigmented cell (FAIN et al. 1988) and some physiological evidence for active H^+ for K^+ exchange in distal colon and renal collecting duct. In the case of the colon, this H^+ for K^+ exchange appears sensitive to mucosal ouabain, which does not inhibit the gastric ATPase (SUSUKI and KANEKO 1989; KAUNITZ and SACHS 1986). In mechanism the gastric ATPase is the only proton pump in mammalian cells that is known to be countertransport pump. Further, the environment of the extracellular face of the gastric ATPase, when stimulated, is 3–4 orders of magnitude more acid than elsewhere in the body.

Inhibitors of the gastric ATPase can therefore be designed which take advantage of the specialized properties of the extracellular domain of the parietal cell acid pump, its unique structure, mechanism, and environment.

Both known classes of inhibitors share the property of being protonatable weak bases. With a pK_a of 5 or less, the acid space of the secreting parietal cell is the only region of the body where these compounds would accumulate. However, the two classes of ATPase inhibitors then diverge in mechanism. One is exemplified by substituted pyridylmethyl-sulfinyl benzimidazoles (e.g., omeprazole) (BORG et al. 1986; SACHS et al. 1988). As discussed later, these compounds are converted in an acid catalyzed reaction to sulfenamides that react covalently with cysteines accessible from the luminal surface of the enzyme. The other class, e.g., protonatable tertiary amines such as SCH 28080, a substituted pyridyl-1,2α-imidazole, act as K^+ competitive antagonists of the ATPase (WALLMARK et al. 1987; IM et al. 1984; NANDI et al. 1983; BROWN et al. 1990; LONG et al. 1983; SCOTT et al. 1987; BEIL et al. 1986). These will be discussed separately. Emphasis, however, will be placed on omeprazole since this compound is in clinical use.

I. Omeprazole

1. Effects on Acid Secretion

Omeprazole, in rat, dog, and man, was found to inhibit both basal and stimulated acid secretion, and inhibition of all stimuli was equipotent with an ED_{50} in man of about 27 mg (BORG et al. 1986; KONTUREK et al. 1984; LARSSON et al. 1983; LIND et al. 1983, 1986).

Omeprazole also inhibited acid secretion in isolated gland or parietal cell preparations, such as rabbit and human gastric glands and cells from pig and guineapig (WALLMARK et al. 1983; ELANDER et al. 1986; MÅRDH et al. 1988; SEWING et al. 1983). In contrast to H_2 blockers, which inhibited only histamine or gastrin stimulated secretion, omeprazole was able to inhibit secretion by these preparations however elicited, e.g., by dbcAMP or even high K^+ solutions.

In permeabilized parietal cells, where acid secretion is dependent upon the addition of exogenous ATP, omeprazole was able to inhibit acid transport; receptor antagonists are without effect (WALLMARK et al. 1983).

The data both in vivo and in vitro are therfore consistent with inhbition of the terminal step of acid secretion by omeprazole.

2. Duration of Action

Omeprazole at 20 mg orally in man inhibited 24-h acidity by about 95% (SHARMA et al. 1984; NAESDAL et al. 1984; LANZON-MILLER et al. 1987). This alone suggests a long duration of action. Following a single dose in dogs and man, 96 h were required for full restoration of maximal acid output following a dose that gave complete inhibition of acid secretion (LARSSON et al. 1983; LIND et al. 1983). The duration of action is somewhat shorter in the rat, being about 48 h (WALLMARK et al. 1988).

With a long acting drug of the omeprazole type, one would expect an increase in the antisecretory effect as a function of repeated administration. A steady state level of inhibition was found after 4 days of once daily dosing (CARLSSON et al. 1986; LIND et al. 1983). Continued treatment for 1 month with omeprazole in man shows no rebound phenomenon (LANZON-MILLER et al. 1987; SHARMA et al. 1987). Following cessation of treatment that had lasted for up to 1 year in the dog, there was a return to control levels of acid secretion within 4 days, the same duration of antisecretory effect as after a single dose (CARLSSON et al. 1986).

Treatment with very high doses in the rat gave rise to gastric hyperplasia due to the high levels of gastrin found in this species. No other organ showed hyperplasia (LARSSON et al. 1988; HÅKANSON et al. 1986). In this type of study, it was found that although plasma gastrin returned to normal 1 week after stopping 3 months' daily treatment, acid and pepsin secretory capacities were concurrently elevated for 3 months, consistent with uniform hyperplasia of parietal and peptic cells (LARSSON et al. 1988).

3. Mechanism of Action

a) Biology

The mechanism of action of omeprazole has been reviewed recently (SACHS et al. 1988; WALLMARK and LINDBERG 1987; LINDBERG et al. 1987).

Radioactive omeprazole was given to a mouse intravenously. Sixteen hours after dose, radioactivity was confined mostly to gastric epithelium and located over the tubulovesicles of the parietal cell (HELANDER et al. 1985). When radioactive omeprazole was administered to rabbits, followed by homogenization of the gastric mucosa and separation of the ATPase vesicles by differential and density gradient separation, the radioactivity was confined to the catalytic subunit of the H^+,K^+-ATPase at about 94kd on a nonreducing gel (FRYKLUND et al. 1988a). These data are shown in Fig. 9.

The relationship of inhibition of acid secretion and ATPase activity following omeprazole administration was studied in both rat and rabbit (WALLMARK et al. 1984b, 1985; FRYKLUND et al. 1988). In the rat there was a parallel decrease in the maximal secretory rate and ATPase activity, with identical IC_{50} values (Fig. 10). A similar parallelism was seen in recovery of acid secretion and ATPase activity following omeprazole inhibition. In rabbit, gastric glands were isolated following omeprazole administration. Acid formation was measured either by accumulation of the weak base ^{14}C-aminopyrine or by oxygen consumption. There was a parallel decrease in these parameters and in ATPase activity.

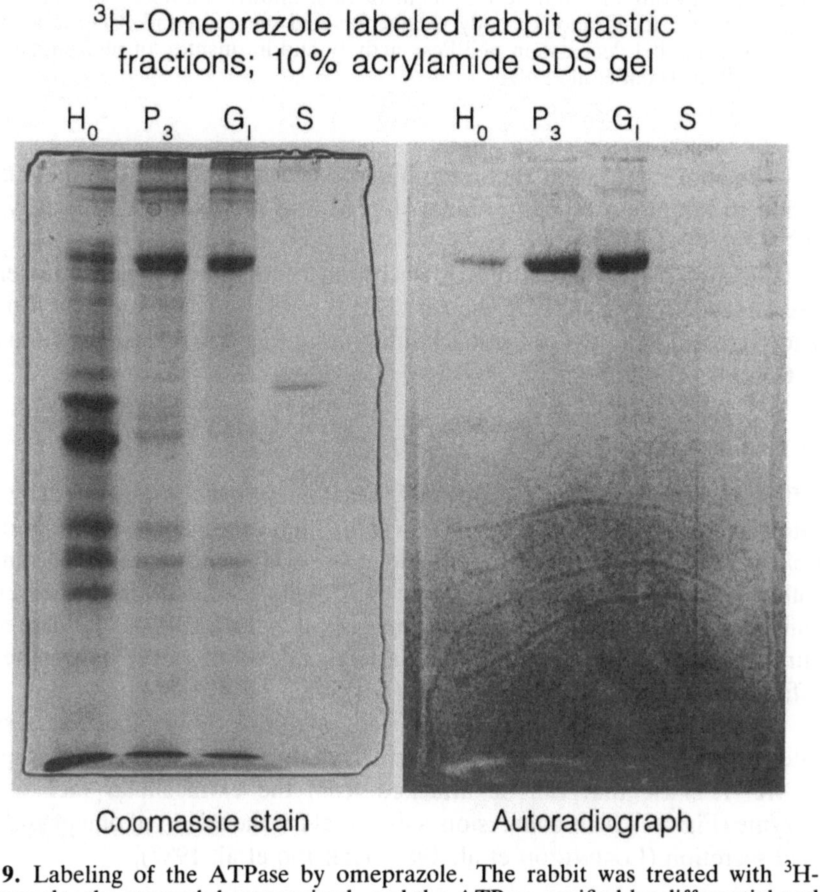

Fig. 9. Labeling of the ATPase by omeprazole. The rabbit was treated with ^3H-omeprazole, the stomach homogenized, and the ATPase purified by differential and gradient centrifugation. On the *left* is the Coomassie stained SDS gel (nonreducing) and on the *right* is the autoradiograph of the omeprazole labeled region. It can be seen that the radioactivity is confined to the region of the catalytic subunit of the H^+,K^+-ATPase (in collaboration with J. FRYKLUND)

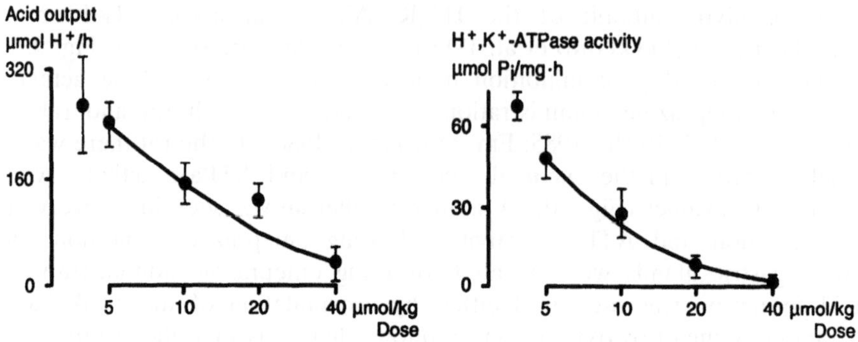

Fig. 10. The relationship between ATPase activity in gastric homogenates and acid secretion following omeprazole treatment of rats. Shown is a dose–response curve ranging from 5 to 40 μmol/kg body weight for acid secretion and ATPase activity. There is a parallel decrease in pNPPase activity and in quantity of phosphoenzyme formed (WALLMARK et al. 1985)

The above data show that the inhibition of acid secretion by omeprazole is due to inhibition of the terminal step of acid secretion, transport by the H^+,K^+-ATPase.

Omeprazole inhibition of acid secretion results in an increase in serum gastrin levels, particularly in the rat. This is entirely due to the inhibition of acid secretion with loss of feedback inhibition of gastrin release, as discussed in Chap. 7.

b) Chemistry

After oral dosing in acid protected form omeprazole is absorbed by the intestine and reaches the parietal cell via the bloodstream. The compound is a lipid-permeable weak base (pK_a 4) and crosses cell membranes. Accordingly, following protonation at the pyridine N, it will accumulate in the secretory canaliculus of the parietal cell by a theoretical factor of 1000. The degree of stimulation of the acid pump in the parietal cell will therefore determine the efficacy of administered omeprazole (DE GRAEF et al. 1986).

Omeprazole also undergoes an acid catalyzed conversion, via a spiro intermediate to a cationic sulfenamide, which then reacts with cysteines in the H^+,K^+-ATPase that can be attacked from the extracellular face of the enzyme (Fig. 11). This conversion is essential for the action of omeprazole on acid secretion (LORENTZON et al. 1987; KEELING et al. 1987).

c) Biochemistry

There are several lines of evidence substantiating the acid dependence of the action of the compound. A sulfide analogue of omeprazole (which does not convert to a sulfenamide) was found to accumulate in isolated rabbit gastric glands when these were stimulated to secrete acid (WALLMARK et al. 1984).

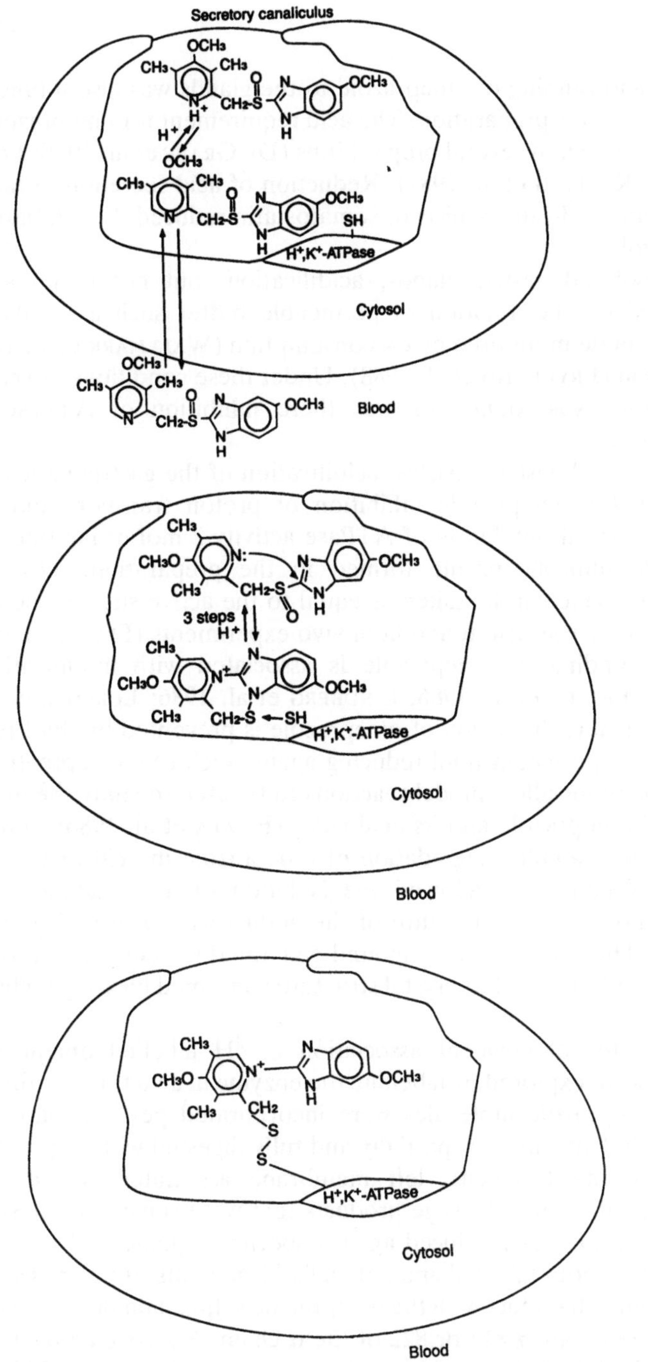

a

b

c

Fig. 11. a Uptake of omeprazole by the secreting parietal cell. The weak base is trapped in this highly acidic space by formation of the charged protonated species. **b** The conversion of omeprazole to the sulfenamide is diagrammed as occurring within the secretory canaliculus, the sulfenamide being a permanent cation. **c** The binding of the sulfenamide to the H^+,K^+-ATPase occurs via disulfide bridges to luminally accessible cysteines in the α or catalytic subunit

Uptake and binding of omeprazole to the glands was also a function of acid secretion by this preparation. The acid requirement for omeprazole inhibition has been shown in several preparations (DE GRAEF et al. 1986; LORENTZON et al. 1987; KEELING et al. 1987). Reduction of acid secretion in rat, rabbit, or dog by either H_2 antagonists or somatostatin reduced the inhibitory action of omeprazole.

In isolated gastric glands, acidification, but not pump activity, was prevented by the addition of permeable buffer such as imidazole. Pump activity can be monitored by O_2 consumption (WALLMARK et al. 1984) or CO_2 production (FRYKLUND et al. 1988). Under these conditions, no conversion of omeprazole was found nor was there inhibition of ATPase dependent metabolism.

In isolated gastric vesicles, acidification of the gastric vesicle lumen was necessary for omeprazole inhibition of proton transport and of ATPase activity. For full inhibition of ATPase activity 2 mol of inhibitor was bound per mole phosphoenzyme formed in the preparation. The quantity of phosphoenzyme can be taken as equal to the active site concentration. This stoichiometry was also found in in vivo experiments (FRYKLUND et al. 1988).

The binding of omeprazole is associated with modification of thiol residues (FIGALA et al. 1986; LINDBERG et al. 1986; LORENTZON et al. 1985, 1987). Further, the action of omeprazole is prevented by thiol reagents and reversed by permeant thiol reducing agents such as mercaptoethanol.

Mercaptans allow model reactions to be used to study the mechanism of action of omeprazole and its analogues (FIGALA et al. 1986; LINDBERG et al. 1986). For example, degradation of omeprazole in acid in the presence of mercaptoethanol has allowed the isolation of a crystalline adduct. This allowed proof of the structure of the adduct as shown in Fig. 11c by x-ray analysis. The rearranged compound generated in acid could also be precipitated in methanol and its crystal structure confirmed by x-ray techniques (Fig. 11b).

The sites of covalent association of ^3H labelled omeprazole to the ATPase were explored by labelling the enzyme in acid transporting vesicles so that 2 omeprazole molecules were incorporated per mol phosphoenzyme. The labelled enzyme was partially and fully digested with trypsin followed by separating the fragments left membrane associated. By determing the sequences of tryptic cleavage products that were separated on SDS gels and by using antibodies produced against specific sequences of the enzyme that reacted with both labelled and unlabelled fragments, it was possible to define the cysteines that react with the omeprazole sulphenamide. The cysteines that certainly react are #813 or 822 of the α chain. No cysteine of the β chain is found to be labelled. The finding that a sequence beginning (LVNE) (amino acid #854) containing cysteine #892 is also perhaps labelled by a luminal, positively charged, reagent suggests that at least an additional pair of membrane spanning sequences is present in this pump, making a total of 10 such domains (Mercier et al. submitted). It may be noted that omeprazole inhibition also inhibits phosphate transfer from ATP and another partial reaction, *p*-nitrophenyl phosphatase activity, as if omeprazole was maintaining the enzyme in an inhibited E_2 form, preventing formation of the E_1 form. Figure 12 diagrams the binding region of omeprazole to the H^+,K^+-ATPase. Binding of the large sulfenamide cation to this extracellular region therefore prevents structural rearrangement in the cytosolic domain that allows ATP binding and phosphorylation. The conformational changes in this pump therefore extend across the membrane spanning sector of the protein. Conformational changes appear to occur over quite large distances.

d) Reversal of Omeprazole Inhibition

Since omeprazole binds covalently to the ATPase, reversal of its action requires either in situ reduction of the disulfide formed or de novo synthesis of the ATPase. Treatment of rats with cycloheximide showed that no reversal of inhibition was obtained in the absence of protein synthesis, arguing that it is de novo synthesis that accounts for restoration of acid secretion (Im et al. 1985a). The relatively short half-life of the pump in man and other species guarantees about 30% restoration of acid secretory capacity every 24 h following a once daily dosage schedule.

The overall mechanism of action of omeprazole is shown diagrammatically in Fig. 13. The overall sequence of events is stated in text and diagrammed in the figure as well.

II. Reversible H^+,K^+-ATPase Inhibitors

No reversible H^+,K^+-ATPase inhibitors have yet been approved for clinical use, but they are nevertheless of interest mechanistically and in terms of future possible therapeutic applications. The best studied of them is SCH 28080 (Fig. 14) but several other types have been described (Im et al. 1984; Wallmark et al. 1987; Brown et al. 1990; Nandi et al. 1983).

A feature of these compounds is that in general they are competitive with respect to K^+ and uncompetitive with respect to ATP or pNPP. Furthermore they bind to either the E_2 or E_2-P forms of the enzyme and exclusively in terms of their competitive inhibition with the extracellular face of the enzyme (Wallmark et al. 1987; Keeling et al. 1988, 1989; Briving et al. 1988). They are all protonatable amines and react with the enzyme in the protonated, charged form.

It has also been shown that SCH 28080 prevents inhibition of the ATPase by omeprazole even in the presence of adequate acidity at the luminal face of the pump (Hersey et al. 1988). This suggests some interaction between the binding site of omeprazole and the binding site of SCH 28080. Both compounds stabilize the E_2 conformer of the enzyme.

With an approach similar to that used for omeprazole, it has been possible to locate one of the regions responsible for binding this K^+

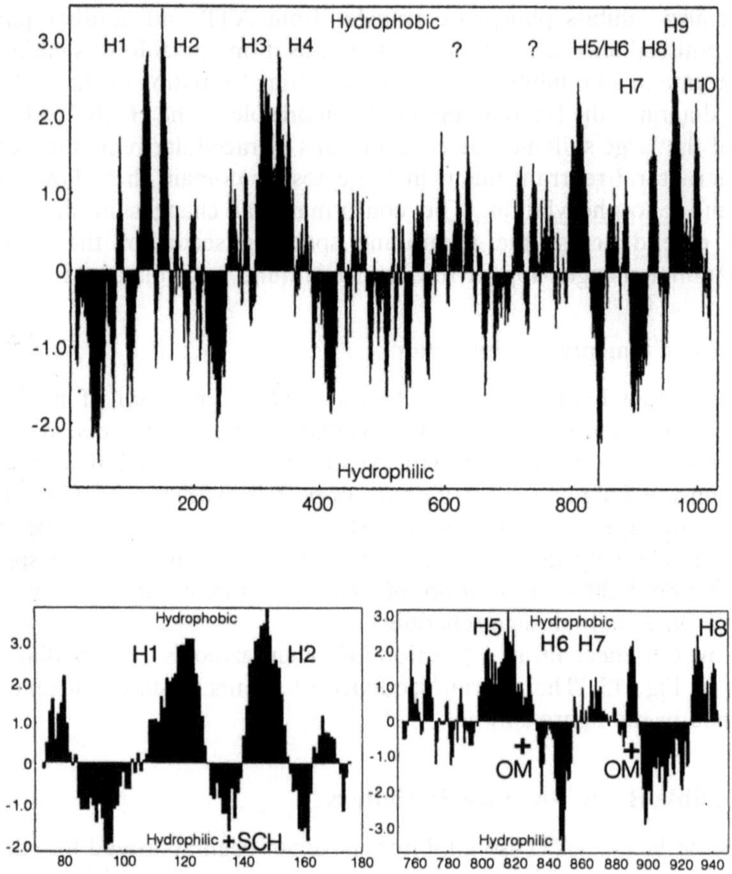

Hydrophobic
Hydrophilic
H1
H2
H3
H4
?
?
H5/H6
H8
H9
H7
H10
3.0
2.0
1.0
0
-1.0
-2.0
200
400
600
800
1000
H1
H2
+SCH
80
100
120
140
160
180
H5
H6 H7
H8
OM
OM
760 780 800 820 840 860 880 900 920 940

a

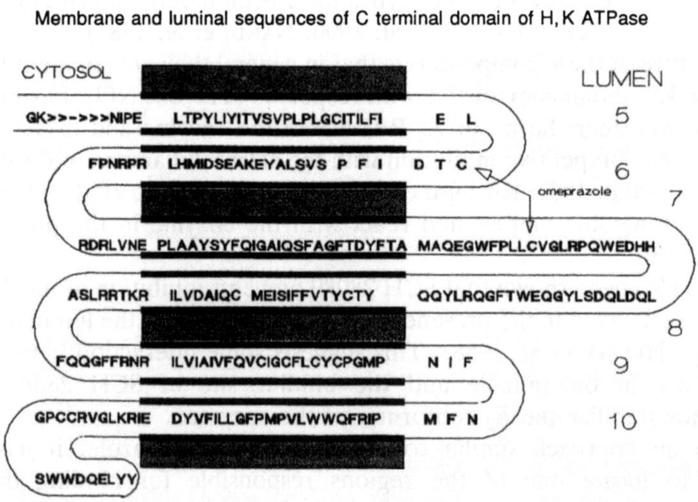

Membrane and luminal sequences of C terminal domain of H, K ATPase
CYTOSOL
LUMEN
GK>>->>>NIPE LTPYLIYITVSVPLPLGCITILFI E L
5
FPNRPR LHMIDSEAKEYALSVS P F I D T C
6
omeprazole
7
RDRLVNE PLAAYSYFQIGAIQSFAGFTDYFTA MAQEGWFPLLCVGLRPQWEDHH
ASLRRTKR ILVDAIQC MEISIFFVTYCTY QQYLRQGFTWEQGYLSDQLDQL
8
FQQGFFRNR ILVIAIVFQVCIGCFLCYCPGMP N I F
9
GPCCRVGLKRIE DYVFILLGFPMPVLWWQFRIP M F N
10
SWWDQELYY

b

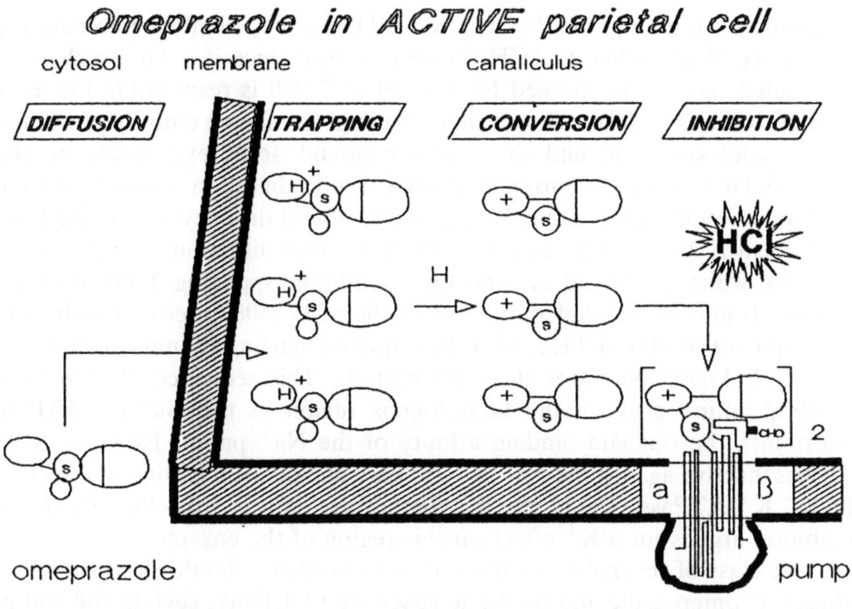

Fig. 13. A diagram of the sequence of action of omeprazole without showing the structural details, emphasizing that this drug is a target activated prodrug

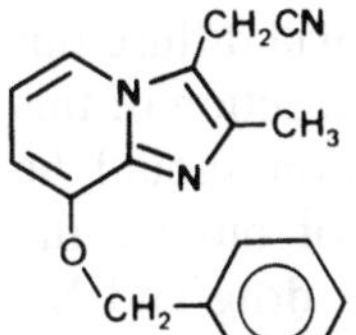

Fig. 14. The structure of SCH 28080, a K^+ competitive antagonist of the H^+,K^+-ATPase. It is only one of several tertiary amines that are highly selective potent inhibitors of this enzyme. Ouabain has a similar selectivity for the Na^+,K^+-ATPase

Fig. 12. a A diagrammatic view of the region of the catalytic subunit that binds omeprazole and SCH 28080. In the upper part of the figure is the hydropathy plot of the catalytic subunit of the H^+,K^+-ATPase, interpretable as composed of 8,10, or even more membrane spanning sectors. In the lower part the C-terminal membrane spanning sequences are illustrated, with the intervening extracellular loops. Omeprazole binds in the H5-H6 and (H7-H8) regions whereas SCH 28080 binds in the H1,H2 region. Both compounds prevent formation of the E_1 form of the enzyme by stabilizing the E_2 form. Omeprazole binds covalently; SCH 28080 is a K^+ competitive antagonist. The binding region of the latter was determined using a photoaffinity analogue of SCH 28080 (MUNSON et al. submitted). **b** The amino acid sequence of the region illustrated above, showing the possible cysteines (*C*) derivatized by omeprazole in the parietal cell. Shown are the a putative membrane spanning sequences and the intervening extracellular loops, as illustrated in the hydropathy plot above

competitive inhibitor of the H^+,K^+-ATPase. A labelled photoaffinity quaternary N derivative of SCH 28080 was used since it is known that the protonated, positively charged form of SCH 28080 is responsible for its K competitive action. It was shown that labelling was almost entirely prevented by the addition of K and that the compound acted exclusively on the extracellular face of the enzyme. Partial tryptic digestion showed that the label was present largely in the N-terminal region of the enzyme running from amino acid E #47 to amino acid R #671. Further digestion gave a labelled sequence which contained the first two membrane spanning domains of the enzyme. It may be concluded that one of the SCH 28080 sites is contained in the loop between H1 and H2, with the sequence starting at amino acid #131, EGDLLTTDDN (MUNSON et al. submitted). This sequence of carboxylic enriched amino acids in the homologous region of the Na^+,K^+-ATPase determines the ouabain binding affinity of the Na^+ pump. However SCH 28080 is inactive against the Na^+,K^+-ATPase and ouabain is without effect on the H^+,K^+-ATPase. The purely K^+ competitive nature of this binding and of inhibition argues for a K^+ effect on this region of the enzyme.

This class of reversible antagonists of the enzyme should show the same efficacy as omeprazole and the same spectrum of activity, such as the ability to inhibit acid secretion irrespective of stimulus. It may be noted that their specificity is largely dependent on their native structure, not acid catalyzed conversion to an active intermediate. The low pH of the parietal cell acid space, however, allows the protonated form to accumulate, increasing the effective concentration of the drug at its site of action. As inhibition progresses and the pH of the canalicular space rises, the drug will diffuse out of the space and, furthermore, K^+ will enter, antagonizing the action of this class of reversible ATPase inhibitor. Their duration of action should be dependent on their plasma concentration, since they do not modify the enzyme covalently. However, given the expected changes in drug and K^+ concentration at the active site strict correlation between plasma levels and effect may be difficult to obtain. The future clinical niche that these compounds will occupy will depend on selectivity of these compounds for the gastric ATPase as compared to any other protein and upon being able to develop compounds of adequate efficacy and duration of action.

III. Clinical Use of Pump Inhibitors

The ability to inhibit the final step of acid secretion, with a relatively long duration of action, has provided a more effective means of suppression of acid secretion by the gastric mucosa. This has allowed more reliable treatment of a variety of acid related disorders as compared to the available short-acting H_2 inhibitors as described in Chap. 7.

References

Allen A, Garner A (1980) Gastric mucus and bicarbonate secretion and their possible role in mucosal protection. Gut 21:249–262

Armstrong JA, Wee SH, Goodwin CS, Wilson DH (1987) Response of *Campylobacter pyloridis* to antibiotics, bismuth and an acid reducing agent in vitro-an ultrastructural study. J Med Microbiol 24:343–350

Bajaj SC, Spenney JG, Sachs G (1977) Properties of gastric antrum. III. Selectivity and modification of shunt conductance. Gastroenterology 72:72–77

Beil W, Hackibarth I, Sewing K-F (1986) Mechanism of gastric antisecretory effect of SCH 28080. Br J Pharmacol 88:19–23

Bergqvist E, Obrink KJ (1979) Gastrin-histamine as a normal sequence in gastrin acid stimulation in the rabbit. Ups J Med Sci 84:145–154

Black JW, Duncan WAM, Durant CJ, Gannellin CR, Parsons ME (1972) Definition and antagonism of histamine H_2 receptors. Nature 236:385–390

Borg KO, Olbe L, Rune SJ, Walan A (eds) (1986) Proceedings of the First International Symposium on Omeprazole. Scand J Gastroenterol 21, Suppl 118

Briving C, Andersson B, Lindberg P, Wallmark B (1988) Inhibition of gastric HK ATPase by substituted imidazol, 2a prydines. Biochim Biophys Acta 346:185–192

Brown TH, Ife RJ, Keeling RJ, Laing SM, Leach CA, Parsons ME, Price CA, Reavill DR, Wiggall KJ (1990) Reversible inhibitors of the gastric HK ATPase: 1, 1-aryl-4-methyl-pyrrolo (3,2-c) quinolines as conformationally restrained analogues of 4 (arylamin) quinolines. J Med Chem (submitted)

Carlsson E, Larsson H, Mattsson H, Ryberg B, Sundell G (1986) Pharmacology and toxicology of omeprazole with special reference to the effects on the gastric mucosa. Scand J Gastroenterol Suppl 118:31–38

Chan CB, Soll AH (1988) Role of cholinergic nervous system in acid secretion. Pharmacology 37, Suppl 1:17–21

Chen MC, Amirian DA, Toomey M, Sanders MJ, Soll A (1988) Prostanoid inhibition of canine parietal cells: mediation by the inhibitory guanosine triphosphate binding protein of adenylate cyclase. Gastroenterology 94:1121–1129

Cheng EH, Bermanski P, Silversmith M, Valenstein P, Kawanishi H (1989) Prevalence of *Campylobacter pylori* in esophagitis gastritis and duodenal disease. Arch Intern Med 148:1373–1375

Chew CS, Brown MR (1986) Release of intracellular Ca and elevation of inositol trisphosphate by secretagogues. Biochim Biophys Acta 846:370–378

Curci S, Debellis L, Fromter E (1987) Evidence for rheogenic sodium bicarbonate cotransport in basolateral membranes of frog oxyntic cell. Pflugers Arch 408:511–514

De Graef J, Woussen-Colle M-C (1986) Influence of the stimulation state of the parietal cells on the inhibitory effect of omeprazole on gastric acid secretion in dogs. Gastroenterology 91:333–337

Demarest JR, Machen TE (1985) Microelectrode measurements from oxyntic cells in intact *Necturus* mucosa. Am J Physiol 249:C535–C540

Demarest JR, Loo DD, Sachs G (1990) Activation of apical chloride channels in the gastric oxyntic cell. Science (in press)

Elander B, Fellenius E, Leth R, Olbe L, Wallmark B (1986) Inhibitory action of omeprazole on acid formation in gastric glands and on H^+,K^+-ATPase isolated from human gastric mucosa. Scand J Gastroenterol 21:268–272

Engel E, Peskoff A, Kauffman GL, Grossman MI (1984) Analysis of hydrogen ion concentration in the gastric gel mucus layer. Am J Physiol 247:G321–G338

Euler AR, Popiela T, Tytgat GN, Kulig J, Lookabaugh JL, Phan TD, Kitt MM (1989) A multicenter trial evaluating arbaprostil (15(R)-15-methyl prostaglandin E_2) as a therapeutic agent for gastric ulcer. Gastroenterology 96:967–971

Fain G, Smolka A, Cilluffo MC, Fain MJ, Lee DA, Brecha NC, Sachs G (1988) Monoclonal antibodies to the HK ATPase of gastric mucosa selectively stained

the non-pigmented cell of the rabbit ciliary epithelium. Invest Opthalmol Vis Sci 29:785–794
Figala V, Klemm K, Kohl B, Krüger U, et al. (1986) Acid activation of H^+,K^+-ATPase inhibiting 2-(2-pyridylmethylsulfinyl) benzimidazoles: isolation and characterization of the thiophillic "active principle" and its reactions. J Chem Soc Chem Commun 129:29
Fimmel CJ, Etienne A, Cilluffo T, von Ritter C, Grasser T, Rey SJ, Blum AL (1985) Long term ambulatory gastric pH monitoring: validation of a new method and effect of H_2 antagonists. Gastroenterology 88:1842–1851
Flemstrom G (1987) Gastric duodenal and mucosal bicarbonate secretion. In: Johnson, LR (ed) Physiology of the gastrointestinal tract. Raven, New York, pp 1011–1030
Fryklund J, Gedda K, Wallmark B (1988a) Specific labelling of gastric H^+,K^+-ATPase by omeprazole. Biochem Pharmacol 37:2543–2549
Fryklund J, Helander HF, Elander B, Wallmark B (1988b) Function and structure of parietal cells after H^+,K^+-ATPase blockade. Am J Physiol 245:G399–G407
Fukui A, Nakazawa S, Goto H, Sugiyama S, Oazawa ,T (1988) Effects of prostaglandin D_2 and omeprazole on indomethacin induced gastric ulcers in rats. Clin Exp Pharmacol Physiol 15:919–926
Gutknecht J (1984) Proton/hydroxide conductance through lipid bilayer membranes. J Membr Biol 82:105–112
Gutknecht J (1988) Proton conductance caused by long chain fatty acids in phospolipid bilayer membranes. J Membr Biol 106:83–93
Håkanson R, Blom H, Carlsson E, Larsson H, Ryberg B, Sundler F (1986) Hypergastrinaemia produces trophic effects in stomach but not in pancreas and intestines. Regul Pept 13:225–230
Hall K, Perz G, Anderson D, Munson K, Guttierez C, Kaplan JH, Hersey SJ, Sachs G (1990) Location of the oligosaccharides in the HK ATPase vesicles of hog gastric mucosa. Biochemistry 29:701–706
Helander HF, Hirschowitz BI (1974) Quantitative ultrastructural studies on inhibited and partly stimulated gastric parietal cells. Gastroenterology 67:447–452
Helander HF, Ramsay C-H, Regårdh C-G (1985) Localization of omeprazole and metabolites in the mouse. Scand J Gastroenterol [Suppl] 108:95–104
Hersey SJ, Steiner L, Mendlein J, Rabon E, Sachs G (1988) SCH 28080 prevents omeprazole inhibition of gastric HK ATPase. Biochim Biophys Acta 956:49–57
Hogben CAM (1955) Active transport of chloride by isolated frog gastric epithelium: origin of gastric mucosal potential. Am J Physiol 180:641–649
Howden CW, Hunt RH (1987) Relationship between gastric secretion and infection. Gut 28:96–107
Hunt TE, Hunt EA (1962) Radioautographic study of proliferation in the stomach of the rat using thymidine H_3 and compound 48/80. Anat Rec 142:505–517
Im WB, Blakeman DP, Mendlein J, Sachs G (1984) Inhibition of HK ATPase and H accumulation in hog gastric membranes by trifluoperazine, verapamil and 8- (*N,N* diethyl amino) octyl 3,4,5 trimethoxy benzoate. Biochim Biophys Acta 770:65–72
Im WB, Blakeman DP, Davis JP (1985a) Irreversible inactivation of the rat gastric H^+,K^+-ATPase in vivo by omeprazole. Biochem Biophys Res Commun 126:78–82
Im WB, Sih JC, Blakeman DP, McGrath JD (1985b) Omeprazole, a specific inhibitor of gastric H^+,K^+-ATPase, is an H-activated oxidizing agent of sulfhydryl groups. J Biol Chem 260:4591–4597
Ito S (1987) Functional gastric morphology. In: Johnson LR (ed) Physiology of the gastrointestinal tract. Raven, New-York, pp 817–852
Johnson LR (1987) Regulation of gastrointestinal growth. In: Johnson LR (ed) Physiology of the gastrointestinal tract. pp 301–333
Kaunitz JD, Sachs G (1986) Identifiction of a vanadate sensitive potassium dependent proton pump from rabbit colon. J Biol Chem 261:14005–14010

Keeling DJ, Fallowfield C, Milliner KJ, Tingley SK, Ife RJ, Underwood AH (1985) Studies on the mechanism of action of omeprazole. Biochem Pharmacol 34:2967–2973
Keeling DJ, Fallowfield C, Underwood AH (1987) The specificity of omeprazole as an H^+,K^+-ATPase inhibitor depends upon the means of its activation. Biochem Pharmacol 36:339–344
Keeling DJ, Laing SM, Senn-Bilfinger J (1988) SCH 28080 is a luminally acting K site inhibitor of the gastric HK ATPase. Biochem Pharmacol 37:2231–2236
Keeling DJ, Fallowfield C, Lawrie KM, Saunders D, Richardson S, Ife RJ (1989) Photoaffinity labeling of the luminal K site of the gastric HK ATPase. J Biol Chem 264:5552–5558
Kondo Y, Fromter E (1987) Axial heterogeneity of sodium bicarbonate cotransport in proximal straight tubules of rabbit kidney. Pflugers Arch 410:481–486
Konturek SJ, Cieszkowski M, Kwiecien N, Konturek J, Tasler J, Bilski J (1984) Effects of omeprazole, a substituted benzamidazole, on gastrointestinal secretion, serum gastrin, and gastrin mucosal blood flow in dogs. Gastroenterology 86:71–77
Lanzon-Miller S, Pounder RE, Hamilton MR, et al. (1987) Twenty-four-hour intragastric acidity and plasma gastrin concentration before and during treatment with either ranitidine or omeprazole. Aliment Pharmacol Ther 1:239–251
Larsson H, Carlsson E, Junggren U, et al. (1983) Inhibition of gastric acid secretion by omeprazole in dog and rat. Gastroenterology 85:900–907
Larsson H, Carlsson E, Ryberg B, Fryklund J, Wallmark B (1988) Rat parietal cell function after prolonged inhibition of gastric acid secretion. Am J Physiol 245:G33–G39
Lind T, Cederberg C, Ekenved G, Haglund U, Olbe L (1983) Effect of omeprazole – a gastric proton pump inhibitor – on pentagastrin stimulated acid secretion in man. Gut 24:270–276
Lind T, Moore M, Olbe L (1986) Intravenous omeprazole: effect on 24-h intragastric pH in duodenal ulcer patients. Digestion 34:78–86
Lindberg P, Nordberg P, Alminger T, Brändström A, Wallmark B (1986) The mechanism of action of the gastric acid secretion inhibitor omeprazole. J Med Chem 29:1327–1329
Lindberg P, Brändström A, Wallmark B (1987) Structure-activity relationships of omeprazole analogues and their mechanism of action. Trends Pharmacol Sci 8:399–402
Long JF, Chui PJS, Derelanko MJ, Steinberg M (1983) Gastric antisecretory and cytoprotective activities of SCH 28080. J Pharmacol Exp Ther 226:114–120
Lorentzon P, Eklundh B, Brändström A, Wallmark B (1985) The mechanism for inhibition of gastric H^+,K^+-ATPase by omeprazole. Biochim Biophys Acta 817:25–32
Lorentzon P, Jackson R, Wallmark B, Sachs G (1987) Inhibition of H^+,K^+-ATPase by omeprazole in isolated gastric vesicles requires proton transport. Biochim Biophys Acta 897:41–51
Machen TE, Paradiso AM (1987) Regulation of intracellular pH in the stomach. Annu Rev Physiol 49:19–33
Maeda M, Ishizaki J, Futai M (1988) cDNA cloning and sequence determination of pig gastric HK ATPase. Biochem Biophys Res Commun 157:203–209
Mårdh S, Song Y-M, Wallmark B (1988) Effects of some antisecretory drugs on acid production, intracellular Ca^{2+} and cyclic AMP production in isolated pig parietal cells. Scand J Gastroenterol 23:977–982
May B (1989) Sucralfate and other non-antisecretory agents in the treatment of peptic ulcer disease. Methods Exp Clin Pharm 11:113–116
Mercier F, Besancon M, Hall K, Sachs G (1991) Location of omeprazole binding to the H^+,K^+-ATPase under transport conditions, J Biol Chem (submitted)
Muallem S, Sachs G (1985) Ca metabolism during cholinergic stimulation of acid secretion. Am J Physiol 248:G216–G228

Muallem S, Burnham C, Blissard D, Berglindh T, Sachs G (1985) Electrolyte transport across the basolateral membrane of the parietal J Biol Chem 260:6641–6653
Muallem S, Fimmel CJ, Pandol SJ, Sachs G (1986) Regulation of free cytosolic Ca in the peptic and parietal cells of the rabbit gastric gland. J Biol Chem 261:2660–2667
Muallem S, Blissard D, Cragoe EM, Sachs G (1988) Activation of Na/H and Cl/HCO_3 exchange by stimulation of acid secretion by the parietal cell. J Biol Chem 263:14703–14711
Munson KB, Gutierrez C, Perez G, Hall K, Sachs G (1990) Labelling of the HK ATPase by a K competitive photoaffinity ligand. evidence for extracellular association of 2 subunits. J Biol Chem (to be published)
Naesdal J, Bodemar G, Walan A (1984) Effect of omeprazole, a substituted benzimidazole, on 24-h intragastric acidity in patients with peptic ulcer disease. Scand J Gastroenterol 19:916–922
Nandi J, Wright MV, Ray TK (1983) Mechanism of gastric antisecretory effects of nolinium bromide. Gastroenterology 85:938–945
Negulescu PA, Machen TE (1988) Intracellular Ca regulation during secretagogue stimulation of the parietal cell. Am J Physiol 254:130–140
Okamoto C, Reenstra WW, Li W, Forte JG (1989) Partial characterisation of a 60–80 kdalton glycoprotein associated with the hog gastric microsomal ATPase. J Cell Biol 107:125a
Paradiso AM, Tsien RY, Demarest JR, Machen TE (1987) Na-H and Cl-HCO_3 exchange in rabbit oxyntic cells using fluorescence microscopy. Am J Physiol 253:C30–C36
Pfeiffer A, Rochlitz H, Herz A, Paumgartner G (1988) Stimulation of acid secretion and phosphoinositol production by rat parietal cell muscarinic M_2 receptors. Am J Physiol 254:G622–G629
Polvani C, Sachs G, Blostein R (1990) Sodium transport by the gastric HK ATPase. J Biol Chem (in press)
Reuben MA, Lasater L, Sachs G (1990) Characterisation of beta subunit of the gastric H,K transporting ATPase. Proc Natl Acad Sci USA 87:6767–6771
Sachs G, Chang HH, Rabon E, Schackmann R, Lewin M, Saccomani G (1976) A non-electrogenic H pump in plasma membranes of hog gastric mucosa. J Biol Chem 251:7690–7698
Sachs G, Spenney JG, Lewin M (1978) H transport: regulation and mechanism in gastric mucosa and membrane vesicles. Physiol Rev 58:106–173
Sachs G, Carlsson E, Lindberg P, Wallmark B (1988) Gastric H^+,K^+-ATPase as a therapeutic target. Annu Rev Pharmacol Toxicol 28:269–284
Sanders MJ, Ayalon A, Roll M, Soll AH (1985) The apical surface of canine chief cells resists H back diffusion. Nature 313:52–54
Schackmann R, Schwartz A, Saccomani G, Sachs G (1977) Cation transport by gastric HK ATPase. J Membr Biol 32:361–381
Scott C, Sundell E, Castroville C (1987) Studies on the mechanism of action of the gastric microsomal H^+,K^+-ATPase inhibitors SCH 32651 and SCH 28080. Biochem Pharmacol 36:97–104
Sewing K-F, Harms P, Schulz G, Hannemann H (1983) Effect of substituted benzimidazoles on acid secretion in isolated and enriched guinea pig parietal cells. Gut 24:557–560
Sharma BK, Walt RP, Pounder RE, Gomes MdeFA, Wood EC, Logan LH (1984) Optimal dose of oral omeprazole for maximal 24 hour decrease of intragastric acidity. Gut 25:957–964
Sharma BK, Axelson M, Pounder RP, et al. (1987) Acid secretory capacity and plasma gastrin concentration after administration of omeprazole to normal subjects. Aliment Pharmacol Ther 1:67–76

Shull GE, Lingrel JB (1986) Molecular cloning of the rat stomach HK ATPase. J Biol Chem 261:16788–16791
Shull GE (1990) cDNA cloning of the β subunit of rat gastric (H^+,K^+)-ATPase, J Biol Chem 265:12123–12126
Silen W (1987) Gastric mucosal defense and repair. In: Johnson LR (ed) Physiology of the gastrointestinal tract. Raven, New York, pp 1055–1070
Smolka A, Helander HF, Sachs G (1983) Monoclonal antibodies against gastric HK ATPase. Am J Physiol 245:G589–G596
Stewart HB, Wallmark B, Sachs G (1981) The interaction of H and K with partial reactions of gastric HK ATPase. J Biol Chem 256:2682–2690
Suzuki Y, Kaneko K (1989) Ouabain sensitive HK exchange mechanism in the apical membranes of guinea pig colon. Am J Physiol 256:G979–G988
Tache Y (1988) CNS peptides and the regulation of gastric acid secretion. Annu Rev Physiol 50:19–39
Townsley MC, Machen TE (1990) Na-HCO_3 cotransport in parietal cells. Am J Physiol (in press)
Urushidani T, Hanzel DK, Forte JG (1987) Protein phosphorylation associated with stimulation of rabbit gastric glands. Biochim Biophys Acta 930:209–219
Wallmark B, Lindberg P (1987) Mechanism of action of omeprazole. In: ISI Atlas of Science: Pharmacology. ISI, London pp 158–161 (ISI atlas of science, vol 1)
Wallmark B, Stewart HB, Rabon E, Saccomani G, Sachs G (1980) The catalytic cycle of the gastric (H^+,K^+)-ATPase. J Biol Chem 255:5313–5319
Wallmark B, Jaresten B-M, Larsson H, Ryberg B, Brändström A, Fellenius E (1983) Differentiation among inhibitory actions of omeprazole, cimetidine, and SCN- on gastric acid secretion. Am J Physiol 245:G64–G71
Wallmark B, Brändström A, Larsson H (1984a) Evidence for acid-induced transformation of omeprazole into an active inhibitor of H^+,K^+-ATPase within the parietal cell. Biochim Biophys Acta 778:549–558
Wallmark B, Jaresten B-M, Lorentzon P, Brändström A (1984b) Inhibition of gastric acid secretion by omeprazole: role of sulfhydryl groups in its inhibitory mechanism. In: Forte JG, Warnock DG, Rector FC Jr (eds) Hydrogen ion transport in epithelia. Wiley, New York; pp 171–183
Wallmark B, Larsson H, Humble L (1985) The relationship between gastric acid secretion and gastric H^+,K^+-ATPase activity. J Biol Chem 260:13681–13684
Wallmark B, Briving C, Fryklund J, Munson K, Jackson R, Mendlein J, Rabon E, Sachs G (1987) Inhibition of H^+,K^+-ATPase and acid secretion by SCH 28080, a substituted pyridyl (1,2a) imidazole. J Biol Chem 262:2077–2084
Walsh JH (1987) Gastrointestinal hormones. In: Johnson LR (ed) Physiology of the gastrointestinal tract. Raven, New York, pp 181–253
Whittle BJR, Vane JR (1987) Prostanoids as regulators of gastrointestinal function. In: Johnson LR (ed) Physiology of the gastrointestinal tract. Raven, New York, pp 142–180
Wilkes J, Kajimura M, Scott DR, Hersey SJ, Sato G (1991) Parietal cell response to muscarinic antagonists. J Membr Biol (in press)
Wolosin JM (1985) Ion transport studies with HK ATPase rich vesicles. Am J Physiol 248:G595–G607
Wolosin JM, Forte JG (1984) Stimulation of oxyntic cell triggers K and Cl conductances in apical HK ATPase membrane. Am J Physiol 246:G537–G545
Wolosin JM, Okamoto C, Forte TM, Forte JG (1983) Actin and associated proteins in gastric epithelial cells. Biochim Biophys Acta 761:171–182

CHAPTER 2

Epidermal Growth Factor

R.V. Nardi, A. Guglietta, and I. Parikh

A. Introduction

Polypeptide growth factors have attracted considerable interest since the initial description of nerve growth factor (NGF) in 1951 (Levi-Montalcini and Hamburger 1951) and, subsequently, the identification of epidermal growth factor (EGF) in 1962 (Cohen 1962). At present, however, the natural roles of these and other peptide growth factors remains a gap in our understanding. In this review we hope to provide some additional perspective from which this gap may be closed.

Epidermal growth factor (EGF) is probably the most widely studied of this group of peptide hormones. As evidenced by the large number of reviews on this compound, a chapter is clearly insufficient to do justice to the large body of information that has been developed. In an effort to focus this chapter, we will review the aspects of EGF pharmacology which make it a potential therapeutic target in the gastrointestinal (GI) tract. Moreover, we will attempt to present EGF as a prototypical ligand both for the "EGF family" itself and for this class of hormones. Consequently, we will not attempt to address whether TGFα is the *in vivo* ligand for the EGF receptor. This is not an attempt to avoid interesting data on this subject but rather it is an attempt to concentrate on pharmacologic mechanisms which may have therapeutic implications. As we will address below the specific ligand that is exploited to achieve the desired therapeutic effect may be dictated by the disease being targeted.

Thus, our topic is focussed on EGF and its role in maintaining the integrity of the gastrointestinal mucosa. To establish a context for this discussion we will briefly review the prevailing concepts regarding the maintenance of mucosal integrity and mucosal disease in the GI tract. Then, we will turn our attention to some of the data on EGF in the GI tract.

B. Perspective on Growth Factors

A few comments about peptide growth factors seem appropriate before focussing on the GI tract. First, it is important to realize that as the list of peptide growth factors has grown so has the appreciation that each of these hormones can influence a broad array of activities. As we will discuss below,

EGF has been shown to affect a broad array of biological activites only some of which actually relate to regulation of cellular growth. It is fair to say that none of the polypeptide growth factors described to date modulates only one biological response. Rather, it is apparent that each of these hormones functions to regulate a variety of biological responses in a number of cell types. Second, it must be emphasized that the growth regulating activities described for growth factors are a byproduct of the biological signaling function these hormones perform. Each of these peptide signals activates a defined set of intracellular signal transduction mechanisms (CARPENTER and COHEN 1990; SPORN and ROBERTS 1990). Consequently, the diversity of actions of the polypeptide hormones is likely the result of the diversity of cell types which possess receptors for these hormones. The different cell types have different biological responses linked to the signal transduction cascades initiated by the receptor-ligand interactions. Finally, peptide growth factors represent a unique set of hormones in that their site(s) of synthesis are as diverse as their target cells. For a better appreciation of the details of this complex group of hormones the reader is referred to a recently published comprehensive treatise (SPORN and ROBERTS 1990).

C. Perspective on Mucosal Disease

Mucosal disease and/or mucosal integrity are commonly represented as a balance between aggressive, offensive factors and defensive factors which appear to play some role in either resisting the aggressive factors or repairing the damage done (Fig. 1). The list of aggressive factors that are ordinarily put on a balance such as this includes acid, pepsin, other enzymes and bile salts. All of these factors can objectively be demonstrated to have the potential for cellular injury. Enzymes can digest the proteins and cell membranes damaging their integrity, as well as damaging the integrity of some other physical barriers that the GI tract possesses. Acids and bile salts can similarly cause cellular damage or damage to the barrier mechanisms. You will note, thromboxanes and other eicosanoids which are arachidonic acid derivatives structurally similar to prostaglandins.

The defensive side of this scale includes a variety of factors that appear to promote the integrity of gastrointestinal mucosa. This defensive side actually has two rather distinct components, the physical barriers to injury and the factors which affect resistance to and repair of mucosal injuries. Obviously, mucous and bicarbonate secretions at cellular surfaces represent the equivalent of direct physical barriers to some of the injuring agents "aggressive factors." Under resistance/repair prostaglandins and peptide growth factors are included. It should be noted that these are not complete lists, nor is it likely that a complete list of factors involved in mucosal integrity could be assembled anytime in the near future. Even more importantly, the factors involved and their quantitative relationships will not be equivalent in all

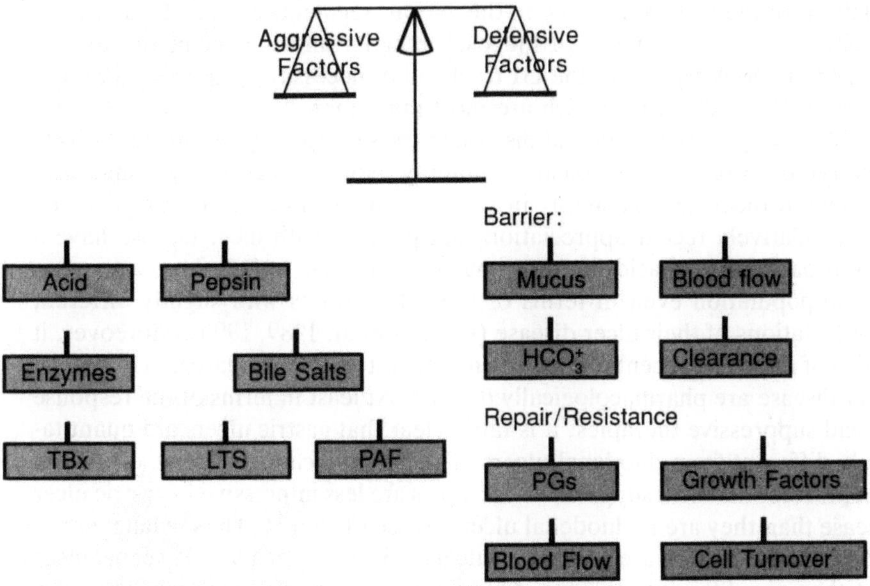

Fig. 1. Balance between aggressive, offensive factors and defensive factors in mucosal disease

segments of the GI tract. For example, clearance of aggressive factors is clearly important in the esophagus (ORR et al. 1981; RICHTER and CASTELL 1982). In contrast, the stomach appears to have a constantly harsh environment and clearance may have less importance. Also, the relative infrequency of gastric ulcers suggests that the stomach is largely resistant to its acidic environment. Moreover, local basic conditions have been shown to cause gastric injury and may be of some relevance in *H. pylori* infections (S. SZABO, Personal Communication). Similarly, acid is probably not a major component among the aggressive factors in lower portions of the GI tract where the predominant luminal environment is either neutral or basic. In the duodenum, however, it is fairly widely accepted that acidification is an important factor in duodenal ulcer disease.

The changing environment in the GI tract is responsible for altering the enzymatic activity that dominates in various segments. Pepsin is essentially only active in the stomach where the pH is <3 and the pancreatic enzymes have a variety of different pH optima that render them optimally active in various segments of the GI tract. Since all of these enzymes are different with respect to their turnover number and the amount of enzymes present, it is not hard to envision the complexity of the quantitative interrelationships that exist in the various regions of the GI tract.

Thus, this balance is actually a multitude of quantitatively different combinations of the factors involved in the various segments of the GI tract. Consequently, the maintenance of mucosal integrity and the repair of mucosal injury in various regions of the GI tract will of necessity be quite different in terms of the mechanisms which are most important.

This complexity of mucosal disease in the GI tract represents a relatively new appreciation in the medical community. Not long ago many would have considered ulcer disease simply in terms of the acid output of the patients. It is a relatively recent appreciation that patients with ulcer disease have a very broad range of acid secretory outputs and that in fact there appear to be sub-population even in terms of the acid outputs with slightly different manifestations of their ulcer disease (COLLEN et al. 1989, 1990). Moreover, it is also of relatively recent appreciation that gastric ulcer disease and duodenal ulcer disease are pharmacologically distinct. At least in terms of the response to acid suppressive therapies, it is fairly clear that gastric ulcers are quantitatively different from duodenal ulcers. The data indicate a pattern, even with omeprazole, that acid suppressive therapies are less impressive in gastric ulcer disease than they are in duodenal ulcer disease (Table 1). Thus, whatever the factors and balances are in gastric ulcer and duodenal ulcer it seems clear that they are different in some respect which is not well understood at this time.

These and other observations prompted researchers to search for the factors other than acid that might be important in mucosal integrity in the gastric mucosa. The work of Robert and others have demonstrated the involvement of prostaglandins in mucosal integrity (ROBERT 1977). However, it seems clear from the efforts that have been made on prostaglandins and acid suppressive therapies that the homeostatic mechanisms responsible for maintaining mucosal integrity extend well beyond these mechanisms. In this context, attention has turned to peptide growth factors and EGF in particular.

Table 1. Pharmacology of duodenal and gastric ulcer disease

		Healing rates (4 weeks)	
		DU	GU
Ranitidine		73%	59%
Cimetidine			(68%)[a]
Omeprazole	(10 mg)	68–86%	–
	(20 mg)	–	(66%)[a]
	(30 mg)	83%	–
	(40 mg)	–	69%
		92–94%	81%
		–	80%

Du, duodenal ulcer; GU, gastric ulcer.
[a] 6-week data.

D. EGF Structure

Stanley Cohen originally described EGF in 1962 (COHEN 1962). The primary and secondary structure of this 53 amino acid polypeptide (6054 daltons) are known from a variety of species (CARPENTER and WAHL 1990) Similarly, the structure of other members of the EGF family are known (CARPENTER and WAHL 1990). While the overall sequence homologies among this group of peptides are greater than 50% in general, the conservation around residues important in the secondary and tertiary structure are more striking. Recently, a consensus sequence has been reported ($X_nCX_7CX_{2-3}GXCX_{10-13}CXCX_3YXGXRCX_4LX_n$) in which the three disulfide bonds create loops which can be somewhat variable in length and amino acid sequence but basically invariant in secondary and tertiary structure (CARPENTER and COHEN 1990). NMR and circular dichroism studies indicate that neither EGF nor TGFα have much helical structure and both polypeptides have two sets of anti-parallel b-sheet structures. (HOLLADAY et al. 1976; MAYO 1984, 1985).

The gene and mRNA sequences for members of the EGF family are also known. All of the members of the EGF family are cleaved from larger precursor proteins which are translated from messages which undergo extensive post-transcriptional processing (MROCZKOWSKI et al. 1989; CARPENTER and WAHL 1990). The EGF precursor seems the most interesting of these proteins. It is a 130,000 dalton protein and contains eight additional amino acid sequences with significant homology to EGF (BELL et al. 1986; SCOTT et al. 1985; GRAY et al. 1983). At present, the understanding of the precursor is limited although it seems energetically wasteful to discard the 970 residue protein that results from the cleavage release of EGF.

E. Structure-Activity Relationships

Since there are several ligands which interact with the EGF receptor it is thought that understanding the common structural features may pinpoint the structural requirements for the ligand-receptor interaction. This research has exploited techniques to modify the polypeptide backbone of EGF either through genetic manipulation, chemical modification or enzymatic digestion. It should be noted that these studies have focussed principally on mitogenic activity or receptor binding as the functional assessments. Such an approach assumes that the diverse responses to EGF have a common receptor-mediated signal transduction mechanism which may activate functional pathways in different cell types.

Site directed mutagenesis studies have demonstrated that the leucine at residue 47, a highly conserved position in the EGF family, can not be altered without dramatic reductions in mitogenic activity (RAY et al. 1988; LAZAR et al. 1988; DUDGEON et al. 1990). Position 23 is also intolerant of the apparently conservative change of leucine to threonine (CAMPION et al. 1989).

Conservative substitutions for the aromatic residues in the second disulfide loop seem tolerated without huge losses in activity (DEFEO-JONES et al. 1989; ENGLER et al. 1988; CAMPION et al. 1989). Nonconservative changes of the charged residues in this second disulfide loop are well tolerated without loss of activity (ENGLER et al. 1988).

The effect of chemical modification of the methionine at position 21 has been somewhat controversial. Several laboratories have found that oxidation of this residue does not appear to change the activity of EGF (HEATH and MERRIfIELD 1986; RIEMAN et al. 1987). Cyanogen bromide treatment to cleave the peptide bond between positions 21 and 22 has been reported to have either drastic (BURGESS et al. 1988) or trivial (SCHECHTER et al. 1979; SCHREIBER et al. 1981) effect on receptor interaction. This later controversy may be related to the efficiency of the CNBr cleavage among these studies. Iodination of tyrosine residues does not apparently alter binding to the receptor in that this is the commonly used radioligand.

A broad array of fragments of EGF have been evaluated for receptor interactions. Some groups have reported receptor binding activity with synthetic peptides corresponding to the mid-portions of the EGF sequence, however, the potencies of these molecules were generally four or more orders of magnitude less than the intact EGF (KOMORIYA et al. 1984; HEATH and MERRIfIELD 1986; DEFEO-JONES et al. 1989). In contrast, additions and deletions to the N- or C-terminus have been shown to retain reasonable receptor interaction and mitogenic activity. N-terminal conjugates of EGF with fluorscein, ferritin, and ricin or diptheria toxin (A chains) exhibited more than 50% of the potency of the unmodified molecule (CHOPRA et al. 1987). Deletion of residues 1–5 does not appear to affect activity. (DEFEO-JONES et al. 1989) Loss of up to five of the C-terminal residues reportedly alters potency by varying amounts but generally within an order of magnitude of EGF (SHOYAB et al. 1989; BURGESS et al. 1988; GREGORY et al. 1988). Interestingly, several of these fragments are present in biological fluids such as plasma, saliva and urine (T. AMARANT et al., in preparation; Fig. 2). Further, EGF1-48 and EGF1-49 are more stable than EGF in gastric juice and trypsin (Fig. 3) although EGF has been reported somewhat resistant to proteolysis (MENEGATTI et al. 1989; BRITTON et al. 1989). EGF1-47 reportedly retains only about 10% of the activity of EGF and shorter fragments displayed even less activity (HOLLENBERG and GREGORY 1980; BURGESS et al. 1988; GREGORY et al. 1988).

F. Biological Effects

EGF was initially discovered while Dr. COHEN was attempting to identify factors that would stimulate neuronal growth. He observed that extracts of mouse submaxillary glands induced precocious eyelid opening and tooth eruption when administered to neonatal rats (COHEN 1962). A 53 amino

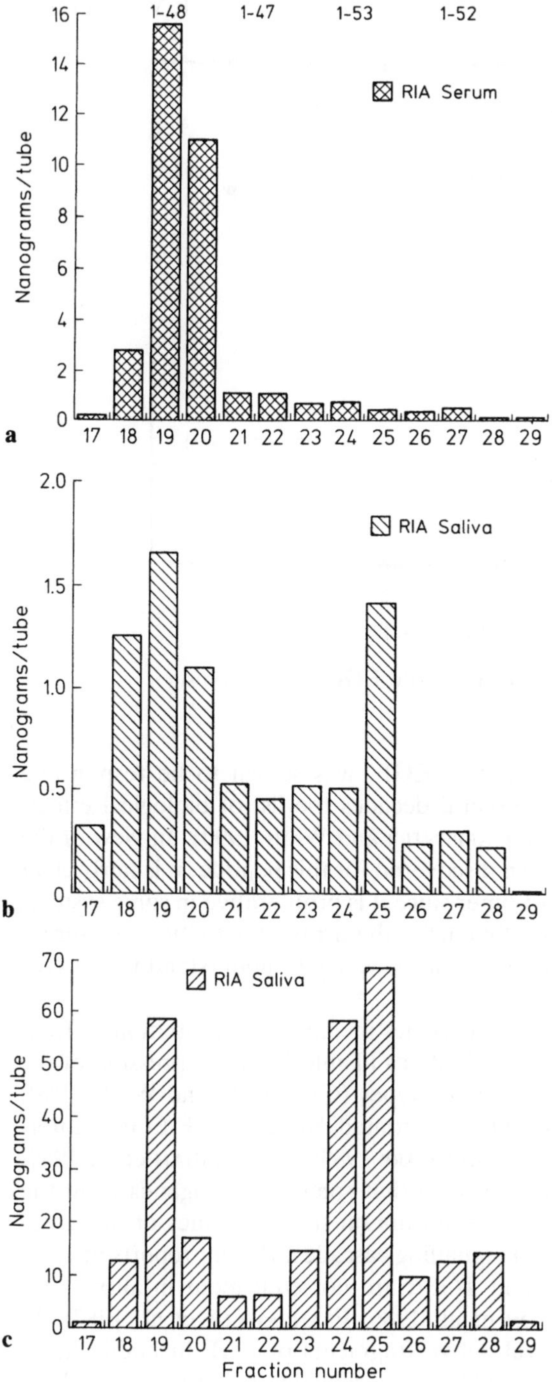

Fig. 2a.–c. EGF fragments present in plasma (**a**), saliva (**b**), and urine (**c**) according to radioimmuno assay (*RIA*)

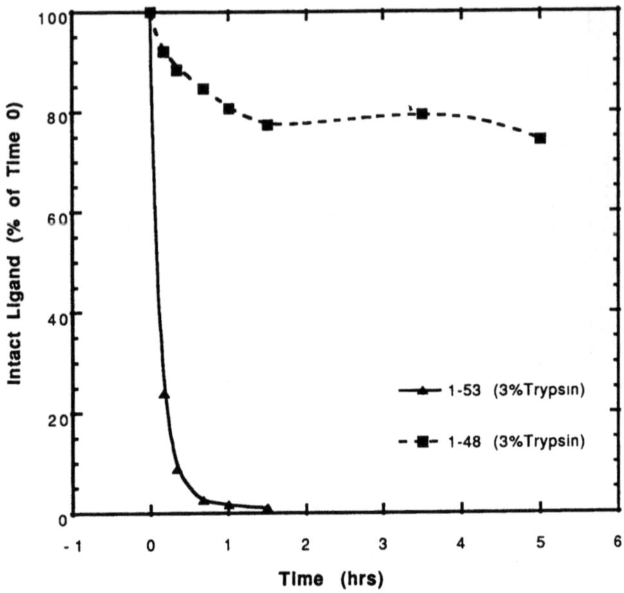

Fig. 3. Degradation of EGF and EGF 1–48 in trypsin

acid polypetide, subsequently dubbed EGF, was shown to be responsible for these effects. Over the last several decades the list of biological effects of EGF has grown (see tables in Carpenter and Wahl 1990). In view of the variety of activities that have been discovered for this peptide, it is fairly clear now that EGF is probably a misnomer since it is proliferative in some systems and antiproliferative in others. Obviously, the array of activities also represents something of a complicating factor as we try to understand the in vivo role of this compound.

The sources of this diversity of activities include the distribution of EGF immunoreactive material among body fluids (Table 2), the expression of the EGF receptors in nearly all adult tissue types (Carpenter and Wahl 1990) and the array of intracellular signals initiated by the EGF-EGFR interaction (Earp et al. 1988; McCune and Earp 1989; Cunningham et al. 1989; Carpenter and Cohen 1990). It may be that some of the ligands from the EGF family preferentially bind to receptors on specific tissues or preferentially activate certain intracellular signalling cascades. Recent reports provide the initial evidence that EGF and TGFα are not equivalent in all systems (Schreiber et al. 1986; Ibbotson et al. 1986; Francavilla et al. 1987). In addition, the presence of several active fragments of EGF in bodily fluids suggests that processing might enable some selective activity among these species (T. Amarant et al., in preparation). It is also possible that promiscuous receptor-ligand interactions may insure that a necessary regulatory signal is not lacking. At present, such issues can not be definitively resolved.

Table 2. Concentrations of EGF in biological fluids

Fluid	Mean (ng/ml)	Reference
Urine	88	STARKEY and ORTH
Saliva	92	1977
Milk	140	
Breast fluid	205	CONNOLLY and ROSE
Brunner's glands	1.6	1988
Pancreatic juice	2.3	
Serum	0.27	KIRKEGAARD et al. 1984
		HIRATA et al. 1982
		OKA and ORTH 1983

Further, it is unknown whether other EGF receptor-like molecules may play a role in generating diversity in the EGF activity profile.

In the context of this diverse activity profile and the questions identified above, we will turn our attention to the current understanding of the activity of EGF in the gastrointestinal tract.

G. Gastrointestinal Activity

As indicated in Table 2, EGF is found in many biological fluids and it is synthesized and secreted from many tissues. From these data it is apparent that the GI tract has a very significant exposure to EGF and other members of the EGF family including naturally occurring fragments of EGF. For the purposes of this discussion the effects of EGF in the GI tract fall into three main categories: developmental; gastric acid secretion; and trophic.

I. Developmental Effects of EGF

In addition to the originally discovered developmental effects, EGF was found to affect a variety of tissues in neonatal mice (COHEN and TAYLOR 1974). In the GI tract, neonatal rats receiving parentral EGF had significantly increased whole stomach weights, increased DNA, RNA and protein content of the mucosa and increased gastric acid secretion (DEMBINSKI and JOHNSON 1985). Duodenal and gastric tissue increases in ornithine decarboxylase activity have been reported for EGF treated mice (FELDMAN et al. 1978). In addition, human fetal tissue organ culture studies have demonstrated that EGF has significant effects on the morphology, proliferation and differentiation of various gastrointestinal tissues (WEAVER and WALKER 1988; MENARD et al. 1988; CHOPRA et al. 1987). Interestingly, the morphological and differentiating effects may be the most important with proliferative activity being affected by other growth regulating hormones (MENARD et al. 1988; CHOPRA et al. 1987).

It has long been recognized that milk contains significant amounts of EGF (Table 2). This has led to investigation into the possible role of ingested EGF in the development of the GI tract. Several reports address the absorption of EGF from the GI tract (WEAVER et al. 1990; THORNBURG et al. 1987). Clearly, EGF in the gastrointestinal lumen was found to interact with the intestinal mucosa. These tissues had 10- to 100-fold higher concentration of the exogenous ligand than other tissues examined. Confirmation that the EGF in the other tissues was the result of absorption of intact EGF was not reported in these studies. EGF administered by gavage to neonatal rats (POLLACK et al. 1987) or rabbits (O'LOUGHLIN et al. 1985) has been found to affect the maturation of the intestinal brush border. Interestingly, parenteral administration showed a different profile of effects (O'LOUGHLIN et al. 1985). In view of the data showing several EGF fragments in biological fluids, these differing profiles may be the result of different ligands interacting with different tissues.

II. Gastric Acid Secretion

Among the gastrointestinal activities that have been reported for EGF are effects on gastric acid secretion. It is notable that human urogastrone, which was subsequently found to be EGF, was isolated using inhibition of gastric acid secretion as the bioassay (GREGORY 1975, 1985). In perfused rat stomach preparations intravenous injection of EGF was found to abolish histamine-stimulated acid secretion (BOWER et al. 1975). In Heidenhain pouch dogs, gastric acid secretion was also suppressed following intravenous administration of EGF (BOWER et al. 1975; GREGORY et al. 1988). S.J. KONTUREK et al. (1984) reported dose-dependent inhibition of pentagastrin stimulated gastric acid secretion in both gastric fistula and Heidenhain pouch dogs. EGF also inhibited histamine and urecholine stimulated gastric acid secretion in these models. EGF did not affect serum gastrin levels. In rats, intravenous administration of EGF suppressed both basal and gastrin stimulated gastric acid secretion (OLSEN et al. 1986a). Fragments of EGF have also been reported to suppress gastric acid secretion (GREGORY et al. 1988; A. GUGLIETTA et al., personal communication) although they may not be as potent as EGF (GREGORY et al. 1988).

It appears that this inhibition of secretion may involve acid production in parietal cells as evidenced by the fact that there appears to be dose-dependent inhibition of aminopyrine accumulation in isolated gastric glands treated with EGF (DEMBINSKI et al. 1986; SHAW et al. 1987; FINKE et al. 1985). Histamine- and cAMP-stimulated aminopyrine accumulation was inhibited but inhibition of the cAMP-stimulated accumulation was only observed at $10^{-4} M$ cAMP or less. In contrast to the in vivo data, carbechol stimulated aminopyrine accumulation was unaffected by EGF (SHAW et al. 1987). It should be noted that these inhibitory activities of EGF are quantitatively less efficacious than proton pump inhibitors under all conditions and less effective than H2 antagonists in histamine-stimulated glands.

These anti-secretory effects have been confirmed in humans following intravenous administration. In volunteers (ELDER et al. 1975; S.J. KONTUREK et al. 1989), patients with a history of duodenal ulcer disease (KOFFMAN et al. 1982) and patients with Zollinger-Ellison syndrome (ELDER et al. 1974) EGF was found to inhibit pentagastrin-stimulated gastric acid secretion. Doses of 1 $\mu g\, kg^{-1}\, h^{-1}$ also inhibited basal acid output (S.J. KONTUREK et al. 1989). Serum gastrin level were reportedly unaffected by the EGF infusions. Secretion of EGF was reportedly stimulated by sham and ordinary feeding although the increased plasma level apparently is not enough to affect gastric acid secretion (S.J. KONTUREK et al. 1989).

Interestingly, in animals intragastric administration of EGF does not appear to affect gastric acid or pepsin secretion (S.J. KONTUREK et al. 1981a; OLSEN et al. 1986). Intraduodenal infusions were also without effect on either basal or pentagastrin-stimulated gastric acid secretion (OLSEN et al. 1986a; KIRKEGAARD et al. 1983). It is notable that these intralumenal administrations were at doses 10- to 100-fold greater than the parenteral doses that produced significant inhibition of acid secretion

III. Trophic Effects

Trophic activity in the intestine has been reported for intravenously administered EGF (GOODLAD et al. 1987). Installation of EGF into the gastrointestinal lumen also has trophic effect. ULSHEN et al. (1986) have demonstrated increases in DNA synthesis and crypt labeling in response to intralumenal infusions of EGF (1.25–15 μg/48 h). These effects were principally local in that ileal infusion had relatively minor upstream effect, while jejunal infusion did have some downstream effects which were significantly less than the local jejunal effects. Similarly, intragastric administration of EGF has been shown to increase organ weight and DNA synthesis in both the stomach and duodenum (DEMBINSKI et al. 1982).

In an attempt to identify whether EGF may have a role in the pathophysiology of the GI tract, a series of studies has been performed to evaluate the effect of salivary secretions and exogenous EGF in the maintenance and restoration of mucosal integrity. Removal of the salivary gland was associated with both gastric lesions and duodenal ulcers in cysteamine-treated rats (OLSEN et al. 1984) while cysteamine-treated controls had only duodenal ulcers. EGF or saliva +EGF reduced the cysteamine damage in sialoadenectomized rats. Sialoadenectomy slowed the healing of cysteamine- and acetic acid-induced lesions in the stomach and duodenum (OLSEN et al. 1986a,b; S.J. KONTUREK et al. 1988). Oral, intragastric, or subcutaneous administration of EGF restored the rate of healing. Further, EGF treatment accelerated the rate of ulcer healing in animals with salivary glands intact. EGF treatment has also been shown to reduce the injury or to accelerate the healing of lesions induced by aspirin (S.J. KONTUREK et al. 1981b).

The mechanism by which EGF stimulates healing appears to be the result of an increased rate of tissue repair. In EGF treated animals, the rate at which the ulcer shrinks (tissue is regenerated) is markedly faster in EFG treated rats or dogs than in animals receiving only saline therapy (NARDI et al. unpublished data, GUGLIETTA et al. unpublished data). This increased healing rate was dose dependent (Figs. 4, 5). Thus, it appears that the effect of EGF in terms of the ulcer healing process is one in which the rate of tissue regeneration is stimulated.

H. Conclusion

The studies on the mechanism of action of EGF in ulcer healing have left a picture of mucosal disease that can be represented as having at least two phases (Fig. 6). There is a period which can be termed the precontracture or pre-healing period during which a mucosal injury may get worse or stay about the same. The events that are ongoing during this time are unclear. During this time period the body must begin the healing process. Subsequently, re-epithelization occurs. EGF can stimulate this reepithelization process. The localization of the EGR receptor to the basolateral membranes of intestinal enterocytes suggests that this repair activity may be precluded except when mucosal injuries exist (SCHEVING et al. 1989).

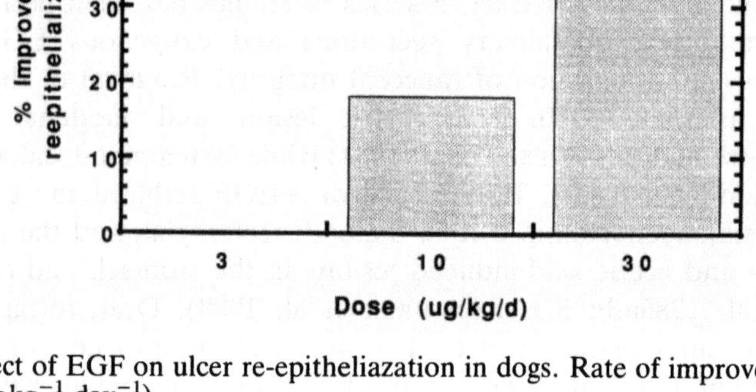

Fig. 4. Effect of EGF on ulcer re-epitheliazation in dogs. Rate of improvement (%) vs. dose ($\mu g\,kg^{-1}\,day^{-1}$)

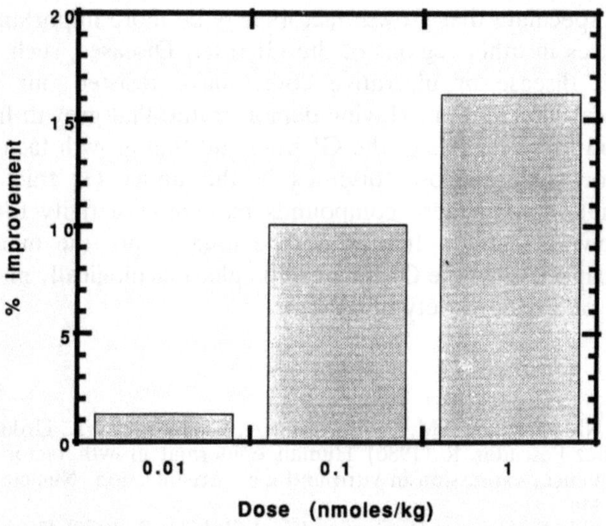

Fig. 5. Effect of EGF on nonsteroidal anti-inflammatory drug (NSAID)-induced gastric damage in the rat. % improvement vs. dose (nmoles/kg)

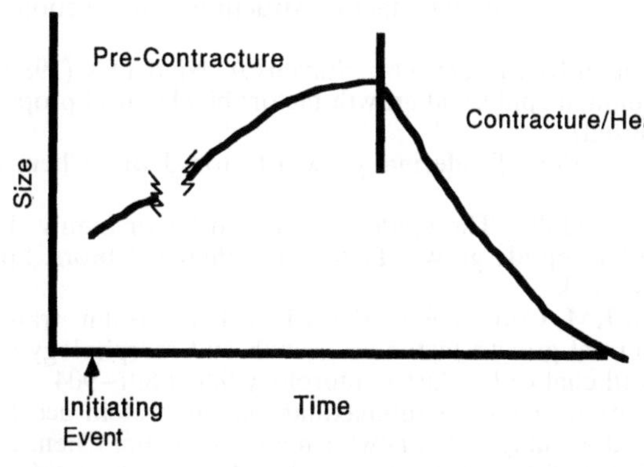

Fig. 6. Ulcer phases

Interestingly, acid suppressive therapies do not appear to effect the rate at which tissue regeneration occurs rather their effects appear during the pre-contracture period (R. De Novo et al. unpublished data).

We are entering an exciting time in terms of our understanding of mucosal disease. It is also fairly clear that acid suppressive therapies may not be the total answer in mucosal diseases of the GI tract. Epidermal growth factor and/or other factors that influence the reepithelization process must be evaluated as additional armamentarium for the physician to use for patients with mucosal diseases that are untreated by or refractory to current therapies. Hopefully, we will be able to identify patient populations who are most in need of the different types of therapies that will become available. It is also interesting to speculate that growth factors may be more important in other mucosal diseases in other regions of the GI tract. Diseases, such as inflammatory bowel disease or ulcerative colitis have resisted our efforts at pharmacological intervention. Having demonstrated that growth factors can have effects on these regions of the GI tract and that growth factors can be therapeutic for some mucosal diseases in the upper GI tract it seems reasonable that in time these compounds may show activity for mucosal diseases in lower GI tract. It may not be long before the maintenance/regenerative capacities of the GI tract can be pharmacologically manipulated to the benefit of a wide variety of patients.

References

Bell GI, Fong NM, Stempie NM, Wormsted MA, Caput D, Ku L, Urdea MS, Rall LB, Sanchez-Pescador R (1986) Human epidermal growth factor precursor: cDNA sequence, expression in vitro and gene organization. Nucleic Acids Res 14:8427–8446

Bower JM, Camble R, Gregory H, Gerring EL, Willshire IR (1975) The inhibition of gastric acid secretion of epidermal growth factor. Experientia 31:825–826

Britton JR, George-Nascimento C, Udall JN, Koldovsky O (1989) Minimal hydrolysis of epidermal growth factor by gastric fluid of preterm infants. Gut 30:327–332

Burgess AW, Lloyd CJ, Smith S, Stanley E, Walker F, Fabri L, Simpsom RJ, Nice EC (1988) Murine epidermal growth factor: structure and function. Biochemistry 27:4977–4985

Campion SR, Matsunami RK, Engler DA, Stevens A, Niyogi SK (1989) Site-directed mutagenesis of human epidermal growth factor: biochemical properties of β-loop mutants. (submitted)

Carpenter G, Cohen S (1990) Epidermal growth factor. J Biol Chem 265(14):7709–7712

Carpenter G, Wahl MI (1990) The epidermal growth factor family. In: Sporn MB, Roberts AB, (eds) Peptide growth factors and their receptors. Springer, Berlin Heidelberg New York

Chopra DP, Siddiqui KM, Cooney RA (1987) Effects of insulin, transferin, cholera toxin, and epidermal growth factor on growth and morphology of human fetal normal colon epithelial cells. Gastroenterology 92(4):891–904

Cohen S (1962) Isolation of mouse submaxillary gland protein accelerating incisor eruption and eylid opening in the newborn animal. J Biol Chem 237:1555–1562

Cohen S, Taylor JM (1974) Epidermal growth factor: chemical and biological characterization. Recent Prog Horm Res 30:533–550

Collen MJ, Stanczak VJ, Ciarleglio CA (1989) Refractory duodenal ulcers (nonhealing duodenal ulcers with standard doses of antisecretory medication). Dig Dis Sci 34:233–237

Collen MJ, Lewis JH, Benjamin SB (1990) Gastric acid hypersecretion in refractory gastroesophageal reflux disease. Gastroenterology 98:654–661

Connolly JM, Rose DP (1988) Epidermal growth factor-like proteins in breast fluid and human milk. Life Sci 42:1751–1756

Cunningham TW, Kuppuswamy D, Pike LJ (1989) Treatment of A431 cells with epidermal growth factor (EGF) induces desensitization of EGF-stimulated phosphatidylinositol. J Biol Chem 264(26):15351–15356

Defeo-Jones D, Tai JY, Vuocolo GA, Wegrzyn RJ, Schofield TL, Riemen MW, Oliff A (1989) Substitution of lysine for arginine at position 42 of human transforming growth factor-α eliminates biological activity without changing internal disulfide bonds. Mol Cell Biol 9(9):4083–4086

Dembinski A, Gregory H, Konturek SJ, Polanski M (1982) Trophic actions of epidermal growth factor on the pancreas and gastroduodenal mucosa in rats. J Physiol (Lond) 325:35–42

Dembinski AB, Johnson LR (1985) Effect of epidermal growth factor on the development of rat gastric mucosa. Endocrinology 116(1):90–94

Dembinski A, Drozdowicz D, Gregory H, Konturek SJ, Warzecha Z (1986) Inhibition of acid formation by epidermal growth factor in the isolated rabbit gastric glands. Physiologie 378:347–357

Dudgeon TJ, Cooke RM, Baron M, Cambell ID, Edwards RM, Fallon A (1990) Structure-function analysis of epidermal growth factor: site-directed mutagenesis and nuclear magnetic reasonance. EBS Lett 261(2):392–396

Earp HS, Hepler JR, Petch LA, Miller A, Berry AR, Harris J, Raymond VW, McCune BK, Lee LW, Grisham JW, Harden TK (1988) Epidermal growth factor (EGF) and hormones stimulate phosphoinositide hydrolsis and increase EGF receptor protein synthesis and mRNA levels in rat liver epithelial cells. J Biol Chem 263(27):13868–13874

Elder JB, Ganguli PC, Gillespie IE, Gerring EL, Gregory H (1974) Effect of urogastrone in Zollinger-Ellison syndrome. Br J Surg 61:916

Elder JB, Ganguli PC, Gillespie IE, Gerring EL, Gregory H (1975) Effect of urogastrone on gastric secretion and plasma gastrin levels in normal subjects. Gut 16:887–893

Engler DA, Rise K, Matsunami RK, Campion SR, Stringer CD, Stevens A, Niyogi SK (1988) Cloning of authentic human epidermal growth factor as a bacterial secretory protein and its initial structure-function analysis by site-directed mutagenesis. J Biol Chem 263:12384–12390

Feldman EJ, Aures D, Grossman MI (1978) Epidermal growth factor stimulates ornithine decarboxylase activity in the digestive tract of mouse. Proc Soc Exp Biol Med 159:400

Finke U, Rutten M, Murphy RA, Silen W (1985) Effects of epidermal growth factor on acid secretion from Guinea pig gastric mucosa: in vitro analysis. Gastroenterology 88(5):1175–1182

Francavilla A, Ove P, Polimeno L, Sciascia C, Coetzee M, Pellici R, Todo S, Kam I, Starzl TE (1987) Different response to epidermal growth factor of hepatocytes in cultures isolated from male or female rat liver. Gastroenterology 93:597–605

Goodlad RA, Wilson TJG, Lenton W, Gregory H, McCullagh KG, Wright NA (1987) Intravenous but not intragastric urogastrone-EGF is trophic to the intestine of parenterally fed rats. Gut 28:573–582

Gray A, Dull TJ, Ullrich A (1983) Nucleotide sequence of epidermal growth factor cDNA predicts a 128 000 molecular weight protein precursor. Nature 303:722–725

Gregory H (1975) Isolation and structure of urogastrone and its relationship to epidermal growth factor. Nature 257:325–327

Gregory H (1985) In vivo aspects of urogastrone-epidermal growth factor. Cell Sci Suppl 3:11–17

Gregory H, Thomas CE, Young JA, Willshire IR, Garner A (1988) The contribution of the C-terminal undecapeptide sequence of urogastrone-epidermal growth factor to its biologcial action. Regul Pept 22:217–226

Heath WF, Merrifield RB (1986) A synthetic approach to structure-function relationships in the murine epidermal growth factor molecule. Proc Natl Acad Sci 83(17):6367–6371

Hirata Y, Uchihashi M, Nakajima M, Fukita T, Matsukura S (1982) Immunoreactive human epidermal growth factor in human pancreatic juice. J Clin Endocrinol Metab 54:1174–1177

Holladay LA, Savage CR, Cohen S, Puett D (1976) Conformation and unfolding thermodynamics of epidermal growth factor and derivatives. Biochemistry 15:2624–2633

Hollenberg M, Gregory H (1980) Epidermal growth factor-urogastrone: biological activity and receptor binding derivatives. Mol Pharmacol 17:314–320
Ibbotson KJ, Twardzik DR, D'Souza S, Smith DD, Winkler ME, Derynck R, Mundy GR (1986) Human recombinant transforming growth factor α stimulates bone resorption and inhibits formation in vitro. Proc Natl Acad Sci USA 83:2228–2232
Kirkegaard P, Olsen PS, Poulsen SS, Nexo E (1983) Epidermal growth factor inhibits cysteamine-induced duodenal ulcers. Gastroenterology 85:1277–1283
Kirkegaard P, Olsen PS, Nexo E, Holst JJ, Poulsen SS (1984) Effect of vasoactive intestinal polypeptide and somatostatin on secretion of epidermal growth factor and bicarbonate from Brunner's glands. Gut 24:1225–1229
Koffman CG, Elder JB, Ganguli PC, Gregory H, Geary CG (1982) Effect of urogastrone on gastric secretion and serum gastrin concentration in patients with duodenal ulceration. Gut 23:951–956
Komoriya A, Hortsch M, Meyers C, Smith M, Kanety H, Schlessinger J (1984) Biologically active synthetic fragments of epidermal growth factor: localization of a major receptor-binding region. Proc Natl Acad Sci USA 81(3):1351–1355
Konturek JW, Bielanski W, Konturek SJ, Bogdal J, Oleksy J (1989) Distribution and release of epidermal growth factor in man. Gut 30:1194–1200
Konturek SJ (1988) Role of epidermal growth factor in gastroprotection and ulcer healing. Scand J Gastroenterol 23:129–133
Konturek SJ, Radecki T, Brzozowski T, Piastucki I, Dembinski A, Dembinska-Kiec A, Amuda A, Gryglewski R, Gregory H (1981a) Gastric cytoprotection by epidermal growth factor. Gastroenterology 81(3):438–443
Konturek SJ, Brzozowski T, Piastucki I, Dembinski A, Radecki T, Dembinska-Kiec A, Zmuda A, Gregory H (1981b) Role of mucosal prostaglandins and DNA synthesis in gastric cytoprotection by luminal epidermal growth factor. Gut 22:927–932
Konturek SJ, Cieszkowski M, Jaworek J, Konturek J, Brzozowski T, Gregory H (1984) Effects of epidermal growth factor on gastrointestinal secretions. Am J Physiol 246:G580–G586
Konturek SJ, Dembinski A, Warzecha Z, Brzozowski T, Gregory H (1988) Role of epidermal growth factor in healing of chronic gastroduodenal ulcers in rats. Gastroenterology 94(6):1300–1307
Konturek SJ, Bielandski W, Konturek JW, Oleksy J, Yamazaki J (1989) Release and action of epidermal growth factor on gastric secretion in humans. Scand J Gastroenterol 24:485–492
Lazar E, Watanabe S, Dalton D, Sporn MB (1988) Transforming growth factor a: mutation of aspartic acid 47 and leucine 48 results in different biological activities. Mol Cell Biol 8:1247–1252
Levi-Montalcini R, Hamburger V (1951) Selective growth stimulating effects of mouse sarcoma on the sensory and sympathetic nervous system of the chick embryo. J Exp Zool 116:233–238
Mayo K (1984) Epidermal growth factor from the mouse. Structural characterization by proton nuclear magnetic resonance and nuclear Overhauser experiments and 500 MHz. Biochemistry 23:3960–3973
Mayo K (1985) Epidermal growth factor from the mouse. Physical evidence for a tiered β-sheet domain: two dimensional NMR correlated spectroscopy and nuclear Overhauser experiments on bacbone amide protons. Biochemistry 24:3783–3794
McCune BK, Earp HS (1989) The epidermal growth factor receptor tyrosine kinase in liver epithelial cells: the effect of ligand-dependent changes in cellular location. J Biol Chem 264(26):15501–15507
Menard D, Arsenault P, Pothier P (1988) Biologic effects of epidermal growth factor in human fetal jejunum. Gastroenterology 94(3):656–663
Menegatti E, Scalia S, Bortolotti F, Ascenzi P, DeMarco A (1989) Controlled proteolysis of mouse epidermal growth factor. Int J Pept Protein Res 34:161–165

Mroczkowski B, Reich M, Chen K, Bell GI (1989) Recombinant human epidermal growth factor precursor is a glycosylated membrane protein with biological activity. (1989) Mol Cell Biol 9(7):2771–2778
Oka Y, Orth DN (1983) Human plasma epidermal growth factor/β-urogastrone is associated with blood platelets. J Clin Invest 72:249–259
O'Loughlin EV, Chung M, Hollenberg M, Hayden J, Zahavi I, Gall DGJ (1985) Effect of epidermal growth factor on ontogeny of the gastrointestinal tract. Am J Physiol 249:G674–G678
Olsen PS, Poulsen SS, Kirkengaard P, Nexo E (1984) Role of submandibular saliva and epidermal growth factor in gastric protection. Gastroenterology 87(1):103–108
Olsen PS, Poulsen SS, Therkelsen K, Nexo E (1986a) Oral administration of synthetic human urogastrone promotes healing of chronic duodenal ulcers in rats. Gastroenterology 90(4):911–917
Olsen PS, Poulsen SS, Therkelsen K, Nexo E (1986b) Effect of sialoadenectomy and synthetic human urogastrone on healing of chronic gastric ulcers in rats. Gut 27:1443–1449
Orr WC, Robinson MG, Johnson LF (1981) Acid clearance during sleep in the pathogenesis of reflux esophagitis. Dig Dis Sci 26:423–427
Pollack PF, Goda T, Colony PC, Edmond J, Thornburg W, Korc M, Koldovsky O (1987) Effects of enterally fed epidermal growth factor on the small and large intestine of the suckling rat. Regul Pept 17:121–132
Ray P, Moy, FJ, Montelione GT, Lui J, Narang SA, Schlerga HA, Wu R (1988) Structure-function studies of murine epidermal growth factor: expression and site-directed mutagenesis of epidermal growth factor gene. Biochemistry 27:7289–7295
Richter JE, Castell DO (1982) Gastroesophageal reflux: pathogenesis, diagnosis and therapy. Ann Intern Med 97:93–103
Rieman MW, Wegrzyn RJ, Baker AE, Hurni WM, Bennett CD, Oliff A, Stein RB (1987) Isolation of multiple biologically active and chemically diverse species of epidermal growth factor. Peptides 8:877–885
Robert A (1977) Cytoprotection of prostaglandins. Gastroenterology 77:761–767
Schechter Y, Hernaez L, Schlessinger J, Cuatrecasas P (1979) Local aggregation of hormone-receptor complexes is required for activation by epidermal growth factor. Nature 278:835–838
Scheving LA, Shiuba RA, Nguyen TD, Gray GM (1989) Epidermal growth factor receptor of the intestinal enterocyte. J Biol Chem 264(3):1735–1741
Schreiber AB, Yarden Y, Schlessinger JA (1981) A non-mitogenic analogue of epidermal growth factor enhances the phosphorylation of endogenous membrane proteins. Biochem Biophys Res Commun 101:517–523
Schreiber AB, Winkler ME, Derynck R (1986) Transforming growth factor α: a more potent angiogenic mediator than epidermal growth factor. Science 232:1250–1253
Scott J, Patterson S, Rall L, Bell GI, Crawford R, Penschow J, Niall H, Coghlan J (1985) The structure and biosynthesis of epidermal growth factor precursor. Cell Sci Suppl 5:19–28
Shaw GP, Hatt JF, Anderson NG, Hanson PJ (1987) Action of epidermal growth factor on acid secretion by rat isolated parietal cells. Biochem J 244:699–704
Shoyab M, Plowman GD, McDonald VL, Bradley JG, Todaro GJ (1989) Structure and function of human amphiregulin: a member of the epidermal growth factor family. Science 243:1074–1076
Sporn MB, Roberts AB (1990) Peptide growth factors and their receptors. Springer, Berlin Heiclelberg New York
Starkey RH, Orth SDN (1977) Radioimmunoassay of human epidermal growth factor (urogastrone). J Clin Endocrinol Metab 45:1144–1153
Thornburg W, Rao RK, Matrisian LM, Magaun BE, Koldovsky O (1987) Effect of maturation on gastrointestinal absorption of epidermal growth factor in rats. Am J Physiol 253:G68–G71

Ulshen MH, Lyn-Cook LE, Raasch RH (1986) Effects of intraluminal epidermal growth factor on mucosal proliferation in the small intestine of adult rats. Gastroenterology 91(5):1134–1140
Weaver LT, Gonnella PA, Israel EJ, Walker WA (1990) Uptake and transport of epidermal growth factor by the small intestinal epithelium of the fetal rat. Gastroenterology 98(4):828–837
Weaver LT, Walker WA (1988) Epidermal growth factor and the developing human gut. Gastroenterology 94(3):845–847

CHAPTER 3

Gastrin and Other Peptide Hormones

J. VAN DAM and M.M. WOLFE

A. Introduction

The existence of a humoral substance involved in the stimulation of gastric acid secretion was first postulated in 1905 by EDKINS, who characterized an antral mucosal extract which he called gastrin. For many years the activity of this substance was confused with that of histamine, casting serious doubt on the existence of gastrin. The studies of KOMAROV in 1938 verified gastrin as a hormone distinct from histamine. In 1964, GREGORY and TRACY succeeded in isolating the peptide from porcine antral mucosa, identifying its amino acid composition, and synthesizing it.

Gastrin, secreted by G (gastrin) cells in the antral mucosa, is the most potent substance known to stimulate gastric acid secretion (WOLFE and McGUIGAN 1984). Following stimulation, the secretion of acid is modulated by a negative feedback loop in which antral acidification inhibits the further release of acid (WALSH and LAM 1980; WOLFE and SOLL 1988). The precise mechanism of this negative feedback loop has not been elucidated, although recent studies suggest the potential involvement of the polypeptide somatostatin (SHORT et al. 1985a). Previous studies (CHAYVIALLE et al. 1978; HARTY et al. 1986) suggest that alterations in the normal relationship between antral gastrin and somatostatin cells may contribute to the gastric acid hypersecretion seen in some ulcer patients; however, the precise role of gastrointestinal regulatory peptides in the pathogenesis of peptic ulcer disease remains unknown.

B. The Molecular Heterogeneity of Gastrin

Gastrointestinal regulatory peptides are generally synthesized as precursors (prohormones), which are subsequently altered by enzymatic cleavage into their bioactive forms. Many peptides exist naturally in several molecular forms which vary by the length of the peptide chain, with the smaller form constituting an integral component of the larger molecule. Although the different forms of the peptide exhibit similar biological properties, their activities may differ with respect to potency or duration of action. In addition to multiple molecular forms of an individual regulatory peptide, many peptides are related, with variable degrees of structural homology in their amino acid sequence. Often these structurally homologous peptides possess similar biological properties, and it has been postulated that such peptides may be derived from a common ancestral form.

As has been observed with other gastrointestinal peptides, gastrin exists in several molecular forms (Fig. 1). The first gastrin peptide discovered was the heptadecapeptide form G17 (Fig. 2), often referred to as "little gastrin" (GREGORY et al. 1979). With the introduction of gastrin radioimmunoassay, a larger, more basic form of the peptide was demonstrated, which was designated "big gastrin." This peptide contains 34 amino acids (G34), including the G17 heptadecapeptide covalently linked at the N-terminal with a structurally distinct heptadecapeptide. Although the precise relationship between these two peptides is not universally accepted, prevailing theories suggest that G17 is generated by sequential tryptic cleavage of G34 (DOCKRAY et al. 1978). Both are derived from a precursor peptide called preprogastrin consisting of 101 amino acid residues, which contains a single copy of the sequence corresponding to G34 (PAUWELS et al. 1986). The gene that directs the synthesis of preprogastrin has been demonstrated in human DNA and consists

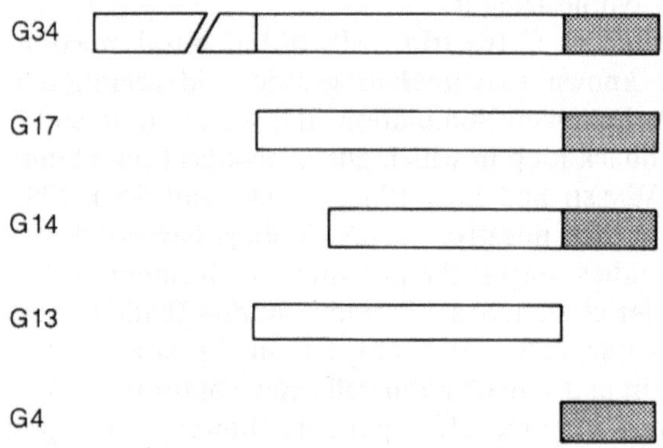

Fig. 1. Major molecular species of gastrin. All except G13 contain the biologically active C-terminal portion (indicated by the *stippled portion*)

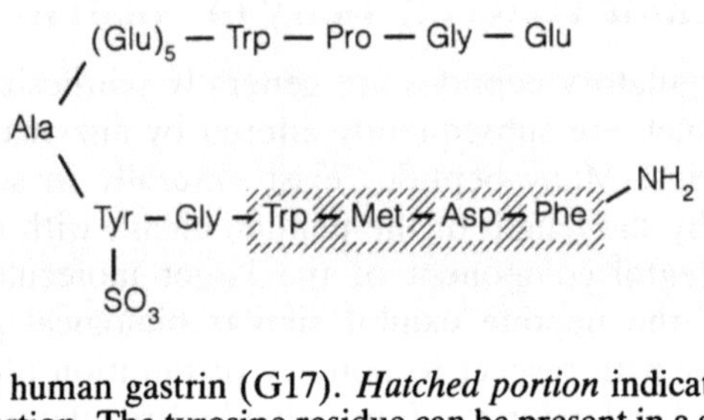

Fig. 2. Structure of human gastrin (G17). *Hatched portion* indicates the biologically active C-terminal portion. The tyrosine residue can be present in a sulfated (as shown) or nonsulfated form.

of approximately 4100 base pairs (WIBORG et al. 1984). Other circulating forms of gastrin have been described which occur in low concentration or do not increase postprandially (WOLFE and MCGUIGAN 1984). The two most prominent of these, previously referred to as "minigastrins," are the C-terminal tetradecapeptide (G14) and N-terminal tridecapeptide (G13). The former is biologically active, while the latter lacks the C-terminal tetrapeptide required for acid secretion (Fig. 1). The smallest biologically active form to be isolated from the stomach is the C-terminal hexapeptide G6 (GREGORY et al. 1979); however, the precise role of this fragment is not yet fully understood. In all, high resolution gel and ion-exchange chromatography have suggested the presence of at least 20 different forms of immunoreactive gastrin (REHFELD 1980).

In antral mucosa, which contains the highest tissue concentration of gastrin, G17 is the predominant molecular form, with only a small proportion of G34 present. In contrast, in the duodenum and proximal jejunum, the ratio of G17 to G34 approaches 1 (LAMERS et al. 1982). Early studies suggested that the potency of circulating G17 in the stimulation of gastric acid secretion was six to eight times that of G34 (WALSH et al. 1976), but more recent studies have demonstrated the two to be equipotent on a molar basis (EYSSELEIN et al. 1984). Therefore, although it was previously felt that the amount of G34 released after a meal did not contribute substantially to the acid secretory response, it is now estimated that due to its longer biological half-life, G34 may account for as much as one-third of the meal-stimulated gastrin release (LAMERS et al. 1982).

C. Gastrin Release

Gastrin release is stimulated by a number of intraluminal substances as well as neural signals and mediators. Food is the most important stimulant of gastrin release and protein the most potent component of food to stimulate acid secretion (RICHARDSON et al. 1976). While some experiments using vagally denervated fundic (Heidenhain) pouches demonstrate that a meat meal potentiates pentagastrin-induced acid secretion by a humoral mechanism (FERNSTROM et al. 1987), most evidence suggests it is the products of proteolysis, such as amino acids and small fragments, that most significantly stimulate gastrin release (ELWIN 1974). Not all amino acids are equipotent in their ability to stimulate gastrin release, and phenylalanine and tryptophan appear to be the most potent in this regard (TAYLOR et al. 1982).

The first step in protein-stimulated gastrin release is the transport of amino acids into the cell. Experiments in isolated rodent G cells demonstrate that the ability of an amino acid to stimulate gastrin release is directly correlated to its lipid solubility, the aromatic and long chain aliphatic amino acids being the most potent (LICHTENBERGER et al. 1982a). The next step in protein-stimulated gastrin release is amino acid decarboxylation to a postulated, intracellular second messenger amine. The requirement of decarboxylation prior to protein-stimulated gastrin release is supported by evidence that inhibitors of decarboxylase activity abolish amino acid-induced gastrin release (LICHTENBERGER et al. 1982a) and that removal of ammonia and amines from the standard diet by lyophylization produces a 50% attenuation in the postprandial release of gastrin (LICHTENBERGER et al. 1982b). Challenge with a protein-rich meal potentiates gastric acid secretion in dogs (KEUPPENS et al. 1976) and in cats (FERNSTROM et al. 1982; REHFELD and UVNAS-WALLENSTEN 1978). Although this potentiation may be stimulated by the absorption of amino acids (FERNSTROM and EMAS 1985; ISENBERG and MAXWELL 1978), other experimental evidence in cats suggests that the mechanism of potentiation of gastric acid secretion in response to a protein meal is humoral in origin and independent of amino acid absorption (FERNSTROM et al. 1987). A novel, nongastrin peptide has been identified in extracts of porcine intestine and has been designated "entero-oxyntin" (VAGNE and MUTT 1980). This peptide has been shown to increase acid secretion in cats prepared with Heidenhain pouches and to enhance the gastric acid secretory response to intravenous pentagastrin. Whether this mechanism exists in humans is unknown.

Secretion of preformed cellular products involves, in part, the transduction of cell surface stimulation into intracellular second messengers. In addition to the intracellular amines discussed previously, calcium may also function as an intracellular second messenger. The precise role for calcium in gastrin release and gastric acid secretion is not yet clear. In vitro experiments using enriched rodent G cells have demonstrated an increase in gastrin release when the calcium channel antagonist verapamil is added to calcium-containing cell medium (LICHTENBERGER et al. 1981). In contrast, studies using rat antral organ culture demonstrated that cAMP-stimulated release of gastrin is, at least in part, calcium dependent, an assertion further supported by the stimulation of gastrin secretion by the calcium ionophore A 23187 (HARTY et al. 1981). Recent studies have also demonstrated that calcium increases gastrin messenger RNA (mRNA) levels in a concentration-dependent manner, an effect which is inhibited significantly by nifedipine and the chelating agent EGTA (KARNIK et al. 1989a). These experiments further showed that the calcium ionophore ionomycin increased steady state levels of gastrin mRNA. Although the involvement of the adenylate cyclase second messenger pathway has been examined extensively in the gastric parietal cell, little information is available regarding its role in the stimulation of the G cell. However, KARNIK et al. (1989a) have demonstrated recently that forskolin, an agent that stimulates adenylate cyclase and thereby increases intracellular cAMP, significantly increases steady state levels of gastrin mRNA.

At the cellular level, the ultrastructural appearance of secretory granules in G cells yields insight into the mechanism of postprandial gastrin release. Electron-dense granules found in G cells of fasting rats are replaced by electron-lucent granules within 5 min of a meal (TRACK et al. 1978). After degranulation and a concomitant rise in immunoreactive serum gastrin levels, subsequent gastrin release may be dependent on either its rapid biosynthesis or its release from cytoplasmic stores.

After a meal, the secretion of gastric acid is modulated by a feedback control mechanism in which antral acidification inhibits the further release of gastrin (Fig. 3). While there is individual variation, postprandial gastrin release may account for up to 90% of meal-stimulated gastric acid release

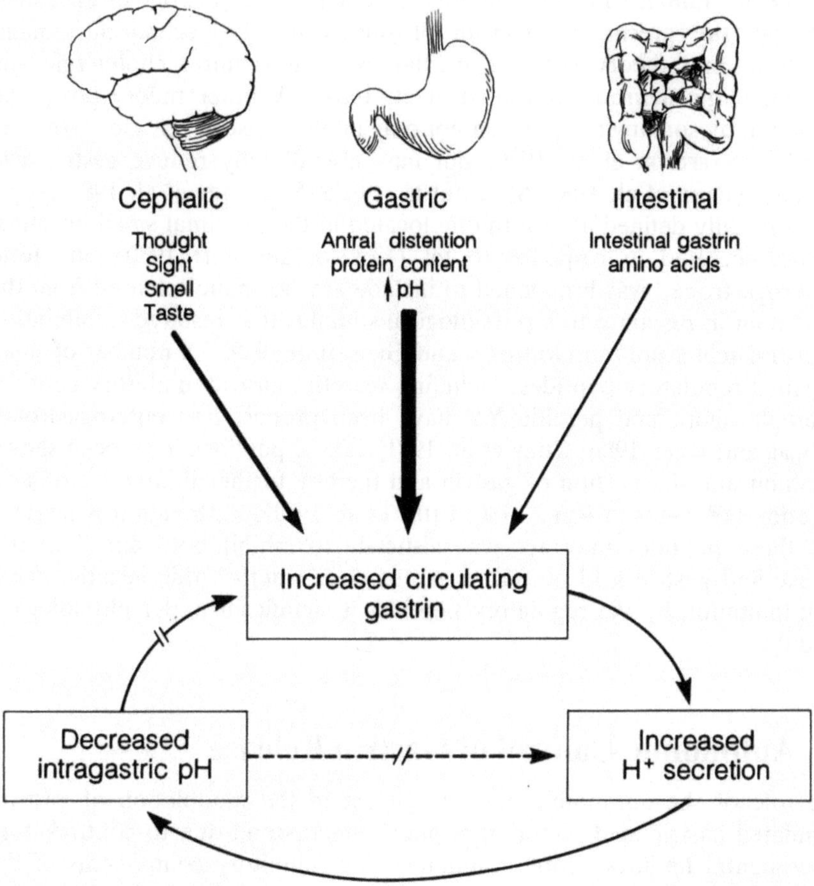

Fig. 3. Mechanisms involved in meal-stimulated gastrin and gastric acid secretion and the negative feedback inhibition of postprandial gastrin release. Following a meal, gastrin release and gastric acid secretion are stimulated, and intragastric pH decreases with time. As the pH approaches 1.5, gastrin release is completely inhibited, completing a negative feedback loop that diminishes further secretion of hydrogen ion. A local feedback mechanism of intraluminal acidity on hydrogen ion secretion may also contribute to this process. As indicated by the *width of the arrows*, the relative contribution to circulating gastrin during the cephalic and intestinal phases of acid secretion is considerably smaller than the amount of gastrin released during the gastric phase of a meal

(BLAIR et al. 1987b). The feedback inhibition of gastrin is well correlated with intragastric pH. Following a meal, gastric pH decreases in response to gastric acid secretion. As the luminal pH approaches 3.5–3.0, gastrin inhibition is observed, and with further acidification to a pH of 1.5, gastrin release is abolished (MCGUIGAN 1974). Conversely, when acid secretion is inhibited by the use of potent antisecretory agents such as the substituted benzimidazole omeprazole, the serum gastrin levels measured in rats increase significantly (ALLEN et al. 1986). Fasting serum gastrin levels have also been shown to increase in human subjects treated with omeprazole (FESTEN et al. 1986). Although the precise mechanism of this feedback mechanism remains unknown, one theory suggests mediation by intramural cholinergic and noncholinergic neurons (SAFFOURI et al. 1984). Another theory postulates mediation by somatostatin, which not only inhibits gastrin release (WOLFE et al. 1984; SAFFOURI et al. 1979) but may also directly reduce gastric acid secretion (PARK et al. 1987; SHORT et al. 1985a; SCHUBERT et al. 1988).

Originally defined as a hormone located in the proximal small intestinal mucosa secreted in response to fat (KOSAKA and LIM 1930), the term "enterogastrone" was broadened to include any hormone released from the duodenum in response to a physiological stimulus that resulted in inhibition of gastric acid secretion (JOHNSON and GROSSMAN 1969). A number of small intestinal regulatory peptides, including secretin, gastric inhibitory peptide, enteroglucagon, and peptide YY have been proposed as enterogastrones (WOLFE and REEL 1986; CHEY et al. 1981). These peptides have been shown to inhibit antral secretion of gastrin and thereby further inhibit gastric acid secretion (WOLFE and REEL 1986; CHEY et al. 1981). Although it is possible that these peptides may act synergistically to inhibit both antral gastrin release and gastric acid output, it is not clear whether this negative feedback inhibition by the regulatory peptides is significant under physiological conditions.

D. Autonomic Control of Gastrin Release

The role of the autonomic nervous system in the modulation of gastrin-stimulated gastric acid secretion is poorly understood due to contradictory experimental findings. Both stimulatory and inhibitory components of the parasympathetic nervous system have been demonstrated to influence gastrin release (WALSH and LAM 1980; GROSSMAN 1979). Specifically, vagally mediated release of gastrin can be elicited by direct vagal stimulation and by insulin-induced hypoglycemia (BRANDSBORG et al. 1975), whereas the hypergastrinemia elicited in response to vagotomy suggests a tonic vagal inhibition of gastrin release (FRIER et al. 1982; HOLLINSHEAD et al. 1985). Postvagotomy hypergastrinemia is evident within 24 h of truncal vagotomy and is not explained by either alterations in serum somatostatin levels or the rapid development of G cell hyperplasia (HOLLINSHEAD et al. 1985).

Studies aimed at examining the effect of cholinergic stimulation on gastrin release have also yielded conflicting results. In one study, although sham feeding stimulated gastrin release and augmented gastric acid secretion by activating efferent vagal pathways to the stomach, the cholinergic agonist bethanechol did not, suggesting the mechanism for gastrin release by sham feeding may not be cholinergic in nature (HIGGS et al. 1976). In contrast, in studies using the isolated vascularly perfused rat stomach which maintains intramural pathways, the axonal blocker tetrodotoxin abolished peptone-stimulated gastrin release (and somatostatin inhibition), suggesting that the regulation of gastrin secretion by intraluminal chemicals is mediated by neural pathways (SAFFOURI et al. 1984). Responses to atropine in the same experimental protocol further defined the intramural neurons as both cholinergic and noncholinergic (SAFFOURI et al. 1984). An enhanced gastrin response to feeding caused by moderate doses of atropine following vagotomy may be attributed to the loss of acid inhibition of gastrin release (DOCKRAY and TRACY 1980). Others have shown that regardless of the state of gastric vagal innervation, atropine infusion reduces food-stimulated gastrin release (HIRSCHOWITZ et al. 1981; KONTUREK et al. 1974; SCHILLER et al. 1982).

Adrenergic receptor agonists with both α and β-adrenergic properties such as epinephrine and norepinephrine have variable effects on both gastrin release and gastric acid production (CHRISTENSEN and STADIL 1976; HARTY et al. 1981; KOOP et al. 1983; DALY 1984). In rats, intravenous injection of isoproterenol (1 mg/kg) causes a fivefold increase in serum gastrin levels (HSU and COOPER 1977). Administration of β-adrenergic blocking agents abolished the response to isoproterenol (STADIL and REHFELD 1973; HSU and COOPER 1977; HAYES et al. 1978), suggesting that the mechanism of gastrin release may involve β-adrenergic receptors. In humans, the selective β_2-adrenergic receptor agonist terbutaline significantly increases serum gastrin concentration, but inhibits pentagastrin-stimulated and food-stimulated gastric acid secretion (THIRLBY et al. 1988). β_2-Adrenergic receptor agonists are known to activate adenylate cyclase and thereby increase intracellular cAMP (THOMPSON et al. 1977). However, cAMP has been shown to stimulate gastric acid secretion (CHEW et al. 1980; SOLL and WOLLIN 1979), suggesting that the mechanism for terbutaline inhibition of gastric acid secretion may not be a direct response. The effect of terbutaline on gastrin release may involve the stimulation of a β-adrenergic receptor on antral gastrin cells (THIRLBY et al. 1988). Alternatively, the effect of terbutaline may be mediated through the release of gastrin-releasing peptide (GRP), since β-adrenergic-stimulated gastrin release in the rat stomach is inhibited by GRP antisera (SHORT et al. 1985b), and because GRP restores the postprandial gastrin response in dogs in which vagal integrity has been interrupted by cryogenic blockade (GREENBERG 1987).

The precise role of distention and its mechanism of action in the acid secretory response and in gastrin release has not been clearly defined, although most studies have found distention to be a potent stimulus for the secretion of gastric acid (PETERS et al. 1982; SCHILLER et al. 1980; HAKANSON et al. 1980). While human studies have demonstrated that acid secretion stimulated by distention is inhibited by the administration of atropine (PETERS et al. 1982) and by vagotomy (HAKANSON et al. 1980), others (SCHILLER et al. 1980) reported that distention-induced gastrin release was enhanced by atropine. PETERS et al. (1982) observed that antral distention stimulated both gastrin release and acid output, and although α-adrenergic blockade had no effect, β-adrenergic blockade with propranolol nearly abolished the gastrin response. Simultaneously, only a small, insignificant decrease in distention-induced acid secretion was observed, leading the authors to conclude that the effect of distention on gastric acid secretion does not involve β-adrenergic pathways and is independent of any effect on gastrin release.

The amino acid γ-aminobutyric acid (GABA) has been identified within the enteric nervous system (KRANTIS 1981; JESSEN 1981) and is capable of stimulating gastrin release from isolated rat antral mucosa (HARTY and FRANKLIN 1983). Hexamethonium, a ganglionic nicotinic recptor antagonist, does not affect GABA-induced gastrin release (RICHTER et al. 1987), suggesting that GABA causes antral gastrin release through direct stimulation of antral postganglionic neurons.

E. Bombesin-Like Peptides

Gastrin-releasing peptide is a neuropeptide which was isolated originally from porcine gastric mucosa. It exists naturally in both 14- and 27-amino acid forms (Fig. 4), with the larger molecule representing an extension at the N-terminal. Based on their structural homology and similar biological properties, GRP is generally regarded as the mammalian counterpart of bombesin, a tetradecapeptide originally isolated from the skin of the discoglossid frog *Bombina bombina* (IMPICCIATORE et al. 1974). Bombesin is a potent stimulant of gastric acid secretion, an effect mediated by gastrin (DELLE FAVE et al. 1980). GRP is found in nerve fibers of the submucosal and myenteric plexus along the entire gastrointestinal tract, pancreatic acini, celiac ganglia, and brain (YANAIHARA et al. 1981; MOGHIMZADEH et al. 1983). Both bombesin and GRP act locally via a neurocrine route following release into the interstitial space surrounding their target cells (COOKE 1986). GRP may mediate vagally stimulated gastrin release by acting as a neurotransmitter within gastric tissue. Evidence for such a mechanism includes experiments showing that vagally induced gastrin release may involve noncholinergic pathways (SCHUBERT and MAKHLOUF 1982; WOLFE et al. 1987) and that vagally mediated gastrin release can be abolished by specific bombesin antisera (SCHUBERT et al. 1985). In addition, isolated canine gastrin cells may be stimulated directly by both bombesin and the cholinergic agonist carbamylcholine, suggesting distinct receptors for each stimulant (SUGANO et al. 1987).

Bombesin
pGlu-Gln-Arg-Leu-Gly-Asn-Gln-Trp-Ala-Val-Gly-His-Leu-Met-NH_2

Gastrin Releasing Peptide 14-27
Met-Tyr-Pro-Arg-Gly-Asn-His-Trp-Ala-Val-Gly-His-Leu-Met-NH_2

Gastrin Releasing Peptide
Lys-Thr-Leu-Val-Thr-Gly-Gly-Gly-Ala-Pro-Leu-Pro-Val
|
Met-Tyr-Pro-Arg-Gly-Asn-His-Trp-Ala-Val-Gly-His-Leu-Met-NH_2

Somatostatin-28
Lys-Arg-Glu-Arg-Pro-Ala-Met-Ala-Pro-Asn-Ser-Asn-Ala-Ser
|
Ala-Gly-Cys-Lys-Asn-Phe-Phe-Trp
| |
Cys-Ser-Thr-Phe-Thr-Lys

Somatostatin-14
Ala-Gly-Cys-Lys-Asn-Phe-Phe-Trp
| |
Cys-Ser-Thr-Phe-Thr-Lys

Fig. 4. Amino acid sequence of bombesin, GRP, and somatostatin. Amino acids *underlined* represent those amino acids that differentiate bombesin from GRP

In addition to stimulating gastrin release, GRP stimulates the release of many peptides, including somatostatin, motilin, neurotensin, cholecystokinin, enteroglucagon, and pancreatic polypeptide. Other biological properties include the stimulation of pancreatic enzyme secretion, gallbladder contraction, and gastric and intestinal motility. Due to the ability of GRP to stimulate the release of other gastrointestinal regulatory peptides, it is unclear whether these actions are direct or mediated through other peptides. No disease states characterized by a deficiency of GRP have been described. However, GRP-like peptides have been isolated in a number of oat cell bronchogenic carcinomas, where they may function as regulatory peptides promoting the growth of these malignancies (MOODY et al. 1988).

In addition to their role in the autonomic nervous system, GRP and other regulatory peptides have been implicated as intercellular messengers within the central nervous system (BROWN and FISHER 1984). Bombesin was shown to act within the brain to inhibit gastric acid secretion in rats (TEPPERMAN and EVERED 1980; TACHÉ et al. 1980). In more recent experiments, synthetic porcine GRP was shown to cause a release of gastrin when given intravenously in rats (TACHÉ et al. 1981). Furthermore, when given intracisternally, but not intravenously, GRP caused a dose-dependent reduction in both the volume and the acidity of gastric secretion (TACHÉ et al. 1981). In a study of the effects of 30 peptides administered intracerebroventricularly on basal and pentagastrin-stimulated gastric acid secretion, none of the peptides studied significantly increased basal acid secretion (LENZ et al. 1986). A number of peptides administered intracerebroventricularly, including porcine GRP and bombesin, significantly decreased pentagastrin-stimulated acid output by 88% and 95%, respectively (LENZ et al. 1986). In the same study, the absence of any significant alteration in the serum gastrin level following intracerebroventricular administration of the peptides investigated suggests that gastrin does not directly contribute to the centrally stimulated inhibition of gastric acid secretion.

F. Somatostatin

Although originally identified in sheep hypothalamus as an inhibitor of growth hormone release (BRAZEAU et al. 1973), somatostatin is a potent physiological inhibitor of several gastrointestinal regulatory peptides (e.g., gastrin, cholecystokinin, secretin), gastric acid secretion, gastrointestinal blood flow, small intestinal and gallbladder motility, and pancreatic enzyme secretion. Somatostatin exists naturally as both somatostatin-14 (a cyclic tetradecapeptide) and somatostatin-28, with the larger molecule representing an N-terminal extension of the smaller form (Fig. 4). The preprohormone from which somatostatin is synthesized has been isolated and its molecular structure sequenced (MONTMINY et al. 1984). Somatostatin-28 was isolated from porcine intestine, purified, and sequenced (PRADAYROL et al. 1980), while somatostatin-14 was purified from a number of tissues, including porcine hypothalamus (SCHALLY et al. 1976) and catfish pancreas (ANDREWS and DIXON 1981). In addition to being localized in several digestive organs, including the stomach, small intestine, and biliary tree, somatostatin has been demonstrated in the retina and hypothalamus, in close proximity to α- and β-islet cells of the pancreas, in the cardiac vagus, and in the glomerulus of the kidney (POLAK and BLOOM 1986). In the gastrointestinal tract, the highest concentrations of somatostatin-containing cells are within the gastric antrum and fundus, and it is somatostatin-14 that is the principal form released.

In the human gastrointestinal tract, the majority of somatostatin is located in the mucosal layer, in specialized endocrine cells designated D cells. Although some differences in antral and fundic D cells exist, both possess long cytoplasmic processes that are fundamental to the local release of somatostatin. Recent experiments have demonstrated that gastric somatostatin exerts inhibitory effects on gastrin release and on hydrogen ion secretion through a paracrine mechanism in which the peptide is released into the immediate interstitial environment of gastrin cells (CHIBA et al. 1981; WOLFE et al. 1984). In these studies, somatostatin-containing cells were found to possess long cytoplasmic processes which extended in close proximity to their target cells (Fig. 5). In experiments using rat antral mucosa in tissue culture, immunoneutralization of endogenous somatostatin with specific antisera resulted in an increase in the gastrin concentration in the culture medium, suggesting that somatostatin exerts a continuous inhibitory effect on the gastrin cell (WOLFE et al. 1984). Although the precise mechanism

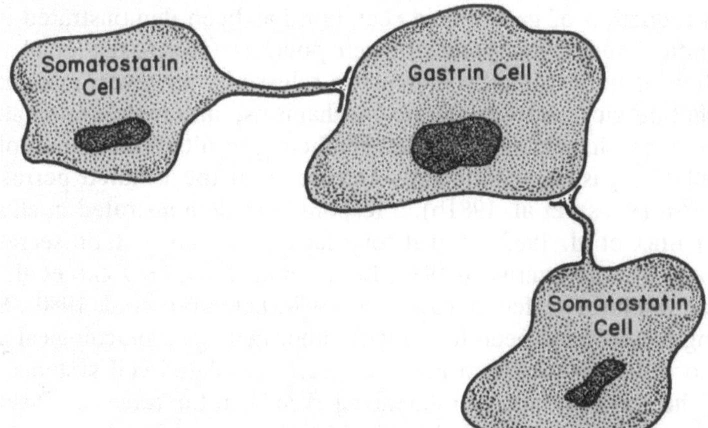

Fig. 5. Schematic depicting the relationship between G and somatostatin cells in the gastric antrum. Somatostatin cells contain long cytoplasmic processes which extend in close proximity to G cells and which secrete somatostatin into the immediate interstitial environment

by which somatostatin inhibits the gastrin cell has yet to be defined, studies at the molecular level have demonstrated that somatostatin inhibition of antral gastrin cells involves not only posttranslational events (HARTY et al. 1985) but also modulation at the pretranslational level (KARNIK et al. 1989b).

There is evidence to suggest that antral D cells may possess chemoreceptors sensitive to changes in gastric pH, and that pH-induced modulation of somatostatin synthesis and secretion mediates a paracrine inhibition on gastrin secretion from adjacent G cells (BRAND and STONE 1988). Specifically, omeprazole-induced achlorhydria reduced D cell activity at the molecular level by producing a significant decrease in antral somatostatin mRNA. In addition, it appears that somatostatin may mediate the inhibitory properties of secretin and other candidate enterogastrones (WOLFE et al. 1983; WOLFE and REEL 1986).

Studies aimed at defining the mechanisms regulating somatostatin release have been difficult due to the very nature of its release. Because of its paracrine mechanism of release and local effects on neighboring target cells, plasma somatostatin levels may not reflect an accurate or sensitive measurement of somatostatin stimulation (LUCEY and YAMADA 1989). Ingestion of a mixed meal stimulates an increase in plasma somatostatin levels in dogs (SCHUSDZIARRA et al. 1978a) and humans (VINIK et al. 1981; COLTURI et al. 1984). Intragastric or intraduodenal instillation of fat, carbohydrates, or protein stimulates an increase in gastric and pancreatic somatostatin (BERELOWITZ et al. 1978; CHAYVIALLE et al. 1980). Acid is another very potent stimulus for somatostatin release, as can be measured following intragastric and intraduodenal administration of acid (SCHUSDZIARRA et al. 1978b).

The inhibitory effect of somatostatin does not require an intact vagus nerve as reduction of gastric acid secretion has been demonstrated in both vagally intact and denervated stomach pouches (KONTUREK et al. 1976). Modulation of postprandial somatostatin release is, however, influenced by vagal, cholinergic, and adrenergic mechanisms, although examination of these neural mechanisms has yielded conflicting results. Stimulation of vagal nerves inhibits gastric somatostatin release from the isolated perfused rat stomach (MCINTOSH et al. 1981b), a response not demonstrated in all similar studies (CHIBA et al. 1982). Vagal tone facilitates somatostatin secretion in humans and dogs (GREENBERG 1987; LUCEY et al. 1985; GUZMAN et al. 1979), but has an inhibitory effect in cats (UVNAS-WALLENSTEN et al. 1980). Similar conflicting results have been found with other neuropharmacological agents, leading to the use of in vitro methods such as isolated cell systems to distinguish the various factors influencing somatostatin release. The use of cultured canine fundic D cells has elucidated at least two stimulatory pathways for somatostatin: a cAMP-dependent system and a cAMP-independent system which may involve intracellular protein kinase C activation (SOLL et al. 1984b, 1985; YAMADA et al. 1984).

Cholinergic regulation of somatostatin release has been studied extensively. In the vascularly perfused rat stomach, gastric inhibitory peptide (GIP)-stimulated somatostatin-like immunoreactivity (SLI) is inhibited by vagal stimulation, an effect mimicked by acetylcholine (MCINTOSH et al. 1981a). Parasympathomimetics have also been shown to inhibit basal SLI secretion (SAFFOURI et al. 1980). The cholinergic influence on fundic somatostatin release appears to be pH dependent (SCHUSDZIARRA et al. 1979). In an acidic environment, the gastric and intestinal phases of a meal activate a cholinergic effect which is primarily inhibitory, while at a neutral pH, the gastric and intestinal phases of a meal cause cholinergic activity which is primarily stimulatory. The infusion of the cholinergic antagonist atropine during gastric or intestinal meals inhibited antral somatostatin release in one study (SCHUSDZIARRA et al. 1979). In another study, the infusion of atropine (0.01 or 0.1 mg/kg) did not inhibit the initial component of somatostatin release, which occurs within 10 min of eating; however, the increase in plasma SLI which normally occurs 60 min after a meal was completely abolished (UVNAS-WALLENSTEN et al. 1982). Further evidence for a cholinergic mechanism in the regulation of somatostatin release has been demonstrated in vitro. In recent studies using rat antral mucosal strips in short-term culture, the addition of the cholinergic agonist carbachol to the incubation medium produced a decrease in somatostatin synthesis and release, consistent with the hypothesis that the increase in gastrin release stimulated by carbachol may be due, at least in part, to the inhibitory effects on antral somatostatin cells (WOLFE et al. 1984). In other studies using rat antral fragments, the addition of atropine to the culture medium prevented GABA-induced inhibition of somatostatin release (HARTY and FRANKLIN 1986).

There is much less controversy regarding adrenergic regulation of somatostatin release. β-Adrenergic mechanisms have been shown to stimulate somatostatin release in the isolated canine pancreas (SAMOLS and WEIR 1979). Furthermore, stimulation of splanchnic nerves caused a release of gastric somatostatin in the isolated rat stomach (MCINTOSH et al. 1981b). Examination of the effect of adrenergic agonists and antagonists in the perfused, isolated rat stomach has demonstrated that the SLI response to adrenergic stimulation is predominately mediated by β receptors, since the two- to sixfold increase in SLI stimulated by isoproterenol, epinephrine, and norepinephrine was completely inhibited by propranolol, but not influenced by phentolamine (KOOP et al. 1983).

Somatostatin exerts a wide range of effects in the gastrointestinal tract, including the inhibition of many regulatory peptides such as gastrin, cholecystokinin, vasoactive intestinal peptide, glucagon, and secretin (REICHLIN 1986; THOMAS 1980). Somatostatin is in turn stimulated by gastrin (as well as by secretin, bombesin, and other regulatory peptides), a process which may contribute to the feedback control mechanism for the regulation of gastric acid secretion. The potent inhibitory effect of somatostatin on gastric acid secretion and the beneficial effects of somatostatin on stress-induced mucosal erosions have raised the possibility that alterations in the physiology of endogenous somatostatin might be implicated in the development of peptic ulcer disease. One proposed mechanism is impaired feedback regulation between gastric acid and antral gastrin secretion (LAMERS 1987), due in part to alterations in endogenous somatostatin secretion (REICHLIN 1983). Support for such a mechanism includes evidence that some patients with peptic ulcer disease have a reduced gastric antral somatostatin content (SUMII et al. 1981; CHAYVIALLE et al.1978). Furthermore, experimental induction of duodenal ulcer by cysteamine is associated with the depletion of immunoreactive somatostatin (SZABO and REICHLIN 1985). In addition, when studied in vitro, antral mucosa from duodenal ulcer patients may have a decreased ability to release somatostatin (HARTY et al. 1986). Conversely, morphological studies, in which the number of D cells per unit area of gastric antrum was measured, revealed no significant difference when peptic ulcer patients were compared with normal subjects (ARNOLD et al. 1982, 1986). Experimental evidence presently available does not permit the conclusion that a deficiency of antral somatostatin, with resultant hyperchlorhydria, represents the primary cause of peptic ulcer disease.

As is the case with all gastrointestinal regulatory peptides, somatostatin has a very short circulatory half-life (<5 min). However, analogues of the peptide have been synthesized which are not only far more potent than the naturally occurring peptide, but which are also more resistant to metabolic clearance. The delay in the disappearance from the circulation and the enhanced potency permit the use of these analogues as pharmacological agents. To date, somatostatin analogues have been used successfully in the treatment of clinical conditions caused by several peptide-secreting tumors, including malignant carcinoid tumors (KVOLS 1986; KVOLS et al. 1986), gastrinomas, glucagonomas, insulinomas (KVOLS et al. 1987; LONGNECKER

1988a,b; VINIK et al. 1988), VIPomas, and acromegaly (due to increased circulating growth hormone levels). Although the analogues do not appear to prevent or impede the progression of metastatic disease, they do lower circulating concentrations of the tumor peptide by inhibiting its release, thereby producing symptomatic relief. For example, the somatostatin analouge octreotide [Sandostatin (SMS-201-995)] has been shown to be efficacious as a therapeutic inhibitor of gastrin release and gastric acid secretion in patients with gastrinoma (BONFILS et al. 1986). There appears, however, to be some loss of efficacy during 1-week administration (25 and 100 µg subcutaneously t.i.d.) in healthy human subjects (LONDONG et al. 1989). Because this agent requires parenteral administration, long-term management of patients with gastric acid hypersecretion will continue to consist in use of the potent oral H_2 antagonists and substituted benzimidazoles. In contrast, in VIPoma patients, in whom no other effective therapy is available, treatment with somatostatin analogues has resulted in marked reductions in plasma VIP levels, as well as almost complete cessation of diarrhea (MATON et al. 1985).

Due to its ability to decrease splanchnic blood flow, somatostatin has also been used with variable success to treat patients with gastrointestinal hemorrhage from ulcer disease. In a prospective study comparing the effects of somatostatin and cimetidine in patients with severe bleeding from peptic lesions, somatostatin was superior to the H_2 antagonist in stopping active bleeding and in reducing transfusion requirements (KAYASSEH et al. 1980). In contrast, however, in a large (534 patients) controlled, double-blind trial of patients with upper gastrointestinal bleeding, there were no significant differences between the group treated with somatostatin and the group given placebo when rates of rebleeding, mean number of blood transfusions required, and operative and mortality rates were compared (SOMERVILLE et al. 1985). A summary of the results of various comparative trials of somatostatin was unable to demonstrate any significant difference between somatostatin and placebo or antacid in the control of acute bleeding due to peptic ulceration (CHRISTIANSEN and YOTIS 1986). These findings are supported by additional studies in patients with bleeding lesions secondary to corticosteroid and nonsteroidal anti-inflammatory therapy (CORAGGIO et al. 1984). Additional controlled prospective studies are therefore needed before the safety and efficacy of somatostatin and somatostatin analogues can be established.

Somatostatin has also been shown to be effective in controlling esophagogastric variceal bleeding. Somatostatin has been demonstrated to be either as effective (KRAVETZ et al. 1984) or significantly more effective (BASSO et al. 1983; JENKINS et al. 1985a) than vasopressin in controlling acute variceal bleeding, and with a lower rate of complications in each case. Comparison of somatostatin with esophageal balloon tamponade has demonstrated somatostatin to be superior in controlling acute variceal bleeding, with significantly fewer complications (AVGERINOS et al. 1989). The precise mechanism by which somatostatin acts to control variceal bleeding is unknown; however, intravenous administration of somatostatin analouge has been shown to reduce intravariceal pressure in patients with portal hypertension (JENKINS et al. 1985b).

G. Mechanism of Gastrin-Induced Gastric Acid Secretion

Gastric acid is secreted by parietal cells located in gastric glands within the oxyntic mucosa. In an early study in 17 patients undergoing partial gastrectomy for proven gastroduodenal disease, a highly significant correlation was found between the number of parietal cells and the estimated "maximum acid output" (CARD and MARKS 1960). A gender difference in gastrin release and parietal cell sensitivity to gastrin was demonstrated in human subjects (FELDMAN et al. 1983): In studies using gastrin-specific antibodies, women responded to meal stimulation with a significantly greater plasma gastrin level than men, but secreted approximately the same amount of acid relative to their maximal secretory capacity. These experiments suggest that although women release greater amounts of gastrin when compared with men, they appear to be less sensitive to the stimulatory properties of gastrin on acid secretion. The number of parietal cells in the stomach is not invariably related to the size of the organ. Parietal cell differentiation from progenitor cells in the mucous neck region of oxyntic glands is stimulated by the trophic effects of gastrin and contributes to the parietal cell hyperplasia that often occurs in patients with hypergastrinemia. In rats treated with high doses of omeprazole, the resultant increased levels of circulating gastrin have been shown to stimulate the proliferation of enterochromaffin-like cells (TIELEMANS et al. 1989).

The parietal cell basolateral membrane has a number of distinct surface receptors which, when activated, stimulate hydrogen ion generation and secretion (Fig. 6). The response of the parietal cell to gastrin varies among species (SOLL and BERGLINDH 1987). Characterization of the gastrin receptor in canine fundic parietal cells has been achieved using the radioactive iodine-labeled gastrin analogue ^{125}I-[Leu^{15}] gastrin (SOLL et al. 1984). Gastrin dose–response curves constructed using gastrin binding sites in highly enriched canine parietal cell fractions demonstrated the ability of the receptor antagonist proglumide to inhibit gastrin (SOLL et al. 1981). Other effects, such as a potentiating effect between histamine and both gastrin and acetylcholine, have also been demonstrated in isolated parietal cell preparations (SOLL and BERGLINDH 1987; BLACK and SHANKLEY 1987).

Gastrin does not enter the parietal cell, but rather appears to exert its stimulatory effect by binding to a receptor on the surface of the parietal cell. Once bound to its surface receptor, gastrin and other agonists activate an intracellular second messenger, which presumably enhances cell function by stimulating the generation of protein kinases. As discussed previously, two of the known intracellular transducing systems are related either to the gen-

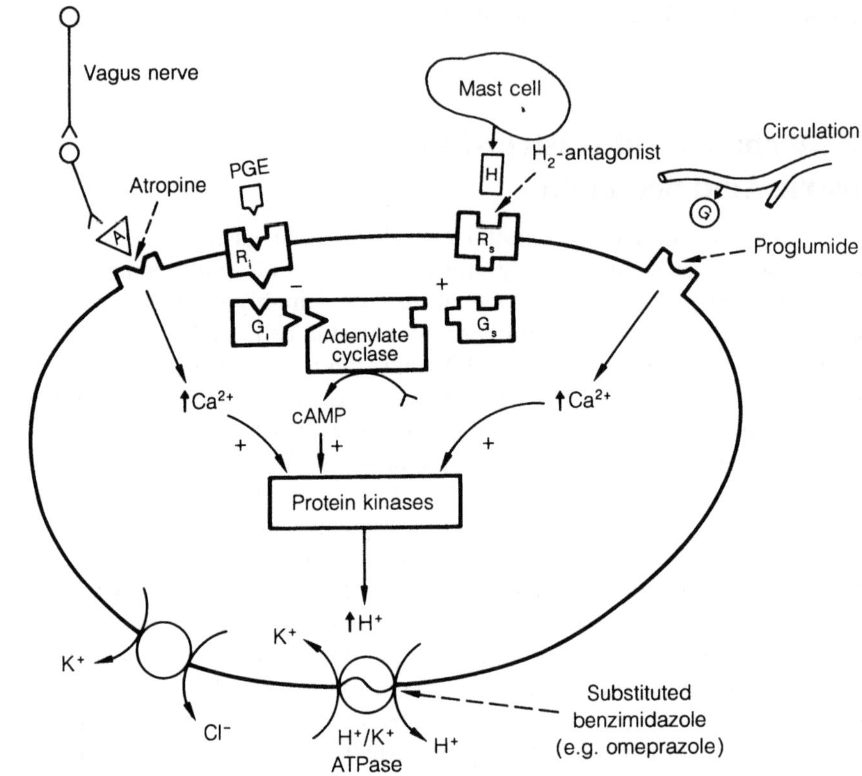

Fig. 6. Schematic representation of a parietal cell and the pathways by which secretagogues stimulate hydrogen ion generation and secretion. Also depicted are sites of action of various antisecretory agents (----). *A*, atropine; *PGE*, E series prostaglandins; *H*, histamine; *G*, gastrin; G_i and G_s, inhibitory and stimulatory catalytic subunits respectively. (WOLFE and SOLL 1988)

eration of cAMP or to alterations in cytosolic calcium concentration. While histamine stimulates parietal cell function by activating adenylate cyclase and increasing cAMP production (SOLL and BERGLINDH 1987), gastrin appears to stimulate the parietal cell by increasing cytosolic calcium (SOLL 1981). Recent reports have demonstrated the importance of cell membrane inositol phospholipid turnover in mediating the regulation of a number of physiological functions (BERRIDGE and IRVINE 1984). Studies using a preparation of isolated canine gastric parietal cells demonstrated that the stimulatory effects of the cholinergic agonist carbachol and gastrin on parietal cells may also be correlated with turnover of cellular inositol phospholipids (CHIBA et al. 1988).

Prostaglandins are a group of long-chain fatty acids, the product of arachidonic acid metabolism in most mammalian tissues. As ubiquitous autocoids, prostaglandins have been shown to modulate a variety of biological functions. In the gastrointestinal tract, prostaglandins have been shown to affect motility, gastric mucosa, blood flow (KONTUREK et al. 1980), and the modulation of gastric acid secretion. In healthy human subjects, intravenous prostaglandin E_1 (PGE_1) inhibited both basal and stimulated gastric acid secretion (CLASSEN et al. 1971). In dogs with denervated fundic (Heidenhain) pouches, intravenous PGE_1 inhibited food-stimulated gastric acid output (BECKER et al. 1973). Although the effect of prostaglandins appeared to be via a direct effect on the parietal cell, in vitro experiments were required to confirm this hypothesis. Studies in isolated gastric mucosa from the bullfrog (*Rana catesbeiana*) demonstrated that the sharp rise in the rate of gastric acid secretion stimulated by gastrin was almost completely blocked by PGE_1 (WAY and DURBIN 1969). Other in vitro studies in isolated canine parietal cells, in which the accumulation of ^{14}C-aminopyrine was used as an index of parietal cell stimulation, demonstrated that PGE_2 and PGI_2 inhibited the response of histamine stimulation (SOLL 1980). These results also suggest a direct effect by prostaglandins on the parietal cell. The intracellular mechanism by which prostaglandins inhibit the parietal cell appears to involve the stimulation of G_i, a GTP-binding protein that inhibits the catalytic subunit of adenylate cyclase, thereby decreasing intracellular levels of cAMP (Fig. 6) (CHEN et al. 1988). Another mechanism by which prostaglandins may modulate gastric acid secretion is through suppression of gastrin release. PGE_2 has been shown to reduce basal gastrin release from the isolated and vascularly perfused rat stomach (SAFFOURI et al. 1980), and may thereby reduce gastric acid secretion.

The stimulation of gastric acid secretion in healthy human subjects given a combined infusion of synthetic human gastrin and calcium gluconate (0.1 mmol Ca^{2+}/kg per hour) does not significantly exceed the response to synthetic human gastrin alone (CHRISTIANSEN et al. 1984). In contrast, patients with duodenal ulcer given a combination infusion of synthetic human gastrin and calcium gluconate respond with significantly greater gastric acid secretion than those given gastrin alone (CHRISTIANSEN et al. 1984). As stated above, gastrin, as well as acetylcholine, appears to stimulate acid secretion by increasing the level of cytosolic calcium in the parietal cell (SOLL 1981). It is not clear whether the increase in calcium is derived from the influx of extracellular calcium or from the mobilization of intracellular calcium stores (CHEW and BROWN 1986; PARADISO et al. 1987; SOLL 1981). It would appear that calcium influx into the cell is important, however, because gastrin-stimulated parietal cell activation is blocked by removing extracellular calcium or by adding lanthanum, a trivalent cation which acts by inhibiting transmembrane fluxes of calcium. If calcium influx does indeed occur through receptor-activated transmembrane channels, these channels differ from those in muscle and nervous tissue since they are not blocked by known calcium channel antagonists such as verapamil or nifedipine (WOLFE and SOLL 1988).

The enzyme H^+,K^+-ATPase activates the mechanism for the secretion of hydrogen ions from the secretory canaliculi of the parietal cell. There is a strong correlation between the activity of gastric H^+,K^+-ATPase and gastric acid secretion (WALLMARK et al. 1985). Substituted benzimidazoles such as omeprazole inhibit gastric acid secretion in vitro and in vivo by interfering with H^+,K^+-ATPase (FELLENIUS et al. 1981). In healthy human subjects, omeprazole produces a dose-dependent inhibition of pentagastrin-stimulated gastric acid secretion (LIND et al. 1983), while fasting serum gastrin levels increase significantly during omeprazole treatment (FESTEN et al. 1986). The effects of omeprazole on antral gastrin cells have also been examined extensively. As stated previously, feedback inhibition of the antral gastrin cell is a function of gastric acidity, and as intragastric pH decreases to 1.5, gastrin release is abolished. Conversely, when acid secretion is inhibited, the feedback inhibitory mechanism is interrupted, and the gastrin cell continues to synthesize and secrete gastrin (BRAND and STONE 1988; WOLFE and SOLL 1988). In rats rendered virtually achlorhydric with high dose omeprazole, plasma and antral concentrations of gastrin become elevated (ALLEN et al. 1986). There is evidence to suggest that the achlorhydria induced by omeprazole stimulates gastrin secretion and gene expression through reduced somatostatin inhibition of G cell activity. Specifically, treatment with omeprazole results in a significant decrease in somatostatin mRNA levels with a concurrent rise in gastrin mRNA (BRAND and STONE 1988).

H. Gastrin and Peptic Ulcer Disease

Contemporary theories of the etiology of peptic ulcer disease suggest an imbalance between aggressive factors, such as acid and pepsin, and mucosal resistance to these aggressive factors. An example of mucosal resistance is the "mucus–bicarbonate barrier" in which mucus provides an "unstirred layer" that concentrates and maintains bicarbonate such that the bicarbonate is able to neutralize hydrogen ions near the gastric luminal surface (FLEMSTROM and TURNBERG 1984). In fact, most patients with duodenal ulcer disease have decreased proximal duodenal mucosal bicarbonate production at rest, in response to hydrochloric acid, and in relation to peak gastric acid secretion (ISENBERG et al. 1987). The role of gastric acid in the pathogenesis of duodenal ulcers is well established and in general, ulcers do not develop in the absence of acid. With the discovery of gastrin, it was originally predicted that the pathophysiology of duodenal ulcer disease would be explained on the basis of an increase in the number of G cells and an elevation in circulating gastrin; however, such has not been the case.

Initial investigation into the relationship between serum gastrin levels and gastric acid secretion demonstrated that fasting serum gastrin concentrations in patients with duodenal ulcer disease were not significantly greater than in control subjects, whereas mean serum gastrin concentrations in patients with gastric ulcer disease were significantly greater than in both control subjects and patients with duodenal ulcer disease (TRUDEAU and MCGUIGAN 1971). The reason for the elevated gastrin levels in gastric ulcer patients has not been completely elucidated. The elevation in serum gastrin levels could be due to the hypochlorhydria often found in gastric ulcer patients (WOLFE and SOLL 1988), which would cause an interruption in acid-gastrin feedback inhibition. Alternatively, it may be related in some way to gastric stasis (DRAGSTEDT 1969). In contrast to studies of gastric emptying in patients with gastric ulcer, a recent study comparing gastric emptying in patients with endoscopically proven duodenal ulcer disease and in matched healthy control subjects was unable to demonstrate a significant difference in mean gastric emptying times (CORINALDESI et al. 1989).

Patients with peptic ulcer disease may have significantly higher fasting and meal-stimulated serum gastrin levels, but a correlation with gastric acid secretion is not obvious. In a large study of duodenal ulcer patients who eventually underwent surgery for their disease, basal and peak postprandial serum gastrin levels were found to be significantly higher than in nondyspeptic volunteers, but no differences in acid secretion were found (POULSEN and AMDRUP 1988). In another examination of basal and food-stimulated serum gastrin concentration in duodenal ulcer patients compared with normal subjects, basal serum gastrin was higher in the ulcer patients; however, increases in serum gastrin after food intake were similar in the two groups (BLAIR et al. 1987a). In addition, basal and peak acid outputs in response to pentagastrin were significantly higher in the duodenal ulcer patients; however, total acid secretion was similar in the two groups when measured following feeding, although the acid secretory response was prolonged in the ulcer group. Therefore, despite significantly greater fasting serum gastrin levels in patients with duodenal ulcer, postprandial gastrin levels appear to increase to the same degree as in normal subjects. This would suggest that increased gastrin release in response to a meal does not likely represent the sole pathogenic factor in peptic ulcer disease.

Some other abnormalities related to gastrin have been found in ulcer patients. For example, under normal conditions when gastric acidity increases ($pH < 3.0$), the release of gastrin is inhibited. Early studies in patients with duodenal ulcers demonstrated an autoregulatory defect whereby gastrin release and acid output were only partially inhibited at a pH of 2.5 (WALSH et al. 1975). While the precise mechanism of this autoregulatory defect remains unknown, one possible mechanism involves a relative deficiency of the peptide somatostatin. As stated previously, the amount of somatostatin released by the antral cells of patients with duodenal ulcer is less than that in control subjects (HARTY et al. 1986). The same is true for the number of somatostatin-containing cells in the antral mucosa of duodenal ulcer patients (CHAYVIALLE et al. 1978). Another possible mechanism involves the relative sensitivity of parietal cells in duodenal ulcer patients. The increased responsiveness of parietal cells of patients with peptic ulcer disease to exogenously administered gastrin and protein meal-stimulated gastrin in some studies (LAM et al. 1980) may explain why some duodenal ulcer patients secrete more gastric acid despite normal basal and postprandial serum gastrin levels.

In other studies, however (ALY and EMAS 1982), the sensitivity of the oxyntic cells to pentagastrin stimulation in duodenal ulcer patients did not differ significantly from age- and gender-matched healthy control subjects.

One final recent hypothesis regarding the mechanism of peptic ulceration suggested that peptic ulcers represent localized areas of mucus rendered susceptible to acid by an autoimmune process (KIRK 1986). This model is based on the stimulatory or destructive immunological effects seen in thyroid disease, in which immune mechanisms produce either destruction of parenchymal cells or excitation by thyroid-stimulating immunoglobulin. The autoimmune hypothesis of peptic ulcer disease suggests that G cell stimulation produces parietal cell hyperplasia predisposing to duodenal ulceration while immune-mediated G cell destruction may reduce trophic effects on the fundic mucosa predisposing to gastric ulceration. The autoimmune model for peptic ulcer disease remains unproven.

J. Hypergastrinemic Syndromes

Two additional disease states characterized by duodenal ulceration and hypersecretion of gastric acid are the Zollinger-Ellison syndrome and antral G cell hyperplasia or hyperfunction. Zollinger-Ellison syndrome, the most striking representation of gastric acid secretion, is characterized by non-β islet cell tumors that secrete gastrin. A complete review of the Zollinger-Ellison syndrome may be found in Chap. 13.

Antral G cell hyperfunction is an unusual entity that is characterized by a moderately elevated fasting serum gastrin concentration and an exaggerated increase in the postprandial serum gastrin levels to more than 200% above the fasting gastrin level (GLOWNIAK et al. 1982; LAMERS and VAN TONGEREN 1979; POLAK et al. 1972). The enhanced gastrin response to feeding in G cell hyperfunction is due to an increased sensitivity to amino acid stimulation, rather than a defective acid inhibitory mechanism (COOPER et al. 1985). While the response of gastrin to a meal is enhanced, provocative testing with intravenous secretin (2 units/kg body weight) results in no appreciable response (FRIESEN and TOMITA 1984). Marked hyperchlorhydria and severe peptic ulceration are commonly observed in antral G cell hyperfunction. There is no sign of gastrin-secreting tumor; however, there may be an increase in the antral G cell density (FRIESEN and Tomita 1981; GANGULI et al. 1974). In a careful investigation of G cell hyperfunction (LEWIN et al. 1984), gastric antral tissue from patients with suspected G cell hyperfunction was compared with antral tissue from 12 control stomachs. G cells were identified by immunohistochemical staining and quantitated in a double-blind manner. The number of G cells in the gastric antrum of the patients with clinically diagnosed primary G cell hyperfunction was significantly greater than the number in control subjects. Other investigators have been unable to confirm this observation (NIELSEN et al. 1981) and as an alternate theory suggest that although a normal number/density of G cells is present, these cells exist in a "hyperfunctional" state and are overly responsive to physiological stimuli (Stave and Brandtzaeg 1978). Yet other investigators find the absolute number/density of antral G cells in duodenal ulcer patients to be highly variable (Keuppens et al. 1980). These authors suggest that preoperative postprandial serum gastrin determinations correlate well with G cell mass and offer this non invasive method for the selection of patients with elevated G cell number. In some instances, antral G cell hyperfunction is familial in origin. In these cases, the mode of inheritance is via a pleiotropic autosomal dominant gene and may be associated with hyperpepsinogenemia I (Taylor et al. 1981). Hypergastrinemia may also be seen in other conditions characterized by the secretion of normal or excessive amounts of gastric acid (Table 1). These include gastric outlet obstruction, chronic renal failure, pheochromocytoma, small intestinal resection, and diabetes mellitus (with or without diabetic gastropathy).

The treatment of duodenal ulcer by the H_2 receptor antagonist cimetidine may occasionally produce mild elevations in postprandial serum gastrin levels (Buchanan et al. 1978) and a small degree of G cell hyperplasia, due to interruption of the pH-dependent negative feedback inhibition of antral G cells (Nielson et al. 1980). These effects on gastrin levels and G cell density may also occur, and be more pronounced, when using more potent antisecre-

Table 1. Conditions associated with hypergastrinemia

- Achlorhydria or hypochlorhydria
  - Chronic atrophic gastritis, with or without autoimmune disorder
    - Pernicious anemia
    - Vitiligo
    - Rheumatoid arthritis
    - Thyrotoxicosis
  - Gastric ulcer
  - Gastric carcinoma
  - Iatrogenic
    - Postvagotomy
    - Drug-induced, e.g., omeprazole
- Hyperchlorhydria or normal acid output
  - Uncertain etiology
    - Chronic renal failure
    - Gastric outlet obstruction
    - Small intestinal resection (transient)
    - Rheumatoid arthritis
    - Diabetes mellitus
  - Associated with increased sympathetic tone
    - Thyrotoxicosis
    - Pheochromocytoma
  - Excluded gastric antrum
  - Antral G cell hyperfunction/hyperplasia
  - Zollinger-Ellison syndrome

tory medications such as famotidine (RYAN et al. 1986), ranitidine, and especially omeprazole (LARSSON et al. 1986). These effects appear to be transient in nature, with gastrin levels and cell density reverting to normal upon the discontinuation of the antisecretory drugs (LARSSON et al. 1988). G cell hyperplasia in humans may also occur with hypercalcemia of diverse etiology, including hyperparathyroidism, sarcoidosis, multiple myeloma, and the hypercalcemia of certain malignancies (DAYAL and WOLFE 1984). The mechanism of this observation has not been defined. Although hypercalcemic patients may show a dramatic 10- to 15-fold increase in absolute G cell number with extension into the intermediate third of the mucosa, these patients do not demonstrate a higher incidence of either hypergastrinemia or peptic ulcer disease.

Another stimulus for antral G cell hyperplasia and resultant hypergastrinemia is truncal vagotomy (ALUMETS et al. 1980; DUNN et al. 1979). Although the precise mechanism for G cell hyperplasia following vagotomy is unknown, theories include (a) reduced luminal acidity following vagotomy with resultant loss of the negative feedback regulation of antral G cells, and (b) loss of a vagally mediated G cell inhibitor other than luminal acid. The effect of reduced antral luminal acidity on the production of G cell proliferation was studied in experimental animals in which the antral mucosa was surgically exposed to nonacidic, gastrointestinal luminal contents (MULHOLLAND et al. 1985). No significant changes in G cell number were observed in antral mucosa exposed to either ileal or jejunal lumina; however, significant G cell hyperplasia was found in antral mucosa exposed to the colonic lumen (55% increase at 2 weeks; further increase at 2 months; sustained at 6 months). The results of this experiment suggest the presence of a trophic substance in the lumen of the colon, but not the small intestine, that induces G cell proliferation. The results also suggest that the lack of luminal acidity alone may not be sufficient to induce G cell hyperplasia.

In contrast to those entities in which hypergastrinemia is associated with hypersecretion of gastric acid, elevated serum gastrin concentrations are more commonly seen in patients with chronic atrophic gastritis, a disorder in which patients are hypo- or achlorhydric (SAFFOURI et al. 1984) (Table 1). As discussed previously, normally when intragastric pH decreases below 3.5–3.0, the release of gastrin is inhibited. However, in patients who do not secrete gastric acid, the gastric pH is unable to fall below 3. As a result, the normal negative feedback mechanism for gastrin release is defective, and such patients develop hyperplasia of G cells (KOOP et al. 1987) and secrete large amounts of the hormone. Many patients with chronic atrophic gastritis also have evidence of concomitant autoimmune disorders, such as pernicious anemia, vitiligo, alopecia areata, rheumatoid arthritis, and thyrotoxicosis.

Patients with hypergastrinemia and achlorhydria may also on occasion exhibit a paradoxical response to secretin provocation, which may lead to the erroneous interpretation of secretin stimulation tests and the diagnosis of the Zollinger-Ellison syndrome in these patients (BRADY et al. 1989;

FELDMAN et al. 1987). False-positive secretin tests have been documented when an impure secretin preparation is used (MCGUIGAN and WOLFE 1980; WOLLMUTH and WAGONFELD 1978), when pure secretin is used but the gastrin antibody cross-reacts with cholecystokinin (WOLFE et al. 1985), and when achlorhydria is present (FELDMAN et al. 1987). It is therefore suggested that gastric acid secretion be measured in hypergastrinemic patients before performing other, more expensive, provocative tests (WOLFE and JENSEN 1987).

K. Conclusion

Since their discovery early this century, peptide hormones have been studied extensively in an attempt to elucidate the mechanisms of gastrointestinal homeostasis, digestion, and absorption. Recent advances in methodology, especially at the molecular level, have yielded additional information and insight into the role of peptide hormones in the pathophysiology of peptic ulcer disease. While many questions remain unanswered, some basic pathways and important feedback control mechanisms involving peptide hormones have been discovered.

References

Allen JM, Bishop AE, Daly MJ, Larsson H, Carlsson E, Polak JM, Bloom SR (1986) Effect of inhibition of acid secretion on the regulatory peptides in the rat stomach. Gastroenterology 90:970–977

Alumets J, El Munshid HA, Hakanson R, Hedenbro J, Liedberg G, Oscarson J, Rehfeld JF, Sundler F, Vallgren S (1980) Gastrin cell proliferation after chronic stimulation: effect of vagal denervation or gastric surgery in the rat. J Physiol (Lond) 298:557–569

Aly A, Emas S (1982) Sensitivity of the oxyntic and peptic cells to pentagastrin in duodenal ulcer patients and healthy subjects with similar secretory capacity. Digestion 25:88–95

Andrews PC, Dixon JE (1981) Isolation and structure of a peptide hormone predicted from a mRNA sequence and second somatostatin from the catfish pancreas. J Biol Chem 256:8267–8270

Arnold R, Hulst MV, Neuhof CH, Schwarting H, Becker HD, Creutzfeldt W (1982) Antral gastrin-producing G-cells and somatostatin-producing D-cells in different states of gastric acid secretion. Gut 23:285–891

Arnold R, Koop H, Schwarting H, Tuch K, Willermer B (1986) Effect of acid inhibition on gastric endocrine cells. Scand J Gastroenterol [Suppl] 125:14–19

Avgerinos A, Klonis C, Rekoumis G, Gouma P, Papadimitriou N (1989) Controlled trial of somatostatin and balloon tamponade in bleeding esophageal varices (Abstr). Gastroenterology 96:A18

Basso N, Bagarani M, Quondamcarlo C, Albertini V, Ziparo V, Anza M, Mari F, Procacciante F, Grassini G, Percoco M, Marocco T, Cucchiara G, Bracci M (1983) Effective control of variceal bleeding by somatostatin: a double-blind, randomized, cross-over study (Abstr). Gastroenterology 84:1100

Becker HD, Reeder DD, Thompson JC (1973) The effect of prostaglandin E_1 on the release of gastrin and gastric acid secretion in dogs. Endocrinology 93:1148–1151

Becker HD, Reeder DD, Thompson JC (1974) Direct measurement of vagal release of gastrin. Surgery 75:101–106

Becker HD, Reeder DD, Thompson JC (1975) Vagal control of gastrin release. In: Thompson JC (ed) Gastrointestinal hormones: a symposium. University of Texas Press, Austin, pp 437–446
Berelowitz M, Kronheim S, Pimstone B, Shapiro B (1978) Somatostatin-like immunoreactivity in rat blood. Characterization, regional differences, and responses to oral and intravenous glucose. J Clin Invest 61:1410–1414
Berridge MJ, Irvine RF (1984) Inositol triphosphate, second messenger in cellular signal transduction. Nature 312:315–321
Black JW, Shankley NP (1987) How does gastrin act to stimulate oxyntic cell secretion? Trends Pharmacol Sci 8:486–890
Blair AJ, Richardson CT, Walsh JH, Feldman M (1985) Acid secretory responsiveness to gastrin heptadecapeptide (G-17) after parietal cell vagotomy (PCV). Clin Res 33:539A
Blair AJ, Feldman M, Barnetic C, Walsh JH, Richardson CT (1987a) Detailed comparison of basal and food-stimulated gastric acid secretion rates and serum gastrin concentrations in duodenal ulcer patients and normal subjects. J Clin Invest 79:582–587
Blair AJ, Richardson CT, Walsh JH, Feldman M (1987b) Variable contribution of gastric acid secretion after a meal in humans. Gastroenterology 92:944–949
Bonfils S, Ruszniewski P, Costil V, Laucournet H, Vatier J, Rene E, Mignon M (1986) Prolonged treatment of Zollinger-Ellison syndrome by long-acting somatostatin. Lancet 1:554–555
Brady CE III, Hyatt JR, Utts SJ (1989) Is the gastrin response to secretin provocation a function of antral G cell mass? Results in the hypergastrinemia of acid hyposecretion. J Clin Gastroenterol 11:27–32
Brand SJ, Stone D (1988) Reciprocal regulation of antral gastrin and somatostatin gene expression by omeprazole-induced achlorhydria. J Clin Invest 82:1059–1066
Brandsborg O, Brandsborg M, Christensen NJ (1975) Plasma adrenaline and serum gastrin: studies in insulin-induced hypoglycemia and other adrenaline infusions. Gastroenterology 68:455–460
Brazeau P, Vale W, Burgus R, Ling N, Butcher M, Rivier J, Guillemin R (1973) Hypothalamic polypeptide that inhibits the secretion of immunoreactive pituitary growth hormone. Science 179:71–79
Brown MR, Fisher LA (1984) Brain peptides as intercellular messengers. JAMA 251:1310–1315
Buchanan KD, Spencer A, Ardill J, Kennedy TL (1978) Hypergastrinaemia due to cimetidine. Gut 19:A437
Bucharth F, Stage JG, Stadil F, Jensen LI, Fischermann K (1979) Localization of gastrinomas by transhepatic portal catheterization and gastrin assay. Gastroenterology 77:444–450
Caldara R, Ferrari C, Romussi M, Bierti L, Gandini S, Curtarelli G (1978) Effect of dopamine infusion on gastric and pancreatic secretion and on gastrin release in man. Gut 19:724–728
Caldara R, Ferrari C, Barbieri C, Romussi M (1980) Effect of four dopaminergic receptor antagonists on gastrin secretion in healthy subjects. Scand J Gastroenterol 15:481–484
Caldara R, Masci E, Barbieri C, Cambielli M, Ferrari C, Tittobello A (1983) Dopaminergic control of gastric acid and gastrin secretion in man: lack of effects after acute oral administration of ibopamine, an analogue of dopamine. Br J Clin Pharmacol 16:112–114
Card WI, Marks IN (1960) The relationship between the acid output of the stomach following "maximal" histamine stimulation and the parietal cell mass. Clin Sci 19:147–163
Chayvialle JAP, Descos F, Bernard C, Martin A, Barbe C, Partensky C (1978) Somatostatin in mucosa of stomach and duodenum in gastroduodenal disease. Gastroenterology 75:13–19

Chayvialle JAP, Miyata M, Rayford P, Thompson JC (1980) Effects of test meal, intragastric nutrients, and intraduodenal bile on plasma concentrations of immunoreactive somatostatin and vasoactive intestinal peptide in dogs. Gastroenterology 79:844–852

Chen MC, Amirian DA, Toomey M, Sanders MJ, Soll AH (1988) Prostanoid inhibition of canine parietal cells: mediation by the inhibitory guanosine triphosphate-binding protein of adenylate cyclase. Gastroenterology 94:1121–1129

Chew CS, Brown MR (1986) Release of intracellular Ca^{2+} and elevation of inositol triphosphate by secretagogues in parietal and chief cells isolated from rabbit gastric mucosa. Biochim Biophys Acta 888:116–125

Chew CS, Hersey SJ, Sachs G, Berglindh T (1980) Histamine responsiveness of isolated gastric glands. Am J Physiol 238:G312–G320

Chey WY, Kim MS, Lee KY, Chang JM (1981) Secretin is an enterogastrone in the dog. Am J Physiol 240:G239–G244

Chiba T, Kadowaki S, Taminato T, Chihara K, Seino Y, Matsukura S, Fujita T (1981) Effect of antisomatostatin γ-globulin on gastrin release in cats. Gastroenterology 81:321–326

Chiba T, Kadowaki S, Taminato T, Kodama H, Chihara K, Seino Y, Fujita T (1982) Proceedings of the 4th International Symposium on Gastrointestinal Hormones, Stockholm

Chiba T, Fisher SK, Park J, Seguin EB, Agranoff BW, Yamada T (1988) Carbamoylcholine and gastrin induce inositol lipid turnover in canine gastric parietal cells. Am J Physiol 255:G99–G105

Christensen KC, Stadil F (1976) Effect of epinephrine and norepinephrine on gastrin release and gastric secretion of acid in man. Scand J Gastoenterol [Suppl] 37:87–92

Christiansen J, Yotis A (1986) The role of somatostatin and a long-acting analogue, SMS 201-995, in acute bleeding due to peptic ulceration. Scand J Gastroenterol 21:109–114

Christiansen J, Kirkegard P, Olsen PS, Petersen B (1984) Interaction of calcium and gastrin on gastric acid secretion in duodenal ulcer patients. Gut 25:174–177

Classen M, Koch H, Bickhardt J, Topf G, Demling L (1971) The effect of prostaglandin E_1 on the pentagastrin-stimulated gastric secretion in man. Digestion 4:333–344

Colturi TJ, Unger RH, Feldman M (1984) Role of circulating somatostatin in regulation of gastric acid secretion, gastrin release, and islet cell function. Studies in healthy subjects and duodenal ulcer patients. J Clin Invest 74:417–423

Cooke HJ (1986) Neurobiology of the intestinal mucosa. Gastroenterology 90:1057–1081

Cooper R, Dockray GJ, Calam J, Walker R (1985) Acid and gastrin responses during intragastric titration in normal subjects and duodenal ulcer patients with G cell hyperfunction. Gut 26:232–236

Coraggio F, Scarpato P, Spina M, Lombardi S (1984) Somatostatin and ranitidine in the control of iatrogenic haemorrhage of the upper gastrointestinal tract. Br Med J 289:224

Corinaldesi R, Stanghellini V, Paparo G, Paternico A, Rusticali AG, Barbara L (1989) Gastric acid secretion and gastric emptying of liquids in 99 male duodenal ulcer patients. Dig Dis Sci 34:251–256

Daly MJ (1984) The classification of adrenoreceptors and their effects on gastric acid secretion. Scand J Gastroenterol [Suppl 89] 19:3–10

Dayal Y, Wolfe HJ (1984) G cell hyperplasia in chronic hypercalcemia: an immunocytochemical and morphometric analysis. Am J Pathol 116:391–397

Debas HT, Seal AM, Cork CA, Soon-Shiong P, Walsh JH (1981) Vagal distribution for stimulation and inhibition of gastrin release. Surg Forum 32:143–145

Debas HT, Hollinshead J, Seal A, Soon-Shiong P, Walsh JH (1984) Vagal control of

gastrin release in the dog: pathways for stimulation and inhibition. Surgery 95:34–37
Delle Fave G, Kohn A, de Magistris L, Mancuso M, Sparvoli C (1980) Effect of bombesin-stimulated gastrin on gastric acid secretion in man. Life Sci 27:993–999
Dockray GJ, Tracy HJ (1980) Atropine does not abolish cephalic vagal stimulation of gastrin release in dogs. J Physiol (Lond) 306:473–80
Dockray GL, Vaillant C, Hopkins CR (1978) Biosynthetic relationships of big and little gastrins. Nature 273:770–772
Dragstedt LR (1969) Peptic ulcer: an abnormality in gastric secretion. Am J Surg 117:143–156
Dunn DH, Decanini CO, Eisenberg MM, Bonsack M, Delaney JP (1979) Mechanism for gastrin cell hyperplasia after truncal vagotomy. Surg Forum 30:376–78
Edkins JS (1905) On the chemical mechanism of gastric secretion. Proc R Soc Lond [Biol] 76:376
Elwin CE (1974) Gastric acid responses to antral application of some amino acids, peptides and isolated fragments of protein hydrolysate. Scand J Gastroenterol 9:239–247
Eysselein VE, Maxwell V, Reedy T, Wunsch E, Walsh JH (1984) Similar acid stimulatory potencies of synthetic human big and little gastrins in man. J Clin Invest 73:1284–1290
Feldman M, Walsh JH, Wong HC, Richardson CT (1978) Role of gastrin heptadecapeptide in the acid secretory response to amino acids in man. J Clin Invest 61:308–313
Feldman M, Richardson CT, Walsh JH (1983) Sex-related differences in gastrin release and parietal cell sensitivity to gastrin in healthy human beings. J Clin Invest 71:715–720
Feldman M, Schiller LR, Walsh JH, Fordtran JS, Richardson CT (1987) Positive intravenous secretin test in patients with achlorhydria-related hypergastrinemia. Gastroenterology 93:59–62
Fellenius E, Berglindh T, Sachs G, Olbe L, Elander B, Sjostrand SE, Wallmark B (1981) Substituted benzimidazoles inhibit gastric acid secretion by blocking (H^+ + K^+)ATPase. Nature 290:159–161
Fernstrom M, Rehfeld JF, Emas S (1982) Postprandial acid secretion and serum gastrin response before and after exclusion of the proximal small intestine in cats. Digestion 24:79–86
Fernstrom M, Emas S (1985) Effect of a protein meal in stomach and jejunum on gastric secretory response to pentagastrin in cats. Dig Dis Sci 30:877–883
Fernstrom M, Uvnas-Moberg K, Emas S (1987) Gastric acid, plasma gastrin, and somatostatin responses to feeding and exogenous gastrin alone and in combination in conscious cats. Dig Dis Sci 32:177–183
Festen HP, Tuynman HA, Defize J, Pals G, Frants RR, Straub JP, Meuwissen SG (1986) Effect of single and repeated doses of oral omeprazole on gastric acid and pepsin secretion and fasting serum gastrin and serum pepsinogen I levels. Dig Dis Sci 31:561–566
Fiddian-Green RG, Vinik AI (1983) The meaning of a gastrin response to a test meal. Surgery 94:1038–1042
Fiddian-Green RG, Pittenger G, Kothary P (1980) Effect of luminal somatostatin on acid secretion and gastrin release. Scand J Gastroenterol 15:305–309
Fiddian-Green RG, Pittenger G, Kothary P, Vinik AI (1983) Role of calcium in the stimulus-secretion coupling of antral gastrin release. Endocrinology 112:753–760
Flemstrom G, Turnberg LA (1984) Gastroduodenal defense mechanisms. In: Isenberg JI, Johansson C (eds) Clinics in gastroenterology. Saunders, Philadelphia, pp 327–354
Frier BM, Corrall RJM, Adrian TE, Bloom SR (1982) The effect of adrenergic and cholinergic mechanisms on the secretion of pancreatic polypeptide and gastrin following hypoglycemia. Clin Endocrinol (Oxf) 17:433–439

Friesen SR, Tomita T (1981) Pseudo-Zollinger-Ellison syndrome: hypergastrinemia, hyperchlorhydria without tumor. Ann Surg 194:481–493
Friesen SR, Tomita T (1984) Further experience with pseudo-Zollinger-Ellison syndrome: its place in the management of neuroendocrine duodenal ulceration. World J Surg 8:552–560
Ganguli PC, Polak JM, Pearse AG, Elder JB, Hegarty M (1974) Antral-gastrin-cell hyperplasia in peptic-ulcer disease. Lancet 1:583–586
Glowniak JV, Shapiro B, Vinik AI, Glaser B, Thompson NW, Cho KJ (1982) Percutaneous transhepatic venous sampling of gastrin: value in sporadic and familial islet-cell tumors and G cell hyperfunction. N Engl J Med 307:293–297
Greenberg GR (1987) Infuence of vagal integrity on gastrin and somatostatin release in dogs. Gastroenterology 93:994–1001
Gregory RA, Tracy HJ, Harris JI, Runswick MJ, Moore S, Kenner GW, Ramage R (1979) Minigastrin: corrected structure and synthesis. Hoppe Seylers Z Physiol Chem 360:73–80
Grossman MI (1979) Neural and hormonal regulation of gastointestinal function: an overview. Annu Rev Physiol 41:27–33
Guzman S, Chayvialle JA, Banks WA, Rayford PL, Thompson JC (1979) Effects of vagal stimulation on pancreatic secretion and on blood levels of gastrin, cholecystokinin, secretin, vasoactive intestinal peptide, and somatostatin. Surgery 86:329–336
Hakanson R, Hedenbro J, Liedberg G, Sundler F, Vallgran S (1980) Mechanisms of gastric acid secretion after pylorus and oesophagus ligation in the rat. J Physiol (Lond) 305:139–149
Harty RF, Franklin PA (1983) GABA affects the release of gastrin and somatostatin from rat antral mucosa. Nature 303:623–624
Harty RF, Franklin PA (1986) Cholinergic mediation of γ-aminobutyric acid-induced gastrin and somatostatin release from rat antrum. Gastroenterology 91:1221–1226
Harty RF, Maico DG, McGuigan JE (1981) Role of calcium in antral gastrin release. Gastroenterology 80:491–497
Harty RF, Maico DG, McGuigan JE (1985) Postreceptor inhibition of antral gastrin release by somatostatin. Gastroenterology 88:675–680
Harty RF, Maico DG, McGuigan JE (1986) Antral release of gastrin and somatostatin in duodenal ulcer and control subjects. Gut 27:652–658
Hayes JR, Ardill J, Shanks RG, Buchanan KD (1978) Effect of catecholamines on gastrin release. Metabolism 27:385–391
Hengels KJ, Muller JE, Scholten T, Fritsch WP (1980) Evidence for the secretion of gastrin into human gastric juice. Gut 21:760–765
Higgs RH, Humphries TJ, Castell DO, McGuigan JE (1976) Lower esophageal sphincter pressures and serum gastrin levels after cholinergic stimulation. Am J Physiol 231:1250–1253
Hirschowitz BI, Gibson R, Molina E (1981) Atropine suppresses gastrin release by food in intact and vagotomized dogs. Gastroenterology 81:838–843
Hollinshead JW, Debas JW, Yamada T, Elashoff J, Osadchey B, Walsh JH (1985) Hypergastrinemia develops within 24 hours of truncal vagotomy in dogs. Gastroenterology 88:35–40
Hsu WH, Cooper CW (1977) Serum gastrin in the rat: cholinergic and adrenergic effects. Proc Soc Exp Biol Med 154:401–406
Impicciatore M, Debas H, Walsh JH (1974) Release of gastrin and stimulation of acid secretion by bombesin in dog. Rend Gastroenterol 6:99–101
Isenberg JI, Maxwell V (1978) Intravenous infusion of amino acids stimulates gastric acid secretion in man. N Engl J Med 298:27–29
Isenberg JI, Selling JA, Hogan DL, Koss MA (1987) Impaired proximal duodenal mucosal bicarbonate secretion in patients with duodenal ulcer. N Engl J Med 316:374–379

Jenkins SA, Baxter JN, Corbett W, Devitt P, Ware J, Shields R (1985a) Efficacy of somatostatin and vasopressin in the control of acute variceal hemorrhage (Letter). Hepatology 5:344–345

Jenkins SA, Baxter JN, Corbett WA, Shields R (1985b) Effects of a somatostatin analogue SMS 201-995 on hepatic haemodynamics in the pig and on intravariceal pressure in man. Br J Surg 72:1009–1012

Jessen KR (1981) GABA in the enteric nervous system – a neurotransmitter function? Mol Cell Biochem 38:69–76

Johnson LR, Grossman MI (1969) Effects of fat, secretin and cholecystokinin on histamine-stimulated gastric secretion. Am J Physiol 216:1176–1179

Karnik PS, Lichtenstein DR, Wolfe MM (1989a) Somatostatin inhibits gastrin gene expression via cAMP and calcium dependent pathways (Abstr). Gastroenterology 96:A249

Karnik PS, Monihan SJ, Wolfe MM (1989b) Inhibition of gastrin gene expression by somatostatin. J Clin Invest 83:367–372

Kayasseh L, Gyr K, Keller U, Stadler GA, Wall M (1980) Somatostatin and cimetidine in peptic ulcer haemorrhage. Lancet 2:844–846

Keuppens F, Bremen J, Woussen-Colle MC, de Graef J (1976) Failure of pentagastrin administration ot restore postprandial acid secretion from Heidenhain pouches after antrectomy in dogs. Surgery 80:586–590

Keuppens F, Willems G, de Graef J, Woussen-Colle MC (1980) Antral gastrin cell hyperplasia in patients with peptic ulcer. Ann Surg 191:276–281

Kirk RM (1986) Could chronic peptic ulcers be localised areas of acid susceptibility generated by autoimmunity? Lancet 1:772–774

Knuhtsen S, Holst JJ, Jensen SL, Knigge U, Nielsen OV (1985) Gastrin releasing peptide: effect upon exocrine secretion, and release from isolated perfused porcine pancreas. Am J Physiol 248:G281–G286

Knuhtsen S, Holst JJ, Baldissera FGA, Skak-Nielsen T, Poulsen SS, Jensen SL, Nielsen OV (1987) Gastrin-releasing peptide in the porcine pancreas. Gastroenterology 92:1153–1158

Komarov SA (1938) Gastrin. Proc Soc Exp Biol Med 38:514–516

Konturek SJ, Biernat J, Olesky J, Rehfeld JF, Stadil F (1974) Effect of atropine on gastrin and gastric acid response to peptone meal. J Clin Invest 54:593–597

Konturek SJ, Tasler J, Cieszkowski M, Coy DH, Schally AV (1976) Effect of growth hormone release-inhibiting hormone on gastric secretion, mucosal blood flow and serum gastrin. Gastroenterology 70:737–741

Konturek SJ, Robert A, Hanchar AJ, Nezamis JE (1980) Comparison of prostacyclin and prostaglandin E_2 on gastric secretion, gastrin release, and mucosal blood flow in dogs. Dig Dis Sci 25:673–679

Konturek SJ, Jaworek J, Bielanski W, Cieszkowski M, Dobrzanska M, Coy DH (1982) Comparison of enkephalin and atropine in the inhibition of vagally stimulated gastric and pancreatic secretion and gastrin and pancreatic polypeptide release in dogs. Peptides 3:601–606

Koop H, Behrens I, Bothe E, Koschwitz H, McIntosh CHS, Pederson RA, Arnold R, Creutzfeldt W (1983) Adrenergic control of rat gastric somatostatin and gastrin release. Scand J Gastroenterol 18:65–71

Koop H, Willemer S, Steinbach F, Eissele R, Tuch K, Arnold R (1987) Influence of chronic drug-induced achlorhydria by substituted benzimidazoles on the endocrine stomach in rats. Gastroenterology 92:406–413

Kosaka T, Lim RKS (1930) Demonstration of the humoral agent in fat inhibition of gastric secretion. Proc Soc Exp Biol Med 27:890–891

Krantis A (1981) GABA in the mammalian enteric nervous system. In: Okada Y, Roberts E (eds) Problems in GABA research. Excerpta Medica New York, pp 128–36

Kravetz D, Bosch J, Teres J, Bruix J, Rimola A, Rodes J (1984) Comparison of intravenous somatostatin and vasopressin infusion in treatment of acute variceal hemorrhage. Hepatology 4:442–446

Kvols LK (1986) Metastatic carcinoid tumors and the carcinoid syndrome. A selective review of chemotherapy and hormonal therapy. Am J Med 81:49–55
Kvols LK, Moertel CG, O'Connell MJ, Schutt AJ, Rubin J, Hahn RG (1986) Treatment of the malignant carcinoid syndrome. Evaluation of a long-acting somatostatin analogue. N Engl J Med 315:663–666
Kvols LK, Buck M, Moertel CG, Schutt AJ, Rubin J, O'Connell MJ, Hahn RG (1987) Treatment of metastatic islet cell carcinoma with a somatostatin analogue (SMS 201-995). Ann Intern Med 107:162–168
Lam SK, Isenberg JI, Grossman MI, Lane WH, Walsh JH (1980) Gastric acid secretion is abnormally sensitive to endogenous gastrin released after peptone test meals in duodenal ulcer patients. J Clin Invest 65:555–562
Lamers CB (1987) Clinical and pathophysiological aspects of somatostatin and the gastrointestinal tract. Acta Endocrinol (Copenh) 286:19–25
Lamers CB, van Tongeren JH (1979) Postprandial serum gastrin levels in patients with combined hypergastrinemia and hyperchlorhydria. Br J Surg 66:547–549
Lamers CB, Walsh JH, Jansen JB, Harrison AR, Ippoliti AF, van Tongeren JH (1982) Evidence that gastrin 34 is preferentially released from the human duodenum. Gastroenterology 83:233–239
Larsson H, Carlsson E, Mattsson H (1986) Plasma gastrin and gastric enterochromaffinlike cell activation and proliferation. Studies with omeprazole and ranitidine in intact and antrectomized rats. Gastroenterology 90:391–399
Larsson H, Carlsson E, Hakanson R, Mattsson H, Nilsson G, Seensalu R, Wallmark B, Sundler F (1988) Time-course of development and reversal of gastric endocrine cell hyperplasia after inhibition of acid secretion. Studies with omeprazole and ranitidine in intact and antrectomized rats. Gastroenterology 95:1477–1486
Lenz HJ, Klapdor R, Hester SE, Webb VJ, Galyean RF, Rivier JE, Brown MR (1986) Inhibition of gastric acid secretion by brain peptides in the dog: role of the autonomic nervous system and gastrin. Gastroenterology 91:905–912
Levine RA, Petokas S, Starr A, Eich R (1983) Effect of verapamil on basal and pentagastrin-stimulated gastric acid secretion. Clin Pharmacol Ther 34:399–402
Lewin KJ, Yang K, Ulich T, Elashoff JD, Walsh JH (1984) Primary gastrin cell hyperplasia: report of five cases and a review of the literature. Am J Surg Pathol 8:821–832
Lichtenberger LM, Shaw LS, Bailey RB (1981) Influence of calcium on the release of gastrin from isolated rodent G cells. Proc Soc Exp Biol Med 166:587–591
Lichtenberger LM, Belansorne R, Graziani LA (1982a) Physiological importance of amino acid uptake and decarboxylation in gastrin release from isolated G cells. Nature 295:698–700
Lichtenberger LM, Graziani LA, Ubinsky WP (1982b) Importance of dietary amines in meal-induced gastrin release. Am J Physiol 6:G341–G347
Lind T, Cederberg C, Ekenved G, Haglund U, Olbe L (1983) Effect of omeprazole – a gastric proton pump inhibitor – on pentagastrin stimulated acid secretion in man. Gut 24:270–276
Londong W, Angerer M, Kutz K, Landgraf R, Londong V (1989) Diminishing efficacy of octreotide (SMS 201-995) on gastric functions of healthy subjects during one-week administration. Gastroenterology 96:713–722
Longnecker SM (1988a) Somatostatin and octreotide: literature review and description of therapeutic activity in pancreatic neoplasia. Drug Intell Clin Pharm 22:99–106
Longnecker SM (1988b) Remission of symptoms of chemotherapy-refractory metastatic insulinomas using octreotide. Drug Intell Clin Pharm 22:136–138
Lucey MR, Yamada T (1989) Biochemistry and physiology of gastrointestinal somatostatin. Dig Dis Sci 34:5s–13s
Lucey MR, Wass JA, Fairclough P, Webb J, Webb S, Medbak S, Rees LH (1985) Autonomic regulation of postprandial plasma somatostatin, gastrin and insulin. Gut 26:683–688

Maton PN, O'Dorisio TM, Howe BA, McArthur KE, Howard JM, Cherner JA, Malarkey TB, Collen MJ, Gardner JD, Jensen RT (1985) Effect of a long-acting somatostatin analogue (SMS 201-995) in a patient with pancreatic cholera. N Engl J Med 312:17–21
McGuigan JE (1974) Gastrin. Vitam Horm 32:47–88
McGuigan JE, Wolfe MM (1980) Secretin injection test in the diagnosis of gastrinoma. Gastroenterology 79:1324–1331
McIntosh C, Pederson RA, Koop H, Brown JC (1981a) Gastric inhibitory polypeptide stimulated secretion of somatostatin-like immunoreactivity from the stomach: inhibition by acetylcholine or vagal stimulation. Can J Physiol Pharmacol 59:468–472
McIntosh C, Pederson R, Muller M, Brown J (1981b) Autonomic nervous control of gastric somatostatin secretion from the perfused rat stomach. Life Sci 29:1477–1483
Meryn S, Straus E (1986) A new rapid gastrin radioimmunoassay. Dig Dis Sci 31:567–570
Moghimzadeh E, Ekman R, Hakanson R, Yanaihara N, Sundler F (1983) Neuronal gastrin-releasing peptide in the mammalian gut pancreas. Neuroscience 10:553–563
Montminy MR, Goodman RH, Horovitch SJ, Habener JF (1984) Primary structure of the gene encoding rat preprosomatostatin. Proc Natl Acad Sci USA 81:3337–3340
Moody TW, Lebovic GS, Carney DN, Korman LY (1988) BN/GRP-like peptides and receptors in small cell lung cancer. Int J Neurosci 40:141–148
Mulholland MW, Magallanes F, Bonsack M, Delaney J (1985) The role of luminal pH in production of gastrin cell hyperplasia in the rat. Surgery 97:308–315
Nielsen HO, Jensen KB, Christiansen LA (1980) The antral gastrin-producing cells in duodenal ulcer patients: a density study before and during treatment with cimetidine. Acta Pathol Microbiol Scand [A] 88:383–386
Nielsen HO, Lauritsen K, Christiansen LA (1981) The antral gastrin-producing cells in duodenal ulcer patients. Acta Pathol Microbiol Scand [A] 89:293–296
Obie JF, Cooper CW (1979) Bombesin stimulates gastrin secretion in the rat without increasing serum calcitonin. Proc Soc Exp Biol Med 162:437–441
Paradiso AM, Tsien RY, Machen TE (1987) Digital image processing of intracellular pH in gastric and chief cells. Nature 325:447–450
Park J, Chiba T, Yamada T (1987) Mechanisms for direct inhibition of canine gastric parietal cells by somatostatin. J Biol Chem 262:14190–14196
Pauwels S, Desmond H, Dimaline R, Dockray GL (1986) Identification of progastrin in gastrinomas, antrum and duodenum by a novel radioimmunoassay. J Clin Invest 77:376–381
Peters MN, Walsh JH, Ferrari J, Feldman M (1982) Adrenergic regulation of distension-induced gastrin release in humans. Gastroenterology 82:659–663
Polak JM, Bloom SR (1986) Somatostatin localization in tissues. Scand J Gastroenterol [Suppl 119] 21:11–21
Polak JM, Stagg B, Pearse AG (1972) Two types of Zollinger-Ellison syndrome: immunofluorescent, cytochemical and ultrastructural studies of the antral and pancreatic gastrin cells in different clinical states. Gut 13:501–512
Polak JM, Bloom SR, Sullivan SN, Pearse AGE (1977) Enkephalin-like immunoreactivity on the human gastrointestinal tract. Lancet 1:972–974
Poulsen J, Amdrup E (1988) The fasting and food-stimulated serum gastrin concentration in 151 duodenal ulcer patients compared to 41 healthy subjects. Regul Pept 21:227–236
Pradayrol L, Jornvall J, Mutt V, Ribet A (1980) N-terminally extended somatostatin: the primary structure of somatostatin-28. FEBS Lett 109:55–58
Primrose JN, Ratcliffe JG, Joffe SN (1980) Assessment of the secretin provocation test in the diagnosis of gastrinoma. Br J Surg 67:744–746

Rehfeld JF (1980) Heterogeneity of gastrointestinal hormones. In: Glass GBJ (ed) Gastrointestinal hormones. Raven, New York, pp 433–449

Rehfeld JF, Uvnas-Wallensten K (1978) Gastrins in cat and dog: evidence for a biosynthetic relationship between the large molecular forms of gastrin and heptadecapeptide gastrin. J Physiol (Lond) 283:379–396

Reichlin S (1983) Somatostatin. N Engl J Med 309:1495–1501, 1556–1563

Reichlin S (1986) Somatostatin: historical aspects. Scand J Gastroenterol [Suppl 119] 21:1–10

Richardson CT, Walsh JH, Hicks MI, Fordtran JS (1976) Studies on the mechanisms of food-stimulated gastric acid secretion in normal human subjects. J Clin Invest 58:623–631

Richter HM, Kelly KA, Go VLW (1987) Proximal gastric vagotomy and mucosal antrectomy: effect on gastric acid secretion, plasma gastrin, and experimental ulcerogenesis in the dog. Surgery 101:623–631

Ryan JR, Vargas R, Chremos AN (1986) Comparison of effects of oral and intravenous famotidine on inhibition of nocturnal gastric acid secretion. Am J Med 81:60–64

Saffouri B, Weir G, Bitar K, Makhlouf G (1979) Stimulation of gastrin secretion from the perfused rat stomach by somatostatin antiserum. Life Sci 25:1749–1753

Saffouri B, Weir GC, Bitar KN, Makhlouf GM (1980) Gastrin and somatostatin secretion by perfused rat stomach. Am J Physiol 238:G495–G501

Saffouri B, DuVal JW, Makhlouf GM (1984) Stimulation of gastrin secretion in vitro by intraluminal chemicals: regulation by intramural cholinergic and noncholinergic neurons. Gastroenterology 87:557–561

Samols E, Weir GC (1979) Adrenergic modulation of pancreatic A, B, and D cells: α-adrenergic suppression and β-adrenergic stimulation of somatostatin secretion, α-adrenergic stimulation of glucagon secretion in the perfused dog pancreas. J Clin Invest 63:230–238

Schally AV, Dupont A, Arimura A, Redding TW, Nishi N, Linthicum GL, Schlesinger DH (1976) Isolation and structure of somatostatin from porcine hypothalami. Biochemistry 15:509–514

Schiller LR, Walsh JH, Feldman M (1980) Distension-induced gastrin release: effects of luminal acidification and intravenous atropine. Gastroenterology 78:912–917

Schiller LR, Walsh JH, Feldman M (1982) Effect of atropine on gastrin release stimulated by an amino acid meal in humans. Gastroenterology 83:267–272

Schubert ML, Makhlouf GM (1982) Regulation of gastrin and somatostatin secretion by intramural neurons: effect of nicotinic receptor stimulation with dimethylphenylpiperazinium. Gastroenterology 83:626–632

Schubert ML, Saffouri B, Walsh JH (1985) Inhibition of neurally mediated gastrin secretion by bombesin antiserum. Am J Physiol 248:G456–G462

Schubert ML, Edwards NF, Makhlouf GM (1988) Regulation of gastric somatostatin secretion in the mouse by luminal acidity: a local feedback mechanism. Gastroenterology 94:317–322

Schusdziarra V (1983) Somatostatin – physiological and pathophysiological aspects. Scand J Gastroenterol 82:69–84

Schusdziarra V, Rouiller D, Harris V, Conlon JM, Unger RH (1978a) The response of plasma somatostatin-like immunoreactivity to nutrients in normal and alloxan diabetic dogs. Endocrinology 103:2264–2273

Schusdziarra V, Harris V, Conlon JM, Arimura A, Unger RH (1978b) Pancreatic and gastric somatostatin release in response to intragastric and intraduodenal nutrients and HCl in the dog. J Clin Invest 62:509–518

Schusdziarra V, Rouiller D, Harris V, Conlon JM, Unger RH (1978a) The response of plasma somatostatin-like immunoreactivity to nutrients in normal and alloxan diabetic dogs. Endocrinology 103:2264–2273

Schusdziarra V, Rouiller D, Harris V, Unger RH (1979) Gastric and pancreatic release of somatostatin-like immunoreactivity during the gastric phase of a meal:

effects of truncal vagotomy and atropine in the anesthetized dog. Diabetes 28:658–663
Short GM, Doyle JW, Wolfe MM (1985a) Effect of antibodies to somatostatin on acid secretion and gastrin release by the isolated perfused rat stomach. Gastroenterology 88:984–988
Short GM, Reel GM, Doyle JW, Wolfe MM (1985b) Effect of GRP on β-adrenergic-stimulated gastrin and somatostatin release in the isolated rat stomach. Am J Physiol 249:G197–G202
Soll AH (1980) Specific inhibition by prostaglandins E_2 and I_2 of histamine-stimulated [^{14}C]aminopyrine accumulation and cyclic adenosine monophosphate generation by isolated canine parietal cells. J Clin Invest 65:1222–1229
Soll AH (1981) Extracellular calcium and cholinergic stimulation of isolated canine parietal cells. J Clin Invest 68:270–278
Soll AH, Berglindh T (1987) Physiology of isolated gastric glands and parietal cells: recpetors and effectors regulating function. In: Johnson LR (ed) Physiology of the gastrointestinal tract, vol 1 2nd edn. Raven, New York, pp 883–909
Soll AH, Wollin A (1979) Histamine and cyclic AMP in isolated canine parietal cells. Am J Physiol 237:E444–E450
Soll AH, Amirian DA, Thomas LP, Reedy TJ, Elashoff JD (1984a) Gastrin receptors on isolated canine parietal cells. J Clin Invest 73:1434–1447
Soll AH, Yamada T, Park J, Thomas LP (1984b) Release of somatostatin-like immunoreactivity from canine fundic mucosal cells in primary culture. Am J Physiol 247:G558–G566
Soll AH, Amirian DA, Park J, Elashoff JD, Yamada T (1985) Cholecystokinin potently releases somatostatin from canine fundic mucosal cells in short-term culture. Am J Physiol 248:G569–G573
Somerville KW, Henry DA, Davies JG, Hine KR, Hawkey CJ, Langman MJ (1985) Somatostatin in treatment of haematemesis and melaena. Lancet 1:130–132
Stadil F, Rehfeld JF (1973) Release of gastrin by epinephrine in man. Gastroenterology 65:210–215
Stave R, Brandtzaeg P (1978) Immunohistochemical investigation of gastrin-producing cells (G cells): estimation of antral density, mucosal distribution and total mass of G cells in resected stomachs from patients with peptic ulcer disease. Scand J Gastroenterol 13:199–203
Steen JH, Steen N, Herning M, Christiansen PM (1982) Relationship between preoperative basal serum gastrin concentration and acid secretion after proximal gastric vagotomy. Scand J Gastroenterol 17:993–995
Stern DH, Walsh JH (1973) Gastrin release in postoperative ulcer patients: evidence for release of duodenal gastrin. Gastroenterology 64:363–369
Sugano K, Park J, Soll AH, Yamada T (1987) Stimulation of gastrin release by bombesin and canine gastrin-releasing peptides: studies with isolated canine G cells in primary culture. J Clin Invest 79:935–942
Sumii K, Fukushima X, Hirata E, Matsumoto Y, Sanuki E, Tsumary S, Sumioka M, Miyoshi A, Miyachi Y (1981) Antral gastrin and somatostatin concentrations in peptic ulcer patients. Peptides [Suppl] 2:281–283
Szabo S, Reichlin S (1985) Somatostatin depletion by cysteamine: mechanism and implication for duodenal ulceration. Fed Proc 44:2540–2545
Taché Y, Vale W, Rivier J, Brown M (1980) Brain regulation of gastric secretion: influence of neuropeptides. Proc Natl Acad Sci USA 77:5515–5519
Taché Y, Marki W, Rivier J, Vale W, Brown M (1981) Central nervous system inhibition of gastric secretion in the rat by gastrin-releasing peptide, a mammalian bombesin. Gastroenterology 81:298–302
Taylor IL, Calam J, Rotter JI, Vaillant C, Samloff IM, Cock A, Simkin E, Dockray GJ (1981) Family studies of hypergastrinemic, hyperpepsinogenemic duodenal ulcer. Ann Intern Med 95:421–425
Taylor IL, Byrne WJ, Christie DL, Ament ME, Walsh JH (1982) Effect of individual

L-amino acid secretion and serum gastrin and pancreatic polypeptide release in humans. Gastroenterology 83:273–278
Tepperman BL, Evered MD (1980) Gastrin injected into the lateral hypothalamus stimulates secretion of gastric acid in rats. Sciences 209:1142–1143
Thirlby RC, Richardson CT, Chew P, Feldman M (1988) Effect of terbutaline, a β_2-adrenoreceptor agonist, on gastric acid secretion and serum gastrin concentrations in humans. Gastroenterology 95:913–919
Thomas WE (1980) Inhibitory effect of somatostatin on gastric acid secretion and serum gastrin in dogs with and without duodenogastric reflux. Gut 21:996–1001
Thompson WJ, Chang LK, Rosenfeld GC, Jacobsen ES (1977) Activation of rat gastric mucosal adenyl cyclase by secretory inhibitors. Gastroenterology 72:251–254
Tielemans Y, Hakanson R, Sunder F, Willems G (1989) Proliferation of enterochromaffinlike cells in omeprazole-treated hypergastrinemic rats. Gastroenterology 96:723–729
Track NS, Creutzfeldt C, Creutzfeldt RA, Creutzfeldt W (1978) The antral gastrin-producing G cell: biochemical and ultrastructural response to feeding. Cell Tissue Res 194:131–139
Trudeau WL, McGuigan JE (1971) Relations between serum gastrin levels and rates of gastric hydrochloric acid secretion. N Engl J Med 284:408–412
Uvnas-Wallensten K, Efendic S, Roovete A, Johansson C (1980) Decreased release of somatostatin into the portal vein following electrical vagal stimulation in the cat. Acta Physiol Scand 109:393–398
Uvnas-Moberg K, Posloncec B, Hagerman M, Castensson S, Rubio C, Uvnas B (1982) Occurrence of an insulin-like peptide in extracts of peripheral nerves of the cat and in extracts of human vagal nerves. Acta Physiol Scand 115:471–477
Vagne M, Mutt V (1980) Entero-oxyntin: a stimulant of gastric acid secretion extracted from porcine intestine. Scand J Gastroenterol 15:17–22
Varner A, Modlin I, Walsh J (1981) High potency of bombesin for stimulation of human gastrin release in gastric acid secretion. Regul Pept 1:289–296
Vinik A, Levitt NS, Primrose B, Wagner LJ (1981) Peripheral plasma somatostatin-like immunoreactive responses to insulin hypoglycemia and a mixed meal in healthy subjects and in noninsulin-dependent maturity-onset diabetics. J Clin Endocrinol Metab 52:330–337
Vinik A, Tsai S, Moattari AR, Cheung P (1988) Somatostatin analogue (SMS 201-995) in patients with gastrinomas. Surgery 104:834–842
Wallmark B, Larsson H, Humble L (1985) The relationship between gastric acid secretion and gastric H^+,K^+-ATPase activity. J Biol Chem 260:13681–13684
Walsh JH, Lam SK (1980) Physiology and pathophysiology of gastrin. Clin Gastroenterol 9:567–591
Walsh JH, Richardson CT, Fordtran JS (1975) pH dependence of acid secretion and gastrin release in normal and ulcer subjects. J Clin Invest 55:462–468
Walsh JH, Isenberg JL, Ansfield J, Grossman V (1976) Clearance and acid-stimulating action of human big and little gastrins in duodenal ulcer subjects. J Clin Invest 57:1125–1131
Way L, Durbin RP (1969) Inhibition of gastric acid secretion in vitro by prostaglandin E_1. Nature 221:874–875
Wiborg O, Berglund L, Boel E, Norris F, Rehfeld JF, Marcker KA, Vuust J (1984) Structure of a human gastrin gene. Proc Natl Acad Sci USA 81:1067–1069
Wolfe MM, Jensen RT (1987) Zollinger-Ellison syndrome. Current concepts in diagnosis and management. N Engl J Med 317:1200–1209
Wolfe MM, McGuigan JE (1984) The immunological characterization of gastrin-like and cholecystokinin-like peptides released in response to a peptone meal. Gastroenterology 87:323–334
Wolfe MM, Reel GM (1986) Inhibition of gastrin release by gastric inhibitory peptide mediated by somatostatin. Am J Physiol 250:G331–G333

Wolfe MM, Soll AH (1988) The physiology of gastric acid secretion. N Engl J Med 319:1707–1715
Wolfe MM, Reel GM, McGuigan JE (1983) Inhibition of gastrin release by secretin is mediated by somatostatin in cultured rat antral mucosa. J Clin Invest 72:1586–1593
Wolfe MM, Jain DK, Reel GM, McGuigan JE (1984) Effects of carbachol on gastrin and somatostatin release in rat antral tissue culture. Gastroenterology 87:86–93
Wolfe MM, Paquet RJ, Reel GM (1985) Specificity of commercially available antibodies used for gastrin measurement. J Lab Clin Med 105:417–421
Wolfe MM, Short GM, McGuigan JE (1987) Beta-adrenergic stimulation of gastrin release mediated by gastrin-releasing peptide in rat antral mucosa. Regul Pept 17:133–142
Wollmuth RL, Wagonfeld JB (1978) False-positive secretin test. Ann Intern Med 88:718–719
Yamada T, Soll AH, Park J, Elashoff J (1984) Autonomic regulation of somatostatin release: studies with primary cultures of canine fundic mucosal cells. Am J Physiol 247:G567–G573
Yanaihara N, Yanaihara C, Mochizuki T, Imura K, Fujita T, Iwanaga T (1981) Immunoreactive GRP. Peptides [Suppl 2] 2:185–192

CHAPTER 4

The Role of Essential Fatty Acids in Gastric and Duodenal Protection and Ulcer Therapy

D. HOLLANDER and A. TARNAWSKI

A. Cytoprotection and Prostaglandins

I. Definition of Cytoprotection

Cytoprotection has been defined as the ability of pharmacological agents to prevent or reduce gastric, duodenal, or intestinal mucosal injury produced by a variety of agents without affecting intragastric acidity. Prostaglandins (PGs) have been shown to protect the gastric mucosa against (a) ulcerogenic insults by aspirin, indomethacin, bile acids, serotonin, and restraint, and (b) damage produced by necrotizing agents such as absolute alcohol, boiling water, 0.6 N HCl, 0.2 N NaOH, and overdistention (ROBERT at al. 1979, 1984; TARNAWSKI 1980; MILLER 1983; MARTI-BONMATI et al. 1980). A demonstration of cytoprotection is the oral or subcutaneous pretreatment of experimental animals (ROBERT et al. 1979, 1884; TARNAWSKI 1980) with a small amount of synthetic or natural PGs prior to the insult, which significantly reduces or even completely prevents mucosal necrosis after exposure to absolute alcohol, boiling water, or other noxious factors.

The key feature of cytoprotection is that protection is accomplished by mechanisms other than reduction of luminal acid (MARTI-BONMATI et al 1980; TARNAWSKI et al. 1985; SZABO et al. 1985). This is clearly indicated by the fact that PGs are able to protect the gastric mucosa at concentrations which do not inhibit gastric acid secretion (ROBERT et al. 1979, 1984; TARNAWSKI 1980; MILLER 1983) and that even complete elimination of acid secretion with cimetidine or ranitidine does not prevent necrosis produced by necrotizing agents (MARTI-BONMATI et al. 1980).

While the cellular mechanisms of PG-induced protection remain unknown, on the tissue level this protective action is attributed to PGs' ability to stimulate mucus and bicarbonate secretion, to protect proliferative zone cells, and to maintain microvascular perfusion and thus preserve delivery of nutrients and oxygen to the glandular cells.

II. Mucosal Sites of Cytoprotection

Sequential analysis of gastric mucosal protection by PGs against absolute alcohol injury has demonstrated that the main morphological feature of PG protection is preservation of the mucosal proliferative zone (TARNAWSKI et al. 1985a). This could be accomplished by two different mechanisms: (a) protection of the mucosal microvasculature in this area, and/or (b) direct protection of the progenitor and glandular cells. It is most likely that both mechanisms are important.

1. Protection of the Mucosal Microvasculature

The gastric mucosal microvasculature is an important target for mucosal injury (SZABO et al. 1985; TARNAWSKI et al. 1985b, 1988; RAINFORD et al. 1984; ROBINS 1980). Damage of endothelial cells occurs early during gastric mucosal injury by ethanol, aspirin, and indomethacin, and precedes glandular cell necrosis. This damage results in formation of thrombi, microvessel rupture, intramucosal hemorrhages, and microvascular stasis. These vascular changes impair oxygen and nutrient transport and add ischemia to the direct injury by offensive agents. PGs prevent or reduce endothelial cell injury and prevent microvascular stasis and hemorrhagic necrosis.

2. Direct Protection of Gastric Mucosal Cells

Studies of gastric epithelial cells in tissue culture and studies of isolated gastric glands indicate that PGs can directly protect gastric epithelial cells in experiments where vascular, neural, and hormonal factors do not play a role. PGs reduce aspirin-induced injury to cultured gastric epithelial cells and significantly reduce or prevent injury by indomethacin and/or ethanol to isolated rat and human gastric glands or dispersed cells (TARNAWSKI et al. 1986a). The protection by PGs of endothelial and glandular cells suggests that PGs have a direct cellular component of protective action (TARNAWSKI et al. 1986a).

III. Metabolism of Natural and Synthetic Prostaglandins

Prostaglandins are synthesized from their precursors – essential fatty acids – by all nucleated cells. The gastrointestinal mucosa is one of the tissues in which this process is very intense (WHITTLE 1977; KONTUREK and PAWLIK 1986). Continuous formation of PGs by the gastrointestinal mucosa most likely represents a physiological process necessary for maintaining cellular integrity of the gastrointestinal mucosa, for which PGs serve as a trophic factor. This is indicated by the fact that when rabbits were immunized against PGE_2 and/or PGI_2, they developed a high incidence of gastrointestinal ulcerations (REDFERN et al. 1987; REDFERN et al. FELDMEN 1989). Pharmacological agents which inhibit the synthesis of PGs [aspirin, indomethacin, and other nonsteroidal anti-inflammatory drugs (NSAIDs)] produce severe damage to the gastrointestinal mucosa, including erosions and ulcerations (WHITTLE 1977; WHITTLE and VANE 1986). The injury coincides with prominent reduction in the mucosal concentration of PGs (WHITTLE 1977; WHITTLE and VANE 1986). Administration of exogenous PGs prevents or reduces mucosal injury produced by aspirin, indomethacin, and other NSAIDs (WHITTLE and VANE 1986).

Natural PGs are generated by enzymatic conversion of their precursors: arachidonic acid (eicosatetraenoic acid), dihomo-γ-linolenic acid (eicosatrienoic acid), and eicosapentanoic acid (KONTUREK and PAWLIK 1986; BAKHLE 1983).

In man arachidonic acid is a predominant precursor, which is converted to PG subscript-2 series (e.g., PGE_2 and PGI_2). Arachidonic acid is derived from dietary linoleic acid or ingested as a constituent of food. After absorption from the gut it is esterified and either constitutes a major component of cell membrane phospholipids or serves as a component of metabolic pool (BAKHLE 1983). Baseline endogenous synthesis of PGs is most likely derived from the metabolic pool of arachidonic acid, while stimulated synthesis (e.g., trauma and chemical or neurohormonal factors) comes from the cell membrane pool (BAKHLE 1983).

Natural PGs are rapidly deactivated by 15-hydroxy PG-dehydrogenase (15 HD), an enzyme which oxidizes C-15OH groups. During a single passage through the lungs (containing a high concentration of this enzyme) 95% of the PGE and PGF series are deactivated. The 15-keto compounds are subsequently reduced by a 3δ-reductase to the 13,14-dihydro δ-3 derivatives, and subsequently undergo β- and ω-oxidation of the side chain and are excreted in the urine as dicarboxylic acid (KONTUREK and PAWLIK 1986; BAKHLE 1983). Both 15 HD and 3δ-reductase are intracellular enzymes. Therefore the substrate has to pass through the cell membrane in order to be reduced. Natural PGE_2 or PGF_2 passes through the membrane and is promptly inactivated. Methylated synthetic PGs (e.g., 16,16dmPGE_2 or misoprostol) also cross the cell membranes but are not inactivated by 15 HD and therefore remain for a prolonged time (hours) in the circulation. Gastrointestinal mucosa and liver rapidly inactivate natural PGs, including the E, F, D, and I types, usually during one passage through portal circulation (KONTUREK and PAWLIK 1986; BAKHLE 1983). Synthetic methylated PGs are not effectively inactivated by 15 HD in gastrointestinal mucosa and in liver and therefore have a much longer biological half-life (hours) compared to natural PGs (minutes) (KONTUREK and PAWLIK 1986) PGs, especially of E or E_2 type, produce systemic side-effects which include diarrhea (approximately 13% of patients), abdominal cramps, bone demineralization, and abortifacient action in pregnant women. These systemic side-effects are most likely due to a slow inactivation of synthetic PGs and therefore prolonged systemic action. In contrast, natural PGs given orally are promptly deactivated during their first passage through the liver or lungs and therefore do not have significant systemic effects.

B. Arachidonic Acid Cascade and Prostaglandin Synthesis by Gastric and Duodenal Mucosa

I. Arachidonic Acid Cascade

Arachidonic acid is a 20-carbon unsaturated fatty acid with four double bonds. Its importance lies in its key role as the precursor of prostanoids, leukotrienes, and a variety of other regulatory and inflammatory compounds. Arachidonic acid is stored in phospholipids in cell membranes and is liberated from phospholipids by the enzymes phospholipase A_2 and C. This hydrolysis reaction results in free arachidonic acid being available for further metabolic transformation into PGs, leukotrienes, and thromboxanes. The hydrolysis of arachidonic acid from phospholipids by phospholipases can be blocked by lipocortin. Lipocortin synthesis can be stimulated by exogenous administration of corticosteroids. Once arachidonic acid is liberated from phospholipids it is available to the cyclooxygenase enzyme system to form prostanoids, which include PGE_2, thromboxanes, and prostacyclines. The cyclooxygenase enzyme system can be blocked by NSAIDs such as indomethacin. The other pathway of arachidonic acid metabolism is the lipoxygenase pathway, which leads to the synthesis of leuckotrienes. The lipoxygenase pathway can be blocked by agents such as benoxaprofen. The metabolic transformation of arachidonic acid to either prostanoids or leukotrienes appears to be substrate limited. That is, as soon as arachidonic acid becomes available through the action of phospholipase on phospholipids, it is converted rapidly by the specific enzyme systems into prostanoids or leukotrienes (RAMWELL 1981).

II. Sources of Arachidonic Acid from Mucosal Pools

Arachidonic acid stored in cell membrane phospholipids is derived from food sources. In the Western diet arachidonic acid, per se, is not a common food constituent. Thus, in Western countries, arachidonic acid is primarily obtained from the conversion of dietary linoleic acid to arachidonic acid by elongation and desaturation of the linoleic acid chain. Thus, in the presence of linoleic acid in the diet, arachidonic acid is not required. In some species, primarily carnivores such as cats, linoleic acid cannot be converted to arachidonic acid, and thus arachidonic acid is required from dietary sources – predominantly animal meats. In humans, arachidonic acid from dietary sources or arachidonic acid synthesized from linoleic acid can be stored in the cell membrane as phospholipids (GALI et al. 1980; VANE and MONCADA 1979).

III. Control of Mucosal Prostaglandin Synthesis

Mucosal synthesis of PGs and leukotrienes appears to be substrate limited. The gastroduodenal mucosa can synthesize either prostanoids or leukotrienes very rapidly as soon as the substrate, arachidonic acid, becomes available. Thus, the limiting factor in mucosal synthesis of PGs is the availability of the precursor arachidonic acid. Therefore, synthesis of prostanoids or leukotrienes is strictly limited by the hydrolysis of phospholipid arachidonic acid to free arachidonic acid by the activity of phospholipases (RAMWELL 1981). As mentioned earlier, the conversion of phospholipid bound arachidonic acid to free arachidonic acid by phospholipases can be blocked by lipocortin.

C. Dietary Sources of Arachidonic and Linoleic Acids

I. Food Sources

The most common dietary source for essential fatty acids in the Western world is linoleic acid from vegetable oils. Humans obtain their essential fatty acids primarily from vegetable oils such as corn oil and safflower oil which contain high concentrations of linoleic acid. Linoleic acid is usually modified by desaturation and chain elongation into arachidonic acid, which is then stored in cell membranes as phospholipids. Arachidonic acid can also be acquired directly from food sources which are predominantly meats and animal oils. This dietary source of arachidonic acid is of lesser importance in the Western diet (HOLLANDER and TARNAWSKI 1986a).

II. Absorption of Dietary Essential Fatty Acids

Both linoleic and arachidonic acids are absorbed primarily in the proximal half of the small intestine (CHOW and HOLLANDER 1978, 1979a). Because of their insolubility in aqueous solutions, bile acids are required in order to dissolve the fatty acids in the luminal fluid by the formation of micellar particles. Once dissolved in micellar particles, the fatty acids are transported across the mucosal unstirred water layer and transferred into the absorptive cell membrane. Transport into the intestinal absorptive cells has a saturable component at low luminal concentrations of the fatty acids which is not energy requiring. This mechanism of transport is defined as facilitated diffusion. This saturable component of the absorption of fatty acids may involve fatty acid binding proteins present in the cell membranes or in the cytosol of the absorptive cells. At high concentrations, both arachidonic and linoleic acids appear to be absorbed by simple passive diffusion which depends on the concentration gradient of the fatty acid (CHOW and HOLLANDER 1979b; HOLLANDER el at. 1984). Once absorbed by the intestinal cells, the fatty acids are reesterified to glycerol forming triglycerides which attach to lipoproteins and are transferred out of the basolateral membrane into either the lymphatic or the portal circulation. More than half of the absorbed fatty acids appear to enter the lymphatic circulation but a significant portion (30%–40%) may enter the portal circulation and reach the liver.

III. Distribution of Absorbed Essential Fatty Acids Between Organs

The essential fatty acids (arachidonic or linoleic) which are absorbed into the lymphatic circulation can reach the systemic circulation attached to either specific lipoprotein fractions or to serum albumin. From the systemic circulation, the essential fatty acids can reach all organs, including the gastrointestinal tract, and are taken up into cell membranes. The fatty acids are stored in cell membranes primarily as phospholipids, with the gastrointestinal tract being a major repository of absorbed fatty acids. Generally, however, all organs contain arachidonic or linoleic acid in their cell membrane phospholipids (NILSSON and MELIN 1988).

The essential fatty acids which are absorbed into the portal circulation reach the liver predominantly and can be stored in liver phospholipids or metabolized directly by the liver into prostanoids. Some of the absorbed phospholipids which enter the portal vein can also be transported as such or as prostanoids or leukotriene metabolites to the lungs, where most of the active metabolites are removed from the circulation during their first pass. Thus, little of the fatty acids or their metabolites which enter the portal vein actually reach the systemic circulation.

IV. The Requirement for Detergents for the Intestinal or Gastric Absorption of Essential Fatty Acids

From the above discussion it should be clear that because of the aqueous insolubility of dietary essential fatty acids their absorption depends on the presence of detergent molecules. Thus, in the small intestine, linoleic or arachidonic acid normally depends on the presence of conjugated bile acids for absorption into the intestinal mucosa (CHOW and HOLLANDER 1978, 1979a,b). Since the concentration of conjugated bile acids in the stomach is minimal and is not sufficient to form micelles, if one wants to enhance the absorption of dietary essential fatty acids into the gastric mucosa one needs to add detergent molecules to the food or to the pharmacologically administered essential fatty acids before they can be solubilized and absorbed by the gastric mucosa. Experimental work done in 1982 and 1983 clearly demonstrated that intragastric administration of detergent solubilized dietary essential fatty acids results in rapid generation of gastric mucosal PGs (HOLLANDER et al. 1982). In the absence of added detergents, there is little evidence for penetration of the fatty acids into the gastric mucosa or the generation of PGs (TARNAWSKI et al. 1983). The most efficient and effective detergent to promote gastric mucosal uptake of dietary essential fatty acids is pluronic F-68. Other detergent molecules do not appear to be able to enhance the gastric mucosal absorption of dietary essential fatty acids.

D. Gastric Mucosal Synthesis of Endogenous Prostanoids from Dietary Essential Fatty Acids

I. The Requirement for Detergents for Absorption of Dietary Essential Fatty Acids into the Gastric Mucosa

When linoleic or arachidonic acid was administered directly into the gastric lumen without detergents no evidence was found for either the generation of mucosal prostaglandins or the ability of these fatty acids to protect the mucosa against acute injury (TARNAWSKI and HOLLANDER, unpublished observations). On the other hand, when the fatty acids were solubilized with the detergent pluronic F-68, a rapid generation and release of PGs into the gastric lumen was seen (HOLLANDER et al. 1982; TARNAWSKI et al. 1983). In addition, following the administration of detergent solubilized essential fatty acids the gastric mucosa was very well protected against acute injury by alcohol or aspirin (HOLLANDER et al. 1982; TARNAWSKI et al. 1988c). The administration of the detergent by itself did not result in either generation of PGs by the gastric mucosa or gastric mucosal protection against injury (HOLLANDER et al. 1982; TARNAWSKI et al. 1983). Likewise, in control experiments the addition of a nonessential fatty acid such as oleic acid (18-carbon monounsaturated fatty acid) did not result in prostanoid generation or mucosal protection even when administered in a solubilized form with pluronic F-68 (TARNAWSKI et al. 1987). These series of experiments clearly indicate that dietary essential fatty acids, when given intragastrically by gavage, have to be administered in a solubilized form using an nonionic detergent such as pluronic F-68. Without solubilizing the fatty acids in detergents there was no evidence of gastric synthesis or release of PGs, nor any evidence for gastric mucosal protection against acute injury by alcohol or salicylates.

II. The Requirement for Direct Gastric Mucosal Contact with Solubilized Essential Fatty Acids for Mucosal Protection

It is well established that most dietary fatty acids are normally absorbed by the proximal small intestine (CHOW and HOLLANDER 1978, 1979a,b). Therefore, the question was raised whether the intragastrically administered essential fatty acids, in their solubilized form, are effective in reducing gastric mucosal injury because of direct contact with the gastric mucosa or perhaps due to subsequent absorption in the jejunum with subsequent access to the gastric mucosa through the systemic circulation. To answer this question we cannulated the proximal jejunum and ligated the pylorus in a group of rats. We then administered the detergent solubilized arachidonic acid intrajejunally while preventing reflux of the material back into the stomach. One hour later we injured the gastric mucosa in a standardized fashion. We found no evidence for protection of the gastric mucosa by intrajejunally administered solubilized dietary essential fatty acids (HOLLANDER et al. 1982; TARNAWSKI et al. 1983). These studies clearly demonstrate that jejunal absorption of solubilized essential fatty acids is not effective in promoting gastric mucosal protection against acute injury. Instead, direct absorption of the solubilized fatty acids by the gastric mucosa is necessary in order to prevent acute injury of the gastric mucosa by alcohol or aspirin. These results are not surprising since we know that jejunally absorbed natural fatty acids will reach the portal or systemic circulations. Their natural PG products are then deactivated and removed from the circulation, usually during their first pass through the liver or lungs. Thus, there is very little reason to suspect that any of the prostanoids generated from jejunal absorption of solubilized fatty acids would ever reach the gastric mucosa in order to protect it against injury. These studies do not answer the question whether chronic ingestion of solubilized dietary fatty acids may not permit them to reach the gastric mucosa eventually and be deposited in the gastric mucosal cell membranes. In fact there is evidence that chronic administration of fatty acids in the solubilized or nonsolubilized form may very well enhance the protective activity of the stomach against injury, signifying long-term accumulation of dietary fatty acids by gastric mucosal cells (TARNAWSKI et al. 1986b).

III. Generation of Prostanoids by the Gastric Mucosa from Solubilized Essential Fatty Acids

Direct administration of detergent solubilized arachidonic acid into the gastric lumen of rats in vivo results in rapid increase in PGE_2 concentrations in the gastric lumen. The concentrations achieved by the administration of a small amount of solubilized arachidonic acid are enormous and reach a few thousand pmoles per milliliter of gastric content (HOLLANDER et al. 1982). In this situation the liberation of prostanoids from the gastric mucosa following arachidonic acid administration can also be blocked by the preadministration of indomethacin to the animals. At this point we do not have information about possible increase in synthesis and/or release of leukotrienes or thromboxanes following administration of solubilized linoleic or arachidonic acid.

E. Gastric Mucosal Protection by Solubilized Essential Fatty Acids

The first experiments to demonstrate the efficacy of dietary essential fatty acids in protecting the gastric mucosa against alcohol injury were done in our laboratory using solubilized arachidonic acid (HOLLANDER et al. 1982; TARNAWSKI et al. 1983). Normally, arachidonic acid is absorbed by the jejunum by a process which requires the presence of biological detergents such as bile acids. In order to solubilize arachidonic acid and make it available for absorption by the gastric mucosal cells, we dissolved it with a nonionic detergent, pluronic F-68. This form of arachidonic acid, when given to rats intragastrically, caused rapid synthesis of PGE_2 with a several thousand fold increase in its luminal concentration within a short time (30 min). Intragastric pretreatment of rats with solubilized arachidonic acid resulted in prevention of gastric mucosal damage by alcohol. Pretreatment of the rats with indomethacin in order to block the conversion of arachidonic acid to PGs abolished 60%–70% of the fatty acid's protective activity. Intragastric pretreatment with 37 mg solubilized arachidonic acid significantly reduced or even completely prevented alcohol induced gross and deep histological gastric mucosal necrosis (gross and histological necrosis <1% of mucosal area compared with 27%–37% and 41%–58% respectively in controls) during the period 15 min-15 h after alcohol administration. Gastric mucosal protection afforded by arachidonic acid was very similar to the mucosal protection provided by PGs in an identical experimental model, with respect to histological, ultrastructural, and functional features. Intrajejunal administration of solubilized arachidonic acid was ineffective in protection of the gastric mucosa against alcohol induced injury, indicating that absorbed PGE_2 was promptly deactivated during portal and pulmonary passage and that a direct contact of the gastric mucosa with solubilized arachidonic acid is required for local generation of protective PGE_2. We also found that once the gastric mucosa is protected by arachidonic acid against alcohol injury, it remains more resistant to subsequent rechallenge with alcohol (Tarnawski et al. 1986b).

In a different study assessing the protective action of solubilized arachidonic acid against acute aspirin induced gastric mucosal injury we found that intragastric pretreatment with 150 mg/kg detergent solubilized arachidonic acid significantly reduced the extent of aspirin induced gross necrosis of gastric oxyntic mucosa (fivefold reduction at 1 h, 12-fold reduction at 4 h, and 20-fold reduction at 18 h). In addition, arachidonic acid reduced deep histological necrosis involving the glandular cells (sixfold reduction at 1 h, 18-fold reduction at 4 h, and 40-fold reduction at 18 h) (Tarnawski et al. 1988c). In control rats pretreated with solubilizer only, aspirin produced significant damage to both superficial and deeper microvessels, consisting of rupture of capillary walls, necrosis of endothelial cells, damage to endothelial organelles, and adherence of platelets and leukocytes to damaged endothelium. Microvascular injury preceded the development of deep necrotic lesions. Microvascular damage and deep mucosal necrosis were significantly reduced by arachidonic acid pretreatment. This study clearly indicated that gastric mucosal microvessels are a major target for aspirin induced injury and arachidonic acid protection (Tarnawski et al. 1988c).

Some authors have evaluated the potential protective action of arachidonic acid against aspirin injury. They were unable to detect a protective action of arachidonic acid. It should be noted, however, that in that study (Rainsford

1978) arachidonic acid was given simultaneously with aspirin and was given either intraperitoneally (therefore PGs could not have been generated, or if generated they were promptly inactivated by liver and lungs and could not have reached gastric mucosa) or intragastrically in a nonsolubilized form and therefore not absorbed by the mucosa.

Solubilized linoleic acid (74 mg), when given as an intragastric pretreatment (60 min before), significantly reduced alcohol induced gross mucosal necrosis (11 to 18-fold reduction, $P < 0.01$ vs solubilizer pretreated rats) and deep histological necrosis (17 to 21-fold reduction vs solubilizer pretreated rats, $P < 0.01$) during 15 min–24 h after alcohol administration (TARNAWSKI et al. 1987).

I. Angiogenic Effect of Essential Fatty Acids

Of major interest is the fact that essential fatty acids – arachidonic acid and linoleic acid – were found to exert a trophic and angiogenic effect on injured gastric mucosa, accelerating new microvessel formation and promoting better quality of mucosal injury repair (TARNAWSKI et al. 1988a, 1989).

F. Dietary Intake of Essential Fatty Acids

I. Animal Studies

So far our discussion has centered on the ability of detergent solubilized fatty acids to offer acute protection against injury by various necrotizing or irritating substances. In order to be effective, dietary essential fatty acids have to be solubilized in detergents in order to penetrate the gastric mucosa and offer protection. The question we will address in this section deals with the issue of nonsolubilized dietary sources of essential fatty acids and their role in gastric or duodenal mucosal protection. That is, are dietary fatty acids present in ingested foods able to offer protection against mucosal injury or against ulcer formation? The latest study which examined this question in an animal model was published by SCHEPP et al. (1988). Three groups of rats were fed diets deficient in (0.3%), sufficient in (3%), or supplemented with (10%) linoleic acid for 8–10 weeks. These diets contained linoleic acid as a natural food constituent and did not contain detergents or other agents to increase the solubility of the fatty acids. The authors found that diets deficient in linoleic acid reduced the release of PGE_2 into the gastric lumen by 77% and increased basal and intragastric stimulated gastric acid secretion. Moreover, when these rats fed diets deficient in linoleic acid were subjected to cold restraint induced gastric mucosal lesions, there was a 280% increase in the area of gastric mucosal damage when compared to controls. Thus, dietary deficiency of linoleic acid in the rat resulted in marked increase in susceptibility of the stomach to injury and an increase in gastric acid secretion. In contrast, when these investigators supplemented the diets with 10% linoleic acid, PGE_2 release into the gastric lumen increased by 106% and acid released into the lumen decreased by 44% in the basal state and 78% in the stimulated state. The rats which were supplemented with a 10% linoleic acid containing diet were able to withstand cold restraint induced mucosal lesions, which were reduced by 80% following dietary supplementation as compared to controls. In addition, pretreatment of the rats with indomethacin (which blocked the cyclooxygenase system) abolished the protective effects of linoleic acid supplemented diets. From this study it is clear that the chronic supplementation of the diet with linoleic acid in a nonsolubilized form does markedly increase the defensive properties of the gastric mucosa and diminishes both basal and stimulated acid secretion. Since we know from previous experiments that dietary fatty acids are primarily absorbed by the proximal half of the small bowel and cannot be absorbed immediately by the stômach in the absence of added detergents, we must conclude from these experiments that the salutary effect of dietary linoleic acid must be due to its absorption by the jejunum and eventual accumulation in membrane phospholipids in the stomach and duodenum. This study in rats provides strong evidence and a scientific basis for the design and execution of human trials with supplemental dietary essential fatty acids. These trials should examine the efficacy of dietary supplementation with essential fatty acids in preventing recurrent gastric or duodenal ulcerations and/or protecting the gastroduodenal mucosa against injury.

II. Human Intake of Dietary Essential Fatty Acids and Its Relationship to Peptic Ulcer Disease

The dietary intake of essential fatty acids in the Western world has been changing drastically over the past 80 years. In assessing the comparative intake of dietary essential fatty acids early this century versus today's intake, it is clear that a recall method would not be appropriate. Therefore, we assessed the intake of dietary essential fatty acids over the past 80 years by relying on governmental statistics and information regarding total population intake of nutrients (HOLLANDER and TARNAWSKI 1986a). Fortunately, both in the United States and in Great Britain, information is available regarding the total population intake of specific food substances. In the United Kingdom, the Ministry of Agriculture, Fisheries and Food does a yearly survey of food ingestion. The same is true in the United States, where the Department of Agriculture provides yearly summaries of nutrient content of the National food supply. Thus, using commercial information of total population food intake and analysis of food constituents, we have been able to obtain accurate information on the intake of lipids per person in the United States and in Britain for the period 1909–1981. During that period the intake of vegetable oils by each person in the United States increased from 21 g/day in 1909 to 68 g/day in 1981. During the same period the ingestion of animal fats did not change and remained at 95–103 g/day (Fig. 1). When we tabulated the specific intake of oleic (nonessential fatty acid) versus linoleic acid, we found a small increase in oleic acid intake from 50 g/day in 1909 to 65 g/day in 1981. The most remarkable increase in intake of fatty acids occurred, however, with linoleic acid. In 1909 the daily ingestion of linoleic acid per person was 9 g/day. In contrast, by 1981 linoleic acid intake increased to 26 g/day in the United States (Fig. 2). This almost threefold increase in intake of linoleic acid was highly significant and showed a marked contrast to the intake of other fatty acids. The enormous increase in dietary ingestion of essential fatty acids since 1909 in the Western world has occurred for commercial and for public health reasons. Commercially, vegetable oils have been cheaper to isolate, produce, and market. In addition, there has been a great deal of public health pressure to switch from animal to vegetable fats in order to reduce the incidence of heart disease.

This enormous increase in the intake of dietary essential fatty acids by the population in the Western world has profound potential implications for changes in gastroduodenal functions and gastroduodenal protection against injury (HOLLANDER and TARNAWSKI 1986a,b). As noted earlier in the chapter, dietary essential fatty acids can provide effective protection against

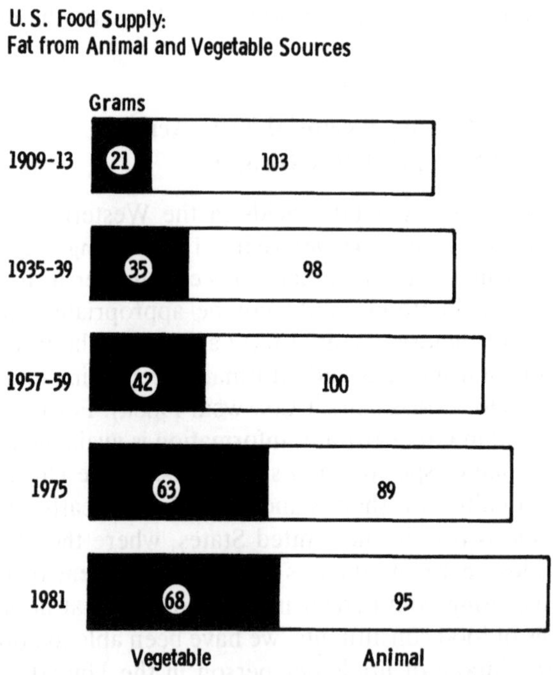

Fig. 1. Changes in vegetable and animal fat intake in the United States from 1909 to 1981. The amounts represent the number of grams of fat available to be ingested per person per day. The data are based on information from RIZEK et al. (1984)

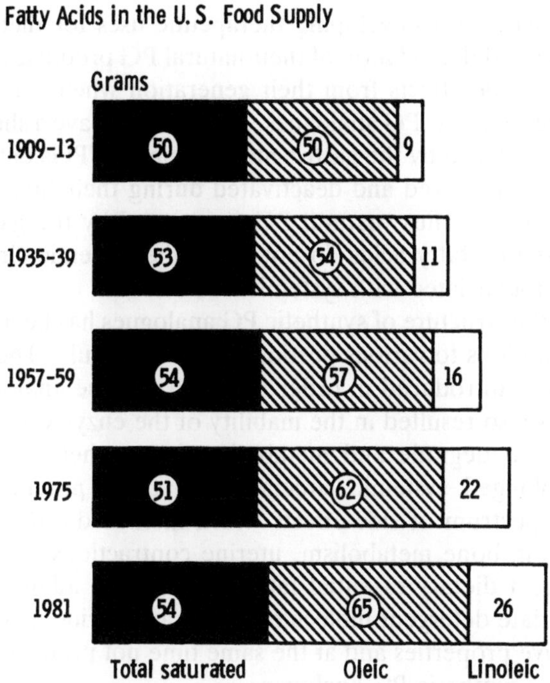

Fig. 2. Changes in saturated fat oleic and linoleic acid intake between 1909 and 1981 in the United States. Amounts represent the number of grams available to be ingested per person per day. Data are based on information from RIZEK et al. (1984)

gastroduodenal mucosal injury in animal models. The chronic ingestion of dietary fatty acid can also result in decreased gastric acid secretion and increased resistance to stress induced injury. Dietary supplementation with essential fatty acids appears to have a cumulative beneficial effect in animal studies. In addition, a solubilized form of dietary fatty acids can also induce changes in the human gastric mucosal ability to secrete hydrochloric acid. Given this information, we propose that the enormous increase in the dietary intake of essential fatty acids could very well be responsible, at least in part, for the decreases observed in the incidence and virulence of peptic ulcer disease over the past 3–4 decades. It could also perhaps account for changes in the underlying resistance of the gastroduodenal mucosa to all forms of injury (SCHEPP et al. 1988; HOLLANDER and TARNAWSKI 1986a).

G. Potential Therapeutic Advantages of Dietary Essential Fatty Acids Over the Synthetic Prostaglandins

Since potent synthetic analogues of natural PGs are available, why should we consider potential therapeutic use of dietary fatty acids as PG precursors?

The major reason for developing therapeutic uses for dietary essential fatty acids is the rapid degradation of their natural PG products and therefore the lack of major side-effects from their generation when compared to the side-effects of the synthetic PG analogues. Natural PGs have a short biological half-life. When produced by the gastric mucosa, natural PGs enter the portal circulation and are removed and deactivated during their first pass through the liver and/or lungs. Thus, natural PGs generated by the gastric mucosa from dietary essential fatty acids do not reach the systemic circulation and therefore are not associated with systemic side-effects.

In contrast, the structure of synthetic PG analogues has been modified by methyl group additions to various portions of the molecule. These structural modifications were introduced in order to stabilize these analogues. Unfortunately, this has also resulted in the inability of the enzyme systems in liver and lung tissues to degrade and metabolize the synthetic PG analogues, resulting in prolonged systemic circulation of these potent compounds, causing a wide spectrum of side-effects which include diarrhea, abdominal cramps, changes in bone metabolism, uterine contractions, and even abortions. Therefore, if dietary essential fatty acids can be administered orally with the appropriate detergent molecule, they may provide us with the ideal mucosal protective properties and at the same time not produce the systemic side-effects of the synthetic PG analogues.

The only exception would be application of dietary essential fatty acids for healing of gastroduodenal mucosal injury during chronic treatment with NSAIDs. Since these drugs inhibit the enzymes converting arachidonic acid to PGs, one cannot expect generation of natural PGs and their protective and healing action by the administration of PG precursor fatty acids. In all other types of acute or chronic gastric mucosal injury (such as prevention of acute alcohol injury, stress ulcerations in critically ill patients, and repair and healing of erosions or ulcerations), essential fatty acids should be as effective as synthetic PGs without their major systemic side-effects.

I. Effect of Short-Term Treatment with Dietary Essential Fatty Acids on the Human Gastric Mucosa

The effects of dietary essential fatty acids on the human stomach were assessed by Palmer and co-workers, who examined this question in normal male volunteers who took 1 g linoleic acid with pluronic F-68 detergent twice daily for 2 weeks (GRANT et al. 1988). At the end of the study, these volunteers were found to have a small reduction in their basal and stimulated acid output, a significant rise in serum gastrin, and a pronounced increase in their intragastric content of PGs. This study demonstrates that solubilized linoleic acid can induce functional changes in the human stomach compatible with the generation of endogenous PGs. It remains to be determined whether the increased generation of PGs will protect the human gastric mucosa against injury or promote the healing of established injury.

H. Summary and Conclusion

Dietary essential fatty acids – arachidonic acid and linoleic acid – serve as constituents of cells' phospholipid membranes and as precursors for synthesis of PGs. In acute experiments they protect the gastric mucosa against numerous damaging factors, including absolute alcohol and aspirin. This protection is accomplished by their local mucosal conversion to cytoprotective PGs by the gastric mucosa.

Chronic feeding of a linoleic acid enriched diet to rats inhibits gastric acid secretion, increases gastric mucosal generation of PGE_2, and reduces cold restraint ulcerations. Inhibition of acid secretion and increased mucosal PGE_2 was also observed in man after 2 weeks' ingestion of linoleic acid.

The use of essential fatty acids for the protection and healing of the gastric mucosa has in many instances clear advantages over the use of synthetic PGs, because natural PGs generated by the gastric mucosa from essential fatty acids exert only topical action and do not reach the systemic circulation. Therefore such treatment is not associated with systemic side-effects. For this reason essential fatty acids may be the treatment of choice in the future for prophylaxis and healing of gastroduodenal mucosal lesions with the only exception of injury produced by NSAIDs.

References

Bakhle YS (1983) Synthesis and catabolism of cyclo-oxygenase products. Br Med Bull 39:214–218

Chow SL, Hollander D (1978) Arachidonic acid intestinal absorption: Mechanism of transport and influence of luminal factors on absorption *in vitro*, Lipids 11: 768–776

Chow SL, Hollander D (1979a) Linoleic acid absorption in the unanesthetized rat: mechanism of transport and influence of luminal factors on absorption rate. Lipids 14:378–385

Chow SL, Hollander D (1979b) A dual, concentration-dependent absorption mechanism of linoleic acid by rat jejunum *in vitro*. J Lipid Res 20:349–356

Gali C, Agrandi E, Petroni A, Tremoli E (1980) Dietary essential fatty acid, tissue fatty acids and prostaglandin synthesis. Prog Fd Nutr Sci 4:1–7

Grant HW, Palmer KR, Kelly RW, Wilson NH, Misiewicz JJ (1988) Dietary linoleic acid gastric acid and prostaglandin secretion. Gastroenterology 94:955–959

Hollander D, Tarnawski A (1986a) Dietary essential fatty acids and the decline in peptic ulcer disease – a hypothesis. Gut 27:239–242

Hollander D, Tarnawski A (1986b) Dietary essential fatty acids and peptic ulcer disease (letter to the editor). Gut 27:1108–1109

Hollander D, Tarnawski A, Ivey KJ, DeZeery A, Zipser RD, McKenzie WN (1982) Arachidonic acid protection of rat gastric mucosa against ethanol injury. J Lab Clin Med 100:296–308

Hollander D, Dadufalza VD, Sletten EG (1984) Does essential fatty acid absorption change with aging? J Lipid Res 25:129–134

Konturek JS, Pawlik W (1986) Physiology and pharmacology of prostaglandins. Dig Dis Sci [Feb Suppl] 31:6s–19s

Marti-Bonmati E, Alino SF, Loris JM et al. (1980) Effects of cimetidine, atropine and

prostaglandin E_2 on rat mucosal erosions produced by intragastric distension. Eur J Pharmacol 68:48–53
Miller T (1983) Protective effects of prostaglandins against gastric mucosal damage: current knowledge and proposed mechanisms. Am J Physiol 245:G601–23
Nilsson A, Melin T (1988) Absorption and metabolism of orally fed arachidonic and linoleic acid in the rat. Am J Physiol 255:G612–618
Rainford KD (1978) The role of aspirin in gastric ulceration. Some factors involved in the development of gastric mucosal damage induced by aspirin in rats exposed to various stress conditions. Am J Digest Dis 23:521–530
Rainford KD, Fox SA, Osborne DJ (1984) Comparative effects of some non-steroidal antiinflammatory drugs on the ultrastructural integrity and prostaglandin levels in the gastric mucosa. Relationship to drug uptake. Scand J Gastroenteroll (Suppl 101) 19:55–68
Ramwell PW (1981) Biologic importance of arachidonic acid. Arch Int Med 141: 275–278
Redfern JS, Feldman M (1989) Role of endogenous prostaglandins in preventing gastrointestinal ulceration: induction of ulcers by antibodies to prostaglandins. Gastroenterology 96:596–605
Redfern JS, Blair AJ, Lee E, Feldman M (1987) Gastrointestinal ulcer formation in rabbits immunized with prostaglandin E_2. Gastroenterology 93:744–752
Rizek RL, Welsh SO, Marston RM (1984) Levels and sources of fat in the US food supply and in diets of individuals. In: Milner J, Perkins EG (eds) Cancer – a molecular event. American oil Chemists' society
Robert A, Nezamis JE, Lancaster C, Hanchar AJ (1979) Cytoprotection by prostaglandins in rats. Prevention of gastric necrosis produced by alcohol, HCl, NaOH, hypertonic NaCl and thermal injury. Gastroenterology 77:433–43
Robert A, Lancaster C, Davis JP et al. (1984) Distinction between antiulcer effect and cytoprotection. Scand J Gastroenterol (Suppl 101) 19:69–72
Robins PG (1980) Ultrastructural observations on the pathogenesis of aspirin induced gastric erosions. Br J Exp Pathol 61:497–504
Schepp W, Steffen B, Ruoff HJ, Schusdziarra V, Classen M (1988) Modulation of rat gastric mucosal prostaglandin E_2 release by dietary linoleic acid: effects on gastric acid secretion and stress-induced mucosal damage. Gastroenterology 95:18–25
Szabo S, Trier JS, Brown A, Schnoor J (1985) Early vascular injury and increased vascular permeability in gastric mucosal injury caused by ethanol in the rat. Gastroenterology 88:228–
Tarnawski A (1980) Cytoprotection. A new fashion or real progress? Pol Arch Med Weswn 64:97–104
Tarnawski A, Hollander D, Stachura J, Krause WJ (1983) Arachidonic acid protection of gastric mucosa against alcohol injury: sequential analysis of morphologic and functional changes. J Lab Clin Med 102:340–351
Tarnawski A, Hollander D, Stachura J et al. (1985a) Prostaglandin protection of the gastric mucosa against alcohol injury – dynamic time related process. The role of the mucosal proliferative zone. Gastroenterology 89:366–74
Tarnawski A, Hollander D, Stachura J (1985b) Ultrastructural changes in the gastric mucosal microvessels after ethanol. Gastroenterol Clin Biol 9 (12 bis):93–7
Tarnawski A, Brzozowski T, Hollander et al. (1986a) Prostaglandin protection of isolated human gastric glands against ethanol-induced injury. Evidence for cytoprotection in vitro (abstract). Gastroenterology 90:1658
Tarnawski A, Hollander D, Stachura J, Dadufalza V, Gergely H (1986b) Is arachidonic acid protected gastric mucosa more resistant to rechallenge with a second dose of ethanol? Klin Wochenschr 64:35–39
Tarnawski A, Hollander D, Gergely H (1987) Protection of gastric mucosa by linoleic acid – a nutrient essential fatty acid. Clin Invest Med 10:132–136
Tarnawski A, Hollander D, Stachura J, Gergely H (1988a) Essential fatty acids – arachidonic and linoleic have trophic and angiogenic effect on the gastric mucosa injured by alcohol. Gastroenterology 94:A455

Tarnawski A, Stachura J, Gergely H, Hollander D (1988b) Microvascular endothelium – a major target for alcohol injury of the human gastric mucosa. Histochemical and ultrastructural study. J Clin Gastroenterol 10(1):554–564

Tarnawski A, Hollander D, Stachura J, Krause WJ, Gergely H (1989a) Protection of the gastric mucosa against aspirin injury by arachidonic acid – a dietary prostaglandin precursor fatty acid. Eur J Clin Invest 19:278–290

Tarnawski A, Hollander D, Stachura J, Sarfeh IJ, Gergely H, Krause WJ (1989) Angiogenic response of gastric mucosa to ethanol injury is abolished by indomethacin. Gastroenterology 96:A505

Vane JR, Moncada S (1979) Polyunsaturated fatty acids as precursors of prostaglandins. Acta Cardiol [Suppl] (Brux) 23:21–37

Whittle BJR (1977) Mechanisms underlying gastric mucosal damage induced by indomethacin and bile salts and the actions of prostaglandins. Br J Pharmacol 60:455–60

Whittle BJR, Vane JR (1986) Prostanoids as regulators of gastrointestinal function. In: Johnson LR (ed) Physiology of the gastrointestinal tract, 2nd edn. Raven, New York, pp 147–180

CHAPTER 5

Helicobacter pylori

G.M.A. Börsch and D.Y. Graham

A. Introduction

The rediscovery of spiral shaped, *Campylobacter*-like gastric bacteria, later termed *Campylobacter pylori* (*C. pylori*), and in October 1989 renamed as *Helicobacter pylori* (*H. pylori*: Goodwin et al. 1989), has suddenly questioned the comprehensiveness of previous pathogenetic concepts in peptic ulcer disease. *H. pylori* finally offers an intriguing explanation to some of the puzzling complexities of this disease, e.g., why virtually all idiopathic, recurrent ulcers occur in the presence of chronic type B gastritis. *H. pylori* leaves other equally perplexing riddles unresolved, e.g., the fact that peptic ulcers are invariably a localized and periodic phenomenon, a finding obviously hard to correlate with a bacterial infection that is both diffuse and stable. Above all and for the first time, however, *H. pylori* has suggested the possibility of obtaining lasting cure rather than mere temporary control of ulcer disease, which would open a completely new era in the medical management of this condition.

This chapter will attempt to describe the role of *H. pylori* in ulcer disease based on the current body of knowledge. We will initially focus on epidemiological aspects and on the pathogenetic role of these bacteria. We will then review the efficacy and safety of present treatment modalities to eradicate *H. pylori*, followed by an analysis of the effects of bacterial eradication on healing and relapse in duodenal and gastric ulcer disease. The irrefutable, important role of *H. pylori* will be emphasized, even though the therapeutic implications may be difficult to exploit given present-day therapeutic possibilities.

B. Clinical Relevance of *Helicobacter pylori*

I. Frequency in the General Population and Association with Chronic Gastritis and Peptic Ulcer Disease

A very strong association of *H. pylori* infection of the upper gastrointestinal tract with chronic type B gastritis, duodenal ulcer disease, and, to a somewhat lesser extent, gastric ulcer disease has been clearly established by

B.J. Marshall in his original work from Western Australia (Marshall and Warren 1984; Marshall et al. 1985; Marshall 1986). These findings were rapidly confirmed by a number of studies from various geographical areas (Rollason et al. 1984; Jones et al. 1984; Steer 1985; Price et al. 1985; Morris et al. 1986; Buck et al. 1986; Burette et al. 1986; Von Wulffen et al. 1986; Bohnen et al. 1986; Hirschl et al. 1987a,c; Hazell et al. 1987; Lamouliatte et al. 1987b; Taylor et al. 1987; Jiang et al. 1987; Raskov et al. 1987; Menge et al. 1987a,b; Malfertheiner et al. 1987; Dickgiesser et al. 1987; Börsch et al. 1988b; Niemelä et al. 1987; Marcheggiano et al. 1987). The same disease associations also exist in the pediatric age group (Czinn et al. 1986, 1989; Drumm et al. 1987; Cadranel et al. 1988; Kilbridge et al. 1988; Eastham et al. 1988; Mahoney et al. 1988; Mahoney and Littlewood 1989).

The frequency of *H. pylori* in chronic type B gastritis is approximately 70% in large series (Steininger et al. 1989). It is even higher in chronic active gastritis (Stolte et al. 1989; Wyatt and Dixon 1988). The exact rate depends on the definition of histological activity, which so far has differed between various investigative groups.

In duodenal ulcer disease, the prevalence of *H. pylori* has consistently been found to be around 95% by investigators using carefully validated diagnostic techniques (Wyatt and Dixon 1988). A meta-analysis of 1054 duodenal ulcer cases published in the literature has yielded a frequency of *H. pylori* in duodenal ulcer disease of only 88% (Börsch 1988b). However, this lower rate is very likely due to methodological inadequacies encountered by some of the earlier studies. Careful note also has to be taken that these figures apply to the prevalence of *H. pylori* in gastric mucosal biopsies of duodenal ulcer patients. It is much more difficult to detect these bacteria in the duodenum, but meticulous histological search has succeeded in demonstrating *H. pylori* in the duodenum with a frequency of 96% of duodenal ulcer cases (Johnston et al. 1988). Gastric metaplasia in the duodenum apparently paves the way for *H. pylori* to colonize the duodenum (Wyatt et al. 1987; Wyatt and Rathbone 1989; Graham 1989a,b), by providing target cells for these bacteria (Malfertheiner et al. 1989).

The prevalence of *H. pylori* in gastric ulcer disease varies more widely, but has most consistently been found to be around 70% (Wyatt and Dixon 1988). A previous meta-analysis of 753 published gastric ulcers revealed *H. pylori* in 64% of the cases only, which, again, may be explained by methodological inadequacies of earlier studies (Börsch 1988b), but also by heterogeneity of the various study groups. *H. pylori* has been found with a much higher frequency of 96% in subgroups with idiopathic gastric ulcers, after exclusion of patients with known causes of their ulcer disease, which is equivalent to the *H. pylori* frequency found in duodenal ulcerations (Rauws et al. 1988).

Comparatively little is known on the prevalence of *H. pylori* in the general population. There is a marked rise in the prevalence of active *H.*

pylori infection (GRAHAM et al. 1988b) or the seroprevalence of *H. pylori* (KOSUNEN et al. 1989; MITCHELL et al. 1988; PEREZ-PEREZ et al. 1988) with increasing age. In a ^{13}C urea breath test study, the frequency of *H. pylori* was 24% in the age group 20–39 years, rising to 36% in persons aged 40–59 years and 82% in the 60–84 year age range, while an association with age was not apparent in patients with peptic ulcer, who had a high *H. pylori* prevalence already in the young age groups (GRAHAM et al. 1988b).

However, the age-adjusted prevalence differs markedly between various geographical areas and ethnic groups (GRAHAM et al. 1988b, 1989a; KOSUNEN et al. 1989; MITCHELL et al. 1988). For example, the frequency of *H. pylori* in a sample of the Saudi population aged 16 years or older has been reported to be 79% (AL-MOAGEL et al. 1989). In Peru, 45% of children 1 year or younger from poor income families harbor *H. pylori* (KLEIN et al. 1989). In contrast, a low *H. pylori* frequency of only 23% has been found in white elderly Virginia women (MARSHALL et al. 1989c). Therefore, any associations of *H. pylori* with disease have to be viewed against the age-adjusted prevalence of *H. pylori* in that specific population. Another important epidemiological finding is the observation that populations with marked differences in their propensity to develop duodenal ulcer disease, such as Ethiopians or Australian aboriginals, also reveal equivalent differences in their *H. pylori* prevalence (DWYER et al. 1988a,b).

II. Causation

1. Chronic Gastritis

Very strong disease associations such as those described for *H. pylori* and duodenal or idiopathic gastric ulcer disease suggest, but by no means prove, causal relationships. Concerning causation, a direct causal relationship primarily exists between *H. pylori* and chronic gastritis. Evidence to support this view includes: (a) various clinical observations such as human experiments studying the sequelae of self-inoculation with *H. pylori* (MARSHALL et al. 1985; MORRIS and NICHOLSON 1987), the repeatedly encountered phenomenon of *H. pylori*-induced epidemic hypochlorhydria in association with acute and chronic gastritis (GRAHAM et al. 1988a), and results of antibacterial treatment leading to resolution of chronic gastritis (RAUWS et al. 1988; RAUWS and TYTGAT 1989; RAUWS 1989; MCNULTY et al. 1986; GLUPCZYNSKI et al. 1988; DOOLEY et al. 1988; ODERDA et al. 1989a; ALPERT et al. 1989); (b) studies in animal models (KRAKOWKA et al. 1987); (c) studies on the local and systemic immune response (RATHBONE et al. 1989; WYATT and RATHBONE 1988); and (d) morphological, microbiological, or biochemical observations, demonstrating mechanisms in *H. pylori* which have previously been established as pathogenic or virulence factors in other bacteria such as enteropathogenic *E. coli* (GOODWIN et al. 1986; RATHBONE et al. 1988; RATHBONE and HEATLEY 1989; FAUCHERE et al. 1989).

The power or inadequacies of these various findings to support causation have been dealt with, among many other aspects of *H. pylori*, by a number of thorough reviews (Goodwin et al. 1986; Marshall 1986; Rathbone et al. 1986; Graham and Klein 1987; Graham 1989a,b; Tytgat and Rauws 1987, 1989; Blaser 1987; Hornick 1987; Bartlett 1988; Dooley and Cohen 1988; Graham 1989b; Börsch 1987, 1989a,b; Stadler and Blum 1989). The notion that *H. pylori* is indeed a direct cause of chronic type B gastritis is now accepted as valid by the scientific community.

2. Peptic Ulcer Disease

It is obvious that such a clear-cut direct causal relationship as has been described between *H. pylori* and chronic gastritis does not exist between *H. pylori* and peptic ulcer disease (Graham 1989a,b). First, *H. pylori* infection is much more prevalent than peptic ulcer disease. Therefore, only a minor fraction of people harboring *H. pylori* (lifetime prevalence approximately 80%) will apparently develop peptic ulcer disease (lifetime prevalence around 10%). Second, peptic ulcer disease is not invariably associated with *H. pylori* infection. Approximately 5% of duodenal and 30% of gastric ulcer patients will not have *H. pylori*. These observations may be taken as an indication that *H. pylori* merely plays the role of a risk factor for peptic ulcer disease in general. Undoubtedly, it does play this role. Indeed, the relative risk in British blood donors harboring *H. pylori* to have peptic ulcer disease is about seven as compared with the baseline ulcer frequency of *H. pylori* negative British donors (Wyatt et al. 1988; Börsch 1988c, 1989a).

However, there is conclusive evidence mainly derived from therapeutic eradication trials indicating a more essential role of *H. pylori* at least in ulcer subgroups. Sustained eradication of *H. pylori* in chronic recurrent, almost invariably also gastritis-associated, duodenal ulcer disease leads to a dramatic fall of 1-year ulcer relapse rates to 0%–20% (see Sect. D), suggesting, at least for a majority of duodenal ulcer relapses, a "no *H. pylori* – no ulcer" relationship (Graham 1989b). Initial observations on recurrence rates in gastric ulcer disease after *H. pylori* eradication suggest an equivalent role of *H. pylori* also in subgroups of gastric ulcer disease (Börsch et al. 1989a,b).

Nevertheless, note has to be taken that the scientific data arguing for a causal role of *H. pylori* in peptic ulcer disease almost exclusively apply to duodenal ulcer relapses in previously established duodenal ulcer cases. It is a tempting speculation that the same would also be true for the initial ulcer manifestion. Evidence to support this assumption has recently been put forward by Sipponen (1990), who has demonstrated that chronic gastritis and thus *H. pylori* precedes the initial manifestation of peptic ulcers, and not vice versa.

To account for the apparent "no *H. pylori* – no ulcer" relationship at least in the majority of duodenal ulcer relapses and to eliminate semantic ambiguities from the debate on causation, the proposition has been advanced to define a gastritis-associated variant of peptic ulcer disease, comprising virtually all cases of chronic (recurrent) duodenal ulcer disease and an as yet poorly defined proportion of gastric ulcers (Börsch 1987, 1989a,b; Graham 1989a,b). For this gastritis-associated variant of ulcer disease, *H. pylori* might be described as a necessary, albeit not sufficient condition, in addition to being a mere risk factor for peptic ulcer disease in general. According to this concept, *H. pylori* then assumes a pathogenetic role equivalent to that of acid and pepsin, both representing another necessary, though by itself not sufficient, set of conditions for peptic ulcer disease (except possibly in the case of Zollinger-Ellison syndrome). Therapeutic interventions to reduce either acid/pepsin or *H. pylori* would then suffice to prevent (or at least markedly diminish) relapses. The previous therapeutic experience with parietal cell vagotomy and long-term maintenance H_2 antagonist therapy for peptic ulcer disease, and the new data on the effect of *H. pylori* eradication (see Sect. D) are compatible with this scheme. Also, healing of peptic ulcers or prevention of relapse despite persistence of *H. pylori* (Hui et al. 1987) is readily explained by this model.

Goodwin's (1988) approach to define *H. pylori* as the major predisposing cause of duodenal ulcer disease, while acid and pepsin would act as precipitating causes, is another semantic way to accommodate previous pathogenetic concepts with present-day experimental findings on *H. pylori*.

In gastric ulcer disease, the situation is made somewhat more complicated by the considerable proportion of cases arising independently of *H. pylori*. It has to be assumed that such patients stay under lifelong risk to acquire a coincidental, but causally unrelated *H. pylori* infection. Also, nonbacterial gastric ulcer causes may affect patients with previously established, asymptomatic *H. pylori* spread. Therefore, it is safe to predict that gastritis- (and *H. pylori*-) associated gastric ulcer disease will be coincidentally associated with, but nevertheless causally unrelated to, *H. pylori* in a considerable, as yet undefined number of cases.

The most stringent definition of *H. pylori* dependent ulcer disease would then be "an *H. pylori* associated recurrent duodenal or gastric ulcer, that does not relapse after eradication of *H. pylori*, unless reinfection by *H. pylori* occurs" (Börsch 1989a). Unfortunately, this is an "a posteriori" definition, based on trial, in all, and error, in some, ulcer patients.

Clearly, such a theoretical concept based on conditional logic does not give additional proof of a causal relationship. It is rather meant to put the apparently significant role of *H. pylori* in the pathogenesis of peptic ulcer disease into a precise and testable perspective. Simultaneously, this model reconciles the evolving bacterial role in ulcer pathogenesis with the long acknowledged place of acid and pepsin and also with the role of other relevant disease modifiers such as smoking, intrinsic, environmental, or genetic elements. These act as variable risk factors and might explain why some *H. pylori*-infected individuals develop peptic ulcers, while others with identical prerequisites in terms of *H. pylori* infection and acid output do not, or why ulcer relapses occur periodically against the background of a fixed gastric secretory capacity and a stable bacterial infection. An alternate view, that bacterial strains may differ in regard to their ulcerogenic potential, has been proposed (GRAHAM and KLEIN 1987; FIGURA et al. 1989), but so far remains unproven. This alternative would also fail to explain the periodic nature of peptic ulcers.

In summary, therefore, evidence is rapidly accumulating to support a role of *H. pylori* as a cocausal factor in previously idiopathic, gastritis-associated ulcer disease, highlighted by the acronym GAUD (BÖRSCH 1987).

C. Attempts to Eradicate *Helicobacter pylori*

If these considerations indeed give an adequate reflection of the pathogenetic role of *H. pylori*, then antibacterial treatment should exert a profound effect on the natural history of peptic ulcer disease. This would assign top clinical priority to research aimed at identifying suitable treatment regimens to eradicate *H. pylori*. However, two decisive prerequisites will have to be met to make any *H. pylori*-oriented therapy useful. First. total eradication of these bacteria from their habitat in the gastric or gastroduodenal environment rather than temporary suppression of the bacterial density will be necessary to exploit the full therapeutic potential of *H. pylori* in peptic ulcer disease. Second, early reinfections from an outside source should be rare events. Otherwise they would tend to make any therapeutic benefit a transitory event and prevent a lasting impact of *H. pylori* therapy on the natural history of peptic ulcer disease.

Therefore, the efficacy of treatment regimens so far applied to eradicate *H. pylori* will be reviewed in this section. Also, an estimate of reinfection rates from outside sources will be given based on data from the literature. In the context of this presentation, eradication will be defined as negative *H. pylori* results by validated, sensitive diagnostic tests, preferentially sensitive culture techniques, obtained not before 3–4 weeks after cessation of the index therapy under study (see also Sect. C.II). Work from Amsterdam has clearly shown that a number of therapeutic regimens lead to negative test results immediately after therapeutic interventions. However, the major proportion of such patients will again convert to a state of *H. pylori* positivity within the next 3–4 weeks (RAUWS et al. 1988; LANGENBERG et al. 1985, 1987). Pre- and posttherapeutic analyses of *H. pylori* DNA have indicated that this is due to regrowth of the original bacterial strain, which had not been completely eradicated, but only temporarily suppressed below the threshold of detection. This regrowth of the initial bacterial strain may be appropriately termed bacterial "recrudescence" (LANGENBERG et al. 1986).

On the contrary, patients still having negative *H. pylori* tests 4 weeks after cessation of therapy tend to stay negative for long periods. Their rare bacterial conversions are not due to recrudescence, but to true reinfections (RAUWS et al. 1988). Reinfection rates per year as initially observed in

Amsterdam by RAUWS et al. (1988) were around 12%, or around 6% as observed in Australia by BORODY et al. (1988, 1989). The reinfection rate in Bochum, West Germany was 5.6% for a mean observation period of 6.9 months (BÖRSCH et al. 1989b) and it was also very infrequent in Virginia, U.S.A. as described by MARSHALL et al. (1989b). There is currently no indication that reinfection rates will rise during the 2nd year of follow-up after *H. pylori* eradication (RAUWS 1989).

However, it is not yet known whether patients with peptic ulcer have increased susceptibility to *H. pylori* infections. Somewhere between 1% and 2% of adults in developed countries contract *H. pylori* each year (see Sect. C.I). If ulcer patients do not have an increased susceptibility, one would expect a comparably low but relatively constant rate of reinfections.

In summary, this section deals with genuine eradication of *H. pylori*. Therefore, only studies reporting follow-up after a posttherapeutic interval of at least 3–4 weeks will be considered, unless the inefficiency of any therapeutic regimen is already demonstrated by persistence of positive *H. pylori* test results immediately after completion of that therapy.

I. Natural History

Any assessment of therapeutic effects must be viewed against the background of the natural history of *H. pylori* infection. All data in the literature, especially the work of LANGENBERG et al. (1988), argue in the direction that *H. pylori* infection is a stable condition (GRAHAM et al. 1989a), with little chance of bacterial clearance to occur spontaneously. Cross-sectional data from the United States, Europe, and Australia indicate that infection of these populations is a rather slow process, occurring gradually with 1%–2% of the population contracting *H. pylori* per year. As mentioned earlier, however, the epidemiology of *H. pylori* may be quite different in Third World countries and areas like Peru or Saudi Arabia, where a high prevalence of *H. pylori* has been observed in childhood and adolescence (KLEIN et al. 1989; AL-MOAGEL et al. 1989).

In summary, the natural history of *H. pylori* infection is that of a stable condition, acquired gradually over time in Western industrialized nations, with a more rapid spread during childhood and adolescence in many other parts of the world. In this regard, the *H. pylori* prevalence closely mirrors the epidemiology of hepatitis A virus or polio infections (GRAHAM 1990). It is against the background of this high degree of stability of *H. pylori* infection that uncontrolled observations can claim some significance, when reporting substantial eradication rates.

II. Eradication of *Helicobacter pylori* Infections

One must recognize that we do not yet know the best method of treating an *H. pylori* infection. Definitions used for "eradication," "recrudescence or

Table 1. Criteria for eradication of *H. pylori*

Laboratory

Invasive:

1. Failure to culture the organism from at least two gastric mucosal biopsies, at least one taken from the antrum
2. Failure to visualize the organism on gastric mucosal biopsy specimens (at least one antral) using sensitive special stains or preferably specific immunohistochemical techniques
3. Continued improvement in the histology of the gastric mucosa with a return to or toward normal and absence of polymorphonuclear infiltration

Noninvasive:

1. Continued fall in titer of specific anti-*H. pylori* antibodies
2. Continued negative urea breath tests

Clinical

1. Absence of duodenal or gastric ulcer recurrence
2. Risk of developing a duodenal or gastric ulcer less than that of a control population (for those who have not had duodenal or gastric ulcer)

relapse," or "reinfection" are still operational and are not based upon results of careful investigations. The current working definition of eradication of the infection is the absence of detectable infection 1 month after stopping treatment. This definition allows for an overestimation of the number of patients who will be free of the infection 1 year after therapy. It is not yet clear which of the 8%–12% of patients in whom infection reappears represent relapse from failure to eradicate the original infection (most likely) or from reinfections acquired either iatrogenically at the time of endoscopy or from the environment.

Eradication of the infection should be associated with continued improvement in the gastric and duodenal histology, a fall in antibody titer, continued urea breath test negativity, and inability to either culture or visualize the organism in gastric mucosal biopsies (Table 1). The best definition of eradication would include having the patient's risk for development of duodenal or gastric ulcer return to (or better still, be less than) that of the general population. This implies that eradication would equate with long-term eradication measured over a period of years instead of weeks or months. Peptic ulcer disease is a relapsing problem of long duration. Thus, a minor change such as a marked reduction in relapse frequency that lasted only 1 or 2 years would have little overall benefit to society compared to what can be obtained now with maintenance H_2 receptor antagonist therapy.

III. Methods to Confirm Eradication of *Helicobacter pylori* Infections

The simplest and least expensive method to confirm eradication of *H. pylori* infections is to identify decreasing titers of specific anti-*H. pylori* antibodies. The many ongoing treatment trials should provide sufficient data to confirm the usefulness of this approach but the lack of standardized reagents and

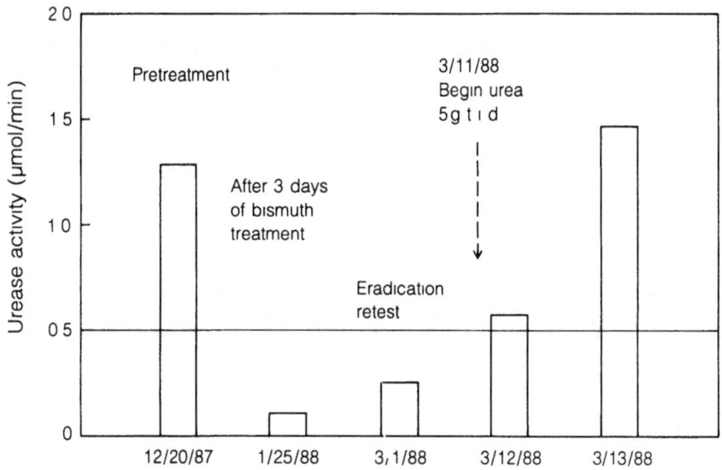

Fig. 1. The result of a provocative urea breath test is shown. Following 3 days of therapy with bismuth subsalicylate, gastric *H. pylori* infection was suppressed such that 2 months later the breath test remained negative. Provocation with oral administration of unlabeled urea resulted in prompt identification of the true status of the infection. (Klein and Graham 1989).

antigens for measuring the immune response will, for a time, restrict its applicability to specific laboratories or research units.

The urea breath test provides semiquantitative information concerning the bacterial load in the stomach. The sensitivity of the urea breath test for detection of eradication of the infection can be enhanced by the provocative urea breath test in which unlabeled urea is fed (approximately 5 g or 1 teaspoon in juice) three times daily for 1 or 2 days prior to performing the diagnostic breath test. This method will increase the amount of urea hydrolyzed (µmol/min) and turn borderline negative tests positive (Fig. 1).

Helicobacter pylori infections are often patchy and can easily be missed in a partially treated patient. Thus, reliance on the results of culture or histological examination of gastric biopsies will lead to an overestimation of the eradication rate. The availability of specific monoclonal antibodies that will identify *H. pylori* in paraffin-fixed sections should improve the sensitivity of histological evaluation of the status of the infection.

IV. Bismuth Salts

Various bismuth salts such as colloidal bismuth subcitrate, bismuth subsalicylate, or bismuth subnitrate, act as bactericidal agents on *H. pylori*. Observations by electron microscopy demonstrate a rapid in vivo destruction of *H. pylori* and its outer cell walls shortly after oral ingestion of bismuth salts (Marshall et al. 1987; Rauws and Tytgat 1987). This in vivo destruction has even been found after treatment with famotidine 40 mg b.i.d. and 650 mg

Table 2. Rates of *H. pylori* eradication obtained by bismuth monotherapy

Author	Drug	Dosage (mg)	Duration (days)	*n*	Indication	Study type	"Eradication" *n* weeks after treatment
Börsch et al. (1988a)	Bismuth subsalicylate	3 × 900	28	17	Gast Ulcer	Pilot	0: 8/17 (47%) 4: 1/15 (7%)
Langenberg et al. (1987)	CBS	4 × 120	28	84	Gast	Pilot	0: 35/84 (42%) 4: 8/84 (10%)
Lambert et al. (1987)	CBS	4 × 120	56	45	DU	Pilot	0: 20/45 (44%) >26: 12/45 (27%)
Wagner et al. (1989)	Bismuth subsalicylate	3 × 600	28	35	Ulcer Gast	Contr	0: 18/35 (51%) 4: 8/51 (23%)
Wagner et al. (1989)	Bismuth subsalicylate	3 × 600	42	12	DU	Contr	0: – 4: 2/12 (17%)
Mannes et al. (1989)	Bismuth subsalicylate	3 × 600	14	12	DU	Contr	0: – 4: 7/12 (58%)
O'Riordan et al. (1989)	CBS	4 × 120	28	23	DU	Contr	0: – 4: 10/23 (43%)
Marshall et al. (1988)	CBS	4 × 120	56	32	DU	RCT	2: 7/22 (32%) 12: 6/22 (27%)
Weil et al. (1988, 1989)	CBS	4 × 120	28–56	26	Gast	Contr	0: 21/26 (81%) 4: 7/26 (27%)
Weil et al. (1988, 1989)	CBS	4 × 240	14	20	Gast	Contr	0: 16/20 (80%) 4: 0/20 (0%)
Lambert et al. (1988)	CBS CBS	4 × 120 4 × 120	28 56	20 20	Gast Gast	Contr Contr	0: 13/20 (65%) 0: 14/20 (70%) 24: 6/20 (30%)
	CBS	2 × 240	56	20	Gast	Contr	0: 6/20 (30%) 24: 3/20 (15%)

Abbreviations: Gast, gastritis; Contr, controlled trial; RCT, randomized controlled trial; CBS, colloidal bismuth subcitrate; DU, duodenal ulcer.

sodium bicarbonate given with each meal (GRAHAM, unpublished observations). In vitro, bismuth acts to devitalize *H. pylori* by apposition of metal ion to bacterial membranes, but bismuth by itself does not provoke bacteriolysis (ARMSTRONG et al. 1987). The development of resistance to bismuth salts by *H. pylori* is unknown (GOODWIN et al. 1989b).

While bismuth salts may effectively suppress *H. pylori* with negative test results immediately after therapy in up to 78% (MCNULTY et al. 1986) or even 83% (MENGE 1988; MENGE et al. 1987a, 1988), the compounds rarely eradicate. The best results of bismuth monotherapy with an eradication rate of 43% have been published by the O'MORAIN group from Dublin, Ireland (O'RIORDAN et al. 1989). Most other authors have reported eradication rates after bismuth monotherapy between 10% and 30% (BÖRSCH 1988a; HIRSCHL and PLETSCHETTE 1989). A compilation of *H. pylori* eradication rates after bismuth therapy as reported by various authors is given in Table 2. Note should also be taken of LAMBERT's recent work, that colloidal bismuth subcitrate given as 2 × 2 tablets is apparently less effective (15% eradication) than in a dose of 4 × 1 tablets (30% eradication: LAMBERT et al. 1988). Also, increasing the doses of colloidal bismuth subcitrate (WEIL et al. 1988, 1989) as well as bismuth subsalicylate (KRAJDEN et al. 1989) will not improve eradication rates.

Besides their antibacterial action, bismuth salts, and in particular colloidal bismuth subcitrate, possess a number of pharmacodynamic properties with a potential to enhance ulcer healing (Table 3). These include, among others, formation of glycoprotein–bismuth complexes with mucus, also providing a protective coating in the ulcer crater, stimulation of prostaglandin E_2 production, and enhancement of lateral epithelial growth leading to reepithelialization (SCARPIGNATO and GALMICHE 1988; WAGSTAFF et al. 1988). Most of these properties have been established by investigating the pharmacodynamic effects of colloidal bismuth subcitrate in experimental models, while the scientific background of other bismuth salts, with the exception of bismuth subsalicylate in travellers' diarrhea, is rather limited.

The many pharmacodynamic properties of colloidal bismuth subcitrate may explain why this drug possesses at least equal efficacy as histamine H_2

Table 3. Pharmacodynamic properties of bismuth salts, and in particular colloidal bismuth subcitrate

1. Binding to ulcer base
2. Inactivation of pepsin
3. Binding of bile acids
4. Stimulation of prostaglandin biosynthesis
5. Suppression of leukotriene biosynthesis
6. Stimulation of and complexation with mucus
7. Inhibition of various enzymes
8. Binding of epithelial growth factor
9. Stimulation of lateral epithelial growth
10. Bactericidal action on *H. pylori*

receptor antagonists in the treatment of peptic ulcer disease (Wagstaff et al. 1988). In addition, this compound has the advantage of lower ulcer relapse rates than those seen after initial healing with the H_2 receptor antagonists. The spontaneous duodenal ulcer relapse rates in the year following healing of the index ulcer differ by approximately 26% (Miller and Faragher 1986; Dobrilla et al. 1988; McLean et al. 1988; Scarpignato and Galmiche 1988), while after the 2nd posttherapeutic year, the proportion of patients with at least one ulcer relapse has again risen to the same level as after H_2 antagonist treatment (Lane and Lee 1988).

This medium-term effect on the natural course of duodenal ulcer disease is best explained by the marginal effect of this drug on the eradication of *H. pylori*. Similar observations, albeit in much smaller patient numbers, have been published on the post-therapeutic course of gastric ulcer disease with colloidal bismuth subcitrate as the active agent (Tytgat 1987). However, regardless of their proven value in the treatment of peptic ulcer disease, bismuth salts can hardly be considered to be effective drugs when the treatment of *H. pylori* is the primary therapeutic goal, in view of their low eradication rates of generally not more than 10%–30%.

V. Antimicrobials as Monotherapy

The same applies to antimicrobial drugs used as monotherapy. Below we summarize studies that have assessed the posttherapeutic *H. pylori* state of treated patients not before 3–4 weeks after cessation of the index therapy, unless the inefficiency of the treatment regimen under study had been sufficiently documented by demonstrating posttherapeutic persistence of *H. pylori* infection immediately after therapy. With very few exceptions – vancomycin, trimethoprim, sulfonamides (Goodwin et al. 1988), cefsulodin (McNulty 1989), and quinolones of the first generation (Simor et al. 1989) –

Table 4. Antimicrobials so far applied and proved ineffective in treating *H. pylori* colonization

Ciprofloxacin	Oral penicillin
Ofloxacin	Bacampicillin
Norfloxacin	Pivmecillinam
Nitrofurantoin	Doxycycline
Furazolidone	Erythromycin
Fusidic acid	Josamycin
Nifuroxazide	Spiramycin
Paromomycin	Rifampicin
Tinidazole	Amoxicillin
Metronidazole	

Table 5. Eradication of *H. pylori*: antimicrobial monotherapy

Author	Drug	Dosage	Duration (days)	*n*	Indication	Study type	"Eradication" *n* weeks after treatment
Hirschl et al. (1987a)	Ciprofloxacin	2 × 500 mg	14	13	DU	Pilot	0: 0/13 (0%)
Stone et al. (1988)	Ciprofloxacin	2 × 500 mg	14	16	Gast	Pilot	0: 5/14 (36%)
Kalenic et al. (1987)	Ofloxacin	NS	7	6	Gast	Pilot	0: 4/6 (67%) 26: 2/6 (33%)
Kalenic et al. (1987)	Metronidazole	NS	10	6	Gast	Pilot	0: 6/6 (100%) 26: 0/2 (0%)
Patey et al. (1989)	Metronidazole	2 × 500 mg	28	9	Gast	Pilot	0: 0/9 (0%)
Marshall et al. (1988)	Tinidazole	2 × 500 mg	10	29	DU	RCT	2: 1/29 (3%) 12: 1/29 (3%)
Glupczynski et al. (1987)	Ofloxacin	2 × 200 mg	21	5	DU	DB, contr	0: 1/5 (20%) 9: 1/5 (20%)
Mertens et al. (1989)	Norfloxacin	2 × 400 mg	28	17	NUD	Pilot	0: 2/17 (12%)
Börsch et al. (1988a)	Nitrofurantoin	3 × 100 mg caps.	10	13	Gast Ulcer	Pilot	0: 0/13 (0%)
Gilman et al. (1987)	Nitrofurantoin	400 mg suspension	14	24	Gast	Contr	0: 19/24 (79%) 6: 4/18 (22%)
Gilman et al. (1987)	Furazolidone	400 mg suspension	14	14	Gast	Contr	0: 13/14 (93%) 6: 4/9 (44%)
Coelho et al. (1989a)	Furazolidone	4 × 100 mg tablets	28–56	15	DU	RCT	0: 3/15 (20%) 24: 2/15 (13%)
Glupczynski et al. (1989a)	Nifuroxazide	3 × 440 mg	21	8	Gast	Contr	0: 1/8 (13%) 4: 0/8 (0%)
Glupczynski et al. (1989a)	Paromomycin	3 × 1 g	14	10	Gast	Contr	0: 0/10 (0%)
Hirschl et al. (1987b)	Penicillin V	3 × 1 Mega	10	25	DU	Pilot	0: 0/25 (0%)

Table 5 (continued)

Author	Drug	Dosage	Duration (days)	*n*	Indication	Study type	"Eradication" *n* weeks after treatment
Hirschl et al. (1987c)	Bacampicillin	2 × 800 mg	21	15	DU	Contr	0: 3/15 (20%)
Morris and Nicholson (1987)	Doxycycline	2 × 100 mg	28	1	Gast	Pilot	0: 0/1 (0%)
Schaub et al. (1987)	Doxycycline	200 mg	10	3	Gast	Pilot	0: 0/3 (0%)
McNulty et al. (1986)	Erythromycin	4 × 500 mg suspension	14	15	Gast	Contr	0: 0/15 (0%)
Lamouliatte et al. (1987a)	Josamycin	2 g	14	9	Gast	Contr	0: 0/9 (0%)
Langenberg et al. (1985)	Spiramycin	3 × 1 g	28	6	Gast Ulcer	Pilot	0: 0/6 (0%)
Wagner et al. (1989)	Amoxicillin	3 × 750 mg	14	6	Gast Ulcer	Contr	0: 3/6 (50%) 4: 1/6 (17%)
Langenberg et al. (1987)	Amoxicillin	3 × 375 mg	28	19	Gast	Pilot	0: 12/19 (63%) 4: 5/19 (26%)
Burette et al. (1987) Glupczynski et al. (1988)	Amoxicillin	2 × 1 g suspension	7	22	Gast	Contr	0: 20/22 (91%) 3: 0/19 (0%)
Burette et al. (1987) Glupczynski et al. (1988)	Amoxicillin	2 × 1 g suspension	14	18	Gast	Pilot	0: 13/72 (18%) 4: 0/8 (0%)
Weil et al. (1988)	Amoxicillin	3 × 250 mg suspension	28	10	Gast	Contr	0: 9/10 (90%) 4: 3/10 (30%)
Unge et al. (1989)	Amoxicillin	2 × 750 mg	15	7	Gast	Contr	0: 5/7 (71%) 4: 1/7 (14%)
	Omeprazole	40 mg	15	8	Gast	Contr	0: 1/8 (13%) 4: 0/8 (0%)
	Amoxicillin + Omeprazole	2 × 750 mg 40 mg	15	8	Gast	Contr	0: 7/8 (88%) 4: 5/8 (63%)

Abbreviations: DB, double blind; NS, not stated; NUD, nonulcer dysplasia; see also Table 2.

antimicrobials are highly active in vitro against *H. pylori* (McNulty et al. 1988). All of these are highly ineffective in vivo in the natural gastric environment, and the reasons for this may reside in the very complex interrelations of topical and systemic actions of these drugs and their pharmacokinetic properties in the wide pH gradient which is so characteristic of the thin epithelial mucous layer (McNulty 1989). A list of antimicrobials, the efficacy of which as monotherapy against *H. pylori* has previously been assessed, is given in Tables 4 and 5.

Of considerable interest are, however, initial Swedish data that describe a beneficial effect of a profound pH modification on the efficacy of antimicrobial monotherapy, communicated by Unge et al. (1989). In the hands of these investigators, amoxicillin 1.5 g/day for 15 days as monotherapy led to bacterial eradication in a meager 14% of patients treated. However, in stomachs rendered anacidic by omeprazole 40 mg/day, there was a promising eradication rate of five out of eight carriers (63%) by amoxicillin alone. This initial finding urgently needs confirmation by larger trials. Omeprazole-induced hypoacidity does not influence the bioavailability of amoxicillin in such patients (Paulsen et al. 1989). Lower omeprazole doses such as 20 mg apparently will not augment the efficacy of amoxicillin therapy (Lamouliatte et al. 1989).

There has been speculation on the antibacterial action of omeprazole itself (Koop et al. 1988; Mainguet et al. 1989), i.e., on the possibility that it eradicates *H. pylori* by allowing a wide array of gut bacteria to colonize an anacidic and thus rather defenseless stomach, making the stomach a bowel-like environment from a bacteriological point of view. Gut bacteria are then said to compete with *H. pylori* for space or rather mucus, finally eradicating these spirals by depriving them of their ecological niche. However, Unge et al. (1989) clearly suggest that this is not so by describing an eradication rate for omeprazole after 2 weeks of treatment of none in eight. Nevertheless, their original observations open the path to a reinvestigation of the whole range of antimicrobials which had previously been proved to be ineffective, but which may behave differently and possibly effectively after profound pH modifications of the natural gastric environment. A direct effect of omeprazole on the bacterial metabolism is unlikely, since omeprazole per se does not influence ^{13}C urea breath tests (Graham et al. 1989b).

VI. Drug Combinations

1. Triple Drug Combinations

Antimicrobial monotherapy and the bismuth work left the *H. pylori* hypothesis with a bacterium with intelligent and elegant pathogenetic models to describe its potential role in gastroduodenal disease, but unfortunately, without any effective therapy. It was against this background of therapeutic impotence that investigators from Australia (Borody et al. 1988, 1989)

Table 6. Eradication of *H. pylori* by oral triple drug therapy

Author	Drug	Dosage (mg)	Duration (days)	*n*	Indication	Study type	Eradication 4 weeks after treatment
O'Riordan et al. (1989)	CBS	4 × 120	28	20	DU	Contr	17/20 (85%)
	Amoxicillin	3 × 500	7				
	Metronidazole	3 × 400	7				
Börsch et al. (1989a)	BSS	3 × 600	7–14	96	Ulcer and/or NUD	Contr	77/96 (80%)
	Metronidazole	3 × 500	7–14				
	Amoxicillin	3 × 500	7–14				
Borody et al. (1988)	CBS	4 × 120	28	100	DU	Pilot	94/100 (94%)
	Tetracycline	4 × 500	28		NUD		
	Metronidazole	4 × 200	14				
McNulty et al. (1989)	CBS	4 × 120[a]	28	30	NUD	Pilot	17/30 (65%)
	Achromomycin	4 × 250	28				
	Metronidazole	4 × 200	14				
McColl et al. (1989)	CBS	3 × 120	28	10	DU	Pilot	5/6 (83%)
	Amoxicillin	3 × 250	28				
	Metronidazole	3 × 400	7				
Coelho et al. (1989b)	Furazolidone	3 × 100	5	6	DU	Pilot	9/10 (90%)
	Amoxicillin	3 × 500	5		Gastr		
	Metronidazole	3 × 250	5				

Abbreviations: BSS, bismuth subsalicylate; see also previous Tables
[a] Swallow tablets.

focused their attention on what had long been standard for the treatment of tuberculosis: oral triple therapy. Amazingly, BORODYS treatment modality with bismuth and tetracycline for 4 weeks plus metronidazole for 2 weeks (Table 6) yielded an eradication rate of 94% in a large population of duodenal ulcer and nonulcer dyspepsia patients, thus giving unequivocal proof that *H. pylori* infection of the upper gastrointestinal tract is indeed a treatable condition, and that high eradication rates can be obtained with a high degree of reliability. MCNULTY et al. (1989) were unable to completely confirm BORODY's high Australian success rates, finding eradication by a British adaption of BORODY's triple therapy in 65% only (Table 6). However, as has been shown by GLUPCZYNSKI et al. (1989b), full drug compliance is exceptionally rare in such patients, especially when treatment has to be taken up to four times daily (CRAMER et al. 1989). Also, swallow tablets as used by MCNULTY et al. (1989) might yield results different from those of other colloidal bismuth subcitrate galenic preparations.

Previous work using bismuth subsalicylate 3 × 600 mg, metronidazole 3 × 500 mg, and amoxicillin 3 × 500 mg for as short as 1 week showed eradication in approximately 80% of patients finishing treatment (BÖRSCH et al. -1989a,b). This has recently been confirmed by O'RIORDAN et al. (1989) for a similar therapeutic regimen. Another investigative group achieved eradication in nine out of ten *H. pylori*-infected duodenal ulcer patients after treatment with colloidal bismuth subcitrate 3 × 120 mg, metronidazole 3 × 400 mg, and amoxicillin 3 × 250 mg, given over a 4-week period (MCCOLL et al. 1989).

Therefore, oral triple therapy in various modifications is effective against *H. pylori*, with eradication rates ranging from 80% to 94%, disregarding MCNULTY's 65% results (1989). However, the safety of oral triple therapy has not been proven in large controlled clinical trials, and at present such therapy is not recommended for routine clinical work.

2. Double Drug Combinations

a) Double Drug Combinations with Bismuth Salts

In a systematic effort to investigate whether or not oral triple therapy is really necessary to effectively eradicate *H. pylori*, O'RIORDAN et al. (1989) have added a week of treatment with amoxicillin 3 × 500 mg, metronidazole 3 × 200 or 3 × 400 mg, or metronidazole plus amoxicillin to a 4-week course of colloidal bismuth subcitrate. Bismuth plus metronidazole 3 × 400 mg gave an eradication rate of 85%, which was the same as the 85% rate observed after triple drug therapy with bismuth plus metronidazole plus amoxicillin. The latter might be superfluous in many or most patients. Prior identification of the 20% primary metronidazole resisters by an in vitro sensitivity analysis of their bacterial strain could likewise help to improve results even further (BURETTE et al. 1989; MARSHALL et al. 1989b).

Table 7. Eradication of *H. pylori*: results of double drug combinations

Author	Drug	Dosage	Duration (days)	*n*	Indication	Study type	"Eradication" *n* weeks after therapy
Rogé et al. (1986)	Tetracycline	0.5–1 g	98	7	Gast	Pilot	0: 0/6 (90%)
	Oleandomycin	0.5–1 g	98				
Oderda et al. (1989b)	Amoxicillin	50 mg/kg	42	32	Children	Pilot	0: –
	Tinidazole	20 mg/kg	42				4: 30/32 (94%)
Börsch et al. (1989a)	Metronidazole	3 × 500 mg	7	9	Ulcer	Contr	0: –
	Amoxicillin	3 × 500 mg	7		NUD		4: 7/9 (78%)
Burette et al. (1989)	Tinidazole	2 × 500 mg	8	25	Gast	Pilot	0: –
	Amoxicillin	4 × 500 mg	8		Ulcer		4: 13/25 (52%)
De Koster et al. (1989a,c)	Nitrofurantoin	4 × 100 mg	7	16	Gast	Pilot	0: –
	Amoxicillin	4 × 500 mg	7		Ulcer		4: 4/16 (25%)
De Koster et al. (1989b,c)	Tinidazole	2 × 500 mg	7	30	Gast	Pilot	0: –
	Amoxicillin	4 × 500 mg	7		Ulcer		4: 17/30 (56%)
Coelho et al. (1989b)	Metronidazole	2 × 250 mg	15	4	Gast	Pilot	0: –
	Furazolidone	4 × 100 mg	15		DU		>4: 2/4 (50%)
Börsch et al. (1988a)	Nitrofurantoin	4 × 100 mg	10	6	Gast	Pilot	0: 1/6 (17%)
	BSS	3 × 600 mg	15		Ulcer		4: 0/6 (0%)

Bayerdörffer et al. (1987b)	BSS Ofloxacin	3 × 600 mg 2 × 200 mg	? 28	14	DU	RCT	0: 11/14 (79%) 4: 3/9 (33%)
Langenberg et al. (1987)	CBS Amoxicillin	4 × 120 mg 3 × 375 mg	28 28	20	Gast	Pilot	0: 19/20 (95%) 4: 10/20 (50%)
Wagner et al. (1989)	BSS Amoxicillin	3 × 600 mg 3 × 750 mg	28 14	20	Gast Ulcer	Contr	0: 12/20 (60%) 4: 5/20 (25%)
Mannes et al. (1989)	BSS Amoxicillin	3 × 600 mg 2 × 1 g	14 14	12	DU	Contr	0: – 4: 7/12 (58%)
Weil et al. (1988, 1989)	CBS Amoxicillin	4 × 120 mg 3 × 250 mg	56 14	24	Gast	Contr	0: 24/24 (100%) 4: 10/24 (42%)
Sabbatini et al. (1989)	CBS Amoxicillin	2 × 240 mg 3 × 500 mg	28 10	80	Gast	Pilot	0: – 4: 38/80 (47%)
Marshall et al. (1988)	CBS Tinidazole	4 × 120 mg 2 × 500 mg	56 10	27	DU	RCT	2: 20/27 (74%) 12: 19/27 (70%)
O'Riordan et al. (1989)	CBS Amoxicillin	4 × 120 mg 3 × 500 mg	28 7	10	DU	Contr	0: – 4: 5/10 (50%)
O'Riordan et al. (1989)	CBS Metronidazole	4 × 120 mg 3 × 200 mg	28 7	23	DU	Contr	0: – 4: 13/23 (57%)
O'Riordan et al. (1989)	CBS Metronidazole	4 × 120 mg 3 × 400 mg	28 7	20	DU	Contr	0: – 4: 17/20 (85%)

Abbreviations: see previous Tables

Therefore, double drug therapy is currently of prime interest for the eradication of *H. pylori*, if such treatment should appear desirable from a clinical point of view in an individual patient. Bismuth plus amoxicillin (Rauws et al. 1988) and bismuth plus ofloxacin (Bayerdörffer and Ottenjann 1988; Bayerdörffer et al. 1987b) are not particularly effective combinations (Table 7). A 2-week course of colloidal bismuth subcitrate 4 × 120 mg plus erythromycin 4 × 500 eliminated *H. pylori* in 11 out of 17 duodenal ulcer patients (65%), but a follow-up of not more than 2 weeks make the data of this study not completely reliable (Goodwin et al. 1988). They are not included in Table 7.

In conclusion, the best results so far with double drug therapy have been achieved by bismuth salts plus metronidazole. A metronidazole dose of 3 × 400 mg may be superior (eradication rate 85%) to 3 × 200 mg (eradication rate 57%: O'Riordan et al. 1989). Giving the drug three times daily may also be advantageous, since Marshall et al. (1988) obtained slightly lower eradication rates of 70% by dosing tinidazole, which is comparable to metronidazole, twice daily 500 mg for 10 days in addition to colloidal bismuth subcitrate for 56 days.

b) Double Drug Combinations without Bismuth Salts

Apparently, bismuth is not an essential part of double therapeutic regimens. Initial data suggest that metronidazole plus amoxicillin for 1 week yield eradication rates of 78% (Börsch et al. 1989b), while Oderda et al. (1989b) obtained, even in children, eradication in 94%, albeit by 6 weeks' treatment with this double drug combination. Such a bismuth-free treatment modality merits attention, first, for countries where bismuth compounds are not licensed for medical usage, and second, for randomized controlled *H. pylori* ulcer trials because the "cytoprotective" effects of bismuth compounds might confound their antibacterial activity, making it difficult to interpret the effects of such therapies from a puristic point of view. Also, bismuth compounds make it more difficult to blind both patients and investigators.

VII. Toxicity of Antimicrobials and Bismuth Salts

Amoxicillin and metronidazole are antimicrobials of well-established efficacy in the treatment of *H. pylori* infection, at least when used as drug combinations. Absorption of amoxicillin from the gastrointestinal tract is superior to the absorption of ampicillin, a closely related aminopenicillin. Identical oral doses of ampicillin and amoxicillin will lead to blood levels that are twice as high for amoxicillin as for ampicillin. Diarrhea and rashes are the most frequent untoward side-effects (Wright and Wilkowske 1987). However, true hypersensitivity reactions are rare events and occur with a frequency of 0.01% in patients treated with any penicillin (Saxon et al. 1987). Pseudomembranous colitis has to be mentioned as another potentially serious complication due to amoxicillin treatment (Borody et al. 1988).

Pseudomembranous colitis is extremely rare after metronidazole, which is not surprising, since metronidazole may be used as a first-line drug to treat this condition. Eighty percent of a metronidazole dose given orally is absorbed via the gastrointestinal tract, and 60%–80% of the absorbed drug is cleared by the kidneys. Metronidazole has been said to induce cancerous lesions in animal models. However, long-term follow-up after metronidazole treatment in 771 women has failed to reveal an increased incidence of malignancies in humans (Beard et al. 1988). In the light of present data, single courses of this drug in standard doses, that is 1–1.5 g/day for 7–10 days, therefore appear to be safe (Rosenblatt and Edson 1987; Scully 1988). The safety of long-term or repeated metronidazole applications, however, remains to be established.

Frequent side-effects of metronidazole observed in 5%–10% of patients treated include nausea, a metallic taste, or a burning sensation of tongue or throat (Table 8). Such a "sore throat" phenomenon has also been observed in 11% of patients completing a course of oral triple *H. pylori* therapy (Börsch et al. 1989a). Peripheral or central neuropathies have been described after long-term usage. Structural similarities with disulfiram give metronidazole antabuse-like properties. Simultaneous consumption of alcohol must be discouraged.

Combined treatment with metronidazole and amoxicillin will lead to increased stool weights, by reducing bacterial degradation of nutritional fibers in the colon (Kurpad and Shetty 1986). In addition, ampicillin inhibits bacterial fermentation of carbohydrates in the colon (Rao et al. 1988). The same will in all likelihood also apply to amoxicillin.

Table 8. Potential side-effects of metronidazole (based on Scully 1988)

Minor
Nausea
Abdominal pain
Metallic taste
Burning sensation of tongue
Reversible neutropenia
Darkening of urine
Rash
Burning sensation of urethra or vagina
Major
Peripheral neuropathy
Seizures
Cerebellar dysfunction
Encephalopathy
Antabuse-like action
Pseudomembranous colitis (extremely rare)

Treatment with bismuth salts in standard doses (below 1.5 g of bismuth ion per day) for periods up to 4 or 8 weeks is a well-established and safe form of therapy (Bader 1987; Tytgat 1987 Menge 1988; Rösch et al. 1989). Bismuth encephalopathy will be an extremely unlikely event unless much higher doses or substantially longer treatment periods are used. This has been extensively reviewed by Bader (1987). Early absorption peaks after a new, swallowable galenic formulation of colloidal bismuth subcitrate (Hespe et al. 1988; Gavey et al. 1989 Nwokolo et al. 1989) have recently been described. The clinical significance of this finding is unclear at present.

Amoxicillin, metronidazole, and bismuth differ in their modes of antibacterial action. Penicillins interfere with the biosynthesis of bacterial cell membranes and eventually lead to lysis of *H. pylori* (Armstrong et al. 1987). Metronidazole exerts bactericidal action by damaging bacterial DNA (Scully 1988; Rosenblatt et al. 1987), leaving *H. pylori* morphologically intact (Armstrong et al. 1987). Bismuth forms metallic deposits at the bacterial membranes and devitalizes *H. pylori*, without inducing bacteriolysis in vitro (Armstrong et al. 1987). The latter apparently is an in vivo phenomenon, which may even be observed after suppression of acid secretion by famotidine 40 mg b.i.d. and 650 mg sodium bicarbonate given with each meal (Graham unpublished observation).

VIII. Experimental Therapeutic Approaches

There are not yet any convincing clinical results concerning interesting experimental approaches such as mucus modifiers or pharmaceutical urease inhibitors. Of course, active *H. pylori* vaccination, if ever possible, could very well prove to virtually eradicate chronic active gastritis and duodenal ulcer disease and, hypothetically, also to modify the prevalence of gastric cancer. However, at issue is mucosal, not systemic, immunity, the induction of which could prove to be extremely difficult.

More practically oriented experimental approaches to treat *H. pylori* presently center around the reinvestigation of antimicrobial efficacy after prior induction of profound pH changes in the gastric environment, for example via omeprazole-induced anacidity (Unge et al. 1989). A list of other substances proved ineffective by their lack of influence on ^{13}C urea breath tests is given in Table 9, based on data provided by Graham et al. (1989b). Trimipramine and other antipsychotic drugs also inhibit *H. pylori* in vitro, but the clinical relevance of this finding is presently unclear (Kristiansen et al. 1989).

The better current therapies were developed by "trial and error" using a brute force approach. There are good possibilities for optimization of these methods. One must remember that the actual protocols are arbitrary. For example, bismuth preparations will remain in the stomach for a longer period and probably be better dispersed if they are administered with or after meals

Table 9. List of substances that lack effect on *H. pylori*, according to results of ^{13}C urea breath tests (based on GRAHAM et al. 1989b)

Ulcer drugs
Cimetidine
Ranitidine
Famotidine
Omeprazole
Misoprostol
Sucralfate
Liquid antacids
Nonsteroidal antirheumatic drugs
Aspirin
Indomethacin
Ibuprofen
Naproxen
Tolmetin
Selected oral antimicrobials
Oral penicillins
Trimethoprim – sulfamethoxazole
Dicloxacillin
Various salts
Lithium
Ferrous sulfate
Gold
Zinc
Various other drugs
Acetaminophen
Phenytoin
Hydrochlorothiazide
Propranolol
Metoprolol
Metoclopramide
Ursodesoxycholic acid

instead of before meals. The antimicrobial will also have longer dwell times in the stomach if given to the fed patient, but one must consider whether there are important food–antimicrobial or bismuth–antimicrobial interactions (e.g., bismuth and tetracycline) that might reduce effectiveness. One would predict that the formulation (tablet, capsule, liquid, powder, enteric coated, etc.) may also have a profound influence on agents that are expected to act topically. Systematic investigations of a variety of possibly important parameters are needed to refine and optimize therapy and to avoid declaring a therapeutic strategy useless because the drug was given at the wrong time or in the wrong formulation.

D. Eradication of *Helicobacter pylori* and Peptic Ulcer Disease

I. Effect on Gastritis

Eradication of *H. pylori* leads to rapid amelioration and in time to resolution of chronic active and chronic type B gastritis (Alpert et al. 1989; Rauws et al. 1988; Dooley et al. 1988; Marshall et al. 1987). The active component of type B gastritis resolves rapidly, while it may take up to 1 or 2 years for the chronic inflammatory changes of the gastric mucosa to regress (Rauws et al. 1988; Rauws 1989; Rauws and Tytgat 1989). This response is a lasting effect, while mere reduction of the bacterial density only leads to a transient amelioration of gastric changes (Glupczynski et al. 1988). Chronic type B gastritis apparently respresents a reversible immune response of the gut-associated mucosal immune system to *H. pylori* antigen(s). Therefore, and contrary to previous concepts, chronic type B gastritis is not an expression of either mucosal aging or wear and tear.

II. Effect on Healing of Duodenal Ulcers

Ulcer treatment has previously, and successfuly, focused on manipulating physiological events such as secretion of acid or pepsin. *H. pylori* has now opened the fundamentally new approach of putting antimicrobials to work in ulcer therapy. In this section, studies on duodenal and gastric ulcer disease that allow correlations of healing and relapse with treatment effects on *H. pylori* will be reviewed. We will consider trials using bismuth salts and/or antimicrobial drug modalities, since conventional ulcer therapy based on H_2 receptor antagonists, antacids, sucralfate, or pirenzepine will in all likelihood not influence a patient's *H. pylori* state. A small number of prior studies have investigated the healing properties of various antimicrobials in peptic ulcers, without addressing the role of *H. pylori*. These studies and also their shortcomings have been analyzed elsewhere (Bianchi Porro and Lazzaroni 1989; Bayerdörffer and Ottenjann 1988; Coghlan et al. 1989) and will also be exempt from this review.

There is at present, however, a dearth of well-conducted, sufficiently large, and adequately published *H. pylori* ulcer trials. The pertinent studies and their location in the literature, as identified by their principal author and the journal of publication of full reports or abstracts, are given in Table 10. Detailed publications are still the exception rather than the rule and are therefore marked by an asterisk.

It is, however, appropriate to point out that acceleration of ulcer healing is not a crucial test for the role of *H. pylori* in ulcer disease, either in theory or in practice. Potential analogies to the inefficiency of cytoprotective prostaglandins, e.g., low dose misoprostol, in promoting ulcer healing (Börsch

Table 10. Studies addressing the effect of the *H. pylori* state on healing and relapse of peptic ulcer disease: principal author and journal of publication

Coghlan et al. (1987)[a]:	Lancet 2:1109
Marshall et al. (1988)[a]:	Lancet 2:1437
Bayerdörffer et al. (1987a)[a]:	Dtsch Med Wochenschr 112:1407
Lambert et al. (1987):	Gastroenterology 92:1489
Borody et al. (1988):	Gastroenterology 94:A43
Smith et al. (1988):	Gastroenterology 94:A431
Graham et al. (1989c):	Gastroenterology 96:A181

[a] Published as formal paper.

1987) have to be pointed out. Factors leading to ulcer formation (e.g., local epithelial breakdown, as it could be envisioned in *H. pylori*-induced gastroduodenitis) might be quite distinct from those that eventually govern ulcer healing e.g., speed and capacity of local epithelial repair).

Therefore, any lack of influence of *H. pylori*-oriented therapeutic regimens on ulcer healing kinetics would certainly not disprove an important pathogenetic role of *H. pylori* in peptic ulcer disease. The influence of treatment on relapse would be much more decisive in this regard. On the other hand, acceleration of ulcer healing by antibacterial therapy would provide further minor support for a causal effect of gastroduodenal *H. pylori* infection on peptic ulcers, even though it will probably be of little or no clinical importance, since existing therapeutic modalities effectively and safely accomplish the goal of rapid ulcer healing.

Studies published by Graham et al. (1989c), Bayerdörffer et al. (1987a), Marshall et al. (1988), and Lambert et al. (1987) have investigated the influence of *H. pylori* on duodenal, ulcer healing. Adding 2 weeks of oral triple therapy, i.e., bismuth subsalicylate, tetracycline 2 g, and metronidazole 750 mg per day, to ranitidine 300 mg alone significantly accelerated healing in the first 39 duodenal ulcer patients of a randomized controlled *H. pylori*-oriented duodenal ulcer trial (Graham et al. 1989c). The 4-week healing rates were 81% after additional triple therapy versus a low 44% after ranitidine alone (Table 11).

Likewise, Bayerdörffer et al. (1987b) have described significantly faster duodenal ulcer healing after adding ofloxacin 2 × 200 mg to ranitidine 300 mg nocte (Table 11). The latter data are somewhat difficult to explain, since ofloxacin rarely eradicates *H. pylori* (Table 5). It may, however, reduce the bacterial density and thus exert some influence on ulcer healing. Since quinolones have the propensity to induce resistant *H. pylori* strains in a high proportion of patients treated, these drugs are presently not considered to be useful agents in the therapy of *H. pylori* infection.

The data of the largest randomized controlled *H. pylori*-oriented trial in duodenal ulcer disease by Marshall et al. (1988) show a tendency for tinidazole to improve 10-week ulcer healing rates above those observed for

Table 11. Effect of adding antimicrobial drugs to standard therapy on the healing kinetics of duodenal ulcers

	Cumulated percent healed					
	2 wk	4 wk	6 wk	8 wk	10 wk	12 wk
[a] Ranitidine	10	44	ND	60	ND	83
R + triple	37	81*	ND	87	ND	100
[b] Ranitidine	44	68	88	96	96	100
R + ofloxacin	80	92	100	ND	ND	ND
[c] Bismuth	ND	ND	ND	ND	68	ND
B + tinidazole	ND	ND	ND	ND	74	ND
[c] Cimetidine	ND	ND	ND	ND	59	ND
C + tinidazole	ND	ND	ND	ND	76	ND

*$P < 0.05$; ND, not done.
[a] Graham et al. (1989c): initial 39 DU patients.
[b] Bayerdörffer et al. (1987a): 50 DU patients.
[c] Marshall et al. (1988): 100 DU patients.

either cimetidine (76% vs 59% healing) or colloidal bismuth subcitrate alone (74% vs 68% healing: Table 11). A further look at the figures also reveals that after bismuth therapy with or without concomitant tinidazole administration, ulcers healed in 10 out of 22 patients (45%) having remained *H. pylori* infected posttherapeutically, but much more frequently in 25 out of those 27 who had turned *H. pylori* negative (93%).

The sole evidence against an influence of the *H. pylori* state on ulcer healing is a brief remark by Lambert et al. (1987), that the *H. pylori* state after 8 weeks of colloidal bismuth subcitrate therapy was unrelated to healing in their uncontrolled ulcer trial. Numbers to allow any scrutiny of this statement are not given in the abstract. All further papers forming the data base of this review (Table 10) fail to address ulcer healing.

Therefore, the amalgamated data on the effect of *H. pylori*-oriented therapy on ulcer healing kinetics suggest that suitable antimicrobial therapy may accelerate healing of duodenal ulcers (Graham et al. 1989c; Bayerdörffer et al. 1987a). This effect may be more pronounced in populations with or after therapeutic regimens leading to low ulcer healing rates. After therapy with bismuth salts, clearance of *H. pylori* is probably associated with faster ulcer healing (Marshall et al. 1988). Due to a current lack of published data, the effect of antimicrobials on healing kinetics of gastric ulcers is presently unknown.

III. Effect on Relapse Rates of Duodenal Ulcers

The posttherapeutic *H. pylori* state has a most profound, almost dramatic, impact on duodenal ulcer relapse rates. Nevertheless, a reservation has to be made insofar as published observations presently cover periods of only up to 12 or 18 months. Also, the studies shaping our knowledge in this field (Table

Table 12. Duodenal ulcer relapses and *H. pylori* state

Author	*n*	Therapy	HP-negative after therapy	Follow-up (months)	Ulcer relapses and posttherapeutic *H. pylori* state	Ulcer relapse rate after 12–18 months	
						HP + patients	HP − patients
Lambert et al. (1987)	45	CBS[a]	12/45 = 27%	12	All relapses HP +	NS	0%
Borody et al. (1988)	21	Triple[a]	94%	18	3/21 (14%), all relapses HP+	NS	0%
Coghlan et al. (1987)	66	CIM vs CBS	4/23 = 17% 12/23 = 52%	12	HP + : 19/24 = 79% HP − : 1/10 = 10%	79%	27% (10%)[b]
Marshall et al. (1988)	100	CIM/TIN CBS CBS/TIN	1/51 = 2% 7/22 = 32% 20/27 = 74%	12	HP + : 37/44 = 84% HP − : 5/24 = 21%	84%	21% (8%)[c]
Smith et al. (1988)	44	RAN vs CBS	0/23 = 0% 16/21 = 76%	18	HP + : 14/18 = 78% HP − : 4/16 = 25% All relapses HP+	78%	25%: all relapses CP +

Abbreviations: CBS, colloidal bismuth subcitrate; CIM, cimetidine; TIN, tinidazole; RAN, ranitidine; HP+, *H. pylori* infected; HP −, *H. pylori* negative; NS, not stated.

[a] uncontrolled study.

[b] 10% refers to the 1-year duodenal ulcer relapse rate of patients with persistent eradication of *H. pylori*, while the 27% figure also includes patients with reinfections.

[c] 8% relates to patients with anatomically proven ulcer craters (Marshall 1989), while the 21% rate includes additional patients with symptomatic but not necessarily anatomical recurrences.

10) remain far from flawless in design, are small in number, and with only three exceptions remain to be published in full detail.

The experimental findings are summarized in Table 12. The data clearly suggest that *H. pylori*-infected patients having their ulcers healed by conventional therapeutic strategies have high 12- to 18-month duodenal ulcer relapse rates approximating 80%, while ulcer relapses in patients maintaining a state of *H. pylori* eradication are extremely rare, probably between 0% and 8%–10%. This certainly comes close to a "no *H. pylori* – no duodenal ulcer" relationship (Graham 1989b). The lower relapse rate of 10% in the study of Coghlan et al. (1987 Table 12) applies to patients remaining persistently *H. pylori* negative, while the relapse rate of 27% involves all patients who were *H. pylori* negative after an index therapy of cimetidine or colloidal bismuth subcitrate and thus includes patients with bacterial reinfections. Likewise, the lower relapse rate of 8% in the Marshall et al. (1988) study applies to *H. pylori* negative patients with anatomically proven duodenal ulcer relapse (Marshall 1989), while the higher rate of 21% relapses includes recurrence of any ulcer-like symptoms, not necessarily being associated with true anatomical ulcer relapses. The ulcer recurrence rates of patients with bacterial suppression after anti-*H. pylori* treatment, but recrudescence of infection within 4 weeks after cessation of the index therapy, merit further study.

Four other trials in this field deserve further comment. A small German study by Eberhardt et al. (1988) in 39 duodenal and three gastric ulcer patients showed higher healing and lower relapse rates for bismuth subsalicylate 3 × 600 mg versus cimetidine 800 mg nocte, but this work is seriously flawed by technical difficulties leading to an *H. pylori* detection rate of only 61% in this small group of ulcer patients. This precludes a meaningful analysis of the influence of *H. pylori* on healing and relapse.

A study by Bianchi Porro and Lazzaroni (1988) comparing ulcer recurrences after healing induced by H_2 receptor antagonists or by colloidal bismuth subcitrate was published as a letter to the editor and reports the posttherapeutic, but not the initial *H. pylori* state. There was a high bacterial clearance, but a low genuine eradication rate after colloidal bismuth subcitrate. Therefore, *H. pylori* was eradicated in too few patients to form a sufficiently large, genuinely *H. pylori*-negative group for follow-up. In this study, 94% of patients were *H. pylori*-infected on ulcer relapse, which clearly supports rather than denies a causal role of *H. pylori* in recurrent duodenal ulcers.

A study by Humphreys et al. (1988) includes cases with duodenal and gastric ulcers in addition to erosions or esophageal lesions, which also precludes a precise analysis. The data are nevertheless interesting insofar as they support a role of *H. pylori* in determining healing rate after therapy with liquid colloidal bismuth subcitrate 4 × 5 ml. Six weeks of this drug induced healing in 82% of *H. pylori*-infected but only 42% of *H. pylori*-negative lesions, while the results of cimetidine treatment were similar in both groups: 70% versus 67%.

Another study by BAYERDÖRFFER et al. (1988) found the addition of ofloxacin 2 × 200 mg to standard H_2 receptor antagonist therapy useful in the management of 12 patients with previously refractory duodenal ulcers that had stayed unhealed despite 3 months of H_2 receptor antagonist treatment. All lesions healed within 6 weeks of adding ofloxacin 2 × 200 mg to the previous therapy. However, these findings were uncontrolled and thus difficult to interpret (BAYERDÖRFFER et al. 1988).

IV. Effect on Relapse Rates of Gastric Ulcers

Concerning relapses in gastric ulcer disease, the assumption has been advanced that many or maybe even most gastric ulcers will behave exactly like duodenal ulcers (BÖRSCH 1989a). This was based on observations of 30 patients with *H. pylori*-associated gastric ulcers treated by oral triple therapy (BÖRSCH et al. 1989b). However, any formal or controlled data on gastric ulcers to prove or disprove this assumption are currently unavailable in the literature. It has already been discussed in Sect. B that the relation between gastric ulcers and *H. pylori* will by necessity be less clear-cut than the relation between duodenal ulcers and *H. pylori*. A number of gastric ulcer will be *H. pylori* associated, but not *H. pylori* induced. Therefore, recurrence of gastric ulcers despite eradication of *H. pylori* may be expected in a considerable proportion of gastric ulcer patients and would not disprove a causal role of *H. pylori* at least for a subgroup of gastric ulcer disease.

E. Whom to Treat and What to Expect?

The decision to initiate anti-*H. pylori* treatment should not be taken lightly. AXON (1990) defined three responsibilities of the physician in relation to treatment of an *H. pylori* infection. These responsibilities are to the patient, to society, and to our medical colleagues. One starts with the knowledge that we currently have a variety of safe and effective medical therapies that both hasten the healing of peptic ulcer and reduce the rate of ulcer relapse. In addition, we have effective surgical therapies; highly selective vagotomy is a very safe operation with minimal morbidity. Current therapies are not without risk. These risks range from side-effects of the antimicrobial therapy such as allergic reactions and pseudomembranous colitis to development of antimicrobial-resistent strains of *H. pylori* such that when a safe and effective therapy is identified, the patient will not be able to be cured. For society, we must not further enhance the spread of the antimicrobial-resistant microorganisms. In this context we are more concerned with the development of antimicrobial-resistant organisms other than *H. pylori*. This could be a particularly significant problem when one considers that there are millions of patients who would qualify for therapy for *H. pylori* infection. The last responsibility, to our colleagues, means that we should not promote therapy of *H. pylori* beyond the current realities, i.e., high dosage of relatively toxic drugs seems to yield modestly good eradication rates but the experience and follow-up are both limited.

The decision to treat carries with it the responsibility to follow up the patient to confirm that eradication of the *H. pylori* infection has occurred. The available data suggest that a course of triple therapy is associated with an alteration in the rate of ulcer relapse, maybe even in those patients in whom the infection recurs. Thus, the fact that a symptomatic ulcer relapse does not occur for 3, 6, or 9 months after therapy does not, by itself, signify that the therapy eradicated the infection. We have little, or no, information about what to do for the previous ulcer patient who has undergone reinfection (or relapse) and remains asymptomatic, or for that matter what to do for those who experience a symptomatic relapse. Does reinfection several years after initial eradication carry with it the same risk of development of recurrent ulcer disease? What is the time interval between infection and ulcer disease? Answers to these questions are required before we can formulate a rational plan to add anti-*H. pylori* therapy to our armamentarium to treat ulcer disease.

F. Summary and Conclusions

Helicobacter pylori is accepted as a direct cause of chronic active type B gastritis. It is without doubt a powerful risk indicator for peptic ulcer disease in general. For a substantial subgroup of ulcer patients with the (previously) idiopathic, gastritis- and thus *H. pylori*-associated disease variant, the more essential role of these bacteria might be described as that of a necessary, albeit by itself not sufficient condition. This assigns *H. pylori* a rank equivalent to that of acid and pepsin in the pathogenesis of such ulcers. Modification of either factor, *H. pylori* or acid/pepsin, would then (and apparently does) suffice to exert a beneficial effect on ulcer disease.

To achieve true eradication of *H. pylori*, however, antimicrobial monotherapy is ineffective (<30%). Bismuth monotherapy is not superior (<30%). Oral triple therapy may be 80%–94% effective, but since it is of yet unproven safety, it should presently not be recommended for routine clinical application. Double therapy with bismuth/metronidazole or amoxicillin/metronidazole as the most suitable candidates presently appears more appealing, especially in the light of initial evidence from Ireland (O'Riordan et al. 1989) and Australia (Marshall et al. 1988) that it may yield results similar to those after oral triple therapy, with eradication rates of 85% or higher. One can also infer from what is known about the safety of metronidazole therapy from its extremely broad application for female genital tract colonizations by *Trichomonas vaginalis* or gram-negative bacteria, that single short-term therapeutic courses of this nitroimidazole will not be hampered by safety considerations (BEARD et al. 1988; ROSENBLATT and EDSON 1989; SCULLY 1988).

A new and highly interesting experimental therapeutic approach presently makes use of profound alterations of gastric pH to improve the in vivo efficacy of antimicrobial monotherapy, but only very limited data are available in this important research field so far.

In summary, effective and reasonably safe regimens to eradicate *H. pylori* now exist. They should suffice to give further clear experimental proof of the *H. pylori* hypothesis by eradicating these organisms safely and predictably in a substantial number of ulcer (and dyspepsia) patients, preferentially entered into large and well-conducted randomized controlled therapeutic trials.

The presently still rather small data base on *H. pylori*-oriented ulcer treatment suggests that suitable antimicrobial therapy may accelerate healing of duodenal ulcers and that clearance of *H. pylori* is associated with faster duodenal ulcer healing after bismuth therapy. Above all, eradication of *H. pylori* will virtually eliminate duodenal ulcer relapses, at least for the 12- to 18-month periods that have so far been prospectively investigated, unless there is bacterial reinfection from outside sources. Somewhere between 1% and 2% of adults in developed countries contract *H. pylori* each year. It is not yet known whether patients with peptic ulcer have increased susceptibility to *H. pylori* infections. If they do not, one would expect a low but relatively constant rate of reinfection. The level of susceptibility, higher, lower, or the same, will eventually dictate the follow-up intervals.

Many or even most gastritis-associated gastric ulcers will probably respond in a similar manner as duodenal ulcers, but controlled data to lend formal proof to this assumption are currently unavailable.

The knowledge of their patients' *H. pylori* state might be of clinical relevance even for clinicians, who refrain from treating ulcer patients with suitable antimicrobial drug combinations for the time being, using bismuth compounds instead. Bismuth-induced healing rates have been reported to be significantly higher in *H. pylori*-associated lesions than in lesions that occur in the absence of *H. pylori* infection (HUMPHREYS et al. 1988), which might influence individual treatment decisions.

It may be concluded, then, that present-day data clearly support a key role for *H. pylori* eradication in attempting cure, and not merely exerting control of the most common, gastritis-associated variant of ulcer disease. The available scientific information is now sufficient for *H. pylori* "believers" to accept the proposition of a potentially lasting termination of previously idiopathic, gastritis-associated ulcer disease as valid. Current *H. pylori* "non-believers" are still entitled to ask for larger patient numbers and better study designs, before finally giving in to the *H. pylori* amendment of the ulcer equation. However, still being "in search of the flawless trial" should not become a permanent excuse for evading a timely personal decision on possibly flawed and imperfect, but nevertheless persuasive experimental *H. pylori* findings.

However, before *H. pylori* eradication will become a standard procedure in ulcer therapy, better treatment regimens, in terms of simplicity, safety, and effectiveness, are urgently needed. Also, many unsettled questions have to be addressed and answered before a rational plan to add anti-*H. pylori* therapy to the present armamentarium for treating ulcer disease can be formulated.

References

Al-Moagel MA, Evans DG, Abdulghani ME, Adam E, Evans DJ Jr, Malaty HM, Klein PD, Graham DY (1989) Comparison of the prevalence of *C. pylori* infection in individuals with and without upper gastrointestinal symptoms. Gastroenterology 96:A10

Alpert LC, Lew GM, Michaletz PA, Graham DY (1989) Effect of eradication of *C. pylori* on gastric function and structure. Gastroenterology 96:A10

Armstrong JA, Wee SH, Goodwin CS, Wilson DH (1987) Response of *Campylobacter pyloridis* to antibiotics, bismuth and an acid-reducing agent in vitro – an ultrastructural study. J Med Microbiol 24:343–350

Axon ATR (1990) Is nonulcer dyspepsia improved by treating Helicobacter pylori infection? In: Ditschuneit H, Malfertheiner P (eds) Helicobacter pylori, gastritis, and peptic ulcer. Springer, Berlin Heidelberg New York Tokyo, pp. 434–437

Bader JP (1987) The safety profile of De-Nol[R]. Digestion [Suppl 2] 37:53–59

Bartlett JG (1988) *Campylobacter pylori*: fact or fancy? Gastroenterology 94:229–238

Bayerdörffer E, Ottenjann R (1988) The role of antibiotics in *Campylobacter pylori* associated peptic ulcer disease. Scand J Gastroenterol [Suppl 142] 23:93–100

Bayerdörffer E, Kasper G, Pirlet T, Sommer A, Ottenjann R (1987a) Ofloxacin in der Therapie *Campylobacter-pylori*-positiver Ulcera duodeni. Dtsch Med Wochenschr 112:1407–1411

Bayerdörffer E, Simon T, Bästlein C, Ottenjann R (1987b) Bismuth/ofloxacin combination for duodenal ulcer. Lancet 2:1467–1468

Bayerdörffer E, Pirlet T, Sommer A, Kasper G, Ottenjann R (1988) Ofloxacin in der Therapie "resistenter" Ulcera duodeni. Eine Pilotstudie. Z Gastroenterol 26:155–159

Beard CM, Noller KL, O'Fallon WMO, Kurland LT, Dahlin DC (1988) Cancer after exposure to metronidazole. Mayo Clin Proc 63:147–153

Bianchi Porro G, Lazzaroni M (1988) *Campylobacter pylori* and ulcer recurrence. Lancet 1:593

Bianchi Porro G, Lazzaroni M (1989) *Campylobacter pylori* and peptic ulcer therapy. Gastroenterol Clin Biol 13:107B-111B

Blaser MJ (1987) Gastric *Campylobacter*-like organisms, gastritis, and peptic ulcer disease. Gastroenterology 93:371–383

Bohnen JMA, Krajden S, Anderson JGD, Kempston JD, Fuksa M, Karmall MA, Osborne A, Babida C (1986) *Campylobacter pyloridis* is associated with acid-peptic disease in Toronto. Can J Surg 29:442–444

Borody T, Cole P, Noonan S, Morgan A, Ossip G, Maysey J, Brandl S (1988) Long-term *Campylobacter pylori* recurrence post-eradication. Gastroenterology 94:A43

Borody T, Noonan S, Cole P, Hyland L, Morgan A, Lenne J, Moore-Jones D, Brandl S (1989) Duodenal ulcer recurrence in patients remaining *C. pylori* (CP) negative long term post-eradication. Gastroenterology 96:A52

Börsch G (1987) *Campylobacter pylori*: new and renewed insights into gastritis-associated ulcer disease (GAUD). Hepato gastroenterology 34:191–193
Börsch G (1988a) Therapie der *Campylobacter pylori*-Infektion. Leber Magen Darm 18:40–45
Börsch G (1988b) Ulcera peptica: Assoziation mit der *Campylobacter pylori*-Besiedlung der Antrum- und Bulbusmukosa. In: Ottenjann R, Schmitt W (eds) Aktuelle Gastroenterologie – *Campylobacter pylori*. Springer, Berlin Heidelberg New York, pp 101–115
Börsch G (1988c) *Campylobacter pylori*, Ulcus und Dyspepsie. Dtsch Med Wochenschr 113:1781–1782
Börsch G (1989a) Ist *Campylobacter pylori* der Erreger der Ulkuskrankheit? Z Gastroenterol 27:121–126
Börsch G (1989b) Clinical significance of *Campylobacter pylori*. Eur J Gastroenterol Hepatol 1:27–33
Börsch G, Mai U, Müller KM (1988a) Monotherapy or polychemotherapy in the treatment of *Campylobacter pylori*-related gastroduodenal disease. Scand J Gastroenterol [Suppl 142] 23:101–106
Börsch G, Schmidt G, Wegener M, Sandmann M, Adamek R, Leverkus F, Reitemeyer E (1988b) *Campylobacter pylori*: prospective analysis of clinical and histological factors associated with colonization of the upper gastrointestinal tract. Eur J Clin Invest 18:133–138
Börsch G, Wegener M, Mai U, Opferkuch W (1989a) Efficiency of oral triple therapy to eradicate *Campylobacter pylori*. In: Mégraud F, Lamouliatte H (eds) Gastroduodenal pathology and *Campylobacter pylori*. Elsevier, Amsterdam, pp 595–598
Börsch G, Wegener M, Reitemeyer E, Mai U, Opferkuch W (1989b) Clinical results and medium term follow-up studies after eradication of *Campylobacter pylori*. In: Mégraud F, Lamouliatte H (eds) Gastroduodenal pathology and *Campylobacter pylori*. Elsevier, Amsterdam, pp 599–603
Buck GE, Gourley WK, Lee WK, Subramanyam K, Latimer JM, DiNuzzo AR (1986) Relation of *Campylobacter pyloridis* to gastritis and peptic ulcer. J Infect Dis 153:664–669
Burette A, Glupczynski Y, Jonas C, de Reuck M, van Gossum M, Deprez C, Tielemans C, Deltenre M (1986) Significance de la présence du *Campylobacter pyloridis* dans l'antre gastrique. Acta Gastroenterol Belg 49:70–83
Burette A, Glupczynski Y, Dereuck M, Labbe M, Deltenre M (1987) *Campylobacter pyloridis* and associated gastritis: investigator blind, placebo controlled trial with amoxicillin (Abstr 28). 4th International Workshop on *Campylobacter* infections, Göteborg
Burette A, Glupczynski Y, Thibaumont F, Deprez C (1989) Evaluation of short-term amoxicillin/tinidazole combination in the treatment of *Campylobacter pylori* infection. Klin Wochenschr [Suppl 18] 67:7–8
Cadranel S, Glupczinsky Y, Labbe M, de Prez C (1988) *Campylobacter pylori* in children. In: Menge H, Gregor M, Tytgat GNJ, Marshall BJ (eds) *Campylobacter pylori*. Springer, Berlin Heidelberg New York, pp 110–115
Coelho LGV, Queiroz DMM, Barbosa AJA, Mendes EN, Rocha GA, Oliveira CA, Lima GF Jr, Passos MCF, Castro LP (1989a) *Campylobacter pylori*, duodenal ulcer and furazolidone treatment. In: Mégraud F, Lamouliatte H (eds) Gastroduodenal pathology and *Campylobacter pylori*. Elsevier, Amsterdam, pp 611–614
Coelho LGV, Passos MCF, Queiroz DMM, Barbosa AJA, Mendes EN, Rocha GA, Oliveira CA, Lima GF Jr, Chausson Y, Castro LP (1989b) Five days triple therapy and 15 days double therapy on *C. pylori* eradication. Klin Wochenschr [Suppl 18] 67:11
Coghlan JG, Gilligan D, Humphreys H, McKenna D, Dooley C, Sweeney E, Keane C, O'Morain C (1987) *Campylobacter pylori* and recurrence of duodenal ulcers – a 12-month follow-up study. Lancet 2:1109–1111

Coghlan JG, Tobin A, O'Morain C (1989) *Campylobacter pylori* and ulcer treatment. In: Rathbone BJ, Heatley RV (eds) *Campylobacter pylori* and gastroduodenal disease. Blackwell, Oxford, pp 232–245

Cramer JA, Mattson RH, Prevey ML, Scheyer RD, Ouellette VL (1989) How often is medication taken as prescribed? A novel assessment technique. JAMA 261: 3272–3277

Czinn SJ, Dahms BB, Jacobs GH, Kaplan B, Rothstein FC (1986) *Campylobacter*-like organisms in association with symptomatic gastritis in children. J Pediatr 109: 80–83

Czinn S, Carr H, Sheffler L, Aronoff S (1989) Serum IgG antibody to the outer membrane proteins of *Campylobacter pylori* in children with gastroduodenal disease. J Infect Dis 159:586–589

De Koster E, Nyst J, Glupczynski Y, Burette A, Deprez C, van Gossum M, Deltenre M (1989a) *Campylobacter pylori*: results of one-week amoxicillin sachets + nitrofurantoin therapy. Klin Wochenschr [Suppl 18] 67:15–16

De Koster E, Nyst J, Glupczynski Y, Deprez C, de Reuck M, Deltenre M (1989b) Treatment of *Campylobacter pylori*: results of one-week amoxicillin sachets + tinidazole therapy. Klin Wochenschr [Suppl 18] 67:16

De Koster E, Nyst J, Glupczynski Y, Deprez C, Jonas C, Deltenre M (1989c) Amoxicillin + tinidazole vs amoxicillin + nitrofurantoin: tinidazole is a key drug in *Campylobacter pylori* treatment. Klin Wochenschr [Suppl 18] 67:16–17

Dickgießer N, Kasper GF, Manegold BC, Jung M, Raute-Kreinsen U (1987) *Campylobacter*ähnliche Bakterien in der Magenschleimhaut. MMW. 129: 420–423

Dobrilla G, Vallerta P, Amplatz S (1988) Influence of ulcer healing agents on ulcer relapse after discontinuation of acute treatment: a pooled estimate of controlled clinical trials. Gut 29:181–187

Dooley CP, Cohen H (1988) The clinical significance of *Campylobacter pylori*. Ann Intern Med 108:70–79

Dooley CP, McKenna D, Humphreys H, Bourke S, Keane CT, Sweeney E, O'Morain C (1988) Histologic gastritis in duodenal ulcer: relationship to *Campylobacter pylori* and effect of ulcer therapy. Am J Gastroenterol 83:278–282

Drumm B, Sherman P, Cutz E, Karmali M (1987) Association of *Campylobacter pylori* on the gastric mucosa with antral gastritis in children. N Engl J Med 316:1557–1561

Dwyer B, Kaldor J, Tee W, Marakowski E, Raios K (1988a) Antibody response to *Campylobacter pylori* in diverse ethnic groups. Scand J Infect Dis 20:349–350

Dwyer B, Nanxiong S, Kaldor J, Tee W, Lambert J, Luppino M, Flannery G (1988b) Antibody response to *Campylobacter pylori* in an ethnic group lacking peptic ulceration. Scand J Gastroenterol 20:63–68

Eastham EJ, Elliott TSJ, Berkeley D, Jones DM (1988) *Campylobacter pylori* infection in children. J Infect 16:77–79

Eberhardt R, Kasper G, Dettmer A, Höchter W, Hagena D (1988) Wirkung von Wismutsubsalicylat versus Cimetidin auf *Campylobacter pylori*, Ulkusheilung und -rezidivrate. Med Klin 83:402–405

Fauchère JL, Rosenau A, Bonneville F (1989) Virulence factors of *Campylobacter pylori*. Gastroenterol Clin Biol 13:59B–64B

Figura N, Guglielmetti P, Rossolini A, Barberi A, Cusi G, Musmanno RA, Russi M, Quaranta S (1989) Cytotoxin production by *Campylobacter pylori* strains isolated from patients with peptic ulcers and from patients with chronic gastritis only. J Clin Immunol 27:225–226

Gavey CJ, Szeto M-L, Nwokolo CU, Sercombe J, Pounder RE (1989) Bismuth accumulates in the body during treatment with tripotassium dicitrato bismuthate. Aliment Pharmacol Ther 3:21–28

Gilman R, Leon-Barua R, Ramirez-Ramos A, Morgan D, Recavarron S, Spira W, Watanabe P, Kraft W, Pearson A (1987) Efficacy of nitrofurans in the treatment of antral gastritis with *Campylobacter pyloridis*. Gastroenterology 92:1405

Glupczynski Y, Labbe M, Burette A, Delmee M, Avesani V, Bruck C (1987) Treatment failure of ofloxacin in *Campylobacter pylori* infection. Lancet 1:1096
Glupczynski Y, Burette A, Labbe M, Deprez C, de Reuck M, Deltenre M (1988) *Campylobacter pylori*-associated gastritis: a double-blind placebo-controlled trial with amoxicillin. Am J Gastroenterol 83:365–372
Glupczynski Y, Burette A, Deprez C, Labbe M (1989a) Evaluation of non-absorbable antibiotics in *Campylobacter pylori* (CP)-associated gastritis. 5th International Workshop on *Campylobacter* Infections, Puerto Vallarta
Glupczynski Y, Nyst JF, Burette A, Vanderlinden MP, Deltenre M (1989b) Lack of antibiotic compliance in patients treated for *Campylobacter pylori*-associated gastritis. 5th International Workshop on *Campylobacter* Infections Puerto Vallarta
Goodwin CS (1988) Duodenal ulcer, *Campylobacter pylori*, and the "leaking roof" concept. Lancet 2:1467–1469
Goodwin CS, Armstrong JA, Marshall BJ (1986) *Campylobacter pyloridis*, gastritis, and peptic ulceration. J Clin Pathol 39:353–365
Goodwin CS, Marshall BJ, Blincow ED, Wilson DH, Blackbourn S, Phillips M (1988) Prevention of nitroimidazole resistance in *Campylobacter pylori* by coadministration of colloidal bismuth subcitrate: clinical and in vitro studies. J Clin Pathol 41:207–210
Goodwin CS, Armstrong JA, Chilvers T, Peters M, Collins MD, Sly L, McConnell W, Harper WE (1989a) Transfer of *Campylobacter pylori* and *Campylobacter mustelae* to *Helicobacter* gen nov as *Helicobacter pylori* comb nov and *Helicobacter mustelae* comb nov, respectively. Int J Syst Bacteriol 39:397–405
Goodwin CS, Bell B, McCullough C, Turner M (1989b) Sensitivity of *Campylobacter pylori* to colloidal bismuth subcitrate. J Clin Pathol 42:216–219
Graham DY (1989a) *Campylobacter pylori* as a pathogenic factor in duodenal ulcer: the case for. Scand J Gastroenterol [Suppl 160] 24:46–52
Graham DY (1989b) *Campylobacter pylori* and peptic ulcer disease. Gastroenterology 96:615–625
Graham DY (1990) *Campylobacter pylori* in human populations: the present and predictions of the future based on the epidemiology of polio. In: Menge H, Gregor M, McNulty CAM, Marshall BJ, Tytgat G (eds) 2nd International Symposium on *Campylobacter pylori*. Springer, Berlin Heidelberg New York (in press)
Graham DY, Klein PD (1987) *Campylobacter pyloridis* gastritis: the past, the present, and speculations about the future. Am J Gastroenterol 82:283–286
Graham DY, Alpert LC, Lacey Smith J, Yoshimura HH (1988a) Iatrogenic *Campylobacter pylori* infection is a cause of epidemic hypochlorhydria. Am J Gastroenterol 83:974–980
Graham DY, Klein DP, Opekun AR, Boutton TW (1988b) Effect of age on the frequency of active *Campylobacter pylori* infection diagnosed by the (13C)urea breath test in normal subjects and patients with peptic ulcer disease. J Infect Dis 157:777–780
Graham DY, Adam E, Klein PD, Evans DJ Jr, Evans DG, Hazell SL, Alpert LC, Michaletz PA, Yoshimura HH (1989a) Epidemiology of *Campylobacter pylori* infection. Gastroenterol Clin Biol 13:84B–89B
Graham DY, Klein PD, Opekun AR, Smith KE, Polasani RR, Evans DJ Jr, Evans DG, Alpert JC, Michaletz PA, Yoshimura HH, Adam (1989b) In vivo susceptibility of *Campylobacter pylori*. Am J Gastroenterol 84:233–238
Graham DY, Lew GM, Michaletz PA (1989c) Randomized controlled trial of the effect of eradication of *C. pylori* on ulcer healing and relapse. Gastroenterology 96:A181
Hazell SL, Hennessy WB, Borody TJ, Carrick J, Ralston M, Brady L, Lee A (1987) *Campylobacter pyloridis* gastritis. II. Distribution of bacteria and associated inflammation in the gastroduodenal environment. Am J Gastroenterol 82: 297–301

Hespe W, Staal HJM, Hall DWR (1988) Bismuth absorption from the colloidal subcitrate. Lancet 2:1258
Hirschl AM, Pletschette M (1989) Antibiotic treatment of *Campylobacter pylori* infection. In: Rathbone BJ, Heatley RV (eds) *Campylobacter pylori* and gastroduodenal disease. Blackwell, Oxford, pp 217–224
Hirschl AM, Stanek G, Rotter M, Hentschel E, Schütze K (1987a) Ulcus duodeni und Antibiotika-Therapie. Dtsch Med Wochenschr 112:781
Hirschl AM, Stanek G, Rotter ML, Hentschel E, Schütze K, Pötzi R, Gangl A (1987b) *Campylobacter pyloridis*: frequency of occurrence, serology and susceptibility to antibiotics and ulcer-drugs (Abstr 64). 4th International Workshop on *Campylobacter* Infections Göteborg
Hirschl AM, Stanek G, Rotter M, Pötzi R, Gangl A, Hentschel E, Schütze K, Holzner HJ, Nemec H (1987c) *Campylobacter pylori*, Gastritis und Ulcus pepticum. Wien Klin Wochenschr 99:493–497
Hornick RB (1987) Peptic ulcer disease: a bacterial infection? N Engl J Med 316: 1598–1600
Hui WM, Lam SK, Chau PY, Ho J, Lui I, Lai CL, Lok ASF, Ng MMT (1987) Persistence of *Campylobacter pyloridis* despite healing of duodenal ulcer and improvement of accompanying duodenitis and gastritis. Dig Dis Sci 32:1255–1260
Humphreys H, Bourke S, Dooley C, McKenna D, Power B, Keane CT, Sweeney EC, O'Morain C (1988) Effect of treatment on *Campylobacter pylori* in peptic disease: a randomised prospective trial. Gut 29:279–283
Jiang SJ, Liu WZ, Zhang DZ, Shi Y, Xiao SD, Zhang ZH, Lu DY (1987) *Campylobacter*-like organisms in chronic gastritis, peptic ulcer, and gastric carcinoma. Scand J Gastroenterol 22:553–558
Johnston BJ, Reed PI, Ali MH (1988) Prevalence of *Campylobacter pylori* in duodenal and gastric mucosa – relationship to inflammation. Scand J Gastroenterol [Suppl 142] 23:69–75
Jones DM, Lessells AM, Eldridge J (1984) *Campylobacter*-like organisms on the gastric mucosa: culture, histological, and serological studies. J Clin Pathol 37:1002–1006
Kalenic S, Falisevac V, Scukanec-Spoljar M, Gmajnicki B, Knezevic S, Vodopija I (1987) Ofloxacin and metronidazole activity on gastritis and peptic ulcer associated with *Campylobacter pylori* (Abstr 75). 4th International Workshop on *Campylobacter* Infections. Göteborg
Kilbridge PM, Dahms BB, Czinn SJ (1988) *Campylobacter pylori*-associated gastritis and peptic ulcer disease in children. Am J Dis Child 142:1149–1152
Klein PD, Graham DY (1989) *Campylobacter pylori* detection by the ^{13}C-urea breath test. In: Rathbone B, Heatley V (eds) *Campylobacter pylori* and gastroduodenal disease. Blackwell, Oxford, pp 94–106
Klein PD, the Gastrointestinal Physiology Working Group of Cayetano Heredia and The Johns Hopkins Universities, Graham DY, Opekun AR, Sekeley S, Evans DG, Evans DJ Jr (1989) High prevalence of *Campylobacter pylori* (CP) infection in poor and rich peruvian children determined by ^{13}C urea breath test (^{13}C-UBT). Gastroenterology 96:A260
Koop H, Stumpf M, Eissele R, Lamberts R, Creutzfeld W, Arnold R (1989) Antral *Campylobacter pylori* in different states of gastric acid secretion. Gastroenterology 96:A267
Kosunen TU, Höök J, Rautelin HI, Myllylä G (1989) Age-dependent increase of *Campylobacter pylori* antibodies in blood donors. Scand J Gastroenterol 24: 110–114
Krajden S, Anderson J, Kempston J, Fuksa M, Matlow A, Skoglund M, Bier D, Marcon N, Kortan P, Haber G, Babida C, Petrea C (1989) Effect of Pepto-Bismol (Bismuth subsalicylate, BSS) dose levels on *C. pylori* clearance. 5th International Workshop on *Campylobacter* Infections, Puerto Vallarta

Krakowka S, Morgan DR, Kraft WG, Leunk RD (1987) Establishment of gastric *Campylobacter pylori* infection in the neonatal gnotobiotic piglet. Infect Immun 55:2789–2796

Kristiansen JE, Justesen T, Hvidberg EF, Andersen LP (1989) Trimipramin and other antipsychotics inhibit *Campylobacter pylori* in vitro. Pharmacol Toxicol 64:386–388

Kurpad AV, Shetty (1986) Effects of antimicrobial therapy on faecal bulking. Gut 27:55–58

Lambert JR, Borromeo M, Korman MG, Hansky J, Eaves ER (1987) Effect of colloidal bismuth (De-Nol) on healing and relapse of duodenal ulcers – role of *Campylobacter pyloridis*. Gastroenterology 92:1489

Lambert JR, Borromeo M, Eaves ER, Hansky J, Korman M (1988) Efficacy of different dosage regimens of bismuth in eradicating *Campylobacter pylori*. Gastroenterology 94:A248

Lamouliatte H, Mégraud F, de Mascarel A, Quinton A (1987a) Placebo-controlled trial of josamycin in *Campylobacter pyloridis* associated gastritis (Abstr 190). 4th International Workshop on *Campylobacter* infections. Göteborg

Lamouliatte H, Megraud F, de Mascarel A, Roux D, Quinton A (1987b) "*Campylobacter pyloridis*" and epigastric pain: endoscopic, histological, and bacteriological correlations. Gastroenterol Clin Biol 11:212–216

Lamouliatte H, Megraud F, de Mascarel A, Barberis C, Bernard PH, Cayla R, Quinton A (1989) Does omeprazole improve amoxicillin therapy directed against *Campylobacter pyloridis*-associated chronic gastritis? Klin Wochenschr [Suppl 18] 67:37

Lane MR, Lee SP (1988) Recurrence of duodenal ulcer after medical treatment. Lancet 1:1147–1149

Langenberg ML, Rauws EAJ, Schipper MEI, Widjojokosumo A, Tytgat GNJ, Rietra PJGM, Zanen HC (1985) The pathogenic role of *Campylobacter pyloridis* studied by attempts to eliminate these organisms. In: Pearson AD, Skirrow MB, Lior H, Rowe B (eds) *Campylobacter* III. PHLS, London, pp 162–163

Langenberg W, Rauws EAJ, Widjojokusumo A, Tytgat GNJ, Zanen HC (1986) Identification of *Campylobacter pyloridis* isolates by restriction endonuclease DNA analysis. J Clin Microbiol 24:414–417

Langenberg W, Rauws EAJ, Houthoff HJ, Oudbier J, Tytgat GJN, Zanen HC (1987) Follow-up of *C. pylori*-associated gastritis (CPG) after treatment with amoxicillin and/or colloidal bismuth (Abstr 94). 4th International workshop on *Campylobacter* infections, Göteborg

Langenberg W, Rauws EAJ, Houthoff HJ, Oudbier JH, van Bohemen CG, Tytgat GNJ, Rietra PJGM (1988) Follow-up study of individuals with untreated *Campylobacter pylori*-associated gastritis and of noninfected persons with non-ulcer dyspepsia. J Infect Dis 157:1245–1249

Mahoney MJ, Littlewood JM (1989) *Campylobacter pylori* in paediatric population. In: Rathbone BJ, Heatley RV (eds) *Campylobacter pylori* and gastroduodenal disease. Blackwell, Oxford, pp 167–175

Mahoney MJ, Wyatt JI, Littlewood JM (1988) *Campylobacter pylori* gastritis. Arch Dis Child 63:654–655

Mainguet P, Delmée M, Debongnie J-C (1989) Omeprazole, *Campylobacter pylori*, and duodenal ulcer. Lancet 2:389–390

Malfertheiner P, Bode G, Vanek E, Stanescu A, Lutz E, Blessing J, Ditschuneit H (1987) *Campylobacter pylori* – besteht ein Zusammenhang mit der peptischen Ulcuskrankheit? Dtsch Med Wochenschr 112:493–497

Malfertheiner P, Stanescu A, Baczako K, Vanek E, Bode G, Ditschuneit H (1988) Wismutsubsalicylat-Behandlung bei *Campylobacter-pylori*-assoziierter chronischer erosiver Gastritis. Dtsch Med Wochenschr 113:923–929

Malfertheiner P, Bode G, Stanescu A, Ditschuneit H (1989) Gastric metaplasia and *Campylobacter pylori* in duodenal ulcer disease: an ultrastructural analysis. Gastroenterol Clin Biol 13:71B–74B

Mannes GA, Bayerdörffer E, Höchter W, Weingart J, Heldwein W, Müller-Lissner S, Oertel H, Blendinger C, Kuntzen O, Bornschein W, Malfertheiner P, Wilkening J, Ruckdeschel G, Pfaller P, von Wulffen H, Köpcke W, Stolte M (1989) Early relapse rate after healing of *C. pylori*-positive duodenal ulcers. Klin Wochenschr [Suppl 18] 67:44

Marcheggiano A, Iannoni C, Agnello M, Paoluzi P, Pallone F (1987) *Campylobacter*-like organisms on the human gastric mucosa. Relation to type and extent of gastritis in different clinical groups. Gastroenterol Clin Biol 11:376–381

Marshall BJ (1986) *Campylobacter pyloridis* and gastritis. J Infect Dis 153:650–657

Marshall BJ (1989) Antimicrobial therapy of duodenal ulcer? Hold off for now. Reply. Gastroenterology 97:510

Marshall BJ, Warren JR (1984) Unidentified curved bacilli in the stomach of patients with gastritis and peptic ulceration. Lancet 1:1311–1315

Marshall BJ, Armstrong JA, McGechie DB, Glancy RJ (1985) Attempt to fulfil Koch's postulates for pyloric *Campylobacter*. Med J Aust 142:436–439

Marshall BJ, Armstrong JA, Francis GJ, Nokes NT, Wee SH (1987) Antibacterial action of bismuth in relation to *Campylobacter pyloridis* colonization and gastritis. Digestion [Suppl 2] 37:16–30

Marshall BJ, Goodwin CS, Warren JR, Murray R, Blincow ED Blackbourn SJ, Phillips M, Waters TE, Sanderson CR (1988) Prospective double-blind trial of duodenal ulcer relapse after eradication of *Campylobacter pylori*. Lancet 2: 1437–1442

Marshall BJ, Barret LJ, McCallum RW, Guerrant RL (1989a) *C. pylori* therapy: is in vitro disc testing with metronidazole worthwhile? 5th International Workshop on *Campylobacter* Infections, Puerto Vallarta

Marshall BJ, Caldwell SH, Hoffman SR, Frierson HF, Guerrant RL, McCallum RW (1989b) Can *C. pylori* be eradicated? Long-term follow-up on 28 successfully treated patients. Gastroenterology 96:A321

Marshall BJ, Caldwell SH, Yu ZJ, Darr F, Chang T, McCallum RW (1989c) Prevalence of *C. pylori* and history of upper GI investigation in healthy Virginians. Gastroenterology 96:A321

McColl KEL, Fullarton GM, El Nujumi AM, MacDonald AM, Brown IL, Hilditch TE (1989) Lowered gastrin and gastric acidity after eradication of *Campylobacter pylori* in duodenal ulcer. Lancet 2:499–500

McLean AJ, Harcourt DM, McNeil JJ (1988) Relapse rate as a major determinant of drug selection in peptic ulcer disease. Drugs 35:329–333

McNulty CAM (1989) Bacteriological and pharmacological basis for the treatment of *Campylobacter pylori* infection. Gastroenterol Clin Biol 13:96B–100B

McNulty CAM, Gearty JC, Crump B, Davis M, Donovan IA, Melikian V, Lister DM, Wise R (1986) *Campylobacter pyloridis* and associated gastritis: investigator blind, placebo controlled trial of bismuth salicylate and erythromycin ethylsuccinate. Br Med J 293:645–649

McNulty CAM, Dent JC, Ford GA, Wilkinson SP (1988) Inhibitory antimicrobial concentrations against *Campylobacter pylori* in gastric mucosa. J Antimicrob Chemother 22:729–738

McNulty CAM, Eyre-Brook IA, Uff JS, Dent JC, Wilkinson SP (1989) Triple therapy is not always 95% effective. 5th International Workshop on *Campylobacter* Infections, Puerto Vallarta

Menge H (1988) Was ist gesichert in der Behandlung der *Campylobacter-pylori*-induzierten Gastritis und des *Campylobacter-pylori*-assoziierten peptischen Ulkus? Internist (Berlin) 29:745–754

Menge H, Hofmann J, Gregor M (1987a) Dosis-Wirkungs-Studien mit Wismutsalzen zur Elimination von *Campylobacter pylori*. Z Gastroenterol [Suppl 4] 25: 44–46

Menge H, Warrelmann M, Loy V, Schmidt H, Gregor M, Skubis R, Hahn H, Riecken EO (1987b) Erste prospektiv erhobene Befunde zum Vorkommen von *Campylobacter pyloridis* in der menschlichen Antrumschleimhaut in der Bundesrepublik Deutschland. Med Klin 82:23–25

Menge H, Hoffmann J, Boenigk U, Gregor M (1988) Attempts to eradicate *Campylobacter pylori* – German experiences. In: Menge H, Gregor M, Tytgat GNJ, Marshall BJ (eds) *Campylobacter pylori*. Springer, Berlin Heidelberg New York, pp 228–230
Mertens JCC, Dekker W, Ligtvoet EEJ, Blok P (1989) Treatment failure of norfloxacin against *Campylobacter pylori* and chronic gastritis in patients with nonulcerative dyspepsia. Antimicrob Agents Chemother 33:256–257
Miller JP, Faragher EB (1986) Relapse of duodenal ulcer: does it matter which drug is used in initial treatment? Br Med J 293:1117–1118
Mitchell HM, Lee A, Berkowicz, J, Borody T (1988) The use of serology to diagnose active *Campylobacter pylori* infection. Med J Aust 149:604–609
Morgan D, Kraft W, Bender M, Pearson A and the Gastrointestinal Physiology Working Group of Cayetano Heredia and The Johns Hopkins Universities (1988) Nitrofurans in the treatment of gastritis associated with *Campylobacter pylori*. Gastroenterology 95:1178–1184
Morris A, Nicholson G (1987) Ingestion of *Campylobacter pyloridis* causes gastritis and raised fasting gastric pH. Am J Gastroenterol 82:192–199
Morris A, Arthur J, Nicholson G (1986) *Campylobacter pyloridis* infection in Auckland patients with gastritis. N Z Med J 99:353–355
Niemelä S, Karttunen T, Lehtola J (1987) *Campylobacter*-like organisms in patients with gastric ulcer. Scand J Gastroenterol 22:487–490
Nwokolo CU, Gavey CJ, Smith JTL, Pounder RE (1989) The absorption of bismuth from oral doses of tripotassium dicitrato bismuthate. Aliment Pharmacol Ther 3:29–39
Oderda G, dell'olio D, Morra I, Ansaldi N (1989a) *Campylobacter pylori* gastritis: long term results of treatment with amoxicillin. Arch Dis Child 64:326–329
Oderda G, Vaira D, Hoton J, Ainley C, Altare F, Ansaldi N (1989b) Amoxicillin plus tinidazole for *Campylobacter pylori* gastritis in children: assessment by serum IgG antibody, pepsinogen I, and gastrin levels. Lancet 1:690–692
O'Riordan T, Tobin A, Beattie S, Sweeney E, Keane C, O'Morain C (1989) Adjuvant antibiotic treatment improves eradication of *Campylobacter pylori* in duodenal ulcer. Gastroenterology 96:A378
Patey O, Chaplain C, Dublanchet A, Malkin JE, Roucayrol AM, Charasz N (1989) Failure of treatment with metronidazole for *Campylobacter pylori* infection. In: Mégraud F, Lamouliatte H (eds) *Campylobacter pylori* and gastroduodenal pathology. Elsevier Amsterdam, pp 629–632
Paulsen O, Höglund P, Walder M (1989) No effect of omeprazole-induced hypoacidity on the bioavailability of amoxicillin or bacampicillin. Scand J Infect Dis 21: 219–223
Perez-Perez GI, Dworkin BM, Chodos JE, Blaser MJ (1988) *Campylobacter pylori* antibodies in humans. Ann Intern Med 109:11–17
Price AB, Levi J, Dolby JM, Dunscombe PL, Smith A, Clark J, Stephenson ML (1985) *Campylobacter pyloridis* in peptic ulcer disease: microbiology, pathology, and scanning electron microscopy. Gut 26:1183–1188
Rao SSC, Edwards CA, Austen CJ, Bruce C, Read NW (1988) Impaired colonic fermentation of carbohydrate after ampicillin. Gastroenterology 94:928–932
Raskov H, Lanng C, Gaarslev K, Fischer Hansen B (1987) Screening for *Campylobacter pyloridis* in patients with upper dyspepsia and the relation to inflammation of the human gastric antrum. Scand J Gastroenterol 22:568–572
Rathbone BJ, Heatley RV (1989) Possible pathogenic mechanisms in *Campylobacter pylori* infection. In: Rathbone BJ, Heatley RV (eds) *Campylobacter pylori* and gastroduodenal disease. Blackwell, Oxford, pp 203
Rathbone BJ, Wyatt JI, Heatley RV (1986) *Campylobacter pyloridis* – a new factor in peptic ulcer disease. Gut 27:635–641
Rathbone BJ, Wyatt JI, Heatley RV (1988) Possible pathogenetic pathways of *Campylobacter pylori* in gastroduodenal disease. Scand J Gastroenterol [Suppl 142] 23:40–43

Rathbone BJ, Wyatt JI, Heatley RV (1989) Local response of the host to *Campylobacter pylori*. Gastroenterol Clin Biol 13:75B–77B
Rauws EAJ (1989) Long term follow-up of *Campylobacter pylori*-associated gastritis after treatment with colloidal bismuth subcitrate and/or amoxicillin. In: Mégraud F, Lamouliatte H (eds) *Campylobacter pylori* and gastroduodenal pathology. Elsevier, Amsterdam, pp 633–636
Rauws EAJ, Tytgat GN (1987) Elektronenmikroskopische Befunde während einer Behandlung *Campylobacter-pylori*-positiver Gastritiden mit Wismutsalzen. Z Gastroenterol [Suppl 4] 25:41–43
Rauws EAJ, Tytgat GN (1989) *Campylobacter pylori*: treatment of gastritis. In: Rathbone BJ, Heatley RV (eds) *Campylobacter pylori* and gastroduodenal disease. Blackwell Oxford, pp 225–231
Rauws EAJ, Langenberg W, Houthoff HJ, Zanen HC, Tytgat GN (1988) *Campylobacter pyloridis*-associated chronic active antral gastritis. A prospective study of its prevalence and the effect of antibacterial and antiulcer treatment. Gastroenterology 94:33–40
Rogé J, Bloch F, Camilleri JP, Tricottet V, Lambert N, Proux MC (1986) Antrites érosives chroniques et "*Campylobacter pyloridis*" – étude histologique et ultrastructurale. Sem Hōp Paris 62:81–89
Rollason TP, Stone J, Rhodes JM (1984) Spiral organisms in endoscopic biopsies of the human stomach. J Clin Pathol 37:23–26
Rösch W, Becker V, Steininger H, Menge H (1989) *Campylobacter-pylori*-assoziierte Gastritis. Therapie mit Wismutsubsalizylat. MMW 130:97–100
Rosenblatt JE, Edson RS (1987) Metronidazole. Mayo Clin Proc 62:1013–1027
Sabbatini F, d'Arienzo A, Piai G, Verre C, Ciacci C, d'Argenio G, Minieri M, Sapio E, Mazzacca G (1989) Influence of blood group and secretor status on *Campylobacter pylori* infection. Gastroenterology 96:A433
Saxon A, Beall GN, Rohr AS, Aldeman DC (1987) Immediate hypersensitivity reactions to betalactam antibiotics. Ann Intern Med 107:204–215
Scarpignato C, Galmiche J-P (1988) Mucosal coating agents: pharmacology and clinical use. In: Bianchi Porro G (ed) Topics in digestive disease. Raven, New York, pp 73–133
Schaub N, Stalder H, Stalder GA, Affolter H, Wegmann W (1987) Versagen von Doxycyclin bei *Campylobacter-pylori*-positiver Gastritis. Dtsch Med Wochenschr 112:117–118
Scully BE (1988) Metronidazole. Med Clin North Am 72:613–621
Simor AE, Ferro S, Low DE (1989) Comparative in vitro activities of six new fluoroquinolones and other oral antimicrobial agents against *Campylobacter pylori*. Antimicrob Agents Chemother 33:108–109
Sipponen P (1990) Risk of peptic ulcer in gastritis. In: Malfertheimer P, Ditschuneit H (eds) Helicobacter pylori, gastritis and peptic ulcer. Springer, Berlin Heidelberg New York Tokyo, pp 223–227
Symposium on *Campylobacter pylori*. Springer, Berlin Heidelberg New York (in press)
Smith AC, Price AB, Borriello P, Levi AJ (1988) A comparison of ranitidine and tripotasssium dicitrato-bismuth (T.D.B.) in relapse rates of duodenal ulcer. The role of *Campylobacter pylori* (C.P.) Gastroenterology 94:A431
Stadler P, Blum AL (1989) Ist *Campylobacter pylori* der Erreger der Ulkuskrankheit? Contra. Z Gastroenterol 27:127–130
Steer HW (1985) The gastroduodenal epithelium in peptic ulceration. J Pathol 146:355–362
Steininger H, Schneider U, Bartz K, Simmler B (1989) *Campylobacter pylori* und Gastritis – Besiedelungsdichte und Grad der Entzündung. Semiquantitative und morphometrische Untersuchung. Leber Magen Darm 19:70–78
Stolte M, Eidt S, Ritter M, Bethke B (1989) *Campylobacter pylori* und Gastritis. Assoziation oder Induktion? Pathologe 10:21–26

Stone JW, Wise R, Donovan IA, Gearty J (1988) Failure of ciprofloxacin to eradicate *Campylobacter pylori* from the stomach. J Antimicrob Chemother 22:92–93

Taylor DE, Hargreaves JA, Lai-King NG, Sherbaniuk W, Jewell LD (1987) Isolation and characterization of *Campylobacter pyloridis* from gastric biopsies. Am J Clin Pathol 87:49–54

Tytgat GNJ (1987) Colloidal bismuth subcitrate in peptic ulcer – a review. Digestion [Suppl 2] 37:31–41

Tytgat GNJ, Rauws EAJ (1987) Significance of *Campylobacter pylori*. Aliment Pharmacol Ther 1:527S–539S

Tytgat GNJ, Rauws A (1989) The role of *Campylobacter pylori* in gastroduodenal disease. A "believer" 's point of view. Gastroenterol Clin Biol 13:118B–121B

Unge P, Olsson J, Gad A, Gnarpe H (1989) Does omeprazole (40 mg O.M.) improve antimicrobial therapy directed towards gastric *Campylobacter pylori* in patients with antral gastritis? A pilot study. In: Mégraud F, Lamouliatte H (eds) Gastroduodenal pathology and *Campylobacter pylori*. Elsevier Amsterdam; pp 641–645

Von Wulffen H, Heesemann J, Bützow G, Löning T, Laufs R (1986) Detection of *Campylobacter pyloridis* in patients with antrum gastritis and peptic ulcers by culture, complement fixation test, and immunoblot. J Clin Microbiol 24:716–720

Wagner S, Freise J, Bär W, Fritsch S, Schmidt FW (1989) Epidemiologie und Therapie der *Campylobacter-pylori*-Infektion. Dtsch Med Wochenschr 114: 407–413

Wagstaff AJ, Benfield P, Monk JP (1988) Colloidal bismuth subcitrate. A review of its pharmacodynamic and pharmacokinetic properties, and its therapeutic use in peptic ulcer disease. Drugs 36:132–157

Weil J, Bell GD, Jones PH, Gant P, Trowell JE, Harrison G (1988) "Eradication" of *Campylobacter pylori*: are we being misled? Lancet 2:1245

Weil J, Bell GD, Harrison G, Trowell JE, Gant P, Jones PH (1989) *Campylobacter pylori* survive high doses bismuth sub-citrate (De-Nol) therapy. In: Mégraud F, Lamouliatte H (eds) Gastroduodenal pathology and *Campylobacter pylori*. Elsevier, Amsterdam, pp 651–653

Wright AJ, Wilkowske CJ (1987) The penicillins. Mayo Clin Proc 62:806–820

Wyatt JI, Dixon MF (1988) Chronic gastritis – a pathogenetic approach. J Pathol 154:113–124

Wyatt JI, Rathbone BJ (1988) Immune response of the gastric mucosa to *Campylobacter pylori*. Scand J Gastroenterol [Suppl 142] 23:44–49

Wyatt JI, Rathbone BJ (1989) Gastric metaplasia in the duodenum and *Campylobacter pylori*. Gastroenterol Clin Biol 13:78B–82B

Wyatt JI, Rathbone BJ, Dixon MF, Heatley RV (1987) *Campylobacter pyloridis* and acid induced gastric metaplasia in the pathogenesis of duodenitis. J Clin Pathol 40:841–848

Wyatt JI, Rathbone BJ, Heatley RV, Losowsky MS (1988) *Campylobacter pylori* and history of dyspepsia in healthy blood donors. Gut 29:706

CHAPTER 6

Development of a New Gastric Antisecretory Drug for Clinical Use

C.W. HOWDEN and R.H. HUNT

A. General Considerations

Antisecretory drugs are widely used in the treatment of peptic ulcer. The term peptic ulcer disease encompasses the conditions of gastric ulcer and duodenal ulcer. In addition, peptic esophagitis and gastroesophageal reflux disease are often included in this generic classification but will not be considered further here. Both duodenal ulceration and gastric ulceration are chronic relapsing conditions. Although often considered together under the general term "peptic ulcer," they differ with respect to pathophysiology, natural history, and response to treatment. Important differences will be outlined.

These disorders are common; it has been estimated that 10%–15% of a population will be affected at some time by peptic ulcer disease (MISIEWICZ and POUNDER 1983). The number of patients admitted to hospital because of peptic ulceration was decreasing (WALT et al. 1986) before the advent of powerful antisecretory drugs, and the true incidence of peptic ulceration may have been decreasing for the past 30 years (LANGMAN 1982). This has also been reflected in a decreased rate of routine hospitalization in the United States (ELASHOFF and GROSSMAN 1980). However, on closer examination of these figures, the decrease in hospital admission has largely been of young people; admission rates for elderly patients are increasing, particularly in elderly women (WALT et al. 1986). An increasing concern is the rise in the rate of ulcer perforation (WALT et al. 1986) and hemorrhage (SOMERVILLE et al. 1986), both of which may be at least partly explained by the use of nonsteroidal anti-inflammatory drugs (NSAIDs) by elderly patients.

B. Etiology and Pathophysiology of Peptic Ulcer

The traditional view of the pathophysiology of peptic ulceration is that an imbalance exists between the aggressive and defensive factors which operate in the upper gastrointestinal tract. The aggressive factors include gastric acid and pepsin, and possibly also bile salts and duodenal contents refluxed into the stomach. The principal defensive factors are mucus and bicarbonate secreted by the gastric and duodenal mucosa, and the inherent ability to increase regional gastroduodenal mucosal blood flow in response to irritation.

Patients with duodenal ulceration tend to have higher levels of gastric acid secretion than age-matched controls. However, there is usually such an overlap between the two groups that this cannot be used as a diagnostic test for the presence of duodenal ulcer.

Using methods of aspiration and intragastric titration, it has been shown that duodenal ulcer patients secrete significantly more acid than controls over a 24-h period (FELDMAN and RICHARDSON 1986). The increased level of acid secretion is present when the stomach is in the resting, unstimulated state and also when the stomach is naturally stimulated by the ingestion of food (FELDMAN and RICHARDSON 1986).

Patients with duodenal ulcer have inappropriately high levels of gastric acid secretion during the night (HENNING and NORPOTH 1932), which may reflect excessive parasympathetic nervous drive in these patients (DRAGSTEDT and OWENS 1943). This important observation is in accord with common clinical experience as patients with duodenal ulceration frequently waken with ulcer pain during the night. Pain may be relieved by food or antacids which buffer the excess acid.

Since there is a wide overlap in levels of acid secretion between patients and controls, this is equivalent to saying that some patients have "normal" levels of acid secretion. This being so, other pathophysiological factors might be involved in the genesis of peptic ulceration. Defects in defensive mechanisms have been suggested: first a reduction in duodenal bicarbonate secretion (ISENBERG et al. 1987) and second, a relative deficiency of local prostaglandins (RACHMILEWITZ et al. 1986). The exact significance of these observations remains unclear, and they require confirmation. For example, the reduction in duodenal bicarbonate secretion might be an effect of duodenal ulceration rather than a cause.

Patients with gastric ulcer have normal or reduced levels of acid secretion when compared with controls (LANZON-MILLER et al. 1987). Gastric ulcer is usually associated with a diffuse gastritis commonly involving the antral and fundic mucosa. This may lead to either reduced acid secretion or increased back-diffusion of acid. The net effect is that levels of intraluminal gastric acid are reduced. Much attention has been focused on impaired mucosal defense in the pathogenesis of gastric ulcer, including reduced mucus and bicarbonate secretion, relative deficiency of mucosal prostaglandins, and local impairment of gastric mucosal blood flow.

The clinical features of duodenal and gastric ulcer are so similar that the two conditions cannot be distinguished by history and physical examination. Pain is the main presenting feature; typically it is episodic rather than constant, is often worse between meals and at night, may waken the patient from sleep, and may be relieved by food, milk, antacids, or occasionally vomiting. However, persistent vomiting is unusual; it may suggest gastric outlet obstruction (a long-term complication of chronic peptic ulceration) or even gastric carcinoma. The recent onset of these symptoms in middle-aged or elderly patients should always be considered seriously and investigated promptly.

Occasionally, peptic ulceration may present with perforation or hemorrhage. Peptic ulceration is the commonest cause of acute upper gastrointestinal bleeding and some patients may have had little or no ulcer pain. This suggests that some peptic ulcers may be "silent" and asymptomatic until they present with a complication. Asymptomatic ulcers are most often found in elderly patients. These patients may be at high risk of perforation or hemorrhage if they are prescribed an NSAID (SOMERVILLE et al. 1986; WALT et al. 1986).

C. Scope for Pharmacological Intervention

Most drugs which are used in the treatment of peptic ulceration act to in some way reduce the quantity or concentration of intraluminal acid. Antacids chemically neutralize acid as they are weak alkalis. They provide symptomatic relief from ulcer pain and can also heal ulcers if taken regularly. Acid secretion by the parietal cells in the stomach can be reduced by specific antagonists of the H_2 receptor (e.g., cimetidine, ranitidine) or the muscarinic cholinergic receptor (e.g., pirenzepine) or the prostaglandin receptor (e.g., misoprostol), or by agents that block the H^+,K^+-ATPase enzyme, which is the active transport site for hydrogen ions (e.g., omeprazole). In simple terms, all these agents act to reduce the aggressive factors involved in peptic ulceration. Some existing drugs for peptic ulcer do not suppress gastric acid secretion and so presumably act by boosting mucosal defenses. Sucralfate and chelated salts of bismuth may act by forming an insoluble plug over an ulcer crater and thereby prevent further digestion by acid and pepsin or alternatively they might act as mild local irritants on the mucosa around the ulcer. This would have the effect of stimulating local endogenous prostaglandin release. Ulcer healing might therefore be the result of increased local prostaglandins.

D. Clinical Development of a New Antisecretory Drug for Peptic Ulcer

Discussion of the clinical pharmacological approach to the development of a new drug for the treatment of peptic ulcer is really only pertinent for drugs with acid-suppressing properties. Such an agent will have been identified as an inhibitor of gastric secretion in animal pharmacology experiments. It might have been the result of a new discovery, or alternatively it could have been developed from the "molecular roulette" of structure–activity relationships practised by the pharmaceutical industry and based on an existing agent.

I. Phase I

The first question to be asked is, "Does the new drug suppress gastric acid secretion in man?" Initially, phase I studies to address this question will be undertaken in human volunteers. It is customary to investigate the effects of the drug on basal acid output (BAO) as well as on acid output in response to stimulation with a variety of secretagogues such as histamine, pentagastrin, and food. In such studies, it is necessary to collect gastric juice for analysis via a nasogastric tube positioned by either fluoroscopy or water recovery (HASSAN and HOBSLEY 1970). The tube should be manipulated so that its tip lies in the most dependent part of the stomach. The stomach is then emptied by hand suction. Under resting conditions, timed collections of gastric juice are made by continuous aspiration using a mechanical pump. For a useful measurement of BAO, this collection is usually made over 1 h. Samples are collected every 15 or 10 min. The volume of each sample is recorded. From each sample, a 1.0 ml aliquot is removed for determination of pH. The titratable acidity of the sample is determined by titrating it to a pH of 7.00 with a known concentration of alkali, usually 0.1 M sodium hydroxide. The acid output of each sample can be calculated from the product of volume and titratable acidity. The acid outputs from the various samples are summated to give the BAO. Conventionally, however, the first two 15-min samples from a 60-min collection are disregarded. BAO is then calculated as the sum of the acid outputs from the last two samples multiplied by 2.

Obviously, studies of BAO may be made before and after treatment with the investigational drug, or alternatively following both the drug and placebo. Using the latter design, it is possible to blind the study and determine the percentage reduction in BAO attributable to the drug. A dose–response relationship can be assessed by studying a range of doses of the drug.

Unfortunately, information on reduction of BAO is not always helpful. BAO shows considerable inter- and intra-subject variability (WHITE and JUNIPER 1973); in some subjects there may be no basal secretion of acid at certain times. In addition, if the mean BAO on placebo is low, it will be very difficult to show a statistically significant reduction due to the drug unless a very large number of subjects is studied. Finally, studies of BAO are of limited relevance; the stomach is not in a true basal state for large parts of a 24-h period.

It is easier to show a significant acid-suppressing effect of a drug when acid secretion is first stimulated with a secretagogue. The agent used most frequently is pentagastrin (Peptavlon). Following intramuscular injection of pentagastrin 6 μg/kg, there is a prompt increase in both the volume and the acidity of gastric juice. This effect usually reaches a peak within 30 min of the injection. The "peak acid output" (PAO) is calculated from the sum of the two consecutive highest acid outputs from 15-min samples multiplied by 2. As for BAO, it is a simple matter to calculate the percentage reduction in PAO attributable to the drug.

Alternatively, the secretagogue may be given by a continuous intravenous infusion. This has the advantage of providing a smoother onset of stimulation of secretion, and an eventual plateau effect. If given intravenously, the response is termed the "plateau acid output." For a more extensive description of tests of acid secretion see BARON (1978).

Other secretagogues apart from pentagastrin include insulin, histamine, and impromidine. Insulin causes hypoglycemia, which stimulates acid secretion via vagal pathways. Its effects are unpleasant and potentially hazardous. There is no indication to continue using it for this type of study. Histamine is a potent and effective stimulant of gastric secretion but with a variety of other pharmacological effects. Although often given with a specific H_1 receptor antagonist to limit its other effects, histamine can be given alone in low doses (e.g., 10 μg/kg i.v.). It is best to avoid the use of H_1 antagonists as they often possess some anticholinergic effect and may therefore directly influence gastric secretion. Impromidine is a specific agonist for the H_2 receptor and therefore a useful pharmacological tool for the assessment of competitive H_2 antagonists (Hunt et al. 1980). Unfortunately, supplies of impromidine are very restricted.

Studies of the effects of a new acid-suppressing drug on basal and stimulated acid secretion can give useful information on the potency of the drug over a variety of doses (e.g., Howden et al. 1987). However, they are of limited value in assessing the effects of a particular drug on the normal patterns of acid secretion during the day. It is in this area that studies of 24-h gastric acidity are of major importance.

The first reported study of an acid-suppressing drug on 24-h intragastric acidity examined the effects of cimetidine in a group of healthy volunteers (Pounder et al. 1976). Since then, the technique has been widely used in the investigation of newer drugs and new dosage schedules of existing drugs. Briefly, such a study attempts to simulate a normal 24-h period of the subject. With a small diameter nasogastric tube in situ and the subjects in an otherwise controlled environment, samples of gastric juice are collected at regular intervals (usually hourly) for determination of pH. Intragastric acidity (equivalent to hydrogen ion activity), $[H^+]$, can be derived according to the formula

$$[H^+] = \frac{1}{\text{antilog pH}} \times 1000$$

and is expressed in mmol/l. Serial measurements of $[H^+]$ plotted against time provide a profile of the intragastric acidity over the 24-h period.

Subjects may be ambulant during such a study. Standardized meals are eaten at set times on each study day with identical meals consumed at the same times on subsequent study days. A description of a standard diet for a 24-h study is now available (Lanzon-Miller et al. 1987). If the patient smokes, the same number of cigarettes must be smoked on each study day at identical timepoints.

During the night it is possible to attempt to collect the entire gastric secretion. First, the stomach is emptied by hand suction; the nasogastric tube is then connected to a mechanical aspiration pump. Gastric juice is collected in hourly samples over a 7- or 8-h period. The pH of each sample is recorded and [H^+] calculated. In addition, the titratable acidity is measured. When this is multiplied by the volume of the sample, acid output is derived. Hence such a study provides information on hydrogen ion activity (intragastric acidity), volume of secretion, and acid output. In addition, small aliquots from each collection may be stored for determination of peptic activity.

In specialized centers, the technique of continuous intragastric pH monitoring using an intragastric electrode has been successfully used in the investigation of antisecretory effect (e.g., MERKI et al. 1987). This methodology has the theoretical advantage that many more data points are generated (pH may be recorded every 5 or 6 s), but equipment is expensive. Continuous intragastric pH monitoring has not become widely available.

Once the intragastric acidity over a 24-h period is plotted for both drug and placebo, or for two different dosage schedules of a drug, it should be possible to estimate visually the effect of the drug. In addition, it should be possible to determine when and for how long the drug is exerting its useful antisecretory effect.

Traditionally, it has been standard practice to calculate the mean intragastric acidity over both the 24-h and the nocturnal period. The effect of an antisecretory drug could then be expressed in terms of percentage reduction of the mean 24-h intragastric acidity on placebo (e.g., HOWDEN et al. 1986a). It has been suggested, however, that it would be more appropriate to report these results in terms of medians (WALT 1986). One advantage of using medians is that the data do not have to be normally distributed. Nonparametric statistical methods may then be applied. However, the median may be less easily computed than the mean, particularly where there are large quantities of data.

Another way to express results is as a percentage reduction in the area under the acidity/time curve (AUC). The AUC can be relatively easily calculated; for example by the linear trapezoidal rule. However, such a calculation does not give much additional information over the percentage reduction in mean intragastric acidity (e.g., HOWDEN et al. 1985b).

Although phase I studies have traditionally been performed in healthy volunteers, it has become apparent to the authors that the pharmaceutical industry would prefer such studies to be carried out in patients with healed duodenal ulcer. While this has some attractions, it has not always been possible for investigative units to have a large enough group of duodenal ulcer patients available who were asymptomatic, on no antiulcer medication, and able to take part in a 24-h study. It is usually much easier to arrange such a study in a group of healthy volunteer subjects. The results of published 24-h studies in both normal healthy volunteers and patients with duodenal ulcer have been compared (HOWDEN et al. 1986b). There is a significant linear relationship between the degree of suppression of acidity in these two populations. It is both practical and appropriate, therefore, that phase I 24-h studies of gastric antisecretory drugs continue to be performed in healthy volunteers. Data derived from these studies may be used to predict the likely degree of suppression of acidity which would be found in duodenal ulcer patients. This should give a good indication of the most appropriate doses and dosage schedules of a new drug to be employed in subsequent phase II and III studies.

II. Phase II

The aim of a phase II study is to assess the likely value of a new drug in the treatment of peptic ulcer in a small group of patients. As well as measuring the ulcer healing rate, it is also necessary to assess the effects of the new agent on ulcer symptoms. It is desirable to have separate studies looking at duodenal ulcer and gastric ulcer. Since the drug will still be at a comparatively early stage of its development, there will be stringent inclusion and exclusion criteria for patients in the study. For example, it may not be considered appropriate to include very young or elderly patients. Likewise it may be necessary to exclude women, particularly those of child-bearing potential. Also excluded would be patients with a recent complication of peptic ulcer, patients who have recently received treatment for an ulcer, patients taking so-called ulcerogenic drugs, including aspirin and NSAIDs, patients with a past history of gastric surgery, and patients with other concomitant serious medical problems. In short, patients suitable for inclusion in a phase II study are likely to constitute a highly selected group.

A phase II study should be designed to identify suitable patients with ulcer symptoms who have an active ulcer seen at endoscopy. Endoscopic evaluation is essential and is the gold standard for assessing ulcer healing in this context; barium radiology is no longer considered acceptable. Once identified, suitable patients are asked for full written consent. They are then recruited to the study and randomized to one or other treatment. Randomization should be double-blinded and may often be stratified for various factors such as smoking.

Exactly what the new drug should be compared with remains a subject of controversy. At the present time, the FDA require placebo-controlled studies of all investigational drugs for peptic ulcer. This effectively means that 50% of suitable patients in such a trial would not be receiving active treatment for their peptic ulcer, the symptoms of which prompted them to seek medical attention. While this raises certain ethical issues, it is apparent that the majority of patients receiving placebo in such trials do not suffer any serious consequences. Additionally, duodenal ulcers will heal in about 42% of these (Howden et al. 1985a; Jones et al. 1987), and a significant proportion will report improvement in symptoms, as part of a placebo effect.

One advantage of placebo-controlled trials is that they allow the investigator to assess the effectiveness of the new agent in alleviating symptoms of dyspepsia. Patients should be questioned directly about symptoms and possible side-effects, and be asked to complete a diary card. A standard antacid is usually issued to all patients; the number of antacid tablets consumed can be taken as an indication of the progress of the patient's symptoms.

Once recruited into a trial, patients are seen at weekly or 2-weekly intervals, which allows for data collection on symptom relief, adverse reactions, and potential toxicology by monitoring hematology and blood chemistry. Endoscopy should be repeated at predetermined timepoints to assess ulcer healing. While it is attractive to have frequent endoscopies, some form of compromise must be reached taking the comfort of the patient into account. A reasonable approach has been to perform endoscopy after 2 and 4 weeks of treatment, or alternatively after 4 and 8 weeks.

Phase II studies should ideally be performed in a small number of institutions, and be closely monitored. As well as measuring healing and symptom relief, it is also possible to obtain valuable additional information on antisecretory effect in duodenal ulcer patients. A good example of such a trial was an early phase II study of omeprazole performed in the United Kingdom (MEYRICK-THOMAS et al. 1984). This study reported on healing rates and antisecretory effects of a range of doses of omeprazole.

III. Phase III

Phase III studies will comprise large, double-blinded, endoscopically controlled trials of the new compound in the treatment of duodenal and gastric ulcer. The initiation of phase III studies will only be justified by the finding of therapeutic efficacy and reasonable safety in the phase II program. Trials are likely to involve a number of centers in order to be certain of recruiting the requisite numbers of patients. The broad outline of the trials is likely to be similar to that of earlier phase II studies. However, since phase III will involve many more patients, there is a much higher chance of detecting a rare but potentially serious adverse effect. Safety testing is therefore very important in the context of these phase III studies.

Obviously, to eliminate bias, these trials should be performed in a randomized double-blind protocol. The question arises again as to what the new drug should be tested against. While in the United States the FDA still favor at least some placebo-controlled studies in the full profile of a new antiulcer drug, elsewhere it has been acceptable to test the new agent against an established treatment. Clearly, it will be comparatively simple to show that a new agent is significantly superior to placebo in healing duodenal ulcer. This is particularly so since the cumulative placebo healing rates in duodenal ulcer apparently reach a plateau after about 4 weeks of treatment (HOWDEN et al. 1986c), although they continue to increase to 12 weeks in gastric ulcer (HOWDEN et al. 1988). Hence, in duodenal ulcer, even if there is no significant advantage of the new drug over placebo at 4 weeks of treatment, there may be a difference in favor of the new agent at 8 weeks since it is likely to go on healing ulcers over that time when placebo will not.

On the other hand, it may be quite difficult to show an advantage in terms of healing rates for a new drug against an already licensed drug. In order to avoid a type II error, it may be necessary to recruit very large numbers of patients in an attempt to show an advantageous healing rate for a new drug. Often, however, pharmaceutical companies will compromise on the numbers of patients and will be content to show that their new drug is equivalent to one already marketed. At the moment, most regulatory authorities are satisfied for a new drug to show "therapeutic equivalence" to existing treatments provided that its safety record is good. It has not yet become necessary for a company to show any specific advantage of its compound over existing treatments in phase III studies for it to be granted a product licence.

IV. Phase IV

As with any new drug, evaluation of a new antisecretory drug for peptic ulcer will continue after a product licence has been granted and the drug marketed. Phase IV studies are also known as postmarketing surveillance studies and are primarily concerned with evaluating the safety profile of the drug and determining the true incidence of any adverse reactions. Cimetidine, for example, has undergone extensive postmarketing surveillance studies (COLIN-JONES et al. 1982, 1983, 1985). These and other studies have helped to define the safety profile of cimetidine and other acid-suppressing drugs. In addition, they have helped to dispel fears that moderate pharmacological suppression of gastric acid secretion might increase the incidence of gastric carcinoma, aroused by some early and poorly documented case reports.

It should be emphasized that there is no uniformly agreed program for phase IV studies, but their importance in the further assessment of drug efficacy and safety is widely acknowledged.

References

Baron JH (1978) Clinical tests of gastric secretion. History, methodology and interpretation. MacMillan, London

Colin-Jones DG, Langman MJS, Lawson DH, Vessey NP (1982) Cimetidine and gastric cancer: preliminary report from post-marketing surveillance study. Br Med J 285:1311–1313

Colin-Jones DG, Langman MJS, Lawson DH, Vessey MP (1983) Post-marketing surveillance of cimetidine: 12 month mortality report. Br Med J 286:1713–1716

Colin-Jones DG, Langman MJS, Lawson DH, Vessey MP (1985) Post-marketing surveillance of the safety of cimetidine: Q J Med 54:253–268

Dragstedt LR, Owens FM (1943) Supradiaphragmatic section of the vagus nerves in the treatment of duodenal ulcer. Proc Soc Exp Biol Med 53:152–154

Elashoff JD, Grossman MI (1980) Trends in hospital admission and death rate for peptic ulcer in the United States from 1970 to 1978. Gastroenterology 78:280–285

Feldman M, Richardson CT (1986) Total 24-hour gastric acid secretion in patients with duodenal ulcer. Comparison with normal subjects and effects of cimetidine and parietal cell vagotomy. Gastroenterology 90:540–544

Hassan N, Hobsley M (1970) Positioning of subject and of nasogastric tube during a gastric secretion study. Br Med J 1:458–460

Henning N, Norpoth L (1932) Die Magensekretion während des Schlafes. Dtsch Arch Klin Med 172:558

Howden CW, Jones DB, Hunt RH (1985a) Nocturnal doses of H_2-receptor antagonists for duodenal ulcer. Lancet 1:647–648

Howden CW, Burget DW, Silletti C, Hunt RH (1985b) Single nocturnal doses of pirenzepine effectively inhibit overnight gastric secretion. Hepatogastroenterology 32:240–242
Howden CW, Derodra JK, Burget DW, Hunt RH (1986a) Effects of low dose omeprazole on gastric secretion and plasma gastrin in patients with healed duodenal ulcer. Hepatogastroenterology 33:267–270
Howden CW, Jones DB, Burget DW, Hunt RH (1986b) Comparison of the effects of gastric antisecretory agents in healthy volunteers and patients with duodenal ulcer. Gut 27:1058–1061
Howden CW, Jones DB, Hunt RH (1986c) Differences in placebo healing rates in duodenal and gastric ulcer: some implications for clinical trials (Abstr). Acta Pharmcol Toxicol [Suppl] (Copenh) 5:201
Howden CW, Burget DW, Silletti C, van Eeden A, Tompkins KB, Hunt RH (1987) Marked suppression of stimulated gastric acid and pepsin secretion by enisoprost, a new PGE_1 analogue. Aliment Pharmacol Ther 1:305–313
Howden CW, Jones DB, Peace KE, Burget DW, Hunt RH (1988) The treatment of gastric ulcer with antisecretory drugs: relationship of pharmacological effect to healing rates. Dig Dis Sci 33(5):619–624
Hunt RH, Mills JG, Beresford J, Billings JA, Burland WL, Milton-Thompson GJ (1980) Gastric secretory studies in humans with impromidine (SK & F 92676) – a specific histamine H_2 receptor agonist. Gastroenterology 78:505–511
Isenberg JI, Selling JA, Hogan DL, Koss MA (1987) Impaired proximal duodenal mucosal bicarbonate secretion in patients with duodenal ulcer. N Engl J Med 316:374–379
Jones DB, Howden CW, Burget DW, Kerr GD, Hunt RH (1987) Acid suppression in duodenal ulcer: a meta-analysis to define optimal dosing with antisecretory drugs. Gut 28:1120–1127
Langman MJS (1982) What is happening to peptic ulcer? Br Med J 284:1063–1064
Lanzon-Miller S, Pounder RE, Hamilton MR, Chronos NAF, Ball S, Merceica JE, Olausson M, Cederberg C (1987) Twenty-four-hour intragastric acidity and plasma gastrin concentration in healthy subjects and patients with duodenal or gastric ulcer or pernicious anaemia. Aliment Pharmacol Ther 1:225–238
Merki HS, Witzel L, Walt RP, Neumann J, Scheurle E, Kaufmann D, Mappes A, Heim J, Rohmel J (1987) Comparison of ranitidine 300 mg twice daily, 300 mg at night and placebo on 24-hour intragastric acidity of duodenal ulcer patients. Aliment Pharmacol Ther 1:217–224
Meyrick-Thomas J, Misiewicz JJ, Trotman IF, Boyd EJS, Wilson JA, Wormsley KG, Pounder RE, Sharma BK, Collier N, Spencer J, Thompson J, Baron JH, Bush A, Cope L, Daly MJ, Howe AL (1984) Omeprazole in duodenal ulceration: acid inhibition, symptom relief, endoscopic healing and recurrence. Br Med J 289: 525–528
Misiewicz JJ, Pounder RE (1983) Peptic ulcer. In: Wetherall DJ, Ledingham JGG, Warrell DA (eds) Oxford textbook of medicine. Oxford University Press, Oxford, pp 12.57–12.70
Pounder RE, Williams JG, Milton-Thompson GJ, Misiewicz JJ (1976) Effect of cimetidine on 24-hour intragastric acidity in normal subjects. Gut 17:133–138
Rachmilewitz D, Ligumsky M, Fich A, Goldin E, Eliakim A, Karmeli F (1986) Role of endogenous gastric prostanoids in the pathogenesis and therapy of duodenal ulcer. Gastroenterology 90:963–969
Somerville K, Faulkner G, Langman M (1986) Non-steroidal anti-inflammatory drugs and bleeding peptic ulcer. Lancet 1:462–464
Walt RP (1986) Twenty four hour intragastric acidity analysis for the future. Gut 27:1–9
Walt RP, Katschinski B, Logan R, Ashley J, Langman M (1986) Rising frequency of ulcer perforation in elderly people in the United Kingdom. Lancet 1:489–492
White WD, Juniper K (1973) Repeatability of gastric analysis. Am J Dig Dis 18:7–13

CHAPTER 7

Therapeutic Use of Omeprazole in Man: Pharmacology, Efficacy, Toxicity, and Comparison with H_2 Receptor Antagonists

P.N. MATON, G. SACHS, and B. WALLMARK

A. Introduction

The inhibition of gastric secretion by altering the activity of the terminal step of acid secretion is a new approach to the therapy of peptic ulcer disease. The active transport of HCl is carried out by a transport enzyme, the H^+,K^+-ATPase. The steps necessary for the formation of acid involve activation of the ATPase in several steps that include (a) insertion of the protein into the canalicular membrane of the parietal cell and (b) activation of KCl permeability of the canalicular membrane so that K^+ can access the luminal surface of the enzyme and enable ATPase activity and hence acid secretion (Fig. 1). The mechanism of acid secretion has been discussed in detail elsewhere in this volume. The clinical use of one inhibitor of the H^+,K^+-APTase, omeprazole, is gaining increasing acceptance worldwide and this review is concerned with published studies of the properities of omeprazole in man.

B. Pharmacology

I. General

The compound omeprazole is by virtue of its chemical properties a selective inhibitor of the gastric H^+,K^+-ATPase and hence an effective inhibitor of acid secretion (SACHS et al. 1988). A description of its pharmacokinetics requires some discussion of its mechanism of action. Omeprazole is a protonatabler weak base of pK_a 4.0. The structure of the compound is shown in Fig. 2. There are two protonatable nitrogens, one on the pyridine ring, the other on the benzimidazole ring. With protonation of the latter, there is a nucleophilic attack by the pyridine nitrogen on the benzimidazole carbon, thereby generating a cationic sulphenamide in a series of reversible reactions as shown in Fig. 2. The sulphenamide is considered to be the species that reacts with thiol (SH) groups accessible from the luminal surface of the H^+,K^+-ATPase (LINDBERG et al. 1986; LORENTZON et al. 1987). The compound omeprazole is therefore a pro-drug activated by the acid secreted by its target enzyme, the H^+,K^+-ATPase. With a pKâ of 4.0, omeprazole is

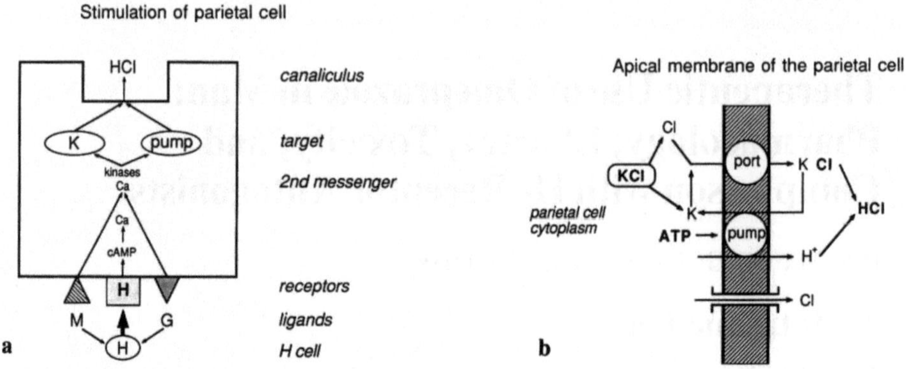

Fig. 1. **a** A model of stimulation of the mammalian parietal cell showing activation of acid secretion by insertion of the acid pump into the canalicula of the parietal cell, and activation of a KCl pathway. **b** A model of the secretory membrane of the parietal cell, showing the presence of the H^+,K^+-ATPase, a Cl conductance, and a KCl pathway to allow H^+ for K^+ exchange by the ATPase

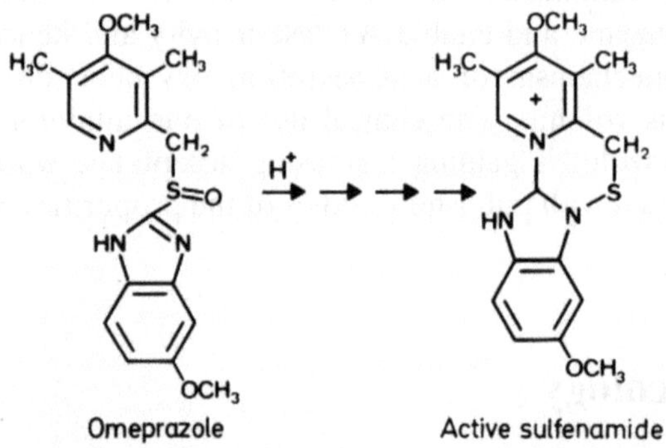

Fig. 2. The chemical conversion of omeprazole, a pro-drug, to its active form by acid in the parietal cell secretory canaliculus. The active sulphenamide reacts with two luminally accessible SH groups in the catalytic subunit of the H^+,K^+-ATPase

concentrated only in the acid spaces of the parietal cell, and being acid labile it must be protected from acid when administered orally. A model of the mechanism of action of omeprazole following oral administration is given in Fig. 3.

II. Plasma Concentrations

Omeprazole is well absorbed from the intestine. Peak plasma concentrations are reached within 2–4 h after oral administration of the encapsulated form of the drug. There are changes in the plasma kinetics of the compound during the first few days of oral administration. The peak plasma concentration is increased by about two fold following 5 days of oral administration, and the

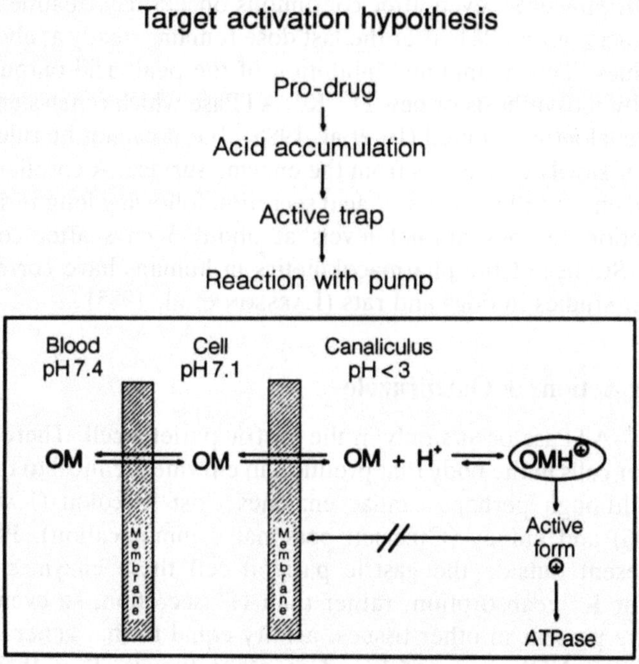

Fig. 3. A schematic representation of the mechanism of action of omeprazole. Omeprazole (*OM*) passes into the parietal cell from the blood and is trapped in the acid spaces of the secreting cell due to the low pH in these spaces. In acid omeprazole is converted into its active form, a cationic sulphenamide, and reacts with the proton pump

terminal half-life is extended from 0.7 to 1.1 h following extended therapy (PRICHARD et al. 1985b).

III. Inhibition of Acid Secretion

The mechanism of inhibition of acid secretion involves the formation of a disulfide bond between the acid-generated sulphenamide of omeprazole and two thiol groups on the H^+,K^+-ATPase. Although the half-life of omeprazole in plasma is about 60 min, the duration of action of omeprazole following a single dose exceeds 24 h due to the stable enzyme inhibitor complex (OLBE et al. 1986). Acid inhibition therefore does not correlate with plasma concentration at any given time point, but with the area under the plasma concentration time curve of omeprazole (LIND et al. 1983). Following a single dose of 20 mg omeprazole, there is marked inhibition of acid secretion for 4–6 h, with moderate inhibition remaining after 24 h (CLISSOLD and CAMPOLI-RICHARDS 1986). With a 20 mg dose repeated over 5 days the inhibition of acid secretion, as monitored by intragastric pH metry, is about 10–100 times more than the inhibition with currently available H_2 receptor antagonists (LIND et al. 1983). However, even after continuous once a day treatment, gastrin-stimulated acid output 24 h after the last dose remains steady at about 35% of control values. This maintained inhibition of the peak acid output could be explained by biosynthesis of new H^+,K^+-ATPase which renews enzyme that has been covalently inhibited (IM et al. 1985), but it cannot be ruled out that the inhibitor slowly dissociates from the enzyme surface. A corollary of this is the time taken for full recovery of acid secretion following long-term therapy. Acid secretion reaches normal levels at about 3 days after cessation of treatment. Studies of the pharmacokinetics in humans have correlated well with similar studies in dogs and rats (LARSSON et al. 1985).

IV. Other Actions of Omeprazole

The H^+,K^+-ATPase occurs only in the gastric parietal cell. There appear to be few other cells in the body that produce an enzyme identical to the H^+,K^+-ATPase, although perhaps similar enzymes exist in colon (KAUNITZ and SACHS 1986) and kidney (GIEBISCH personal communication). Physiologically, if present outside the gastric parietal cell these enzymes would be designed for K^+ reabsorption, rather than H^+ secretion, so even if similar enzymes are present in other tissues, acidity equal to that generated by the gastric H^+,K^+-ATPase is not found in other tissues. It is therefore not surprising that specific extragastric effects of omeprazole have not been found. However, as well as secreting acid, the parietal cell secretes intrinsic factor, and gastric acid is required for activation of pepsinogen to pepsin. Furthermore, inhibition of acid secretion also results in failure to suppress gastrin secretion stimulated by meals.

1. Effect on Secretion of Intrinsic Factor and Vitamin B_{12} Absorption

Studies examining the effect of omeprazole treatment on both intrinsic factor secretion and B_{12} absorption showed that omeprazole had no effect on either parameter (KITTANG et al. 1985, 1987). Omeprazole does not inhibit the morphological change seen in parietal cells after stimulation which involves transfer of tubulovesicles into the microvilli of the secretory canaliculus. It may be presumed therefore that it is the formation of the stimulated state that is correlated with intrinsic factor secretion, rather than the acid secretion produced by the H^+,K^+-ATPase (KITTANG et al. 1985, 1987).

2. Effect on Pepsin

Pepsin is secreted by the chief cells of the gastric gland as the zymogen, pepsinogen. For secretion to appear in the gastrin lumen and to be measurable as pepsin, both acid and volume flow have to be present. In fact, pepsin output is reduced by about 40% by omeprazole treatment, while acid secretion was reduced in these studies by 75% (PEDERSEN et al. 1987). It appears, therefore, that omeprazole has no direct effect on chief cell function.

3. Effects on Motility

Studies of the effect of omeprazole on lower esophageal sphincter pressure (PEDERSEN et al. 1987), gastric emptying of either a liquid or solid meal (HOROWITZ et al. 1984), and the migrating motor complex (PEDERSEN et al. 1987) have shown that omeprazole has no action on upper gastrointestinal motility.

4. Effects on Gastric Endocrine Function

As mentioned above, acid secretion that reaches the G cell in the gastric antrum inhibits gastrin release. Gastrin release is stimulated by a variety of amino acids in gastric contents. Inhibition of acid secretion with a meal should then increase plasma gastrin concentrations. Indeed, a dose of 20 mg omeprazole daily for 4 weeks (which markedly inhibits gastric acid secretion) increased serum gastrin from 10 to 22 pg/ml, but it fell to normal values in 2 weeks after treatment (ARNOLD et al. 1986). Antral gastrin concentration did not differ from that in controls given placebo and the volume densities of G cells and D cells in gastric mucosa were unchanged.

In Sprague-Dawley rats given high doses of omeprazole therapy there is hyperplasia of the neuroendocrine cells in the oxyntic mucosa enterochromaffin-like (ECL) cells which correlates with increases in gastrin levels (SUNDLER et al. 1986), and prolonged omeprazole administration leads to the formation of gastric carcinoids (CARLSSON et al. 1986). These changes are not seen in man, dogs, or mice. Indeed, the two- to fourfold increases in levels of gastrin reached with omeprazole therapy in humans (LANZON-MILLER et al. 1987; KOOP et al. 1987; BRUNNER et al. 1988) are much less than those seen

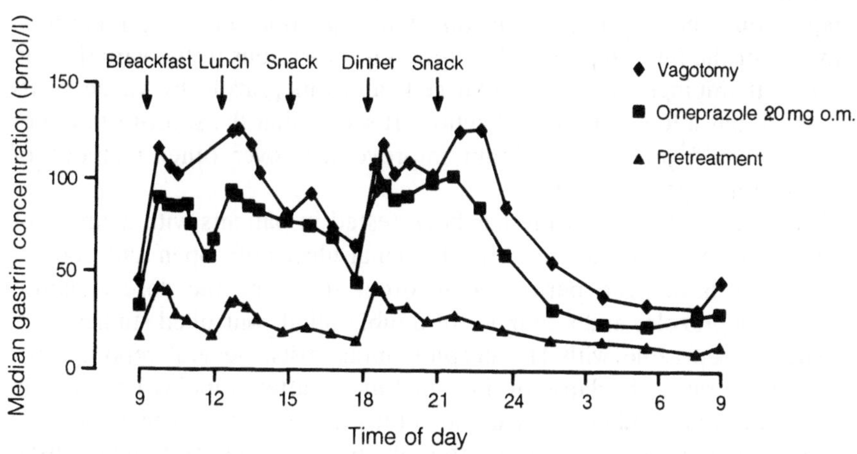

Fig. 4. Plasma gastrin levels in duodenal ulcer patients following highly selective vagotomy and chronic omeprazole treatment, showing equivalence of gastrin levels in the two treatments as compared to control (courtesy of L. OLBE, Gothenburg)

in pernicious anemia and are the same as found after selective vagotomy (Fig. 4). (OLBE personal communication). There appears to be no risk to the gastric endocrine cell population with the use of omeprazole in man in short-term treatment of acid-peptic diseases. The effects of chronic treatment with omeprazole await evaluation. However, after continuous therapy over a 3-year perriod with large doses of omeprazole of 40 mg/day no significant changes in the endocrine population have been found in man (LAMBERTS et al. 1988).

C. Therapeutic Trials in Acid-Peptic Diseases

I. Overview

The inhibition of acid secretion by surgical or chemical means has been the best available therapy to date for the treatment of acid-peptic diseases. Alternative therapies such as sucralfate (mechanism unknown) or treatment of infection by *Helicobacter pylori* perhaps have application in duodenal ulcer disease but show lesser benefits in gastric or esophageal lesions. Inhibition of acid secretion must reach a certain plateau to result in healing and prevention of ulcers. Because the neutralizing capacity of the duodenum exceeds that of the stomach, which in turn exceeds that of the esophagus, progressively greater inhibition is required in treatment of duodenal ulcer, gastric ulcer, and reflux esophagitis. Furthermore, in diseases of acid hypersecretion such as Zollinger-Ellison syndrome and in damage caused by nonsteroidal anti-inflammatory drugs, marked inhibition of acid secretion is required to ensure mucosal integrity.

The range of stimuli that affect the parietal cell is large, and the duration of action of available receptor antagonists is short. It seems therefore that therapy would be improved with longer acting, more effective inhibitors. Inhibition of the final step of acid secretion is impervious to the variations in stimuli that impinge on the parietal cell, and omeprazole by virtue of its mechanism has a long duration of action. It seems that the short-term use of this drug would provide significant improvement over other methods of treatment for peptic diseases.

The efficacy of omeprazole has been tested in patients with avariety of acid-peptic disease. In patients with duodenal ulcer both open and double-blind studies have been performed in order to define the dose–response range of omeprazole, and a number of double-blind controlled studies have compared omeprazole with H_2 receptor antagonists. Several reports have examined the rates of relapse of duodenal ulcers after stopping omeprazole therapy, and some studies have examined the effect of omeprazole in patients with duodenal ulcers resistant to therapy with H_2 receptor antagonists. Similar types of studies have been performed in patients with gastric ulcer and in patients with reflux esophagitits. Finally, omeprazole has been used in a number of open studies in patients with Zollinger-Ellison syndrome, and the effects of omeprazole on symptoms, mucosal disease, and acid secretory rates have been examined. These therapeutic trials in more than 13000 patients have generated a considerable amount of short-term, and also long-term toxicity data.

II. Duodenal Ulcer

1. Effect of Different Doses of Omeprazole

A number of studies have examined the effects of different doses of omeprazole in patients with duodenal ulcer (Table 1). These studies have been of three types: open studies which examined the efficacy of a single dose of omeprazole, double-blind trials that compared the effects of two or more doses of omeprazole, and one double-blind study of omeprazole versus placebo. As the results in these three types of studies are virtually the same, the results of these studies will be discussed together. In all these studies the patients had duodenal ulcers (in most studies at least 0.5 cm in diameter) documented at endoscopy, and in the double-blind studies randomization produced comparable groups of patients. Omeprazole was administered once per day in all the studies.

The doses of omeprazole used varied from 10 to 60 mg/day. In every study there was rapid relief of symptoms. In studies in which symptoms were monitored after 1 week of therapy, there was a marked reduction in the number of patients with symptoms and a reduction in the severity of the symptoms in those patients with remaining symptoms (GUSTAVSSON et al. 1983; NAESDAL et al. 1985; British Cooperative Study 1984; PRICHARD et al. 1985a). In three studies where symptoms were assessed after 2 weeks of therapy all symptoms had resolved (RINETTI et al. 1986; Scandinavian Multicentre Study 1984) and in all nine studies, nearly all patients were symptom-free after 4 weeks of therapy. In those studies in which antacid consumption was monitored, use of antacids declined markedly and rapidly during omeprazole therapy (NAESDAL et al. 1985; British Cooperative Study 1984; PRICHARD et al. 1985).

In the studies that examined the effects of different doses of omeprazole (GUSTAVSSON et al. 1983; PRICHARD et al. 1985; HÜTTEMANN et al. 1986; Belgian Multicentre Group 1986) there were no significant differences between the rates and degree of symptom relief in the different groups of patients.

The effect of different doses of omeprazole on healing of duodenal ulcers is shown in Table 1. In two studies that used omeprazole 10 mg/day, 83% of all ulcers were healed after 4 weeks of therapy (LAURITSEN et al. 1989; PRICHARD et al. 1985), while in all the other studies using 20–60 mg/day, healing rates were 90% – 100% after 4 weeks. Thus, there was little or no gain in ulcer healing :ates after 4 weeks by using more than 20 mg omeprazole

Table 1. Effects of different doses of omeprazole on ulcer healing in patients with duodenal ulcer

Reference	Type of study	Patients (*n*)	Omeprazole dose (mg)	Percentage of patients with healed ulcers	
				After 2 weeks	After 4 weeks
Gustavsson et al. (1983)	DB	32	20 60	63 100*	93 100
Bader et al. (1986)	O	65	30	83	98
British Cooperative Study (1984)	O	43	20 30 40 60	– – – –	90 100 90 100
Scandinavian Multicentre Study (1984)	O	27	40	–	96
Prichard et al. (1985a)	DB	66	10 30	50 78*	83 94
Naesdal et al. (1985)	DB[a]	44	40	93	100
Hütteman et al. (1986)	DB	115	20 30	79 73	97 93
Belgian Multicentre Group (1986)	DB	62	30 60	75 57	100 97
Karvonen et al. (1986)	O	18	40	–	100
Rinetti et al. (1986)	O	16	30	88	100
Graham et al. (1988)	DB	102 51	20 Placebo	41** 13	75** 27
Lauritsen et al. (1989)	DB	77 78	10 20	48 74**	75 91**

* Significantly different, $P < 0.05$; ** significantly different, $P < 0.001$
Abbreviations: O, open; DB, double-blind.
[a] Half the patients were given 80 mg omeprazole on day 1, followed by 40 mg/day. There were no differences between healing rates in the two groups.

daily. However, when healing rates of duodenal ulcers after 2 weeks of therapy were examined there were significant differences between the results with various doses. Gustavsson et al. (1983) found healing rates of 63% in patients who took 20 mg/day and 100% in patients who took 60 mg/day ($P < 0.05$), and Prichard et al. (1985a) found healing rates of 50% in patients who took 10 mg/day and 78% in patients who took 30 mg/day ($P < 0.05$). Summarizing all the data on healing rates at 2 weeks in the studies shown in Table 1, it appears that there is a progressive increase in healing rates at 2 weeks from 50% to >90% when the dose of omeprazole is increased from 10 to 40 mg/day. However, when comparing 20 and 30 mg in the same study no difference in healing rate was found.

A number of subgroups of patients with duodenal ulcer were identified in these studies in whom ulcer healing rates differed. Three studies demonstrated that smaller ulcers healed more quickly than larger ulcers (Belgian Multicentre Group 1986; HÜTTEMANN et al. 1986; NAESDAL et al. 1985), and one study demonstrated faster healing in males and in those older than 55 years (HUTTEMANN et al. 1986). Duodenal ulcers that occur in patients who smoke are known to be more resistant to therapy with H_2 receptor antagonists than ulcers occurring in nonsmokers (ELASHOF and GROSSMAN 1980; KORMAN et al. 1983). PRICHARD et al. (1985a) found that in nonsmokers there was no difference in ulcer healing rates when taking 10 or 30 mg omeprazole daily but that 30 mg/day produced significantly greater healing rates than 10 mg/day in smokers after both 2 and 4 weeks of therapy. In two other studies there was no significant difference in healing rates between smokers and nonsmokers, but all the patients with unhealed ulcers after 4 weeks of therapy were smokers (GUSTAVSSON et al. 1983; HÜTTEMANN et al. 1986).

These studies using different doses of omeprazole clearly establish that the drug is effective in producing symptom relief and healing the majority of patients with duodenal ulcers. Some have argued that since 20 mg/day heals 90% of all ulcers after 4 weeks of therapy there is no need to use larger doses [though possibly bigger doses will be needed in the United States (GRAHAM et al. 1988)]. Others suggest that as healing of duodenal ulcers is not checked routinely by follow-up endoscopy, the dose of omeprazole used should be the maximally effective dose in order to heal "all" ulcers. However, as occasional patients with duodenal ulcers prescribed omeprazole 60 mg/day have failed to achieve ulcer healing after 4 weeks of therapy (Belgian Multicentre Group 1986), a dose of omeprazole that heals all ulcers may not be practicable.

2. Comparative Studies of Omeprazole and H_2 Receptor Antagonists

Eleven double-blind studies have compared the efficacy of omeprazole in doses of 10–40 mg/day with conventional doses of H_2 antagonists (cimetidine 400–600 mg b.i.d., or ranitidine 150 mg b.i.d. or 300 mg at night) (Table 2). In all but one study, data are available on symptom relief. Five studies demonstrated significant advantages for omeprazole over H_2 receptor antagonists in alleviating symptoms. BARDHAN et al. (1986) and BIGARD et al. (1987) noted that omeprazole was superior to H_2 antagonists at improving daytime pain ($P < 0.01$) but there was no significant difference in the effect of the two drugs on nocturnal pain or other symptoms. Studies by ARCHAMBAULT et al. (1988), MARKS et al. (1988), and DAHLGREN et al. (1988) noted that after 2 weeks' therapy significantly fewer patients taking omeprazole had symptoms than the H_2 antagonist-treated group ($P < 0.01$). Other studies demonstrated a trend for omeprazole to improve symptoms faster and more effectively but the differences did not reach statistical significance (LAURITSEN et al. 1985; HUI et al. 1987; GUSTAVSSON et al. 1987; VAN DEVENTER et al. 1988). One

Table 2. Double-blind controlled trials comparing the efficacy of omeprazole and H_2* receptor antagonists in inducing ulcer healing in patients with duodenal ulcer

Reference	Drug dose (mg/day)	Patients (n)	Percentage of patients with healed ulcers	
			After 2 weeks	After 4 weeks
LAURITSEN et al. (1985)	O 30	67	73**	92*
	C 1000	65	46	74
CLASSEN et al. (1985a)	O 20	146	72*	96
	R 300	160	59	92
BARDHAN et al. (1986)	O 20	33	83*	97*
	O 40	36	83*	100*
	R 300	33	53	82
HETZEL et al. (1988)	O 40	41	82**	100*
	C 800	47	49	80
HUI et al. (1987)	O 10	88	75*	92
	O 20	90	81**	92
	R 300	89	62	89
GUSTAVSSON et al. (1987)[a]	O 40	45	76**	98**
	C 800	42	40	71
BIGARD et al. (1987)	O 20	124	64**	90*
	C 800	131	44	79
ARCHAMBAULT et al. (1988)	O 20	80	58	84
	C 1200	79	46	80
MARKS et al. (1988)	O 20	69	65*	97*
	R 300	66	39	81
VAN DEVENTER et al. (1988)	O 20	151	42**	82**
	R 300	158	34	63
DAHLGREN et al. (1988)	O 30	79	66*	97*
	C 800	73	45	84

* $P < 0.05$; ** $P < 0.001$ compared with H_2 receptor antagonist.
Abbreviations: O, omeprazole; C, cimetidine; R, rantidine.
[a] Study included 17 patients with prepyloric ulcers. Data not given separately.

study found that patients taking omeprazole consumed less antacids than patients taking ranitidine (BARDHAN et al. 1986), but three other studies found no differences in antacid consumption in omeprazoletreated and H_2 antagonist-treated groups (BIGARD et al. 1987; ARCHAMBAULT et al. 1988; MARKS et al. 1988).

The results of these comparative studies on ulcer healing are shown in Table 2. In general healing rates in patients taking omeprazole were similar to those in the noncomparative studies (see above), except that in Chinese patients 10 mg/day was as effective as 20 mg/day (HUI et al. 1987), and in Canadian and U.S. patients 20 mg/day produced lower healing rates than other studies (ARCHAMBAULT et al. 1988; VAN DEVENTER et al. 1987). Similarly, healing rates of ulcers in those patients treated with cimetidine or ranitidine were similar to results obtained previously with these drugs (BROGDEN et al. 1978, 1985). All the comparative studies but one (ARCHAMBAULT et al. 1988) showed significantly greater healing rates in patients taking omeprazole after 2 weeks of therapy. The therapeutic advantage for omeprazole over H_2 antagonists varied from 8% to 36% (mean 23%), as shown in Table 2. After 4 weeks of therapy omeprazole produced significantly higher healing rates than H_2 antagonists in eight of the studies (LAURITSEN et al. 1985; BARDHAN et al. 1986; HETZEL et al. 1986; GUSTAVSSON et al. 1987; BIGARD et al. 1987; MARKS et al. 1988, VAN DEVENTER et al. 1988; DAHLGREN et al. 1988). In two other studies healing rates in omeprazole-treated and H_2 antagonist-treated groups were around 90%, thus obscuring significant differences between the patient groups (CLASSEN et al. 1985a; HUI et al. 1987). In no study was there a therapeutic advantage for the H_2 antagonist at any time point, though the advantage for omeprazole over H_2 antagonists was less after 4 weeks (4%–27%, mean 14%) than after 2 weeks of therapy (Table 2).

Three of the comparative studies examined healing of ulcers after 6 weeks (DAHLGREN et al. 1988; GUSTAVSSON et al. 1987; ARCHAMBAULT et al. 1988) and one (BARDHAN et al. 1986) after 8 weeks of therapy. In only one case (DAHLGREN et al. 1988) was there a significant difference between the omeprazole and H_2 receptor antagonist groups, because after 6–8 weeks of therapy about 90% of all ulcers had healed in all treatment groups.

As exhibited in the noncomparative studies, in the studies comparing omeprazole with H_2 antagonists, differences in healing rates were observed in subgroups of patients. Three studies found that ulcer healing was delayed in smokers taking omeprazole and H_2 antagonists (CLASSEN et al. 1985a; HUI et al. 1987; DAHLGREN et al. 1988), but others (LAURITSEN et al. 1985; ARCHAMBAULT et al. 1988; MARKS et al. 1988) found that smoking had no effect on ulcer healing in any patient group. CLASSEN et al. (1985a) found that smaller ulcers healed faster than large ones, and HUI et al. (1987) found that ulcer healing was delayed in patients less than 30 years old, those with increased acid secretion, and those with remissions of less than 5 months.

Overall it appears from these comparative studies that omeprazole in doses of 20–40 mg heals ulcers faster than conventional doses of H_2 antagonists. This difference is clear at 2 weeks, is less evident at 4 weeks, and is no longer demonstrable after 6–8 weeks of therapy. Although H_2 antagonists and omeprazole produce rapid and effective resolution of symptoms, omeprazole seems to produce somewhat faster and more complete improvement than does ranitidine or cimetidine.

3. Relapse After Stopping Omeprazole Therapy

In patients with duodenal ulcers that have healed with H_2 receptor antagonist therapy, relapse rates of 50%–60% 6 months after stopping therapy have been reported (BARDHAN et al. 1986; BROGDEN et al. 1982). Two noncomparative studies of the use of omeprazole have examined relapse rates after stopping therapy. NAESDAL et al. (1985) observed that in 44 patients whose ulcers had healed on omeprazole, 18 had a symptomatic relapse within 6 months (range 2–23 weeks, mean 14). Of these, 15 patients were endoscoped and eight had duodenal ulcers, indicating a recurrence rate of up to 23%. In the British Cooperative Study (1984) 44% of 36 patients developed symptomatic relapses, and duodenal ulcers were found in 11, a relapse rate in 6 months of 31%. In a study comparing omeprazole with ranitidine, GUSTAVSSON et al. (1987) found an 8-week relapse rate of 26% in patients whose ulcers were healed with omeprazole, and a 58% relapse rate in patients whose ulcers were healed with cimetidine ($P < 0.05$). BARDHAN et al. (1986) followed patients after the ulcers had been healed, and endoscoped them at 3 and 6 months, or sooner if they developed symptoms. After 6 months 58% of patients whose ulcers had healed with 20 mg omeprazole, 83% of patients who had taken 40 mg omeprazole, and 60% of those who had taken ranitidine had developed recurrent duodenal ulceration. LAURITSEN et al. (1985) followed 91 patients whose duodenal ulcers had been healed. Forty-five percent of those healed with omeprazole relapsed within 6 months, as compared with 59% of those healed with cimetidine (NS). DAHLGREN et al. (1988) found a 54% relapse rate in patients who had stopped omeprazole and a 56% rate in those who had stopped cimetidine therapy (NS). Overall, these studies indicate that relapse rates of duodenal ulcers are probably similar whether the ulcers have been healed by omeprazole or H_2 receptor antagonists. Thus although omeprazole does not confer any advantage in preventing relapse, the more rapid healing with omeprazole therapy is not associated with a more rapid relapse rate.

4. Omeprazole Treatment for Ulcers Resistant to H_2 Receptor Antagonists

Several studies have determined the efficacy of omeprazole in healing duodenal ulcers resistant to conventional or larger doses of H_2 receptor antagonists. Three of these studies (TYTGAT et al. 1987; PEN et al. 1988; BRUNNER et al. 1988) simply switched the patients to omeprazole and examined healing rates, while three other studies (BARDHAN et al. 1988a,b; French Cooperative Study 1987) randomized the patients to omeprazole or H_2 receptor antagonists and compared the ability of the two regimens to heal ulcers.

TYTGAT et al. (1987) studied 18 patients of whom 14 had duodenal or jejunal ulcers. All ulcers had failed to heal on at least 6 months of H_2 receptor antagonist therapy with or without pirenzepine or mucosal protective agents. When the patients were switched to omeprazole 40 mg/day all the ulcers healed, usually within 2 weeks, and all within 8 weeks. Patients were then put on cimetidine or ranitidine but 12 of the 15 patients (80%) had relapsed by 1 year. PEN et al. (1988) gave omeprazole 40 mg/day to 11 patients whose duodenal ulcers had not healed after 6 months of full dose H_2 receptor antagonist therapy. All ulcers healed after 4–8 weeks of omeprazole, and when eight patients were put on maintenance therapy of omeprazole 20 mg/

day there was only one relapse at 9 months. BRUNNER et al. (1988) gave omeprazole 40 mg/day to 11 patients with duodenal ulcers that had not healed after at least 3 months of ranitidine 450–600 mg/day. All the ulcers healed after 4 weeks of omeprazole, and on omeprazole 40 mg/day as maintenance there were no relapses.

The French Cooperative Study (1987) examined 151 patients with duodenal ulcers that had failed to heal on at least 6 weeks of cimetidine 800 mg/day or ranitidine 300 mg/day. The patients were randomized to omeprazole 20 mg daily or ranitidine 150 mg b.i.d. There was rapid symptomatic relief in both groups, and healing rates were similar at 4 weeks (48% for the omeprazole and 46% for the ranitidine group) and 8 weeks (80% and 75%). In a study of similar design BARDHAN et al. (1988b) randomized 119 patients with ulcers (88% duodenal ulcers) that had failed to heal on at least 8 weeks of cimetidine 800–1000 mg/day or ranitidine 300 mg/day, to either omeprazole 40 mg/day or continuation of the H_2 receptor antagonist. After 4 weeks the healing rate of the omeprazole group was 87% and that of the H_2 receptor antagonist group, 39% ($P < 0.001$), and after 8 weeks' therapy the rates were 98% and 60% ($P < 0.001$). Omeprazole was also significantly better than H_2 receptor antagonists at producing pain relief. In a further study BARDHAN et al. (1988b) tested omeprazole in a group of patients with so-called ultra-resistant ulcers that had failed to heal after at least 3 months of cimetidine 2000 mg or 3000 mg/day. Patients were randomized to continue with cimetidine or receive omeprazole 40 mg/day for 8 weeks, after which those patients with ulcers that had failed to heal were crossed over to the other therapy. Of the patients that received omeprazole, 24 of 26 healed. When the failures on cimetidine were given omeprazole, seven of eight healed but neither of the two failures on omeprazole healed. Overall, 31 of 33 patients healed with omeprazole and 16 of 24 healed with cimetidine – a significant difference.

Including both the open and the comparative trials, five of the six studies demonstrate that omeprazole can heal a large proportion of duodenal ulcers that are resistant to H_2 receptor antagonists, and that omeprazole 40 mg/day is probably superior to continuing the H_2 receptor antagonist. Only the French study failed to demonstrate any difference between omeprazole and ranitidine, both drugs healing the majority of ulcers, and that study had the least stringent definition of resistance i.e., failure to heal after only 6 weeks of H_2 receptor antagonists in conventional doses and used only 20 mg/day of omeprazole. It may be that the more "resistant" the ulcers are, the more likely they are to be healed only by omeprazole.

III. Gastric Ulcer

1. Noncomparative Studies of Omeprazole

Two open studies examined the efficacy of omeprazole 30 mg/day in patients with gastric ulcer. HÜTTEMANN et al. (1986) studied 32 patients and found

Table 3. Double-blind controlled trials comparing the efficacy of omeprazole and ranitidine in inducing ulcer healing in patients with gastric ulcer

Reference	Drug (mg/day)	Patients (n)	Percentage of patients with healed ulcers		
			After 2 weeks	After 4 weeks	After 6–8 weeks
CLASSEN et al.	O 20	184	43	81	95
(1985b)	R 300	45	45	80	90
BARBARA et al.	O 20	80	35*	74*	96*
(1987)	R 300	80	9	53	85
BATE et al.	O 20	105	–	73*	84
(1988)	C 800	92	–	55	74
LAURITSEN et al.	O 30	82	54*[a]	81	86
(1988)	C 1000	78	39	73	78
WALAN et al.	O 20	203	–	69**	89
(1989)	O 40	195	–	80**	96**
	R 300	205	–	59	85

* $P < 0.05$; ** $P < 0.001$ compared with H_2 receptor antagonist.
Abbreviations: O, omeprazole; C, cimetidine; R, ranitidine.
[a] Significant only on intention to treat figures.

more than 70% to be free of symptoms after 14 days' therapy. Healing rates were 22% after 2 weeks' and 72% after 4 weeks' treatment, similar results to those obtained in previous studies of H_2 receptor antagonists (BROGDEN et al. 1978, 1982). DARLE et al. (1986) gave omeprazole 30 mg/day to 27 patients and found healing rates of 69% after 2 weeks and 92% after 6 weeks of treatment.

2. Comparative Studies of Omeprazole and Ranitidine

Four double-blind studies have compared the efficacy of omeprazole and ranitidine in patients with ulcers of the gastric body and antrum, and one study examined a group of patients with prepyloric ulcers (LAURITSEN et al. 1988) (Table 3). One of the studies that included both antral and gastric body ulcers found no significant differences in symptoms on the two drugs (CLASSEN et al. 1985b), but two other studies found that symptoms resolved faster in the omeprazole-treated group. BARBARA et al. (1987), WALAN et al. (1989), and BATE et al. (1988) found that after 4 weeks' therapy significantly more omeprazole-treated patients were symptom-free (81% vs 60%, $P < 0.01$) and the omeprazole group consumed less antacid. The study of prepyloric ulcers (LAURITSEN et al. 1988) found that after the 1st week significantly more omeprazole-treated patients were symptom-free than in the ranitidine group, but overall, the number of hours of pain in the two groups was not significantly different. In these studies healing of ulcers was assessed at 2, (CLASSEN et al.

1985b; BARBARA et al. 1987; LAURITSEN et al. 1988), 4, and 6 or at 4 and 8 weeks (Table 3). One study showed no significant difference between omeprazole and ranitidine at any time point (CLASSEN et al. 1985b). In the other studies the rates of healing on omeprazole were significantly greater than those on ranitidine or cimetidine after 4 weeks' therapy (BARBARA et al. 1987; WALAN et al. 1989; BATE et al. 1988), with 40 mg omeprazole being more effective than 20 mg omeprazole in the one study where two doses were given (WALAN et al. 1989). In only two of the four studies was omeprazole superior to ranitidine after 6–8 weeks' therapy (BARBARA et al. 1987; WALAN et al. 1989). In the study of prepyloric ulcers, omeprazole was superior to ranitidine in producing ulcer healing after 2 weeks of therapy, but thereafter the drugs were equally efficacious (LAURITSEN et al. 1988). These studies contained subgroups of patients whose ulcers healed more slowly than others. CLASSEN et al. (1985b) and WALAN et al. (1989) found that large ulcers healed more slowly than small ones, and CLASSEN et al. (1985b) but not WALAN et al. (1989) that ulcers in the gastric body healed more slowly than prepyloric ulcers. In the studies by CLASSEN et al. (1985b) and WALAN et al. (1989) smoking had no effect on ulcer healing; the effects of smoking were not examined in the other studies.

In summary, comparative trials of omeprazole and H_2 receptor antagonists have demonstrated that omeprazole 20–40 mg produces faster, and in some cases greater healing rates than does ranitidine 150 b.i.d. or cimetidine 400 mg b.i.d. Omeprazole is effective for ulcers of both the gastric body and the antrum. The reasons for the failure of the study of CLASSEN et al. (1985b) to demonstrate any advantage of omeprazole over ranitidine is not clear but could be related to the fact that patients will small (<5 cm) ulcers were included, and in that study there was a greater response to ranitidine than in the other studies (Table 3).

3. Relapse After Stopping Omeprazole Therapy

In the study by WALAN et al. (1989) those patients whose ulcers were healed were then followed for 6 months. The patients whose ulcers had been healed by omeprazole had significantly fewer symptomatic relapses and recurrent ulcers than the patients whose ulcers had been healed with ranitidine. However, another study (Danish Multicentre Study Group 1988) of 218 patients whose gastric ulcers had been healed with 30 mg omeprazole or 1000 mg cimetidine per day found no difference between recurrence rate of symptoms or ulcers in a 6-month period after cessation of therapy. They did note, however, that relapses were more likely to occur in patients who were smokers and in those who had prepyloric ulcers.

4. Omeprazole Treatment for Ulcers Resistant to H_2 Receptor Antagonists

BARDHAN et al. (1988b) treated 19 patients with gastric ulcers as part of a group of 99 patients with peptic ulcers that had failed to heal on cimetidine

800–1000 mg/day or ranitidine 300 mg/day. Patients were randomized to continue with the H_2 receptor antagonist or take omeprazole 40 mg/day. After 8 weeks of therapy 98% of the omeprazole group had healed, but only 60% of the H_2 receptor antagonist group ($P < 0.001$). The study by TYTGAT et al. (1987) included three patients with gastric ulcers that had failed to heal with 6 months' therapy with H_2 receptor antagonists. All three ulcers healed with omeprazole 40 mg/day within 8 weeks. BRUNNER et al. (1988) treated 43 patients with gastric ulcers that had failed to heal with 3 months or more of ranitidine 450–600 mg/day. In all but two cases omeprazole 40 mg/day healed the ulcers within 8 weeks.

As with duodenal ulcer, omeprazole is capable of healing most gastric ulcers that have failed to heal with H_2 receptor antagonists. These data further suggest that small amounts of gastric acid are a major factor in the failure of some gastric ulcers to heal – a suggestion that has been disputed in the past.

IV. Reflux Esophagitis

1. Effect of Different Doses of Omeprazole

The only trials of different doses of omeprazole in patients with reflux esophagitis, other than the studies comparing omeprazole with ranitidine, come from Australia (Table 4). An open pilot study of omeprazole 30 mg/day in eight patients demonstrated complete symptom relief in seven patients after 2 weeks, and impressive healing rates of 75% at 4 weeks and 88% at 8 weeks (DENT et al. 1987). These data compared with previously published rates of healing of esophagitis by H_2 receptor antagonists of about 60% at 8 weeks (RICHTER 1986). A subsequent double-blind trial of omeprazole 20 or 40 mg/day compared with placebo confirmed the effectiveness of omeprazole therapy in abolishing heartburn (this was achieved in 81% of patients com-

Table 4. Effect of different doses of omeprazole on the healing of reflux esophagitis

Reference	Drug dose (mg/day)	Patients (n)	Type of study	Percentage of patients with healed esophagitis	
				After 4 weeks	After 8 weeks
DENT et al. (1987)	30	8	Open	75	88
HETZEL et al. (1988)	20	82	Double-blind	70	79
	40	82		82*	85
	Placebo	32		6**	

* $P < 0.05$ compared with other omeprazole-treated groups.
** $P < 0.001$ compared with omeprazole-treated groups.

pared with 6% on placebo: $P < 0.001$) and in healing esophagitis (HETZEL et al. 1988). The same gruop subsequently compared 20 and 40 mg omeprazole daily in 164 patients in a double-blind study and found that while 40 mg/day produced significantly greater healing rates after 4 weeks' treatment, by 8 weeks both treatment groups were comparable (HETZEL et al. 1988). When the patient groups were analyzed on the basis of severity of esophagitis, the benefits of 40 mg omeprazole compared to 20 mg were significant for grades 2 and 3 but not grade 4 after 4 weeks of therapy. With respect to symptoms, heartburn was abolished in 57% of patients taking omeprazole 20 mg/day and 72% of those taking to 40 mg/day ($P < 0.05$) but by 4 weeks of therapy there was no difference between the groups (HETZEL et al. 1988).

These studies established that omeprazole effectively treated heartburn and produced healing of esophagitis when used in doses of 20–40 mg/day. The 40 mg/day produced faster resolution of symptoms and healing of esophagitis, but 20 and 40 mg/day were equally effective after 8 weeks of therapy.

2. Comparative Studies of Omeprazole and H_2 Receptor Antagonists

Seven studies have compared the effectiveness of omeprazole 20–60my/day with ranitidine 150 mg b.i.d. and one with cimetidine 400 mg q.i.d. in healing reflux esophagitis (Table 5). All these studies were double-blind and had adequate numbers of comparable patients in the different treatment groups. In all but one study symptoms and mucosal healing were assessed after 4 and 8 weeks of therapy; in the other, assessments were made after 3 and 6 weeks (Table 5).

Every study found omeprazole to be superior to ranitidine in producing symptom relief. Four studies found that after 4 weeks of therapy omeprazole abolished heartburn in 71%–92% of patients, whereas ranitidine or cimetidine abolished heartburn in 24%–59% of cases ($P < 0.01$ in each study) (SANDMARK et al. 1988; VANTRAPPEN et al. 1988; ZEITOUN et al. 1987; DEHN et al. 1988). The other studies all found that omeprazole caused resolution of heartburn more rapidly and to a greater extent than did ranitidine (DAMANN et al. 1986; KLINKENBERG-KNOLL et al. 1987; HAVELUND et al. 1988) ($P < 0.001$). KLINKENBERG-KNOL et al. (1987) found omeprazole to be superior to ranitidine in resolving regurgitation or dysphagia, and antacid consumption was less in patients taking omeprazole but the differences were not significant. However, HAVELUND et al. (1988) found patients taking omeprazole did require less antacid.

As shown in Table 5, each of the comparative studies demonstrated that omeprazole healed reflux esophagitis more rapidly and more effectively than did ranitidine. After 4 weeks of therapy omeprazole healed 67%–85% of patients with esophagitis, and ranitidine healed 27%–45% ($P < 0.001$). Comparable figures after 8 weeks of therapy were 85%–95% healing by omeprazole and 38%–65% healing by ranitidine (Table 5). In general, these

Table 5. Double-blind controlled trials comparing the efficacy of omeprazole and ranitidine in inducing healing of reflux esophagitis

Reference	Drug dose (mg/day)	Patients (n)	Percentage of patients with healed esophagitis	
			After 4 weeks[a]	After 8 weeks[a]
DAMMAN et al. (1986)	O 40	98/19[b]	60*	84*
	R 300	89/20	50*	45
KLINKENBERG KNOL et al. (1987)	O 60	25	76**	88**
	R 300	26	27	38
VAN TRAPPEN et al. (1988)	O 40	31	85**	95**
	R 300	30	40	52
ZEITOUN et al. (1987)	O 20	62	81**	95**
	R 300	69	45	65
SANDMARK et al. (1988)	O 20	152	67**	85**
	R 300		31	50
HAVELUND et al. (1988)[c]	O 40	162	75**	85**
	R 300		26	44
DEHN et al. (1988)	O 40	36	57**	74**
	C 1600	31	29	28

* $P < 0.005$; ** $P < 0.001$ compared with H_2 receptor antagonist.
Abbreviations: O, omeprazole; R, ranitidine.
[a] Except for study 1, in which patients were assessed after 3 and 6 weeks.
[b] Study stopped when animal toxicity data became available; 164 patients assessed after 3 weeks and 39 after 6 weeks.
[c] Data are included only for grades 2/3; higher rates of healing were observed in grade 1.

comparative studies confirmed the results of the noncomparative studies with omeprazole (see above) and the trials of H_2 receptor antagonists (RICHTER 1986) in healing esophagitis. Most studies included only patients with erosive esophagitis but in one study that stratified cases into grade 1 and grade 2/3 esophagitis, the benefits of omeprazole over ranitidine were particularly marked in the patients with more severe esophagitis (grades 2/3) (HAVELUND et al. 1988).

3. Relapse After Stopping Omeprazole Therapy

Very few data on relapse of esophagitis after cessation of therapy are available. HETZEL et al. (1988) monitored 107 patients in whom esophagitis had healed; if symptoms of reflux recurred the patients were endoscoped and all patients were endoscoped after 6 months. Of these 107 patients, 25% were found to have relapsed 1 month and 82% 6 months after stopping omeprazole.

4. Omeprazole Treatment for Reflux Esophagitis Resistant to H_2 Receptor Antagonists

FAUSA et al. (1987) studied four patients in whom more than 3 months of cimetidine 1200 mg/day or ranitidine 300 mg/day had failed to heal esophagitis.

When given omeprazole 40 mg/day, three of the patients had healed by 4 weeks, and all four by 8 weeks of therapy, and none relapsed when put on maintenance of omeprazole 20 mg/day. HETZEL et al. (1986) described a single patient with severe hemorrhagic esophagitis unresponsive to ranitidine 300 mg b.i.d. which showed a dramatic response to omeprazole 40 mg/day, and then maintenance with 20 mg/day. BARDHAN et al. (1987) gave omeprazole 40 mg/day to 38 patients whose esophagitis had failed to heal after more than 3 months of cimetidine 3200 mg/ady. Symptoms were abolished or improved in 90%, and complete or near complete healing occurred in 87% after 8 weeks of omeprazole therapy. BRUNNER et al. (1988) treated 28 patients with esophagitis that had failed to heal after at least 3 months of ranitidine 450–600 mg/day. All 28 healed after 4–12 weeks of omeprazole 40 mg/day. In the double-blind study of omeprazole versus ranitidine listed above, KLINKENBERG-KNOL et al. (1987) switched drug in those patients in whom 8 weeks of therapy had not produced healing. Thirteen patients who had not healed on ranitidine 150 mg b.i.d. haled on omeprazole 60 mg/day for 8 weeks. Of the three patients who failed to heal on omeprazole 60 mg/day, one healed after 8 weeks of ranitidine 150 mg b.i.d. KLINKENBERG-KNOL et al. (1988) also studied a group of patients who had failed to respond to more than 3 months of therapy with 1600 mg cimetidine or 600 mg ranitidine daily. Of 73 patients, 30 of whom had had complications of esophagitis, and 27 previous surgery, all had complete healing of esophagitis after 4–12 weeks of omeprazole 40 mg/day. When these patients were put on omeprazole 20 mg/day as maintenance, 81% were still healed at 6 months and of 14 who relapsed, 12 responded to omeprazole 40 mg/day and two to 60 mg/day. Clearly omeprazole will heal esophagitis in patients who are resistant to conventional or even larger doses of H_2 receptor antagonists.

V. Zollinger-Ellison Syndrome

A relatively large number of patients with Zollinger-Ellison syndrome have been treated with omeprazole (Table 6). In every case these have been open studies and in most reports the patients were given omeprazole because either their symptoms or acid outputs, or both, were resistant to "large" doses of H_2 receptor antagonists, cimetidine, ranitidine, or famotidine. However, this resistance is relative. As one group have shown in several studies over more than 10 years, gastric acid output can be safely reduced, and symptoms and mucosal disease resolved, with any of the H_2 receptor antagonists, provided sufficient drug is given (JENSEN et al. 1986). However, in the only studies in patients given omeprazole in whom symtoms and mucosal disease were controlled prior to therapy (MCARTHUR et al. 1985; MATON et al. 1989) as much as 12 g cimetidine or 9.2 g ranitidine daily was required in certain patients.

In most of these studies patients with Zollinger-Ellison syndrome had symptoms and mucosal disease prior to therapy. Omeprazole was given usually as 60 mg once per day initially and subsequent dose adjustments were

Table 6. Open studies of the effects of omeprazole in patients with Zollinger-Ellison syndrome

Study	Patients (*n*)	Previous H_2 dose (g/day)[a]	Control of symptoms	Healed mucosa	Omeprazole dose (mg)	Acid output <10 mEq/h[b]	Duration (months; mean in parentheses)	Dose increases (*n*)
Blanchi et al. (1982)	1	1.2 + P	1	1	80 b.i.d.	1	12	0
Oberg and Lindström (1983)	2	0.5	2	NA	60–80	2	1	0
Lamers et al. (1984)	7	0.3 – 1.2	7	7	30–60 b.i.d.	7	8–19 (14)	3
Vezzadini et al. (1984)	1	1.2 + P	1	1	20 b.i.d.	1	4	0
Bardram and Stadil (1986)	9	1.2 – 2.7	9	9	20–80	9	0–24 (12)	9
Delchier et al. (1986)	7	0.6–1.2	7	7	60–80 b.i.d.	7	4–24 (15)	2
Lloyd-Davies et al. (1988)[c]	80	0.45 – 1.2 + P	80% ±	90% ±	20–120 t.i.d.	90% ±	0–48 (19)	19
Hirschowitz et al. (1988)	31	NA	87%	39%	20–160	31	0–18 (NA)	NA
Corleto et al. (1988)	9	0.6 – 3.2	NA	9	20–40	NA	6–16 (NA)	0
Maton et al. (1989, 1990)[d]	40	1.2 – 9.2 + P	37	40	40–60 b.i.d.	40	15–6 (29)	9

Abbreviations: C, cimetidine; R, ranitidine; P, probanthine; NA, no available data.
[a] Expressed as ranitidine equivalents calculated from Howard et al. (1985).
[b] Acid output measured in the last hour before the next dose of drug. ± Data not available on all patients in the study.
[c] Includes patients in Bianchi et al. (1982), Oberg and Lindström (1983), Lamers et al. (1984), Vezzadini et al. (1984), Bardram et al. (1986), and Delchier et al. (1986).
[d] All patients controlled adequately on H_2 receptor antagonists prior to switching to omeprazole (includes patients in McArthur et al. 1985).

made principally on the basis of assessment of acid output in the last hour before the next dose of drug. Reducing acid to <10 mEq/h has been shown to be a safe criterion for management of patients with Zollinger-Ellison syndrome (JENSEN et al. 1986) and safer than assessment of symptoms (RAUFMAN et al. 1983). However, patients with Zollinger-Ellison syndrome and a previous partial gastrectomy (MATON et al. 1988) or those with reflux esophagitis (MILLER et al. 1988) may require acid to be reduced to <1 mEq/h to heal mucosal disease. Doses of omeprazole required in the studies of patients with Zollinger-Ellison syndrome varied from 20 mg once per day to as high as 120 mg every 8 h (Table 6). In the two largest studies the median daily dose was 65–75 mg once per day. In each of these studies the dose was split into 12 hourly doses when the daily dose reached 120 mg/day. Thirty percent of patients required the dose to be split into two 12-hourly doses to achieve adequate control of acid output (LLOYD-DAVIES et al. 1988; MATON et al. 1988). Splitting 120 mg every 24 h into two 60-mg 12-hourly doses lowers acid output considerably (MATON et al. 1989) and thus avoids an increase in daily dose.

In most studies only a minority of patients have required an increase in dose of omeprazole to maintain acid outputs <10 mEq/h, a situation which contrasts with the use of H_2 antagonists in patients with Zollinger-Ellison syndrome, whereby most patients will require one dose increase per year (JENSEN et al. 1986). The stability of the dose of omeprazole is seen most clearly in the studies of LLOYD-DAVIES et al. (1988) and MATON et al. (1989), in which patients required an average of less than 0.25 increases in dose per patient per year.

In those studies in which patients had symptoms dispite H_2 antagonists, omeprazole produced prompt resolution of symptoms (Table 6). Similarly, in the studies where H_2 antagonists had produced adequate symptomatic response, omeprazole maintained patients symptom-free (MC-ARTHUR et al. 1985; MATON et al. 1989), and in all the studies patients preferred omeprazole to the H_2 receptor antagonist. In one study (LLOYD-Davies et al. 1988) omeprazole resolved or markedly improved all symptoms except those due to esophageal stricture, or pyloric or duodenal stenosis. One other study found that omeprazole, when given in sufficiently large dosage to render the patient virtually achlorhydric, was capable of resolving or markedly improving structure formation after initial dilation, when H_2 receptor antagonists had been unable to improve the dysphagia (MILLER et al. 1988).

In the majority of studies patients had mucosal disease prior to starting omeprazole, and omeprazole healed all or the majority of these mucosal lesions. In one study although most mucosal lesions healed, all esophageal strictures and ulcers in three patients failed to heal (LLOYD-DAVIES et al. 1988). It may be that the ulcers were at the gastrojejunectomy site in patients how had had a partial gastrectomy, an ulcer that has been shown to be particularly resistant to therapy in patients with Zollinger-Ellison syndrome and may require sufficient omeprazole to render the patient virtually achlorydric to heal (MATON et al. 1988). In another study only 39% of 18 patients endoscoped after 6 weeks to 6 months of omeprazole therapy had a normal endoscopy, despite acid outputs being <10 mEq/h. The reasons for this are not clear as insufficient data are available to assess this finding (HIRSCHOWITZ et al. 1988).

These studies demonstrate that omeprazole is highly effective therapy for control of acid hypersecretion and acid-related symptoms in patients with Zollinger-Ellison syndrome. Although in nearly all patients with Zollinger-Ellison syndrome acid outputs can be brought within safe limits and symptoms resolved with H_2 receptor antagonists, very large large doses administered every 8, 6, or 4 h may be required. Omeprazole therapy is simpler and more effective, and is preferred by the patients. Omeprazole is now the drug of choice in patients with Zollinger-Ellison syndrome.

VI. Side-Effects and Toxicity

Since the first studies of the use of omeprazole in patients with duodenal ulcer in 1983 more than 13000 patients in clinical trials have been given the drug. Most studies have, however, been short term, and only a relatively smal percentage of patients, those with Zollinger-Ellison syndrome or peptic diseases resistant to H_2 receptor antagonists, have been given the drug for longer than a few weeks.

No significant clinical side-effects of omeprazole have been described in any of the studies. Furthermore, although omeprazole has been shown to inhibit the oxidative metabolism of some drugs in a dose-dependent manner (CLISSOLD and CIAMPOLI-RICHARDS 1986), no drug interactions of clinical importance have been reported. However, clinical experience is limited and patients receiving concomitant therapy with phenytoin or anticoagulants should be closely monitored. There have been no consistent abnormalities in laboratory measurements reported in patients receiving omeprazole.

Long-term data on safety of omeprazole are limited, in part because of concern over the long-term administration of omeprazole to rats, which resulted in gastric endocrine cell hyperplasia and gastric carcinoid tumors (CARLSSON et al. 1986). Further studies have demonstrated that omeprazole (and other powerful inhibitors of gastric acid secretion) can cause carcinoid formation in rats due to drug-induced achlorhydria and hypergastrinemia (CREUTZFELD 1988). Hypergastrinemia stimulates proliferation of gastric endocrine cells, and if sufficiently powerful and prolonged tends to cause carcinoid formation. In therapeutic doses in man omeprazole causes only modest increases in plasma concentrations of gastrin (ARNOLD et al. 1986). Furthermore, although established hypergastrinemic states in man (gastric atrophy with achlorhydria and Zollinger-Ellison syndrome) are associated with an increased risk of the development of gastric carcinoids, this risk appears to be small (SOLCIA et al. 1986).

In a number of patients with idiopathic peptic diseases who have received omeprazole, 40–60 mg for up to 3 years, plasma concentrations of gastrin have remained elevated about four fold (LAMBERTS et al. 1988; KLINKENBERG-KNOL et al. 1988), but no increases in gastric endocrine cells have been observed and no gastric carcinoids have been described (LAMBERTS et al. 1988). Patients with Zollinger-Ellison syndrome have increased numbers of gastric endocrine cells due to tumor-induced hypergastrinemia (HELANDER 1986; MATON et al. 1988; LAMBERTS et al. 1988). However, therapy with omeprazole did not increase plasma concentrations of gastrin in two studies (MATON et al. 1989; LLOYD-DAVIES et al. 1988), although it did increase gastrin concentrations in one other study (CADIOT et al. 1988). Gastric endocrine cells did not increase when patients were treated for up to 3 years (MATON et al. 1988; LEHY et al. 1989). Carcinoids of the stomach have been observed in patients with Zollinger-Ellison syndrome, usually as part of multiple endocrine neoplasia type I (SOLCIA et al. 1988), who received H_2 receptor antagonists and omeprazole, but whether this was due entirely to the hypergastrinemia of Zollinger-Ellison syndrome or due in part to the drug therapy cannot be answered definitively. Further monitoring of long-term omeprazole therapy will be required.

D. Probable Role of Omeprazole in Acid-Peptic Diseases

In stort-term studies omeprazole has proved to be an extremely effective and safe drug. It heals duodenal and gastric ulcers more quickly than conventional doses of H_2 receptor antagonists. Omeprazole is capable of healing ulcers that are resistant to conventional or even larger doses of H_2 receptor antagonists, is more effective than H_2 receptor antagonists in the treatment of reflux esophagitis, and is the best drug available for the management of gastric acid hypersecretory states such as Zollinger-Ellison syndrome. However, it is likely that most or all the patients who require omeprazole because of failure of H_2 receptor antagonists will relapse when omeprazole therapy is stopped, and thus, such patients are likely to require omeprazole long term. The limited long-term data that are available are reassuring, but continued careful surveillance of patients taking omeprazole will be required before the risks, if any, of long-term therapy can be quantified.

References

Archambault AP, Pare P, Bailey RJ, Navert H, Williams CN, Freeman HJ, Baker SJ, Marcon NE, Hunt RH, Sutherland L, Kepkay DL, Saibil FG, Hawken K, Farley A, Levesque D, Ferguson J, Westin J-A (1988) Omeprazole (20 mg daily) versus cimetidine (1200 mg daily) in duodenal ulcer healing and pain relief. Gastroenterology 94:1130–1134

Arnold R, Koop H, Schwarting H, Tuch K, Willemer B (1986) Effect of acid inhibition on gastric endocrine cells. Scand J Gastroenterology [Suppl 125] 21:14–19

Bader J-P, Modigliani R, Soule JC, Delchier JC, Morin T, Pariente EA, Bitoun A, Roterberg A, Blanchi A (1986) An open trial of omeprazole in short-term treatment of duodenal ulcer. Scand J Gastroenterology [Suppl 118] 21:177–178

Barbara L, Saggioro A, Olsson J, Cisternino M, Franceschi M (1987) Omeprazole 20 mg om and ranitidine 150 mg bd in the healing of benign gastric ulcers – an Italian multicentre study. Gut 28:A1341

Bardhan KD, Bianchi Porro G, Bose K, Daly M, Hinchliffe RFC, Jonsson E, Lazzaroni M, Naesdal J, Rikner L, Walan A (1986) A comparison of two different doses of omeprazole versus ranitidine in treatment of duodenal ulcers. J Clin Gastroenterol 8:408–413

Bardhan KD, Morris P, Thompson M, Dhande DS, Hinchliffe RFC, Daly MJ, Carroll NJH, Krakowczyk C (1987) Value of omeprazole in the management of erosive oesophagitis refractory to high dose cimetidine. Gut 28:A1375

Bardhan KD, Dhande D, Hinchliffe RFC, Morris P, Thompson M, Carroll NJH, Daly MJ (1988a) Omeprazole in the treatment of ultra refractory duodenal ulcer. Gastroenterology 94:A22

Bardhan KD, Naesdal J, Bianchi Porro G, Lazzaroni M, Hinchliffe RFC, Thompson M, Morris P, Daly MJ, Carroll NJH, Walen A, Rikner L (1988b) Omeprazole (OM) in the treatment of refractory pepticulcer (RPU). Gastroenterology 94:A22

Bardram L, Stadil F (1986) Omeprazole in Zollinger-Ellison syndrome. Scand J Gastroenterol 21:374–378

Bate CM, Bradby GVH, Wilkinson SP, Bateson MC, Hislop WS, Crowe JP, Willoughby CP, Peers EM, Richardson PDI (1988) Omeprazole provides faster ulcer healing and symptom relief than cimetidine in the treatment of gastric ulcer. Gut 29:A1440–A1441

Belgian Multicentre Group (1986) Rate of duodenal ulcer healing during treatment with omeprazole. A double-blind comparison of a daily dose of 30 mg versus 60 mg. Scand J Gastroenterol [Suppl 118] 21:175–176

Bigard MA, Isal JP, Galmiche JP, Ebrard F, Bader JP (1987) Omeprazole versus cimetidine in short-term treatment of acute duodenal ulcer. Gastroenterol Clin Biol 11:753–757

Blanchi A, Delchier J-C, Soule J-C, Payen D, Bader J-P (1982) Control of acute Zollinger-Ellison syndrome with intravenous omeprazole. Lancet 2:1223–1224

Bordi C, d'Abba T, Pilato FP, Ferrari C (1987) Carcinoid (ECL cell) tumor of the oxyntic nucosa of the stomach: a hormone-dependent neoplasm. Prog Surg Pathol 8:117–195

British Cooperative Study (1984) Omeprazole in duodenal ulceration: acid inhibition, symptom relief, endoscopic healing, and recurrence. Br Med J 289:525–528

Brogden RN, Heel TC, Speight TM, Avery GS (1978) Cimetidine: a review of its pharmacology and efficacy in peptic ulcer disease. Drugs 15:93–131

Brogden RN, Carmine AA, Heel RC, Speight TM, Avery GS (1982) Ranitidine: a review of its pharmacology and therapeutic use in peptic ulcer disease and other allied diseases. Drugs 24:267–303

Brunner G, Creutzfeldt W, Harke U, Lamberts R (1988) Therapy with omeprazole in patients with peptic ulcerations resistant to extended high-dose ranitidine treatment. Digestion 39:80–90

Cadiot G, Lehy T, Mignon M, Ruszniewski P, Elouaer-Blanc L, Bonfils S, Lewin M (1988) Comparative behavior of gastric endocdrine cells and serum gastrin levels in Zollinger-Ellison (ZE) patients during long-term treatment with omeprazole or H_2-receptor antagonists. Gastroenterology 94:A56

Carlsson E, Larsson H, Mattsson H, Ryberg B, Sundell G (1986) Pharmacology and toxicology of omeprazole – with special reference to the effects on the gastric mucosa. Scand J Gastroenterol [Suppl 118] 21:31–38

Classen M, Dammann HG, Domschke W, Hengels KJ, Hüttemann W, Londong W, Rehner M, Simon B, Witzel L, Berger J (1985a) Short duration treatment of duodenal ulcer with omeprazole and ranitidine: results of a multicentre trial. Dtsch Med Wochenschr 110:210–215

Classen M, Dammann HG, Domschke W, Hüttemann W, Londong W, Rehner M, Scholten T, Simon B, Witzel L, Berger J (1985b) Healing rate of gastric ulcer after treatment with omeprazole or ranitidine: results of a German multicentre trial. Dtsch Med Wochenschr 110:628–633

Clissold SP, Campoli-Richards DM (1986) Omeprazole. A preliminary review of its pharmacodynamic and pharmacokinetic properties, and therapeutic potential in peptic ulcer disease and Zollinger-Ellison syndrome. Drugs 32:15–47

Corleto V, Puoti M, Annibale B, Saggioro A, Ambra GD, di Paolo M, delle Fave G (1988) Loss of efficacy of famotidine (FMT) in the control of gastric acid secretion in patients with Zollinger-Ellison syndrome (ZES) reversed by omeprazole (OMP). Gastroenterology 94:A79

Creutzfeldt W (1988) The achlorhydria-carcinoid sequence: role of gastrin. Digestion 39:61–79

Dahlgren S, Domellöf L, Hradsky M, Norryd C, Brunkwall J, Svensson G, Svensson J-O, Karlsson J, Knutson U, Gasslander T, Lindhagen J, Arbman G, Jansson R, Sandström R, Huldt B, Pettersson B-G, Janunger K-G, Sjölund B, Herngvist H (1988) The effects of omeprazole and cimetidine on duodenal ulcer healing and the relief of symptoms. Aliment Pharmacol Ther 2:483–492

Dammann HG, Blum AL, Lux G, Rehner M, Riecken EO, Schiessel R, Wienbeck M, Witzel L, Berger J (1986) Differences in healing tendency of reflux oesophagitis with omeprazol and ranitidine. Results of an Austrian-German-Swiss multicenter trial. Dtsch Med Wochenschr 111:123–128

Danish Multicentre Study Group (1988) Gastric ulcer recurrence after six weeks treatment with omeprazole and cimetidine – six months double blind comparative follow-up study. Gut 29:A1441

Darle N, Falk A, Haglund U, Lind T, Walan A, Naesdal J, Andersen O, Bergsaker-Aspoy J, Halvorsen L, Farup P, Offergaard S, Qvigstad P (1986) Rate of healing of benign gastric ulcer during treatment with omeprazole. Scand J Gastroenterol [Suppl 118] 21:180

Dehn TCB, Shepherd HA, Colin-Jones D, Kettlewell MGW (1988) Double blind comparative study of omeprazole (40 mg od) vs cimetidine (400 mg qds) in the treatment of erosive reflux oesophagitis. Gut 29:A1440

Delchier J-C, Soule J-C, Mignon M, Goldfain D, Cortot A, Travers B, Isal J-P, Bader J-P (1986) Effectiveness of omeprazole in seven patients with Zollinger-Ellison syndrome resistant to histamine H_2-receptor antagonists. Dig Dis Sci 31:693–699

Dent J, Downton J, Heddle R, Buckle PJ, Toouli J, Mackinnon AM, Wyman JB (1987) Effects of omeprazole on peptic oesophagitis and oesophageal motility and pH. Scand J Gastroenterol [Suppl 118] 21:181

Elashof JD, Grossman MI (1980) Smoking and duodenal ulcer. Gastroenterology 79:181

Fausa O, Aadland E, Lotveit T (1987) Omeprazole in the treatment of patients with severe erosive oesophagitis resisant to treatment with H_2-receptor antagonists. Scand J Gastroenterol [Suppl 135] 22:38

French Cooperative Study (1987) Omeprazole versus ranitidine in duodenal ulcer patients unhealed after six weeks treatment with H_2-receptor antagonists. Gut 27:A1341

Goldfain D, LeBrodic MF, Lavergne A, Galian A, Modigliani R (1989) Gastric carcinoid tumors in patients with Zollinger-Ellison syndrome on long-term omeprazole (Letter). Lancet 1:776–777

Graham DY, McCullough A, Sklar M, Sontag S, Roufail W, Stone RC, Bishop RH, Gitlin N, Wong D, Kiss K, Cagliola AJ, Berman AS, Humphries TJ (1988) Omeprazole in duodenal ulcer: the U.S. experience. Gastroenterology 94:A152

Gustavsson S, Adami H-O, Lööf L, Nyberg A, Nyrén O (1983) Rapid healing of duodenal ulcers with omeprazole: double-blind dose-comparative trial. Lancet 2:124–125

Gustavsson S, Nyrén O, Adami H-O, Forhaug K, Knutsson L, Lööf L, Nyberg A, Wollert S (1987) Omeprazole heals duodenal and prepyloric ulcers faster than cimetidine – a single-centre trial. Gastroenterology 92:1420

Havelund T, Laursen LS, Skoubo-Kristensen E, Andersen BN, Pedersen SA, Jensen KB, Fenger C, Hanberg-Sorensen F, Lauritsen K (1988) Omeprazole and ranitidine in treatment of reflux oesophagitis: double blind comparative trial. Br Med J 296:89–92

Helander HF (1986) Oxyntic mucosa histology in omeprazole-treated patients suffering from duodenal ulcer or Zollinger-Ellison syndrome. Digestion [Suppl 1] 35:123–129

Hetzel DJ, Bonnin M (1986) Long term management of hemorrhagic esophagitis with cimetidine and omeprazole. Aust N Z J Med 16:226–228

Hetzel DJ, Korman MG, Hansky J, Eaves ER, Shearman DJC, Ellard K, Piper DW (1986) A double blind multicentre comparison of omeprazole and cimetidine in the treatment of duodenal ulcer. Aust N Z J Med [Suppl 3] 16:595

Hetzel DJ, Dent J, Reed WD, Narielvala FM, Mackinnon M, McCarthy JH, Mitchell B, Beveridge BR, Laurence BH, Gibson GG, Grant AK, Shearman DJC, Whitehead R, Buckle PJ (1988) Healing and relapse of severe peptic esophagitis after treatment with omeprazole. Gastroenterology 95:903–912

Hirschowitz BI, Deren J, Raufman JP, LaMont B, Berman R, Humphries T (1988) A multicenter U.S. study of omeprazole treatment of Zollinger-Ellison syndrome (ZES). Gastroenterology 94:A188

Horowitz M, Hetzel DJ, Buckle PJ, Chatterton BE, Shearman DJC (1984) The effect of omeprazole on gastric emptying in patients with duodenal ulcer disease. Br J Clin Pharmacol 18:791–794

Howard JM, Chremos AN, Collen MJ, McArthur KE, Cherner JA, Maton PN, Ciarleglio CA, Cornelius MJ, Gardner JD, Jensen RT (1985) Famotidine, a new potent long-acting histamine H_2-receptor antagonist: comparison with cimetidine and ranitidine in the treatment of Zollinger-Ellison syndrome. Gastroenterology 88:1026–1033

Howden CW, Payton CD, Meredith PA, Hughes DMA, Macdougall AI, Reid JL, Forrest JAH (1985) Antisecretory effect and oral pharmacokinetics of omeprazole in patients with chronic renal failure. Eur J Clin Pharmacol 28: 637–640

Hui WM, Lam SK, Lau WY, Branicki FJ, Lai CL, Lok ASF, Ng MMT, Poon KP, Fok PJ (1987) Omeprazole (OME) vs ranitidine (RAN) for duadenal ulcer (DU) – one-week, low-dose regimens and factors affecting healing. Gastroenterology 94:A1443

Hüttemann W (1986) Short-term treatment of gastric ulcer with once daily omeprazole. Scand J Gastroenterol [Suppl 118] 21:179

Hüttemann W, Rohner HG, du Bosque G, Rehner M, Hebbeln H, Martens W, Horstkotte W, Dammann HG (1986) 20 versus 30 mg omeprazole once daily: effect on healing rates in 115 duodenal ulcer patients. Digestion 33:117–120

Im WB, Blakeman DP, Davis JP (1985) Irreversible inactivation of rat gastric HK ATPase in vivo by omeprazole. Biochem Biophys Res Commun 126:78–82

Jensen RT, Maton PN, Gardner JD (1986) Current management of Zollinger-Ellison syndrome. Drugs 32:188–196

Karvonen A-L, Keyriläinen O, Uusitalo A, Salaspuro M, Tarpila S, Andrén K,

Helander HF (1986) Effects of omeprazole in duodenal ulcer patients. Scand J Gastroenterol 21:449–454
Kaunitz JD, Sachs G (1986) Identification of a vanadate sensitive potassium dependent proton pump from rabbit colon. J Biol Chem 261:14005–14010
Kittang E, Aadland E, Schünsby H (1985) Effect of omeprazole on the secretion of intrinsic factor gastric acid and pepsin in man. Gut 26:594–598
Kittang E, Aadland E, Schjünsby H, Rohss K (1987) The effect of omeprazole on gastric acidity and absorption of liver cobalamins. Scand J Gastroenterol 22: 156–160
Klinkenberg-Knol EC, Jansen JMBJ, Festen HPM, Meuwissen SGM, Lamers CBHW (1987a) Double-blind multicentre comparison of omeprazole and ranitidine in the treatment of reflux oesophagitis. Lancet 1:349–351
Klinkenberg-Knol EC, Jansen JMBJ, Lamers CBHW, ten Kate RW, Meuwissen SGM (1987b) Effect of long term omeprazole on fasting serum gastrin levels in reflux esophagitis. Gastroenterology 92:1471
Klinkenberg-Knol EC, Jansen JBMJ, de Bruyne JW, Nelis GF, Festen HPM, Snel P, Meuwissen SGM (1988) Longterm efficacy and safety of omeprazole (OME) on healing and prevention of resistant reflux esophagitis. Gastroenterology 94: A230
Koop H, Schwarting H, Knorrmarin MA, Willhardt C, Moser T, Arnold R (1987) Influence of chronic omeprazole treatment in gastric endocrine function. Klin Wochenschr 65:169–173
Korman MG, Hansky J, Eaves ER, Schmidt GT (1983) Influence cigarette smoking on healing and relapse in duodenal ulcer disease. Gastroenterology 83:871–874
Lamberts R, Creutzfeldt W, Stöckmann F, Jacubaschke U, Maas S, Brunner G (1988) Long-term omeprazole treatment in man: effects on gastric endocrine cell populations. Digestion 39:126–135
Lamers CBHW, Lind T, Moberg S, Jansen JBMJ, Olbe L (1984) Omeprazole in Zollinger-Ellison syndrome. Effects of a single dose and of long-term treatment in patients resistant to histamine H_2-receptor antagonists. N Engl J Med 310: 758–61
Lanzon-Miller S, Pounder RE, Hamilton MR, Ball S, Chronos NAF, Raymond F, Olouson M, Cederberg C (1987) Twenty four hour intragastric acidity and plasma gastrin concentration before and during treatment with either ranitidine or omeprazole. Aliment Pharmacol Ther 1:239–252
Larsson H, Mattson H, Sundell G, Carlsson E (1985) Animal pharmacodynamics of omeprazole. A survey of its pharmacological properties in vivo. Scand J Gastroenterology [Suppl 108] 21:23–25
Lauritsen K, Rune SJ, Bytzer P, Kelbaek H, Jensen KG, Rask-Madsen J, Bendtsen F, Linde J, Hojlund M, Andersen HH, Mollmann K-M, Nissen VR, Ovesen L, Schlichting P, Tage-Jensen U, Wulff HR (1985) Effect of omeprazole and cimetidine on duodenal ulcer. A double-blind comparative trial. N Engl J Med 312:958–961
Lauritsen K, Rune SJ, Wulff HR, Olsen JH, Laursen LS, Havelund T, Astrup L, Bendtsen F, Linde J, Bytzer P, Tage-Jensen U, Gluud C, Andersen HH, Schlichting P, Skovbjerg H, Mertz-Nielsen A, Rask-Madsen J (1988) Effect of omeprazole and cimetidine on prepyloric gastric ulcer: double blind comparative trial. Gut 29:249–253
Lauritsen, Andersen BN, Havelund T, Laursen LS, Hansen J, Eriksen J, Jorgensen T, Rask-Madsen J (1989) Effect of 10 mg and 20 mg omeprazole daily on duodenal ulcer: double blind comparative trial. Aliment Pharmacol Ther 3:59–67
Lehy T, Mignon M, Cadiot G, Elouer-Blanc E, Ruszniewski P, Lewin MJM, Bonfils S (1989) Gastric endocrine cell behavior in Zollinger-Ellison syndrome patients upon long term potent antisecretory treatment. Gastroenterology 96:1029–1040
Lind T, Cederberg C, Ekenved G, Haglund U, Olbe L (1983) Effect of omeprazole – a gastric proton pump inhibitor – on pentagastrin stimulated acid secretion in man. Gut 24:270–276

Lindberg P, Nordberg P, Alinger T, Brandstrom A, Wallmark B (1986) The mechanism of action of the gastric acid secretion inhibitor, omeprazole. J Med Chem 29:1327–1329

Lloyd-Davies KA, Rutgersson K, Sölvell L (1988) Omeprazole in the treatment of Zollinger-Ellison syndrome: a 4 year international study. Aliment Pharmacol Ther 2:13–32

Lorentzon P, Jackson R, Wallmark B, Sachs G (1987) Inhibition of the HK ATPase by omeprazole in isolated vesicles requires proton transport. Biochim Biophys Acta 897:41–51

Marks IN, Winter TA, Lucke W, Wright JP, Newton KA, O'Keefe SJ, Marotta F (1988) Omeprazole and ranitidine in duodenal ulcer healing. S Afr Med J 54–6.

Maton PN, Frucht H, Vinayek R, Wank SA, Gardner JD, Jensen RT (1988a) Medical management of patients with Zollinger-Ellison syndrome who have had previous gastric surgery: a prospective study. Gastroenterology 94:294–299

Maton PN, Vinayek R, Frucht H, McArthur KE, Miller LS, Saeed ZA, Gardner JD, Jensen RT (1989) Long term efficacy and safety of omeprazole in patients with Zollinger-Ellison syndrome. Gastroenterology 97:827–836

Maton PN, Lack EE, Collen MJ, Cornelius MJ, David E, Gardner JD, Jensen RT (1990) The effect of Zollinger-Ellison syndrome and omeprazole therapy on gastric oxyntic endorine cells. Gastroenterology 99:943–950

McArthur KE, Collen MJ, Maton PN, Cherner JA, Howard JM, Ciarleglio CA, Cornelius MJ, Jensen RT, Gardner JD (1985) Omeprazole: effective, convenient therapy for Zollinger-Ellison syndrome. Gastroenterology 88:939–944

Mignon M, Lehy T, Bonnefond A, Ruszniewski P, Labeille D, Bonfils S (1986) Development of gastric argyrophil carcinoid tumors in a case of Zollinger-Ellison syndrome with primary hyperparathyroidism during long-term antisecretory treatment. Cancer 59:1959–1962

Miller LS, Frucht M, Saeed ZA, Stark H, Gardner JD, Jensen RT, Maton PN (1988) Esophageal involvement in Zollinger-Ellison syndrome. Gastroenterology 94:A303

Naesdal J, Lind T, Bergsaker-Aspöy J, Bernklev T, Farup PG, Gillberg R, Halvorsen L, Kilander A, Offergaard S, Walan A, Lloyd-Davies KA (1985) The rate of healing of duodenal ulcers during omeprazole treatment. Scand J Gastroenterol 20:691–695

Oberg K, Lindström H (1983) Reduction of gastric hypersecretion in Zollinger-Ellison syndrome with omeprazole. Lancet 1:66–67

Olbe L, Lind T, Cederberg C, Ekenved G (1986) Effect of omeprazole on gastric acid secretion in man. Scand J Gastroenterol [Suppl 118] 21:105–107

Pedersen SA, Kraglund K, Vinter-Jensen L (1987) The effects of omeprazole on gastro-esophageal pressure, intragastric pH and the migrating motor complex in fasting healthy subjects. Scand J Gastroenterol 22:725–730

Pen JH, Michielsen PP, Pelckmans PA, van Maercke YM (1988) Omeprazole in the treatment of H_2-resistant gastro-duodenal ulcers. Gastroenterology 94:A348

Prichard PJ, Rubinstein D, Jones DB, Dudley FJ, Smallwood RA, Louis WJ, Yeomans ND (1985a) Double blind comparative study of omeprazole 10 mg and 30 mg daily for healing duodenal ulcers. Br Med J 290:601–603

Prichard PJ, Yeoman ND, Mihaly GW, Jones DB, Buckle PJ, Smallwood RA, Louis WJ (1985b) Omeprazole: a study of its inhibition of gastric pH and oral pharmacokinetics after morning or evening dosage. Gastroenterology 88:64–69

Raufman J-P, Collins SM, Pandol SJ, Korman LY, Collen MJ, Cornelius MJ, Feld MK, McCarthy DM, Gardner JD, Jensen RT (1983) Reliability of symptoms in assessing control of gastric acid secretion of patients with Zollinger-Ellison syndrome. Gastroenterology 84:108–113

Richter JE (1986) A critical review of current medical therapy for gastroesophageal reflux disease. J Clin Gastroenterol [Suppl 1] 8:72–80

Rinetti M, Vezzadini P, Jonsson E, Tomasetti P, Labo G (1986) Effect and tolerability of omeprazole in the treatment of duodenal ulcer disease. Drugs Expt Clin Res 7:701–705

Sachs G, Carlsson E, Lindberg P, Wallmark B (1988) The gastric HK ATPase as a therapeutic target. Annu Rev Pharmacol Toxicol 28:269–284

Sandmark S, Carlsson R, Fausa O, Lundell L (1988) Omeprazole or ranitidine in the treatment of reflux esophagitis. Results of a double blind randomized Scandinavian Multicentre Study. Scand J Gastroenterol 23:P625–P632

Scandinavian Multicentre Study (1984) Gastric acid secretion and duodenal ulcer healing during treatment with omeprazole. Scand J Gastroenterol 19:882–884

Solcia E, Capella C, Sessa F, Rindi G, Cornaggia M, Riva C, Villani L (1986) Gastric carcinoids and related endocrine growths. Digestion [Suppl 1] 35:3–22

Solcia E, Bordi C, Creutzfeld W, Dayal Y, Dayan AD, Falkmer S, Grimelius L, Havu N (1988) Histopathological classification of non antral gastric endocrine growths in man. Digestion 41:185–200

Sundler F, Carlsson E, Hakanson R, Larsson H, Mattsson H (1986) Inhibition of gastric acid secretion by omeprazole and ranitidine. Effects on plasma gastrin and gastric histamine, histidine decarboxylase activity and ECL density in normal and antrectomised rats. Scand J Gastroenterol [Suppl 118] 21:39–45

Tytgat GNJ, Lamers CBHW, Hameeteman W, Jansen JMBJ, Wilson JA (1987) Omeprazole in peptic ulcers resistant to histamine H_2-receptor antagonists. Aliment Pharmacol Ther 1:31–38

Van Deventer GM, Cagliola A, Whipple J, Humphries T (1988) Duodenal ulcer healing with omeprazole: a multicenter study. Gastroenterology 94:A476

Vantrappen G, Rutgeerts L, Schurmans P, Coenegrachts J-L (1988) Omeprazole (40 mg) is superior to ranitidine in short-term treatment of ulcerative reflux esophagitis. Dig Dis Sci 33:523–529

Vezzadini P, Tomassetti P, Toni R, Bonora G, Labo G (1984) Omeprazole in the medical treatment of Zollinger-Ellison syndrome. Curr Res 35:772–776

Walan A, Bader J-P, Classen M, Lamers CBHW, Piper DW, Rutgersson K, Eriksson S (1989) Effect of omeprazole and ranitidine on ulcer healing and relapse rates in patients with benign gastric ulcer. N Engl J Med 320:69–75

Zeitoun P, Desjars de Keraurone N, Isbal J-P (1987) Omeprazole versus ranitidine in erosive oesophagitis. Lancet 2:621–622

CHAPTER 8

Hypothesis of Peptic Ulcer: A Modern Classification of a Multifactorial Disease

S.H. CALDWELL and R.W. McCALLUM

A. Introduction

There is little doubt that peptic ulcer disease is a complex and multifactorial disease. The literature dealing with this subject is vast. New observations and ideas regarding its pathogenesis and treatment are being published almost monthly. Our goal in the following pages will be to formulate and discuss a hypothesis of peptic ulcer disease. We have attempted to review both the old and new literature in this regard and offer a working classification for the understanding of this complex entity. Many of the areas discussed are further amplified in different sections of this text.

No single mechanism adequately explains the variety of ulcers encountered clinically from chronic, relapsing ulcer to drug-induced ulcer or to acute stress-related ulceration. A number of factors, however, tie these various subsets together. First, the obvious similarity in geographic distribution and gross appearance leads to similar diagnostic strategies. Likewise, clinical symptoms, complications, and medical or surgical management are often similar and therefore make a unifying concept of pathogenesis more appealing.

Underlying each of the various types of peptic ulcer is the widely accepted concept of an essential imbalance between aggressive factors and mucosal defenses with an end result of mucosal ulceration (Fig. 1). Schwarz first proposed this at the turn of the century (SCHWARZ 1910). Although his original statement has been reduced to "no acid – no ulcer", it has recently been pointed out that the actual translation was much broader – "Peptic ulcer is a product of self-digestion; it results from an excess of autopeptic power of gastric juice over the defensive power of gastric (and intestinal) mucosa" (SAMLOFF 1989). Within this general framework, we will begin with some definitions and then discuss the various aggressive and defensive factors, their regulation, and the major types of peptic ulcer. A simple, working classification is discussed with an emphasis on chronic relapsing ulcer.

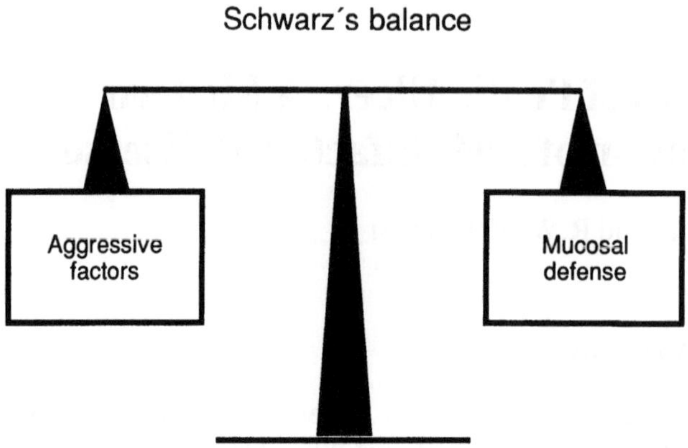

Fig. 1. "Peptic ulcer is a product of self-digestion; it results from an excess of autopeptic power of gastric juice over the defensive power of gastric [and intestinal] mucosa" (SCHWARZ 1910; translated by SAMLOFF 1989)

B. Histopathology of Peptic Ulcer

I. Ulcer Histology

Ulceration of the gastroduodenal mucosa is defined as any breach of the epithelial layer which extends through the muscularis mucosa. Erosions are defined as more shallow disruptions of the epithelium and are often difficult to distinguish from true ulceration at endoscopy (McCARTHY 1989). Erosions are frequently seen together with ulceration and may form a continuum with them. For example, a recent study of duodenal ulcer relapse showed that the presence of erosions in the duodenal bulb at follow-up endoscopy was predictive of eventual relapse of active ulcer (VAN DEVENTER et al. 1989).

Chronic relapsing gastric ulcers, unassociated with drug ingestion, tend to occur along the lesser curvature at the border zone between normal body mucosa in areas of histologic gastritis intermixed with glandular atrophy and intestinal metaplasia (GEAR et al. 1971). The gastritic changes are not limited to the area just surrounding the ulcer (STADELMANN et al. 1971) although the inflammatory changes may be patchy and the greater curvature aspect of the gastric body is often less involved. Gastritic changes usually persist after ulcer healing (GEAR et al. 1971).

Duodenal ulcers are similarly often found in the setting of histologic inflammation (GREENLAW et al. 1980) which persists after ulcer healing (FULLMAN et al. 1985) and, like common gastric ulcer, duodenal ulcers are virtually always associated with type B antral gastritis (MEIKLE et al. 1976; SCHRAGER et al. 1967). The complex interaction of gastric metaplasia of the duodenal bulb, *Helicobacter pylori* infection, histologic duodenitis, and ulceration is further discussed in a later section of this chapter.

II. Gastritis – Definitions

As mentioned, histologic (type B) gastritis is a frequent finding in both gastric and duodenal ulcer. A notable exception to this relationship has been observed in the setting of nonsteroidal anti-inflammatory drug (NSAID)-induced ulcers (MacDonald 1973). Because of the strong association between most non-drug-associated peptic ulcers and gastritis, it will be helpful to briefly review some of the familiar terms used in this context.

1. Endoscopic Gastritis

The broad definition of "gastritis" is sometimes a source of confusion. *Endoscopic gastritis* is often used to describe grossly visible lesions of the mucosa consisting of variable degrees of redness, hyperemia, friability, and hemorrhage. Because of the poor correlation between endoscopic and histologic findings in the stomach (Johnston et al. 1986a), we prefer the less presumptive term *gastropathy* for these lesions. Often what appears to be frankly inflamed mucosa at endoscopy is found on biopsy to be normal mucosa or to have minimal vascular congestion without a prominent inflammatory component. Conversely, endoscopically normal mucosa often is histologically inflamed (Price et al. 1985). A similar discrepancy between gross appearance and histologic findings has been observed in experimental animals exposed to gastric irritants in the presence of protective prostaglandins. The gross appearance in this setting has been interpreted as being free of injury when microscopy has revealed significant damage (Lacy and Ito 1982). A better correlation may exist between the endoscopic and histologic diagnosis of duodenal inflammation (McCallum et al. 1979) and gastric atrophy (Varis 1988). However, improvements in our understanding of ulcer pathogenesis over the next few years will likely depend on very careful assessment of the histologic rather than endoscopic character of the gastroduodenum in ulcer disease.

2. Histologic Gastritis

Histologic gastritis is broadly divided into two main categories, autoimmune (type A) and nonautoimmune (type B). Although both may be associated with extensive atrophy of the mucosa and hypochlorhydria, there are several distinguishing attributes of each (Strickland and Mackay 1973). Autoimmune gastritis is commonly associated with antibodies to parietal cells and intrinsic factor whereas nonautoimmune gastritis is not. Additionally, other autoimmune diseases are often found to coexist with the former but not with the latter. More recently, *H. pylori* has been shown to be causally related to type B gastritis (Warren and Marshall 1983; Rauws et al. 1988; Graham 1989a) but is uncommon in autoimmune gastritis (Flejou et al. 1989).

Beyond the simple division of histologic gastritis into type A and type B, the classification of common, "garden variety" gastritis becomes much more complex. Type B gastritis (the type commonly found among peptic ulcer patients) comprises several distinct but often overlapping subtypes (WHITEHEAD et al. 1972; CORREA 1988). Characteristically, the inflammatory changes involve the antrum but the patchy nature of the lesion and associated *H. pylori* infection has been a well-described problem for investigators in this area (BAYERDORLLER et al. 1989).

Active gastritis refers to the presence of polymorphonuclear cells infiltrating the superficial epithelium, gastric pits, and related lamina propria. *Chronic gastritis* refers to the progression of the inflammatory infiltrates (especially mononuclear cells) into the deeper mucosal layers associated with dropout of the glands, while *gastric atrophy* is described as having minimal inflammation but marked loss of mucosal glands. *Intestinal metaplasia* is often associated with type B gastritis particularly, but not exclusively, in advanced stages. It refers to the replacement of normal gastric epithelial cells with cells that share many properties (particularly staining characteristics) with intestinal epithelial and goblet cells.

Prior to the discovery of *H. pylori*, it was observed that chronic gastritis (type B gastritis) first developed in the antrum and progressed over years into more proximal areas of the stomach (OTTENJAN 1970). This progression appears to be more rapid among gastric ulcer patients than those who have not had a documented ulcer (MAAROOS et al. 1985) and is predominantly along the lesser curvature. Among duodenal ulcer patients, a similar progression occurs in some and is predictive of the development of subsequent gastric ulcer (TATSUTA et al. 1986). With extension of the inflammatory process, there is increasing atrophy and intestinal metaplasia (MAAROOS et al. 1985; OTTENJAN 1970). Although the most common cause of type B gastritis now appears to be *H. pylori*, the factors governing progression of the disease are not yet understood. Indeed, no longitudinal studies have yet clearly demonstrated that the *progression* of chronic active gastritis related to *H. pylori* is the same process that investigators noted prior to the discovery of the organism although such a relationship seems likely (HAZELL et al. 1987).

C. Schwarz's Balance

One of the functions of the normal stomach is to partially digest ingested nutrients. It does so by both mechanical and chemical means. The most important chemical factors are acid (elaborated by the parietal cells) and pepsinogens (elaborated by the chief cells). Gastric pH often drops as low as 1 while proximal duodenal pH may drop as low as 2. Along with acid and pepsin, ulcerogenic drugs and possibly bile constitute some of the proven or suspected aggressive factors to which the gastric and duodenal mucosa is regularly exposed. Some might include *H. pylori* as an aggressive factor. However, it appears that *H. pylori* acts more as a permissive factor to acid-mediated peptic ulceration. This hypothesis, proposed by MARSHALL et al. in 1985a, has recently been dubbed the "leaking roof" theory of ulcer pathogenesis (GOODWIN 1988) and is discussed later.

I. Mucosal Defenses

Mucosal defenses can be conceptually viewed as consisting of four major components (SHORROCK and REES 1988): (a) an unstirred gel layer across which is established a pH gradient (b) the epithelial cells which themselves form a barrier and which elaborate bicarbonate (c) the regenerative capacity of the epithelium, and (d) mucosal bloodflow which nourishes the whole process and serves to sweep away any hydrogen ion that may cross the barrier. The central role of prostaglandins and possibly epidermal growth factor as regulators of this process is discussed below.

1. Measurement of the Barrier

The integrity of the mucosal defenses can be measured in several ways. One of the oldest methods is measurement of the transmucosal potential difference (GEALL et al. 1970). It can be demonstrated both in vitro and in vivo by comparing the electrical potential between the lumen or luminal surface and a reference electrode in a peripheral vein or (in vitro) on the serosal surface. Normally, the mucosa of the stomach and, to a lesser extent, the duodenum, maintain a potential difference (PD) of 30–50 mV (lumen negative).

The PD is an *indirect* measure of the ability of the barrier to control flow of cations (hydrogen, sodium, and potassium ions) across the epithelium (DAVENPORT 1972). In humans, the application of acetylsalicylic acid, alcohol, or alkaline duodenal contents causes a significant drop in PD which is thought to reflect influx of hydrogen ion into the tissue (KAUFFMAN 1985). Regional variations in PD have been described within the stomach, with the crests of mucosal folds having lower PDs than the troughs (MERSEREAU and HINCHEY 1982). This pattern may explain the typical linear pattern of injury induced by some noxious agents (LACY 1985). However, the PD is not an absolute indicator of the adequacy of mucosal protection. For instance, recovery of the PD occurs soon after acute ingestion of aspirin despite the persistence of visible mucosal injury (GRAHAM and SMITH 1986). Furthermore, mucosal erosions have been observed after indomethacin ingestion in humans without a concomitant change in the PD (GRAHAM and SMITH 1986). Thus the PD is only an approximation of the barrier.

2. The Mucus Gel and pH Gradient

The thickness of the overlying mucus gel layer in the human gastroduodenum ranges from 50 to 450 μm with a median of 180 μm (KERSS et al. 1982). Normally, it is composed of 95% water and is impermeable to pepsin and to some extent hydrogen ion. Besides water, it is composed mostly of glycoprotein subunits linked by disulfide bonds and admixed with variable amounts of immunoglobulins, serum proteins, and the remains of spent cells (ALLEN and CARROLL 1985). It is susceptible to proteolysis by pepsin (active at pH below 5) and by a protease elaborated by *H. pylori* (active at pH above 5) (SAROSIEK et al. 1989). The thickness of the layer is markedly diminished in chronic active gastritis associated with *H. pylori* but returns to a normal thickness after eradication of the organism (MARSHALL et al. 1985a).

A pH gradient exists across the gel layer in both humans and animals with near neutral pH at the epithelial surface (BAHARI et al. 1982; TURNBERG and ROSS 1984). Agents which lower the PD across the mucosa are also known to disrupt this gradient (TURNBERG and ROSS 1984). It is maintained via the active transport of bicarbonate by the epithelial cells at a rate of 5%–10% of maximal acid output (ALLEN and GARNER 1980). Specific receptors in part mediate the process which, like mucus secretion, is stimulated by prostaglandin administration (see below). Other stimulants of epithelial bicarbonate secretion include luminal acidification and vagal stimuli (seen during the cephalic phase of gastric secretion).

3. Mucosal Healing

Healing of the gastric mucosa appears to be mediated in experimental animals by both a slow process of regeneration from glandular neck cells (1–2 days) and a more rapid process of restitution (SILEN and ITO 1985). Restitution occurs in a matter of hours and involves the ameba-like migration of neighboring intact cells to cover areas of denuded epithelium. The process occurs underneath a mucoid cap consisting of mucus, denuded cells, and cell debris (WALLACE and WHITTLE 1986). It is independent of mucosal bloodflow (RUTTEN and ITO 1983), unlike most of the other defense mechanisms. It has been likened to an "everyday" phenomenon in response to the ingestion of food and the mechanical grinding of digestion. Its role in common peptic ulcer is unknown.

4. Mucosal Bloodflow

The integrity of the mucosal barrier in preventing hydrogen ion back-diffusion is important but no more so than the ability of the tissue, via its microcirculation, to neutralize and remove the acid. Mucosal perfusion prevents local tissue acidosis after experimental noxious agent exposure (KAUFFMAN 1985; SCHOEN and VENDER 1989). Clinically, the role of ischemia in common ulcer pathogenesis is less clear. However, abnormal circulation may be particularly significant in certain situations. For instance, refractory peptic ulcer has been described in the setting of mesenteric ischemia (CHERRY et al. 1986), and acute stress ulcers may involve primarily a microvascular dysfunction (see below). Additionally, blood flow may be of central importance in ulcer healing, as shown by a recent study using reflectance spectrophotometry. The authors of that study demonstrated a relationship between local oxygen saturation (which in part will depend on blood flow) and the likelihood of duodenal ulcer healing (LEUNG et al. 1989).

5. Other Mechanisms of Defense

The property of surface hydrophobicity was initially described in experimental animals (HILLS et al. 1983). The term denotes the presence, within the plasma membrane of epithelial cells, of compounds such as lysophosphotidylcholine and sphingomyelin which retard the passage of hydrogen ion. Both aspirin and bile salts, which increase permeability of hydrogen ion, impair surface hydrophobicity (SHORROCK and REES 1988; GODDARD et al. 1987). Exogenous prostaglandins are known to increase surface hydrophobicity (KAUFFMAN 1985). Interestingly, *H. pylori* has recently been shown to elaborate lipolytic enzymes which may be capable of impairing surface hydrophobicity through the degradation of phospholipids (SLOMIANY et al. 1989). Endogenous sulfhydryl containing compounds have also been proposed as possible mucosal protective agents although their exact role is not known. Sulfhydryls appear to be essential for prostaglandin synthesis and may act via this mechanism to exert a protective effect after ethanol exposure (SZABO et al. 1981).

II. Aggressive Factors

Acid is the foremost aggressive factor with which the mucosal defenses must contend. Except for malignant ulceration, hydrogen ion is probably a common thread to all types of peptic ulcer. The rarity of mucosal ulcer in conditions of achlorhydria (GOLDSCHMIEDT et al. 1989) supports this. However, all normal humans are exposed to significant luminal acid yet only 5%–10% of adults in Western countries develop peptic ulcer. Even among patients with Zollinger-Ellison syndrome, peptic ulcer is by no means universal. Therefore, acid appears to be essential but not sufficient for most benign ulcers.

1. Hydrogen Ion

The majority of duodenal ulcer patients do in fact produce larger amounts of acid than normal controls (BARON 1963; MERKI et al. 1988). This excess is paralleled by an increased parietal cell mass. Hyperchlorhydria is most evident when stimulated maximal acid output is measured. Both nocturnal and daytime acid production are increased when acid is measured by 24-h pH probe (MERKI et al. 1988) although nocturnal, unbuffered acid production seems to be particularly elevated (DRAGSTEDT 1967; MERKI et al. 1988). Postprandial peak acid output on the other hand is not different in duodenal ulcer patients (FELDMAN and RICHARDSON 1986) although the duration after meals of low intragastric pH is prolonged (MALAGELADA et al. 1977).

However, these findings are not universal and a significant minority of duodenal ulcer patients produce normal amounts of acid.

Distal gastric ulcers behave similarly to duodenal ulcers and are usually characterized by acid hypersecretion (JOHNSON 1965). More proximal gastric ulcers, however, are associated with normal or low fasting (JOHNSON 1965) and stimulated (KAUFFMAN 1985) acid production. Nonetheless, gastric ulcer in the absence of acid is strongly suspicious for malignancy and, as in more distal gastric and duodenal ulcers, hydrogen ion is an important factor in proximal gastric ulcers.

Once secreted by the parietal cell, hydrogen ion is handled in several ways. A portion is neutralized by gastric contents. However, the majority is emptied into the duodenum where it is neutralized by mucosal bicarbonate, pancreatic juice, and possibly Brunner's gland secretions. A small amount inevitably undergoes what has become known as "back-diffusion" or permeation into the epithelium and lamina propria.

At a luminal pH of 2, the normal gradient of hydrogen ion across the mucus gel layer approximates 10^5 (KAUFFMAN 1985). It has been shown that when hydrogen ion crosses the normal barrier in sufficient quantities to produce intramucosal acidosis, visible damage occurs (KAUFFMAN 1985). The amount of damage, however, is not directly proportional to the magnitude of ion flux as other factors such as acid disposal (by mucosal blood flow for instance) can attenuate the effect. Markedly diminished blood flow, systemic acidosis, and absence of an alkaline tide (due to inhibition of acid secretion) all can exacerbate tissue acidosis and resultant injury (SILEN 1985).

2. Aspartic Proteinases

The aspartic proteinases, of which the pepsinogens are best known, constitute the second major aggressive factor. The pepsinogens are secreted principally by the gastric chief cells – pepsinogen I almost exclusively so and pepsinogen II by the pyloric and Brunner's glands as well (SAMLOFF and LIEBMAN 1973). In addition to pepsinogen I and II, the human stomach contains other lesser known aspartic proteinases now known as cathepsins E and D (SAMLOFF 1989). The secretion of pepsinogens parallels that of parietal cell acid secretion with a few notable exceptions. For instance, omeprazole causes a relative dissociation between pepsinogen and acid secretion (THOMPSON et al. 1985) and epidemic achlorhydria, now thought to be often caused by acute *H. pylori* infection (GRAHAM et al. 1988a), is also associated with a relative dissociation of these two functions (RAMSEY et al. 1979). All of the aspartic proteinases are active only below a pH of 5.

The mucus gel layer is susceptible to proteolysis by pepsin (PEARSON et al. 1980) and gastric juice from both duodenal and gastric ulcer patients has been shown to have increased mucolytic activity (ALLEN and CARROLL 1985). On the other hand, bile, aspirin, and acid are not able to dissolve the gel. In relation to the increased mucolytic activity of gastric juice, luminal pepsin I activity is also increased in duodenal ulcer patients (WALKER and TAYLOR 1980).

Hyperpepsinogenemia I, possibly inherited as an autosomal dominant trait, appears to be a risk factor for duodenal ulcer relapse (ROTTER et al. 1979). Interestingly, serum pepsinogen I levels appear to be more important than levels of gastric acid production in predicting ulcer relapse (PETERSON et al. 1985). The relationship, if any, of these factors to *H. pylori* infection is unknown but it is pertinent that *H. pylori* (almost universal among duodenal ulcer patients) can elaborate mucolytic enzymes (SAROSIEK et al. 1988, 1989) and is also a strong predictor of duodenal ulcer relapse (MARSHALL et al. 1988a; COGHLAN et al. 1987). Additionally, gastric histology, which reflects to a large extent the presence or absence of *H. pylori*, is known to correlate with changes in serum pepsinogen levels (SAMLOFF 1989). The significance of these relations has yet to be fully investigated.

3. Bile Acids

Fasting gastric juice bile acid concentrations in gastric ulcer patients have been shown to be higher than in controls and this may relate to abnormal fasting motility (MIRANDA et al. 1985). Reflux of duodenal contents into the stomach has been demonstrated by a variety of methods. Scintigraphy has shown increased reflux of isotope excreted with the bile among peptic ulcer patients (THOMAS 1984). Such reflux has been proposed as a cause of histologic gastritis (LAWSON 1964), but more recent work does not support this (see below). Bile acids and lysolecithin are, however, able to produce significant mucosal injury under experimental conditions and may potentiate back-diffusion of hydrogen ion (DAVENPORT 1968). Furthermore, diversion of bile into the fundus can experimentally produce *fundic* inflammatory changes (DELANEY et al. 1975). The relationship of chronic type B histologic gastritis, bile reflux, and garden variety relapsing gastric ulcer is less clear.

Does bile reflux correlate with chronic active gastritis? Among patients undergoing antrectomy for peptic ulcer disease, persistent histologic gastritis is common (LOFFELD et al. 1988); however, diversion of bile by Roux-en-Y does little to change the degree of inflammation (MALAGELADA et al. 1985). On the other hand, absence of *H. pylori* in this setting is associated with absence of histologic inflammation (O'CONNER et al. 1986; CALDWELL et al. 1989a). The residual changes observed are characterized by foveolar hyperplasia (DIXON et al. 1986; CORREA 1988). The inference is that while bile appears capable of acutely breaking the mucosal barrier and chronically altering mucosal histology (foveolar hyperplasia), it does not appear to be a causative agent in chronic, active gastritis. Its role as a potentiator of ulcer is, however, entirely conceivable given the frequent occurrence of bile reflux in gastric ulcer patients. It has been proposed that gastric ulcer in the absence of typical chronic active gastritis, *H. pylori*, and NSAID ingestion constitutes a distinct subset of bile-related gastric ulcer (O'CONNER et al. 1987).

4. Oxygen Free Radicals

Oxygen free radicals and their relationship to gastric injury has recently been reviewed (PARKS 1989). It is not clear that these highly reactive oxygen metabolites are common factors in mucosal injury. However, there is experimental evidence in animals that such oxidants, produced by the activity of xanthine oxidase, potentiate gastric injury due to hemorrhagic shock (SMITH et al. 1987). This suggests a possible role for these agents in at least stress ulcer pathogenesis. In addition, there is evidence that NSAID-induced injury may in part be mediated by oxygen free radical formation (DEL SOLDATO et al. 1984).

III. Risk Factors as Modifiers of Mucosal Defense

The epidemiology of peptic ulcer disease is beyond the scope of this chapter. However, to the extent that certain risk factors may modulate a given individual's mucosal defenses or their reaction to various aggressive factors, we will briefly discuss two of the well-known risk factors for peptic ulcer disease.

1. Blood Groups

Blood group status has long been known to bear a relation to peptic ulcer disease. Group O type is more common among duodenal ulcer patients and among patients with both a duodenal ulcer and a gastric ulcer (JOHNSON et al. 1964). Similarly, blood group O was more common among a group of rheumatoid arthritic patients with presumed NSAID-induced gastric ulcer (SEMBLE et al. 1987) although classically, proximal (hypocholrhydric) gastric ulcers have been associated with group A blood type (JOHNSON et al. 1964). The significance of these observations remains unknown and by no means are the relations absolute. It can be surmised that, in some way, the absence or presence of blood group antigens in gastric secretions modulates either defensive or aggressive mechanisms or that the association is merely a marker of some other process. Along these lines, the recently described glycerolipid receptor for *H. pylori* was not shown to be significantly more or less common with different blood groups (LINGWOOD et al. 1989).

2. Tobacco Use

Tobacco use imparts a marked risk of duodenal ulcer relapse although the mechanism is not known (SONTAG 1988). Smoking transiently depresses prostaglandin synthesis in the antrum, the fundus, and, to a lesser extent, the duodenum (QUIMBY 1986). Sucralfate therapy appears to attenuate the effect of tobacco on ulcer relapse (LAM et al. 1987) and this may be mediated by stimulated mucosal prostaglandin synthesis (COHEN et al. 1989). Together these two observations support an effect of tobacco on prostaglandin metabolism. A similar effect on tobacco use and ulcer risks has been noted after *H. pylori* eradication (MARSHALL et al. 1988c). Eradication of the organism tends to diminish the risk of relapse regardless of smoking status. In this regard, it was recently shown that among a group of patients with histologic gastritis, there was no difference in tissue prostaglandin levels between smokers and nonsmokers (FUNG et al. 1982). Perhaps *H. pylori*-related gastritis diminishes mucosal prostaglandins to a similar extent as smoking; however, this hypothesis has not been directly tested. Early work in this area has not demonstrated a clear effect of *H. pylori* on mucosal prostaglandins (TAHA et al. 1990), although some effect seems likely.

IV. Regulation of Mucosal Defenses: Prostaglandins and Epidermal Growth Factor

Prostaglandins constitute a family of compounds that consist of 20 carbon-long fatty acid chains arranged in a cyclopentane ring with two side chains. Based on the structure of the ring, prostaglandins are divided into six groups, A through F. Depending on which fatty acid serves as the source of the prostaglandin, the groups are further divided into series, one through three. The series vary in the number of side chain double bonds (SONTAG et al. 1986). E-type prostaglandins predominate in the stomach. Acid secretion is probably not to any great extent controlled or affected by endogenous prostaglandins (MOGARD et al. 1987) although exogenous prostaglandins can suppress acid secretion, probably via cAMP (SOLL 1980; WOOLFE and SOLL 1988). In terms of dose equivalency, 800 μg misoprostol (a synthetic PGE_1) per day has a similar degree of acid suppression as cimetidine at a dose of 1200 mg per day (GRAHAM 1989b).

Prostaglandin metabolism is closely linked to many of the mucosal defense mechanisms disussed above. Many of the data in this area derive from experimental work involving gastric injury induced by noxious agents such as aspirin, acidified bile, ethanol, and hypertonic solutions. Except perhaps for bile, these experiments are best suited to studies of drug-induced ulcers. Their applicability to other types of ulcer is less certain. However, such studies have proven important in experimentally defining the effect of prostaglandins on the mucosal defenses.

1. Role of Prostaglandins in Mucosal Defense

The term "cytoprotection" was originally coined to describe the effect of exogenous prostaglandins in prevention of gross mucosal lesions induced by alcohol, hydrochloric acid, sodium hydroxide, hypertonic saline, and thermal injury (ROBERT et al. 1979). It is now apparent that this protection involves only the deeper vascular injuries induced by these agents (LACY and ITO 1982), which suggests that exogenous and perhaps endogenous prostaglandins modulate to some extent vascular integrity. Superficial, microscopic injury is not prevented by pretreatment with these agents. However, healing of these superficial injuries (by restitution) may be accelerated by prostaglandin pretreatment (LACY and ITO 1984). The mechanism is unknown, but it has been suggested that prostaglandins retard cell senescence (WAGNER 1985). Similarly, prostaglandins may increase overall mucosal thickness (JOHANSSON et al. 1982), perhaps by the same mechanism.

In addition, prostaglandins appear to stimulate gastric and duodenal epithelial mucus production (WILSON et al. 1984), possibly by increasing the number of mucus producing cells (through delayed senescence). Furthermore, hydrogen ion back-diffusion is decreased (DAJANI et al. 1978) and epithelial bicarbonate production is increased (SELLING et al. 1985), as is mucosal blood flow (LEUNG et al. 1985). There is evidence that prostaglandins, in addition, modulate surface hydrophobicity (LICHTENBERG et al. 1983). Although much of the above applies to exogenous prostaglandins, a role for maintenance of the barrier by endogenous prostaglandins is suspected. Recent work with antibodies which depleted the endogenous stores of prostaglandins and produced mucosal ulceration lends credence to this hypothesis (REDFERN et al. 1987).

Deficiency of mucosal prostaglandins has been described in both gastric (WRIGHT et al. 1982) and duodenal (SMITH and HILLIER 1985) ulcer, although high levels have also been described in gastric ulcer (SCHLEGEL et al. 1977). (Perhaps the latter observation represents sampling error as stomachs of gastric ulcer patients often have areas of extensive metaplasia with variable degrees of inflammation, *H. pylori* infection, and atrophy.) In addition, mucosal production of prostaglandins is decreased in response to luminal acid among duodenal ulcer patients (ALQUIST et al. 1983). The cause and relative importance of these abnormalities is not known. Exogenous prostaglandins are no better than placebo in terms of ulcer healing at doses which fail to suppress gastric acid (HAWKEY and WALT 1986) and are not effective in preventing stress ulcers (SKILLMAN et al. 1984). On the other hand, exogenous prostaglandins significantly protect the mucosa from NSAID-induced ulceration in clinical trials (see below).

2. Epidermal Growth Factor and Other Factors

Many other interacting factors are involved in the process of regulation of the mucosal barrier. Secretin reportedly stimulates duodenal mucus production (MILLER 1988) while morphine and vasoactive intestinal peptide stimulate duodenal bicarbonate production in mammals (FLEMSTROM et al. 1985). Gastrin exerts trophic effects not only on the parietal cell mass but on duodenal proliferative activity as well (JOHNSON 1977). Epidermal growth factor (EGF, formerly known as urogastrone) also has trophic effects on the gastric mucosa (JOHNSON and GUTHRIE 1980). EGF is a low molecular weight polypeptide derived from both salivary and duodenal Brunner's glands (MARTI et al. 1989) and is resistant to gastric proteases. Decreased levels of

Table 1. Working classification of peptic ulcer

I. *Chronic relapsing peptic ulcers*
  A. *Drug-related* (NSAIDs, steroids? ethanol?):
  Unless there is coexistent *H. pylori* infection, inflammation is usually minimal and vascular changes such as microscopic hemorrhage are common.
  B. *H. Pylori-positive ulcers:*
  Ulcers with chronic (mononuclear cell) and active (polymorphonuclear cell) inflammation of the antrum and in areas of gastric metaplasia of the duodenum associated with *H. pylori* infection. Gastritis commonly extends into the gastric body.
    1. Gastric ulvers: usually along the lesser curvature and associated with more extensive inflammation, atrophy, and hypochlorhydria.
    2. Duodenal ulcers: gastritic changes are more localized to the antrum with distal extension into metaplastic areas of the duodenum. Hyperchlorhydria is common.
  C. *Hypersecretory states* (Zollinger-Ellison):
  Ulcers develop as a result of massive acid overproduction. *H. pylori* appears to be uncommon. In the absence of *H. pylori* or NSAID ingestion, endocrinologic hypersecretory states should be excluded by specific testing.
  D. *Malignancy:*
  Neoplastic gastric ulcer often masquerades as a benign ulcer. It occurrs in a similar background histology as *H. pylori*-related gastric ulcer although the possible relation is essentially unexplored. Hypochlorhydria is common.
  E. *Other associations* (occult NSAIDs? bile?):
  In some patients an extensive evaluation will fail to reveal any obvious clues as to the underlying pathophysiology. Occult NSAID use, vascular disease, motility disorders, or bile reflux may be relatively more important in this setting.

II. *Acute, stress-related ulcers*
  Vascular insult results in an inability of the mucosal barrier to resist hydrogen ion-mediated ulceration. The majority of lesions are nonulcerating hemorrhages rather than true ulcers.

this substance have been described in the saliva of gastric ulcer patients (Marti et al. 1989). It may exert control over gastroduodenal cell renewal, which normally occurs roughly every 2 or 3 days.

D. Classification of Peptic Ulcer Disease

Because of the complex and normally balanced system of mucosal defense and regulation, it is not surprising that there are a number of ways in which mucosal ulceration can develop. Table 1 illustrates our current working classification of peptic ulcer disease. We have divided peptic ulcer into two broad categories, chronic relapsing ulcers and acute, stress-related ulcers, which appear to involve fundamentally different mechanisms. Within the category of chronic relapsing peptic ulcer, the two major divisions are ulcer in the setting of *H. pylori* and ulcers associated with NSAID ingestion.

Several points regarding this working classification of peptic ulcer disease should be made before proceeding to a discussion of the various types. First of all, there is undoubtedly a good deal of overlap between the various categories. For instance, the elderly patient who may have *H. pylori*-related gastritis might also be ingesting NSAIDs on a regular basis. Secondly, we mean to imply nothing about direct causation within any of the categories. *H. pylori* certainly does not cause ulceration alone (nor does acid). However, together with hydrogen ion, pepsin, and a susceptible individual, it does appear to impart a significant risk of ulcer disease. In fact, it may be the single most common thread tying together histologic gastritis, duodenitis, and frank mucosal ulceration (MARSHALL et al. 1985a; GRAHAM 1989a). The best evidence in support of this hypothesis comes from studies of ulcer relapse. Preliminary studies (discussed below) suggest that eradication of *H. pylori* not only cures histologic gastritis but more significantly alters the natural history of duodenal (and possibly gastric) ulcer disease.

Implicit within this working classification is the concept that most non-drug-induced gastric and duodenal ulcers form a continuum and are fundamentally the same disease (KIRK 1981; GREENLAW et al. 1980). Few would argue that the pylorus serves as a poor boundary for classifying ulcers because of the uncertain border zones between intestinal, pyloric, and fundic type epithelium. Simultaneous duodenal ulcers have been reported in 7%–64% of gastric ulcer patients (RICHARDSON 1989). Among patients who suffer both duodenal and gastric ulcer, the duodenal ulcer often appears chronologically earlier than the gastric ulcer. Both types of ulcer tend to occur in histologically "ill" tissue and progression of the histologic inflammation from the antrum to more proximal areas of the stomach is predictive of the development of gastric ulcer among duodenal ulcer patients (TATSUTA et al. 1986). The proximal progression of histologic gastritis with time is paralleled by changes in acid production such that a gradient exists which correlates with ulcer location (KIRK 1981). Thus acid production ranges from hyperchlorhydria (associated with parietal cell excess) in duodenal ulcer and younger patients to hypochlorhydria (associated with parietal cell loss) in proximal gastric ulcer and older patients. NSAID-induced ulcers are a separate but sometimes superimposed variety of ulcer which share with "gastritic" ulcer (i.e., associated with histologic gastritis) a common pathway of acid-mediated mucosal damage.

E. Drug-Induced Ulcer Disease

I. Nonsteroidal Anti-Inflammatory Drugs and Aspirin

Approximately 10% of patients using NSAIDs chronically have *gastric* ulcers (GRAHAM 1989b). As many as one-third of those with ulcers are asymptomatic (SILVOSO et al. 1979). The absence of symptoms appears to be paralleled by a characteristic absence of diffuse inflammation (MacDonald 1973; Hamilton and Yardley 1980) in many patients. Perhaps both findings are, in part, related to the anti-inflammatory and analgesic properties of these medications. An increased risk of *duodenal* ulcer after chronic NSAID ingestion is suspected by some but is less certain (Soll et al. 1989; Ehsanullah et al. 1988). Mucosal lesions of the duodenum short of frank ulcerations have been documented by endoscopic studies (Ehsanullah et al. 1988). However, some authors have suggested that the role of NSAIDs in duodenal ulcers may be more that of an antagonist to preexisting and unrelated duodenal disease (Graham 1988b). The risk for gastric ulcer is much more obvious, with an estimated 46-fold greater chance of finding a gastric ulcer among NSAID users than among the general population (McCarthy 1989). The mortality risk from NSAID-related peptic ulcers seems particularly high among the elderly (Griffin et al. 1988). Although there does not appear to be a "safe" NSAID in terms of relative toxicity, newer agents are generally less toxic than plain aspirin as judged by endoscopically scored injury (Lanza 1984).

1. Mechanisms of NSAID-Induced Injury

The mechanism by which NSAIDs cause mucosal injury is complex. Recent studies have demonstrated a protective effect in humans of exogenous prostaglandin in terms of gastric ulcer formation among NSAID users (Graham et al. 1988b). This suggests that, among the potential modes of NSAID-induced mucosal toxicity, cyclooxygenase inhibition and resultant prostaglandin deficiency are relatively significant (Table 2). These "cyclooxygenase-dependent" mechanisms include adverse effects not only upon endogenous prostaglandin formation (Hansen et al. 1983), but also secondarily on epithelial bicarbonate and mucus secretion (Kauffman 1989), on surface hydrophobicity (Goddard et al. 1987), and perhaps most importantly on mucosal blood flow (Kitahora and Guth 1987). Oral aspirin administration appears to lead to an early rise in mucosal blood flow due to a local irritant effect; however, this is quickly followed by a subsequent fall in blood flow as cyclooxygenase is inhibited (Kitahora and Guth 1987). The result is an impairment of the ability of the tissue to adequately handle the increased flow of hydrogen ion through the barrier.

Acid plays an integral role in NSAID-related mucosal injury under experimental conditions (Kauffman 1989). The "one-two punch" of aspirin

Table 2. Effects of aspirin on mucosal defenses which are predominantly mediated by cyclooxygenase inhibition

1. Impaired prostaglandin synthesis
2. Diminished blood flow
3. Decreased epithelial bicarbonate
4. Decreased mucus secretion
5. Diminished hydrophobicity

in this setting involves first a topical injury which results in increased hydrogen ion back-diffusion and a concomitant fall in the transmural potential difference. The "second punch" results from prostaglandin depletion and loss of vascular integrity with a failure to clear and neutralize the acid. Clinically, the role of hydrogen ion is less obvious. With the possible exception of duodenal ulcer (EHSANULLA et al. 1988), no beneficial effect of H_2 receptor blockade has been clearly demonstrated in clinical trials of NSAID-induced injury prevention (MCCARTHY 1989). Nonetheless, the extensive body of literature involving animal studies strongly supports a role for acid and tissue acidosis in most NSAID-related injury (IVEY 1988).

Whether or not NSAID-induced mucosal injury is *mainly* topical or systemic is controversial. Both aspirin (KAUFFMAN 1989) and the other NSAIDs (IVEY 1988) appear to be able to cause topical injury. However, *parenteral* administration of aspirin has been reported to produce mucosal damage in cats given aspirin infusion over 7 days (BUGAT et al. 1976). In man, acute administration of parenteral aspirin failed to produce a change in transmucosal potential difference or in gastric histology (IVEY et al. 1980). On the other hand, at least one report has revealed a dose-dependent occurrence of antral ulcers in volunteers given parenteral doses of the NSAID ketorolac tromethamine (LANZA et al. 1987). Thus the issue is not resolved although it seems likely, given the apparent central role of cyclooxygenase inhibition and vascular integrity, that the effect of parenteral administration is little different than that of oral administration.

2. Lesions Associated with NSAID Ingestion

Submucosal hemorrhage is a prominent form of injury after NSAID ingestion (GRAHAM and SMITH 1986; WEISS et al. 1961). It is the main form of injury prevented by the preadministration of prostaglandins in short-term studies (LANZA et al. 1988). The etiology of these lesions may involve vascular microthrombi which have been observed to precede the hemorrhagic lesions induced by luminal aspirin administration (KITAHORA and GUTH 1987). The formation of microthrombi appears to result from vasoconstriction of small arterioles. Clinically, petechiae are seen early after acute aspirin administration (GRAHAM and SMITH 1986). Deeper hemorrhages and erosions follow formation of the petechiae as some lesions coalesce. Subsequently, erosions appear to progress to ulceration.

The factors that govern progression of hemorrhages to erosions to ulceration are not known. Indeed, it is only circumstantial inference that such ulcers evolve through these various stages. Nonetheless, the close association between hemorrhages and erosions (GRAHAM and SMITH 1986) and erosions and ulcers (SILVOSO et al. 1979) suggests that most NSAID-induced ulcers of the stomach follow this pattern. Modifiers are numerous and include simultaneous use of other drugs or alcohol, the patient's underlying vascular system, and perhaps the patient's acid secretory capacity. *H. pylori* is of doubtful significance in this setting.

With continued NSAID exposure, "gastric adaptation" occurs in healthy volunteers over a period of 1 week (GRAHAM et al. 1983). The mechanism is unknown. It involves a disappearance of hemorrhagic injury despite continued NSAID use and thus probably represents a recovery of vascular function through compensatory mechanisms.

3. *Helicobacter pylori* and NSAID Ingestion

Little is known about the coexistence of *H. pylori* infection of the stomach and chronic NSAID ingestion. Most of the studies involving NSAIDs and peptic ulcer to date have not taken this potentially confounding factor into account in either patient or control groups. However, several relevant observations have recently been made. NSAIDs do not appear to change the character of the inflammatory reaction to *H. pylori* over a short-term course of 1 week nor was peptic ulcer particularly evident (PETERSON et al. 1988). The effect of misoprostol therapy on antral histology in peptic ulcer disease has been variably reported (WAGNER 1985; HUI et al. 1986). Although some improvement may occur (HUI et al. 1986), resolution of the inflammation as may be seen with eradication of *H. pylori* has not been reported with misoprostol therapy. Finally, among dyspeptic patients, frank mucosal ulceration appears to be uncommon in the absence of either NSAID use or positive serology for *H. pylori* infection (MARTIN et al. 1989). The clinical implications of this observation are discussed later.

II. Drug-Induced Ulcers – Alcohol

1. Mechanisms of Injury

Although not often considered an ulcer-inducing drug, we have included alcohol in our discussion for several reasons. Both clinically and experimentally, alcohol has been shown to affect the mucosal barrier and more importantly the mucosal histology. It may play an indirect role in ulcer pathogenesis through its effect on these variables, as discussed below. For instance, ethanol lowers the potential difference across the gastric mucosa in humans within minutes of ingestion of 20% or 40% solutions (GEALL et al. 1970). The magnitude of the change varies with the concentration ingested. Animal studies have demonstrated that this change reflects enhanced ionic diffusion into the mucosa (DAVENPORT 1967), and high concentrations of ethanol (greater than 40%) dehydrate gastric mucus and break it down although lesser concentrations may actually stimulate mucus output (ALLEN and CARROLL 1985).

Morphologically, animal studies have shown that alcohol-induced injury, like that of NSAIDs, can be divided into superficial epithelial cell injury and deeper, necrotizing vascular injury (LACY and ITO 1982). These two types of injury appear to be unrelated as pretreatment with prostaglandins can prevent the deeper vascular damage (LACY and ITO 1982). Both types occur within minutes of alcohol exposure (OATES and HAKKINEN, 1988). Under experimental conditions, the superficial injury involves mostly the interfoveolar epithelium and gastric pits and heals rapidly by restitution. The deeper lesions involve intramucosal hemorrhage and superficial vascular engorgement (GUTH et al. 1984) and tend to occur in a linear pattern corresponding to vagal folds (possibly due to regional differences in the microvasculature). Exquisite casting studies of the mucosal vasculature have clearly demonstrated the extent of this type of injury (O'BRIAN et al. 1986).

2. Ethanol and Ulcers

Chronic, active gastritis has been variously associated with chronic alcohol ingestion (GOTTFRIED et al. 1978; PARL et al. 1979). Overall, chronic gastritis appears to be increased among alcoholic patients and this has been related to the early development of atrophic gastritis (PARL et al. 1979; DINOSO et al. 1972). Glandular atrophy may relate directly to chronic alcohol exposure as suggested by animal studies (CHEY et al. 1970). Chronic inflammatory changes are, however, likely related to coexistent *H. pylori* infection, which is common among chronic alcoholics (LAINE et al. 1988).

Despite the extensive body of literature involving the injurious effects of alcohol on the gastric mucosa and the common occurrence of bacterial (*H. pylori*) gastritis in alcoholics, there is no clear association between alcohol and *gastric ulcer*. Likewise, ethanol use does not appear to be a major risk factor for the development of *duodenal ulcer* (FREIDMAN et al. 1974). On the other hand, ethanol use has been related to failure of *duodenal ulcers* to heal (REYNOLDS 1989). This may relate to the effects of ethanol as an acid secretagogue (LENZ et al. 1983). Alternatively, chronic alcoholism has been related to the presence of gastric metaplasia in the duodenum (LEV et al. 1980). Whether this observation is the result of sampling error in duodenal biopsies, excess acid exposure, or a direct effect of alcohol, is not known. The role of gastric metaplasia in the duodenum and duodenal ulcer is discussed later.

III. Drug-Induced Ulcers – Steroids

1. Corticosteroids and Ulcers

The relationship between exogenous steroid therapy and peptic ulcer is controversial. Suspicion that corticosteroids may play some role in ulceration arose from the early observation regarding elevated ACTH levels in stress situations wherein ulcers were quite common (SPIRO 1983). Two large, retrospective meta-analytical studies have been published which reached opposite conclusions regarding the prevalence of peptic ulcer among patients using chronic corticosteroids (CONN and BLITZER 1976; MESSER et al. 1983). Both studies suffered shortcomings (SPIRO 1983); however, it is notable that in both there was an increase (albeit slight in both and of no statistical significance in one) in the risk of peptic ulcer among patients using steroids.

2. Effects of Corticosteroids on the Mucosa

Acute ingestion of corticosteroids has been associated with endoscopically visible gastroduodenal lesions in humans ranging from gastric ulcer to gastric or duodenal erosions (OKADA et al. 1985). In this small, uncontrolled trial, 25 patients about to begin oral steroid therapy for a variety of reasons were endoscoped. None had significant lesions prior to therapy but ten developed erosions of the stomach or duodenum and one developed a gastric ulcer at 2 and 4 weeks after beginning therapy. Gastroduodenal histology was not reported. As has been seen in NSAID-associated ulcers (POUNDER 1989), symptoms were notably absent among those patients with endoscopic lesions.

Physiologically, glucocorticoids exert a number of effects on the gastroduodenal mucosa, including stimulation of gastric secretion (GRAY et al. 1951), Gcell hyperplasia (DELANEY et al. 1979), diminished gastric mucus production (MENGUY and MASTERS 1963), alteration of cell kinetics (LOEB and STERNSCHEIN 1973), and possibly altered prostaglandin metabolism. The effect of exogenous steroid therapy on *H. pylori* is unknown. In our experience with an asthmatic patient on chronic steroid therapy, *H. pylori* seemed no more prolific than we commonly have seen and inflammatory changes were notably present (unpublished observation).

F. *Helicobacter pylori* and Peptic Ulcer

1. *Helicobacter pylori*

Helicobacter pylori is a spiral-shaped, gram-negative organism measuring 2.5 by 0.5 μm. First isolated in 1982 (WARREN and MARSHALL 1983), the organism has now been identified on all continents. The bacterium shows a distinct propensity to infect only gastric-type epithelial cells (LEE and HAZELL 1988) although it is well known to infect such tissue when it exists outside the stomach proper, as in gastric metaplasia of the duodenum (MARSHALL et al. 1985a; WYATT et al. 1987). Outside of the human gastrointestinal tract, *H. pylori* has only been cultured from primate stomachs although a similar spiral organism has been described in the stomachs of lower animals (LEE and HAZELL 1988).

The organisms exist in the mucus gel layer and attached to the epithelial cells, especially at the intercellular junctions (HAZELL et al. 1986). Attachment of *H. pylori* alters the cell surface, causing exposure of sialic acid residues (BODE et al. 1988). Specific receptors on the gastric-type cells are thought to exist and probably explain the specificity of *H. pylori* for these cells. A unique glycerolipid has recently been isolated from human gastric mucosa which recognizes and binds viable *H. pylori* organisms (LINGWOOD et al. 1989). Swarming of the organism at the intercellular junctions may represent either receptor localization or greater nutrient availability (HAZELL et at. 1986). Urease, present in the outer membrane of the organism, may serve to recycle host urea as a nitrogen source through the presence of another enzyme, glutamate dehydrogenase (FERRERO et al. 1988). A fibrillar *N*-acetylneuraminyllactose-binding hemaglutinin has also been identified on some strains of *H. pylori* (EVANS et al. 1989) and may potentiate attachment of the organism.

H. pylori is probably one of the most common infections of humans. Prevalence rates vary widely but most studies agree that infection rates increase with age (PEREZ-PEREZ et al. 1988; MARSHALL et al. 1989). The source of human infection is unknown but much circumstantial evidence points toward human-to-human spread. Thus, increased rates of infection have been reported among the spouses of infected patients (MARSHALL et al. 1988b) and among institutionalized persons (BERKOWICZ and LEE 1987). The possibility that *H. pylori* is also a zoonosis is suggested by the presence of the organism in some primates and, more importantly, by an increased prevalence of seropositivity among slaughterhouse workers in Italy (VAIRA et al. 1988).

2. The Effect of *Helicobacter pylori* on the Mucosa and the Host Response

Two volunteer studies have established *H. pylori* as a cause of histologic gastritis (MARSHALL et al. 1985b; MORRIS and NICHOLSON 1987). Numerous other studies have established the almost uniform presence of *H. pylori* in the setting of histologic, chronic, active gastritis and resolution of the lesion with eradication of the organism (MARSHALL et al. 1985; DOOLEY et al. 1988; RAUWS et al. 1988; LANZA et al. 1989). Although it was initially thought that permanent eradication of the organism was difficult or impossible, it is now apparent that complete cure can be achieved through combination therapy using metronidazole and bismuth compounds to which over 70% of isolates are sensitive (MARSHALL et al. 1988). After eradication, the mucosa slowly returns to normal over a period of several months.

Histologically, *H. pylori* infection has a patchy distribution but most often involves the antrum, particularly early in the disease. Subsequently, it appears to spread to more proximal locations along the lesser curvature although definitive longitudinal studies are not yet available (HAZELL et al. 1987). Colonization, without inflammation, may precede the spread (Bayerdorffer et al. 1989) of more active inflammation. Lymphoid follicles can be seen (WYATT and RATHBONE 1988) but marked polymorphonuclear cell infiltration amid mixtures of lymphocytes and plasma cells is more characteristic. Parietal cell invasion can be seen in early, acute infections when impairment of acid secretion has been noted (MORRIS and NICHOLSON 1987). A nontoxic inhibitor of hydrogen ion secretion may be involved (CAVE and VARGAS 1989). Areas of intestinal metaplasia are characteristically free of organisms, presumably due to absence of specific receptors.

The virulence of chronic *H. pylori* infection in any given individual probably depends on two fundamental aspects of the disease. One relates to the virulence of the organism and the other to the host's immune reaction. Mucin depletion of involved antral mucosa was one of the earliest findings regarding *H. pylori* infection (MARSHALL et al. 1985) and may result from the production by *H. pylori* of a mucolytic protease (SAROSIEK et al. 1988). Eradication of the organism is associated with repletion of the mucus layer (MARSHALL et al. 1985a; LANZA et al. 1989). Infected cells typically assume a cuboidal shape and are depleted of their mucin droplet (MALFERTHEINER and DITSCHUNEIT 1988). The cause of these changes is not known. In addition to mucolytic proteins, some strains of *H. pylori* are capable of toxin production as demonstrated on Chinese hamster cell cultures (GUERRANT, unpublished data). Other strains have been reported to produce a protein known as nonlethal vacuolation factor (LEUNK et al. 1988) and virtually all *H. pylori* produce urease. Whether or not these factors are directly or indirectly injurious to the mucosa is unknown.

There is a significant humoral reaction to *H. pylori* infection which has provided a useful, indirect diagnostic test (PEREZ-PEREZ et al. 1988). Specific serum immunoglobulins of the A and G type are elevated during chronic infection and antibodies can also be found in gastric secretions (RATHBONE et al. 1986). Many of these have marked activity against *H. pylori* urease. Activity has also been demonstrated against the nonlethal vacuolation factor and to a possible colonization factor antigen (GRAHAM 1989a). Despite this extensive immunologic reaction on the part of the host, many, if not most, infected individuals appear unable to spontaneously resolve the infection [although spontaneous resolution has been documented in one volunteer study (MARSHALL et al. 1985b)].

3. *Helicobacter pylori*-Associated Gastroduodenal Ulcers

The association of chronic, active gastritis and *H. pylori* infection with peptic ulcer is quite strong. Table 3 from a recent review summarizes the results from several studies regarding the prevalence of *H. pylori* in various conditions (WYATT 1989). From 70% to 100% of patients with duodenal ulcer have *H. pylori* infection of the stomach. When sought, *H. pylori* can be identified near the crater in the majority of duodenal ulcer patients (MARSHALL et al. 1988a). There it infects metaplastic foci of gastric foveolar cells which are common in duodenal ulcer. No direct evidence confirms a causal relationship between *H. pylori* and peptic ulcer, although circumstantial evidence is mounting. The best evidence that *H. pylori* is more than just an innocent bystander in ulcer disease comes from studies of ulcer relapse.

In the early 1980s it became apparent that the initial type of therapy (i.e., bismuth salts versus acid suppressing medications) given to acute duodenal

Table 3. The prevalence of *H. pylori* infection in patients with peptic ulcer and gastritis in different countries (WYATT 1989)

Country	Duodenal ulcer	Gastric ulcer	Gastritis (histologic)	Normal histology
Netherlands	100% (36)	96% (27)	99% (235)	5% (102)
Australia	90% (70)	67% (40)	99% (95)	5% (20)
Italy	76% (37)	65% (31)	–	16% (27)
China	86% (14)	86% (21)	80% (131)	20% (15)
United States	86% (14)[a]		65% (52)	28% (7)
Denmark	71% (17)	67% (9)	86% (69)	20% (50)
United Kingdom	70% (53)	97% (36)	89% (83)	0% (58)

[a] Including gastric and duodenal ulcers.

ulcer patients could significantly alter the disease's natural history. Some forms of therapy, particularly with bismuth compounds, decreased the rate of ulcer relapse. This observation later led to the discovery that bismuth salts exerted antibacterial effects on *H. pylori*. Two studies have further investigated this effect of bismuth on ulcer relapse and its relation to *H. pylori*. In one, 100 consecutive patients were assigned to receive either cimetidine 400 mg b.i.d. or colloidal bismuth subcitrate one tablet q.i.d. for 8 weeks. In addition, each was given either an antibiotic or placebo for the first 10 days of therapy. Of the 72 patients with persistent *H. pylori* infection 2 weeks after the initial treatment, 61% healed the acute ulcer and the relapse rate at 1 year (on no maintenance therapy) was 81%. This compared to an initial healing rate of 92% and a relapse rate at 1 year of 21% among the patients initially cleared of the infection (MARSHALL et al. 1988a). A similar study has shown a 1 year relapse rate of 79% among patients not cleared of the infection, compared to a rate of 27% when the infection was eradicated (COGHLAN et al. 1987). Additional studies to confirm or refute these results are in progress.

a) Gastric Ulcer

In the absence of drug ingestion, chronic benign relapsing gastric ulcers tend to occur along the lesser curvature of the stomach at the junction between inflamed antral-type mucosa and more normal oxyntic mucosa (OI et al. 1959). The propensity for gastric ulcer occurrence at this site is as yet unexplained. Certain anatomical differences are likely to be important. These include the presence of large muscle bundles which underlie the angulus (OI et al. 1969) and may in some way change the susceptibility of the overlying gastritic mucosa to ulceration. In addition, differences in the anatomical blood supply between the lesser and greater curvatures are known to exist – the lesser curvature lacks the rich submucosal vascular plexus found in most other areas of the stomach (BARLOW et al. 1951). Together with varying mixtures of histologic gastritis and atrophy, these local factors probably interact in a complex process to produce episodic ulceration. (KIRK 1986).

Histologic gastritis among patients with gastric ulcer is regional. Sampling from four sites within the stomach, GEAR et al. (1971) found the same grade of inflammatory changes in all four sites in only two of 35 gastric ulcer patients studied. The greater curvature tends most often to be spared while the lesser curvature is almost invariably marked by inflammatory and atrophic changes (GEAR et al. 1971; TATSUTA et al. 1985). Proximal gastric ulcers are associated with more extensive mucosal disease and variable amounts of atrophy and intestinal metaplasia (TATSUTA and OKUDA 1975). Distal, prepyloric ulcers are associated with more localized antral inflammatory changes (GEAR et al. 1971; TATSUTA and OKUDA 1975). As mentioned previously, the distribution of inflammatory change, atrophy, and metaplasia correlates to the site of ulcers and parallels the relation between the site and gastric acid production. More distal gastric ulcers with less extensive inflammation are associated (like duodenal ulcer) with high or normal acid output while proximal gastric ulcers are associated with more extensive inflammation and diminished secretory capacities (GEAR et al. 1971; TATSUTA and OKUDA 1975; STADELMANN et al. 1971).

The natural history of histologic gastritis associated with gastric ulcer differs from that of the ulcer itself. Chromoendoscopic stains have been utilized to study this process. The benefit of this technique is reduced sampling error incurred on biopsy study alone. Using congo red dye to demonstrate acid secreting areas of the stomach, TATSUTA et al. (1985) demonstrated a more rapid proximal progression of inflammatory gastritis over several years among gastric ulcer patients compared to controls. This progression has been associated with an increasing propensity for the ulcer to heal (TATSUTA et al. 1985; MAAROOS et al. 1985; TATSUTA and OKUDA 1975) and is probably a reflection of diminishing acid production as parietal cells drop out. Additionally, it is amply demonstrated that gastritis tends to persist or even progress after ulcer healing (GEAR et al. 1971; MOORE et al. 1986). Why histologic gastritis behaves differently in different individuals is not known.

Additional factors in gastric ulcer pathogenesis have been described by other investigators. *Fasting* gastric motility appears to be impaired in gastric ulcer patients (MIRANDA et al. 1985). *Postprandial* motility has also been observed to be diminished even after the acute ulcer has healed (MOORE et al. 1986). The relationships between inflammatory changes, atrophy, metaplasia, and gastric hypomotility are not known. *H. pylori* antral gastritis in the absence of gastric ulcer does not appear to delay solid phase gastric emptying (CALDWELL et al. 1989b) although there are conflicting reports (BARRILLEAUX et al. 1988). Diminished gastric motility could predispose to peptic ulcer in several ways (RICHARDSON 1989). For instance, incompetence of the pyloric sphincter may promote bilious reflux. Additionally, antral stasis may delay clearance of gastric acid and food retention may, via gastrin stimulation, cause prolonged postprandial acid secretion.

b) Duodenal Ulcer

Neutralization of acid in the duodenal bulb is accomplished in a number of ways. Basal pH in the bulb of duodenal ulcer patients is lower than in normal controls (RUME 1973). Pancreatic bicarbonate production, however, is normal (ISENBERG et al. 1977). Mucosal epithelial becarbonate production, on the other hand, is impaired among duodenal ulcer patients in the absence of an active ulcer (ISENBERG et al. 1987). The cause of this deficiency is unknown. Several possibilities are suggested from the literature, including impaired prostaglandin metabolism or regulation (HILLIER et al. 1985), disease of the mucus-producing Brunner's glands (KIRKEGAARD et al. 1984), and possibly related to the first two, gastric metaplasia of the duodenal bulb (see below).

Like the term "gastritis," duodenitis has been variously defined in the past. In general, there has been good correlation between the endoscopic appearance (redness, hyperemia, friability, and erosions) and the histologic presence of inflammatory infiltrates (VENABLES 1985; MCCALLUM et al. 1979). However, *histologic duodenitis* has a very patchy distribution with a resulting potential for marked sampling error in biopsy studies (GREENLAW et al. 1980; FRIERSON et al. 1990). Recently, a close association between the presence of chronic, active histologic duodenitis and gastric metaplasia has been demonstrated (SHOUSHA et al. 1983). Furthermore, chromoendoscopic studies using methylene blue (not taken up by metaplastic gastric-type cells in the duodenum) have confirmed the irregular distribution of this complex lesion in the bulb (HARA et al. 1988).

Gastric metaplasia in association with duodenal ulcer was first described by JAMES in 1964. The metaplastic cells usually occur in clusters at the end of blunted villi (JAMES 1964; HARA et al. 1988). Mucin droplets in the apex impart a pale appearance on hematoxylin and eosin stains and the normally present brush border is absent. Alcian blue and periodic acid–Schiff stains have been shown to be superior to hematoxylin and eosin in detecting this lesion (FRIERSON et al. 1990). Little is known about its etiology or natural history. Several lines of evidence have suggested that it is a response to the irritant effects of acid. RHODES (1964) demonstrated the occurrence of gastric metaplasia in the duodenum of cats injected repeatedly with an acid secretagogue. FLOREY et al. (1939) created a duodenal fistula exposed to concentrated gastric juice in pigs and observed the subsequent development of gastric metaplasia in the duodenum. Furthermore, WYATT et al. (1987) recently noted a correlation between a gastric pH less than 2.5 and the extent of gastric metaplasia in the duodenal bulb of humans, and JAMES (1964) in his original description of gastric metaplasia, noted the extension of the lesion more distally in association with the Zollinger-Ellison syndrome. Thus, several observations support the concept that gastric metaplasia in humans is a response to excess duodenal acidification; however, this is as yet unproven.

The origin of the metaplastic cells in the duodenum is also uncertain. Histochemical stains have refuted the notion that the cells represent hyperplasia of Brunner's glands (HARA et al. 1988), as had been suggested (RHODES 1964). It is not known whether the lesion is static, cyclic, or perhaps congenital. Alcohol and male sex have been associated with an increased extent of the lesion (SHOUSHA et al. 1983; LEV et al. 1980). Perhaps of greater importance is the close association of neutrophilic inflammation, gastric metaplasia, and *H. pylori* infection (WYATT et al. 1987; FRIERSON et al. 1990). Inflammation of foci of gastric metaplasia in the bulb is uncommon in the absence of coexistent *H. pylori* infection.

In patients with duodenal ulcer, *H. pylori* has been detected in 28% of single biopsies from the duodenal bulb and 52% of single biopsies from ulcer borders (MARSHALL et al. 1988a). Others have reported a frequency as high as 96% of duodenal organisms among duodenal ulcer patients (JOHNSTON et al. 1986b). Always, the organisms are found on or near areas of metaplasia and with an attendant neutrophilic infiltrate. Essentially, these observations represent an extension of "gastritis" into the duodenum. As with gastric ulcer, all of the governing factors are not yet known and certainly ulcers are not inevitable in the presence of duodenal infection. Nontheless, histologic and therapeutic studies support a role for *H. pylori* in duodenal ulcer – a process most likely mediated by increased acid permeability of the mucosa to acid and pepsin. GOODWIN (1988) has coined the term "leaking roof" to describe the interaction of gastric metaplasia, *H. pylori*, and increased acid permeability (Fig. 2).

G. Ulcers Associated with Hypersecretory States

In keeping with the fundamental theory of ulcer pathogenesis, i.e., an imbalance of defensive and aggressive factors, it is not surprising that peptic ulcer has been observed among patients with Zollinger-Ellison syndrome in the absence of *H. pylori* infection (GRAHAM 1989a). However, as yet no systematic study has been reported regarding the role of gastric metaplasia, *H. pylori* infection, and gastroduodenitis in Zollinger-Ellison syndrome or the other hypersecretory states.

JAMES (1964) described gastric metaplasia extending distally in the setting of gastric acid hypersecretion due to Zollinger-Ellison syndrome. Inflammatory changes and gastric metaplasia were also observed commonly in distal duodenal biopsies of a group of gastrinoma patients suffering steatorrhea (SHIMODA et al. 1968). *H. pylori* infection is infrequent, however, in this setting. In our opinion, peptic ulcer in states of marked gastric acid hypersecretion is most likely the result of an overwhelming assault on normal

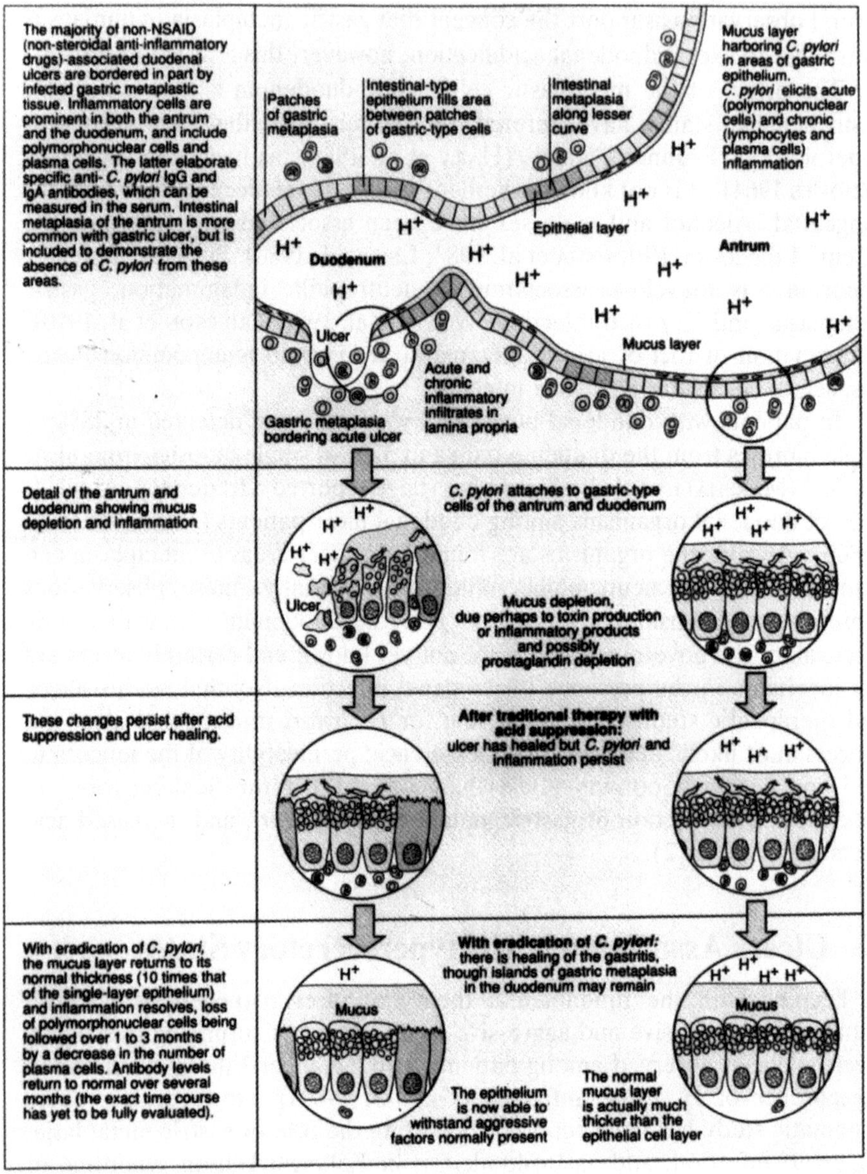

Fig. 2. *Helicobacter pylori* (formerly *Campylobacter pylori*) and the natural history of gastroduodenitis after ulcer healing with and without eradication of *H. pylori* infection (CALDWELL and MCCALLUM 1989)

mucosal defenses although this remains to be proven. The clinical significance of this relationship involves the evaluation of patients with recurrent peptic ulcer in the absence of histologic or serologic evidence of *H. pylori* infection and without a history of NSAID ingestion. Such patients, in our opinion, should undergo more aggressive measures (such as gastric analysis and gastrin testing) to rule out an endocrine-mediated hypersecretory state.

H. Malignant Ulcers

On the surface, malignant gastric ulcer would seem to bear little relationship to the other varieties of gastric ulcer outside of the obvious similarities and sometimes deceptive appearance through the endoscope. The frequent, although not uniform, association with fasting achlorhydria and the obvious explanation of ulceration associated with malignancy of any type, suggest that the mechanisms involved are fundamentally different. On the other hand, several similarities and pertinent points bear brief discussion.

It is of interest that some of the earliest reports of spiral organisms in human stomachs were in association with ulcerating gastric malignancy (Kreinitz 1906). This may be merely coincidental; however, several lines of evidence suggest that gastritis, *H. pylori*, and gastric cancer may in some way be associated (Fox et al. 1989). Gastric cancers are most common in the distal stomach and lesser curvature (Richardson 1989). Malignancy usually occurs in a background histology quite similar to chronic relapsing benign gastric ulcer, i.e., in the setting of various degrees of inflammation, atrophy, and intestinal metaplasia. The trigger for malignant transformation of a chronically inflamed and metaplastic mucosa is not known if indeed this is the mechanism involved. Nitrate metabolism by intestinal bacteria has been proposed in the past as a possible contributing factor in the development of gastric cancer. In this context, it is of note that *H. pylori* does not appear capable of active nitrate reduction (Dooley and Cohen 1988).

J. Other Types of Chronic Relapsing Peptic Ulcer

Although we feel that the majority of non-stress-related ulcers can be explained by one or more of the factors that we have just discussed, there remains a group of patients in whom none of these mechanisms appear to apply. It is likely that over the next few years, as more is learned about *Helicobacter pylori* and peptic ulcer, it will become apparent that a small percentage of patients who have documented ulcer will have no evidence of active *H. pylori* infection or of NSAID ingestion. As mentioned previously, some of these patients may fall into the category of gastric ulcer as a result of bile reflux (O'Conner et al. 1987) and others may have occult hypersecretory conditions. In addition, recurrent gastric ulcers have been reported in a small group of women suffering from mesenteric vascular insufficiency (Cherry et al. 1986). Finally, the accuracy of the medical history will at times have to be questioned in the face of chronic, recurring gastric ulcer without identifiable risk factors. Occult use of salicylates was recently reported in five patients with chronic relapsing and refractory ulcers (PERRAULT et al. 1988). These patients had measurable, often therapeutic, serum salicylate levels, despite a negative history of aspirin use on the initial interview.

K. Acute Mucosal Stress Ulceration

Severe, life-threatening illnesses have long been known to impart a significant risk for gastroduodenal mucosal ulceration. The common situations in which stress ulcers occur include major trauma, severe head injury, extensive burns, sepsis, and major surgical procedures. Diminished mucosal blood flow, as a result of systemic hypotension (or head injury in the absence of systemic hypotension), is a common underlying factor (WILCOX and SPENNEY 1988). Reflectance spectrophotometry has revealed a relationship between the degree of mucosal blood flow impairment and likelihood of subsequent ulcer development (KAMADA et al. 1982).

There is little detailed knowledge regarding the background histology of these ulcers. Endoscopic studies have revealed hemorrhagic and erosive changes within hours of the acute insult although their relation to true ulcer is not known (CZAJA et al. 1974). Unlike chronic relapsing ulcer, the majority of endoscopically visible lesions in the acute setting occur in the fundus or corpus of the stomach. Discrete ulcers are less common than hemorrhages. In one recent series of 44 patients who underwent endoscopy within 24 h of a head injury, only two patients had actual ulcers at the time of the endoscopy (BROWN et al. 1989), while hemorrhagic and erosive lesions were much more common (90% of patients). Whether or not hemorrhagic lesions evolve into true ulcerations is not known.

Although gastric acid secretion during stress is usually normal or decreased (SILEN et al. 1981), hydrogen ion appears to be a significant factor in the pathogenesis of mucosal injury in this setting (MILLER 1987). Localized tissue acidosis occurs (FIDDIAN-GREEN et al. 1983) and possibly results from the inability of the ischemic tissue to handle even small amounts of gastric acid back-diffusion. The relationship of acute stress ulcer to chronic relapsing ulcer is uncertain. Whether antecedent histologic gastritis increases the risk of developing injury or influences its severity remains to be determined.

L. Summary

Peptic ulcer is a heterogeneous and multifactorial disease (Fig. 3). In virtually all of the types of mucosal ulceration there is an acute or sustained loss of equilibrium between aggressive factors (particularly gastric acid) and mucosal defenses. Clinically and pathophysiologically, peptic ulcers can be divided

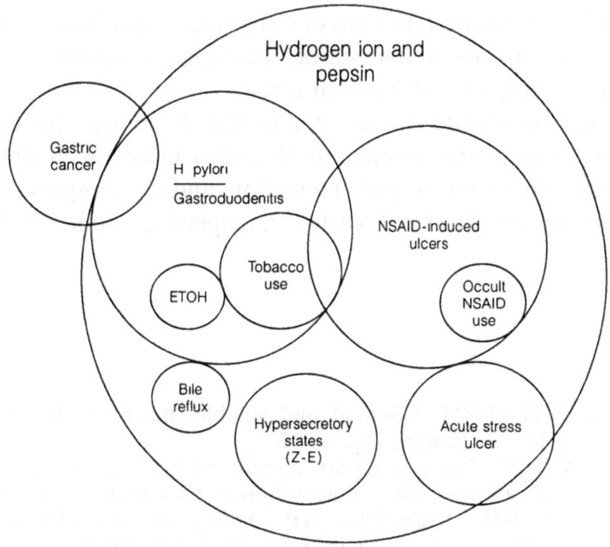

Fig. 3. Conceptual diagram of the relationships between various ulcer etiologies and associated factors. With rare exceptions, acid appears to be common to most forms of gastroduodenal ulcers. NSAID-induced ulcers and *H. pylori*-associated ulcers constitute the major divisions of chronic relapsing ulcer. We have included gastric cancer as overlapping with *H. pylori* infection because of the often common histologic background although no relationship has as yet been proven. Alcohol (*ETOH*) is included within the *H. pylori* group because of its possible relationship to gastric metaplasia of the duodenum and adverse effects on duodenal ulcer healing. *Z-E*, Zollinger-Ellison

into the broad categories of chronic relapsing ulcer and acute stress-related ulcer. The vast majority of ulcers encountered by the practitioner will fall into the category of chronic relapsing peptic ulcer. Within this category exist two major and sometimes overlapping divisions, chronic NSAID ingestion and *H. pylori*-related histologic gastroduodenitis. Outside of malignancy which may at times masquerade as benign ulceration, hydrogen ion plays a crucial role in most forms of peptic ulcers. In the absence of either *H. pylori* infection or known NSAID use, a search should be made for occult NSAID ingestion or a hypersecretory state such as Zollinger-Ellison syndrome.

Acute stress ulcers appear to result fundamentally from deranged mucosal blood flow. Likewise, NSAIDs appear to impair vascular integrity, probably as a result of prostaglandin inhibition. Prostaglandin inhibition appears also to lead to a compromised mucosal barrier in other ways such as impaired mucus production and bicarbonate secretion. Although there is a paucity of data, the available literature would suggest that NSAID-related ulcers often occur in the absence of chronic histologic gastritis. This, along with their clinical silence, may reflect analgesic and anti-inflammatory properties of these medications. In contrast, the majority of relapsing gastroduodenal ulcers occur in the setting of diffuse histologic inflammation.

H. pylori infection of gastric-type cells of either the stomach or the duodenum is the major cause of these inflammatory changes and imparts a significant although not inevitable risk of mucosal ulceration.

Future research should better define the histologic background of NSAID-related ulcer in the absence of *H. pylori* infection, further explore prostaglandin metabolism in *H. pylori* infection, and most importantly, define the natural history of duodenal gastric metaplasia, about which little is known.

References

Allen A, Carroll NJH (1985) Adherent and soluble mucus in the stomach and duodenum. Dig Dis Sci [Suppl] 30:55s–62s

Allen A, Garner A (1980) Progress report: mucus and bicarbonate secretion in the stomach and their possible role in mucosal protection. Gut 21:249–262

Alquist DA, Dozois RR, Zinsmeister AR, Malagelada JR (1983) Duodenal prostaglandin synthesis and acid load in health and in duodenal ulcer disease. Gastroenterology 85:522–528

Bahari HMM, Ross IN, Turnberg LA (1982) Demonstration of a pH gradient across the mucus layer on the surface of human gastric mucosa in vitro. Gut 23: 513–516

Barlow TE, Bentley FH, Waldren DN (1951) Arteries, veins and arteriovenous anastomoses in the human stomach. Surg Gynecol Obstet 93:657–671

Baron JH (1963) The relationship between basal and maximum acid output in normal subjects and patients with duodenal ulcer. Clin Sci 24:357–370

Barrilleaux CN, Jackson ME, Juchau SV, Bauman JM, Leib RC, Goldner F (1988) Influence of *Campylobacter pylori* associated non-ulcer gastritis on solid-phase gastric emptying (abstract). Am J Gastroenterol 83:1029

Bayerdorffer E, Oertel H, Lehn N, Kasper G, Mannes GA, Sauerbruch T, Stolte M (1989) Topographic association between active gastritis and *Campylobacter pylori* colonisation. J Clin Pathol 42:834–839

Berkowicz J, Lee A (1987) Person-to-person transmission of *Campylobacter pylori.* Lancet 2:680–681

Bode GP, Malfertheiner P, Ditschuneit H (1988) Pathogenetic implications of ultrastructural findings in *Campylobacter pylori* related gastroduodenal disease. Scand J Gastroenterol [Suppl] 23:25–39

Brooks FP (1985) The pathophysiology of peptic ulcer disease. Dig Dis Sci [Suppl] 30:15s–29s

Brown TH, Davidson PF, Larson GM (1989) Acute gastritis occurring within 24 hours of severe head injury. Gastrointest Endosc 35:37–40

Bugat R, Thompson MR, Aures D (1976) Gastric mucosal lesions produced by intravenous infusion of aspirin in cats. Gastroenterology 71:754–759

Caldwell SH, McCallum RW (1989) Peptic ulcer disease and *Campylobacter pylori*:new insights into an old disease. Triangle 27:165–177

Caldwell SH, Marshall BJ, Plankey MW, Frierson HF, Hoffman SR, McCallum RW (1989a) *Campylobacter pylori* gastritis after ulcer surgery (Abstr). Va Med 116:515–516

Caldwell SH, Valenzuela G, Marshall BJ, Dye KR, Hoffman SR, Plankey MW, McCallum RW (1989b) *Campylobacter pylori* gastritis does not slow solid phase Tc99 gastric emptying (abstract). Am J Gastroenterol 84:1155

Cave DR, Vargas M (1989) Effect of a *Campylobacter pylori* protein on acid secretion by parietal cells. Lancet 2:187–189

Cherry RD, Jabbari M, Goresky CA, Herba M, Reich D, Blundell PE (1986) Chronic

mesenteric vascular insufficiency with gastric ulceration. Gastroenterology 91:1548–1552
Chey WY, Kosay S, Lorber SH (1970) Effect of ethanol on gastric secretion and histology of the gastric mucosa in dogs (Abstr). Fed Proc 29:255
Coghlan JG, Humphries H, Dooley C, Keane C, Gilligan D, McKenna D, Sweeney E, O'Morain C (1987) *Campylobacter pylori* and recurrence of duodenal ulcers – a twelve month follow-up study. Lancet 2:1109–1111
Cohen MM, Boudler R, Gervais P, Morris GP, Wang H-K (1989) Sucralfate protection of human gastric mucosa against acute ethanol injury. Gastroenterology 96:292–298
Conn HO, Blitzer BL (1976) Non-association of adrenocorticoid therapy and peptic ulcer. N Engl J Med 294:473–479
Correa P (1988) Chronic gastritis: a clinico-pathological classification. Am J Gastroenterol 83:504–509
Czaja AJ, McAlhaney JG, Pruitt BA (1974) Acute gastroduodenal disease after thermal injury. An endoscopic evaluation of incidence and natural history. N Engl J Med 291:925–929
Dajani EZ, Callison DA, Bertermann RE (1978) Effects of E prostaglandins on canine gastric potential difference. Dig Dis Sci 23:436–442
Davenport HW (1967) Ethanol damage to canine oxyntic glandular mucosa. Proc Soc Exp Biol Med 126:657–662
Davenport HW (1968) Destruction of the gastric mucosal barrier by detergents and urea. Gastroenterology 54:175–181
Davenport HW (1972) The gastric mucosal barrier. Digestion 5:162–165
Del Soldato P, Daniotti S, Scarpignato C (1984) Free radical scavenger compounds inhibit indomethacin induced gastrointestinal damage in the rat. J Pharmacol 15:536
Delaney JP, Broadie TA, Robbins PL (1975) Pyloric reflux gastritis: the offending agent. Surgery 77:764–768
Delaney JP, Michel HM, Bensack ME, Eisenberg MH, Dunn DH (1979) Adrenal corticosteroids cause gastrin cell hyperplasia. Gastroenterology 76:913–916
Desai HG, Antia FP (1969) Spontaneous achlorhydria with atrophic gastritis in the Zollinger-Ellison syndrome. Gut 10:935–939
Dinoso VP, Chey WY, Baverman SP, Rosen SP, Ottenberg D, Lorber SH (1972) Gastric secretion and gastric mucosal morphology in chronic alcoholics. Arch Intern Med 130:715–719
Dixon MF, O'Conner HJ, Axon ATR, King RFJG, Johnston D (1986) Reflux gastritis: a distinct histopathological entity. J Clin Pathol 39:524–527
Dooley CP, Cohen H (1988) The clinical significance of *Campylobacter pylori*. Ann Intern Med 108:70–79
Dooley CP, McKenna D, Humphries H, Bourke S, Keane CT, Sweeney E, O'Morain C (1988) Histologic gastritis in duodenal ulcer: relationship to *Campylobacter pylori* and effect of ulcer therapy. Am J Gastroenterol 83:278–282
Dragstedt LR (1967) Gastric secretion tests. Gastroenterology 52:587–589
Ehsanullah RSB, Page MC, Tildesley G, Wood JR (1988) Prevention of gastroduodenal damage induced by NSAIDS: controlled trial of ranitidine. Br Med J 297:1017–1021
Evans DG, Evans DJ, Graham DY (1989) Receptor-mediated adherence of *Campylobacter pylori* to mouse Y-1 adrenal cell monolayers. Infect Immun 57:2272–2278
Feldman M, Richardson CT (1986) Total 24-hour gastric acid secretion in patients with duodenal ulcer. Gastroenterology 90:540–544
Ferrero RL, Hazell SL, Lee A (1988) The urease enzymes of *Campylobacter pylori* and a related bacterium. J Med Microbiol 27:33–40
Fiddian-Green RG, McGough E, Pittenger G, Rothman E (1983) Predictive value of intramural pH and other risk factors for massive bleeding from stress ulceration. Gastroenterology 85:613–620

Flejou JF, Bahame P, Smith AC, Stockbrugger RW, Rode J, Price AB, (1989) Pernicious anaemia and *Campylobacter*-like organisms: is the gastric antrum resistant to colonisation? Gut 30:60–64
Flemstrom G, Kovilaakso E, Briden S, Nylander O, Jedstedt G (1985) Gastroduodenal bicarbonate secretion in mucosal protection. Dig Dis Sci [Suppl] 30:63s–68s
Florey HW, Jennings MA, Jennings DA, O'Conner RC (1939) The reaction of the intestine of the pig to gastric juice. J Pathol Bacteriol 49:105–123
Fox JG, Correa P, Taylor NS, Zavala D, Fantham E, Janney F, Rodriguez E, Hunter F, Diavolitsis S (1989) *Campylobacter pylori*-associated gastritis and immune response in a population at increased risk of gastric carcinoma. Am J Gastroenterol 84:775–781
Freidman GD, Sieglaub AB, Seltzer CC (1974) Cigarettes, alcohol, coffee, and peptic ulcer. N Engl J Med 290:469–473
Frierson HF, Caldwell SH, Marshall BJ (1990) Duodenal bulb biopsy findings in patients with non-ulcer dyspepsia with or without *Campylobacter pylori* gastritis. Modern Pathol (in press)
Fullman H, van Deventer G, Schneidman D, Walsh G, Elashoff J, Weinstein W (1985) "Healed" duodenal ulcers are histologically ill (Abstr). Gastroenterology 88:1390
Fung WP, Mahoney DP, Beilin LJ (1982) The effect of cigarette smoking on gastric secretion of 6-keto prostaglandin F1 alpha. Aust NZ J Med 12:206–210
Geall MG, Phillips SF, Summerskill WHJ (1970) Profile of gastric potential difference in man. Gastroenterology 58:437–443
Gear MWL, Truelove SC, Whitehead R (1971) Gastric ulcer and gastritis. Gut 12:639–645
Goddard PJ, Hills BA, Lichtenberger LM (1987) Does aspirin damage canine gastric mucosa by reducing its surface hydrophobicity? Am J Physiol 252:G421–G430
Goldschmiedt M, Peterson WL, Vuitch F, Feldman M, (1989) Postbulbar duodenal ulcer in a patient with pentagastrin-fast achlorhydria. Gastroenterology 97:771–774
Goodwin CS (1988) Duodenal ulcer, *Campylobacter pylori*, and the "leaking roof" concept. Lancet 2:1467–1469
Gottfried EB, Korsten MA, Lieber CS (1978) Alcohol-induced gastric and duodenal lesions in man. Am J Gastroenterol 70:587–592
Graham DY (1989a) *Campylobacter pylori* and peptic ulcer disease. Gastroenterology [Suppl] 96:615–625
Graham DY (1989b) Prevention of gastroduodenal injury induced by chronic nonsteroidal anti-inflammatory drug therapy. Gastroenterology [Suppl] 96:675–681
Graham DY, Smith JL (1986) Aspirin and the stomach. Ann Intern Med 104:390–398
Graham DY, Smith LJ, Dobbs SM (1983) Gastric adaptation occurs with aspirin administration in man. Dig Dis Sci 28:1–6
Graham DY, Alpert LC, Smith GL, Yoshimura HH (1988a) Iatrogenic *Campylobacter pylori* infection is a cause of epidemic achlorhydria. Am J Gastroenterol 83:974–980
Graham DY, Agrawal NM, Roth SH (1988b) Prevention of NSAID-induced gastric ulcer with misoprostol: multicentre, double-blind, placebo-controlled trial. Lancet 2:1277–1280
Gray SJ, Bensen JA, Reifenstein RW, Spiro HM (1951) Chronic stress and peptic ulcer. I effect of corticotropin (ACTH) and cortisone on gastric secretion. JAMA 147:1529–1537
Greenlaw R, Sheahan DG, DeLuca V, Miller D, Myerson D, Myerson P (1980) Gastroduodenitis: a broader concept of peptic ulcer disease. Dig Dis Sci 25:660–672
Griffin M, Ray WA, Schaffner W (1988) Nonsteroidal anti-inflammatory drug use and death from peptic ulcer in elderly patients. Ann Intern Med 109:359–363

Guth PH, Paulsen G, Nagata H (1984) Histologic and microcirculatory changes in alcohol-induced gastric lesions in the rat: effect of prostaglandin cytoprotection. Gastroenterology 87:1083–1090
Hamilton SR, Yardley JH (1980) Endoscopic biopsy diagnosis of aspirin associated chronic gastric ulcers (Abstr). Gastroenterology 78:A1178
Hansen D, Salman JA, Whittle BJR (1983) Ulcerogenesis and prostanoid inhibition in the cat gastric antrum induced by parenteral aspirin but not salicylate. Br J Pharmacol 80:602–605
Hara M, Harasawa S, Tani N, Miwa T, Tsutsumi Y (1988) Gastric metaplasia in duodenal ulcer. Acta Pathol Jpn 38:1011–1018
Hawkey CJ, Walt RP (1986) Prostaglandins for peptic ulcer: a promise unfulfilled. Lancet 2:1084–1087
Hazell SL, Lee A, Brady L, Hennessey W (1986) *Campylobacter pyloridis* and gastritis: association with intracellular spaces and adaptation to an environment of mucus as important factors in colonization of the gastric epithelium. J Infect Dis 153:658–663
Hazell SL, Hennessy WB, Borody TJ, Carrick J, Ralston M, Brady L, Lee A (1987) *Campylobacter pyloridis* gastritis II: distribution of bacteria and associated inflammation in the gastroduodenal environment. Am J Gastroenterol 82:297–301
Hillier K, Smith CL, Jewell R, Arthur MJP, Ross G (1985) Duodenal mucosa synthesis of prostaglandins in duodenal ulcer disease. Gut 26:237–240
Hills BA, Butler BD, Lichtenberger LM (1983) Gastric mucosal barrier: hydrophobic lining of the lumen of the stomach. Am J Physiol 244:G561–G568
Hui W-M, Lam S-K, Ho J, Ng MMT, Lui I, Lai CL, Lok ASF, Lau WY, Poon GP, Choi S, Choi TK (1986) Chronic antral gastritis in duodenal ulcer. Natural history and treatment with prostaglandin E_1. Gastroenterology 91:1095–1101
Isenberg JI, Cano R, Bloom SR (1977) Effect of graded amounts of acid instilled into the duodenum on pancreatic bicarbonate secretion and plasma secretin in duodenal ulcer patients and normal subjects. Gastroenterology 72:6–8
Isenberg JI, Selling JA, Hogan DL, Koss MA (1987) Impaired proximal duodenal mucosa bicarbonate secretion in patients with duodenal ulcer. N Engl J Med 316:374–379
Ivey KJ (1988) Mechanisms of nonsteroidal anti-inflammatory drug-induced gastric damage. Am J Med [Suppl 2a] 84:41–48
Ivey KJ, Paone DB, Krause WJ (1980) Acute effect of systemic aspirin on gastric mucosa in man. Dig Dis Sci 25:97–99
James AH (1964) Gastric epithelium in the duodenum. Gut 5:285–294
Johansson C, Aly A, Kollberg B, Rubio C, Erkoinen T, Helander H (1982) Oral E2 prostaglandins stimulate growth of the rat stomach, small intestine and colon. Scand J Gastroenterol 17:42–45
Johnson HD (1965) Gastric ulcer: classification, blood group characteristics, secretion patterns and pathogenesis. Ann Surg 162:996–1004
Johnson HD, Love AHG, Rogers NC, Wyatt AP (1964) Gastric ulcers, blood groups and acid secretion. Gut 5:402–411
Johnson LR (1977) New aspects of the trophic action of gastrointestinal hormones. Gastroenterology 72:788–792
Johnson LR, Guthrie PD (1980) Stimulation of rat oxyntic gland mucosal growth by epidermal growth factor. Am J Physio 238:G45–G49
Johnston BJ, Reed PI, Ali MH (1986a) Correlation between endoscopic appearances and histologic diagnosis of antral and duodenal inflammation (abstract). Gastroenterology 90:1480
Johnston BJ, Reed PI, Ali MH (1986b) *Campylobacter*-like organisms in duodenal and antral endoscopic biopsies: relationship to inflammation. Gut 27:1132–1137
Kamada T, Sato N, Kawano S, Fusamoto H, Abe H (1982) Gastric mucosal hemodynamics after thermal or head injury: a clinical application of reflectance spectrophotometry. Gastroenterology 83:535–540

Kauffman GL (1985) The gastric mucosal barrier. Dig Dis Sci [Suppl] 30:69s–76s
Kauffman GL (1989) Aspirin-induced gastric mucosal injury: lessons learned from animal models. Gastroenterology [Suppl] 96:606–614
Kerss S, Allen A, Garner A (1982) A simple method for measuring thickness of the mucus gel layer adherent to rat, frog and human gastric mucosa: influence of feeding, prostaglandins, *N*-acetylcysteine and other agents. Clin Sci 63:187–195
Kirk RM (1981) Are gastric and duodenal ulcers separate diseases or do they form a continuum? Dig Dis Sci 26:149–154
Kirk RM (1986) Could chronic peptic ulcers be localised areas of acid susceptibility generated by autoimmunity. Lancet 1:772–775
Kirkegaard P, Olsen PS, Poulsen SS, Holst J, Schaffalitzky de Mucadell OB, Christiansen J (1984) Effect of secretin and glucagon on Brunner's gland secretion in the rat. Gut 25:264–268
Kitahora T, Guth PH (1987) Effect of aspirin plus hydrochloric acid on the gastric mucosal microcirculation. Gastroenterology 93:810–817
Kreinitz W (1906) Ueber das Auftreten von Spirochaeten verschiedener Form im Mageninhalt bei Carcinoma ventriculi. Dtsch Med Wochenshr 32:872–874
Kreuning J, Bosman FT, Kuiper G, Wal AM, Lindeman J (1978) Gastric and duodenal mucosa in "healthy" individuals. J Clin Pathol 31:69–77
Lacy ER (1985) Prostaglandins and histologic changes in the gastric mucosa. Dig Dis Sci [Suppl] 30:83s–94s
Lacy ER, Ito S (1982) Microscopic analysis of ethanol damage to rat gastric mucosa after treatment with a prostaglandin. Gastroenterology 83:619–625
Lacy ER, Ito S (1984) Ethanol-induced insult to the superficial rat gastric epithelium: a study of damage and rapid repair. In: Allen A, Flemstrom G, Garner A, Silen W, Turnberg LA (eds) Mechanisms of mucosal protection in the upper gastrointestinal tract. Raven, New York, pp 49–56
Laine L, Marin-Sorensen M, Weinstein WM (1988) *Campylobacter pylori* in alcoholic hemorrhagic and erosive gastritis (Abstr). Gastroenterology 94:A246
Lam SK, Hui WM, Lau WY, Branicki FJ, Lai CL, Lok ASF, Ng MMT, Fok PJ, Poon GP, Choi TK (1987) Sucralfate overcomes adverse effect of cigarette smoking on duodenal ulcer healing and prolongs subsequent remission. Gastroenterology 92:1193–1201
Lanza FL (1984) Endoscopic studies of gastric and duodenal injury after the use of ibuprofen, aspirin and other NSAIDs. Am J Med [Suppl 1a] 77:19–24
Lanza FL, Karlin DA, Yee JP (1987) A double-blind placebo controlled endoscopic study comparing the mucosal injury seen with orally and parenterally administered nonsteroidal analgesic ketorolac tromethamine at therapeutic and supratherapeutic doses (Abstr). Am J Gastroenterol 82:939
Lanza FL, Aspinall RL, Swabb EA, Davis RE, Rock MF, Rubin A (1988) Double-blind placebo-controlled endoscopic comparison of the mucosal protective effects of misoprostol versus cimetidine on tolmetin-induced mucosal injury to the stomach. Gastroenterology 95:289–294
Lanza FL, Skoglund ML, Rock MF, Yardley JH (1989) The effect of bismuth subsalicylate on the histologic gastritis seen with *Campylobacter pylori*: a placebo-controlled randomized study. Am J Gastroenterol 84:1060–1064
Lawson HH (1964) Effect of duodenal contents on the gastric mucosa under experimental conditions. Lancet 1:469–472
Lee A, Hazell SL (1988) *Campylobacter pylori* in health and disease: an ecological perspective. Microb Health Dis 1:1–16
Lenz HJ, Ferrari-Taylor J, Isenberg JI (1983) Wine and five percent ethanol are potent stimulants of gastric acid secretion in humans. Gastroenterology 85:1082–1087
Leung FW, Itoh M, Hirabayaski K, Guth PH (1985) Role of blood flow in gastric and duodenal mucosal injury in the rat. Gastroenterology 88:281–289

Leung FW, Reedy TJ, van Deventer GM, Guth PH (1989) Reduction in index of oxygen saturation at margin of active duodenal ulcers may lead to slow healing. Dig Dis Sci 34:417–423
Leunk RD, Johnson PT, David BC, Kraft WG, Morgan DR (1988) Cytotoxic activity in broth-culture filtrates of *Campylobacter pylori*. J Med Microbiol 26:93–99
Lev R, Thomas E, Parl FF, Pitchumoni CS (1980) Pathologic and histomorphometric study of the effects of alcohol on the human duodenum. Digestion 20:207–213
Lichtenberg LM, Graziani LA, Dial EJ, Butler BD, Hills BA (1983) Role of surface-active phospholipids in gastric cytoprotection. Science 219:1327–1329
Lingwood CA, Pellizzari A, Law H, Sherman P, Drumm B (1989) Gastric glycerolipid as a receptor for *Campylobacter pylori*. Lancet 2:238–241
Loeb JN, Sternschein MJ (1973) Suppression of thymidine incorporation into the gastric mucosa of cortisone-treated rats: possible relation to glucocorticoid-induced gastric ulceration. Endocrinology 92:1322–1327
Loffeld RJLF, Loffeld BCA, Arends JW, Flendrig JA, van Spreeuwel JP (1988) Retrospective study of *Campylobacter-like* organisms in patients undergoing partial gastrectomy. J Clin Pathol 41:1313–1315
Maaroos H-I, Salupere V, Uibo R, Kekki M, Sipponen P (1985) Seven-year follow-up study of chronic gastritis in gastric ulcer patients. Scand J Gastroenterol 20:198–204
MacDonald WC (1973) Correlation of mucosal histology and aspirin intake in chronic gastric ulcer. Gastroenterology 65:381–389
Malagelada JR, Longstreth GF, Deering TB, Summerskill WHJ, Go VLW (1977) Gastric secretion and emptying after ordinary meals in duodenal ulcer. Gastroenterology 73:989–994
Malagelada JR, Phillips SF, Shorter RG, Higgins JA, Magrina C, van Heerden JA, Adson MA (1985) Postoperative reflux gastritis: pathophysiology and long-term outcome after Roux-en-Y diversion. Ann Intern Med 103:178–185
Malfertheiner P, Ditschuneit H (1988) Pathogenetic implication of ultrastructural findings in *Campylobacter pylori* related gastroduodenal disease. Scand J Gastroenterol [Suppl 142] 23:25–39
Marshall BJ, McGechie DB, Rogers PA, Glancy RJ (1985a) Pyloric *Campylobacter* infection and gastroduodenal disease. Med J Aust 142:439–444
Marshall BJ, Armstrong JA, McGechie DB, Glancy RJ (1985b) Attempts to fulfill Koch's postulates for pyloric *Campylobacter*. Med J Aust 142:436–439
Marshall BJ, Warren JR, Blincow ED, Phillips M, Goodwin CS, Murray R, Blackbourn SJ, Waters TE (1988a) Prospective double-blind trial of duodenal ulcer relapse after eradication of *Campylobacter pylori*. Lancet 2:1438–1469
Marshall BJ, Dye KR, Hoffman SR, Plankey M, Guerrant RL, McCallum RW (1988b) The prevalence of *Campylobacter pylori* infection in the spouses of infected patients (Abstr). Am J Gastroenterol 83:1036
Marshall BJ, Dye KR, Plankey M, Frierson HF, Hoffman SR, Guerrant RL, McCallum RW (1988c) Eradication of *Campylobacter pylori* infection with bismuth subsalicylate and antibiotic combinations (Abstr). Am J Gastroenterol 83:1035
Marshall BJ, Caldwell SH, Yu ZJ, Darr F, Chang T, McCallum RW (1989) Prevalence of *C. pylori* and history of upper G.I. investigation in healthy Virginians (Abstr). Gastroenterology 96:A321
Marti U, Burwen SJ, Jones AL (1989) Biological effects of epidermal growth factor with emphasis on the gastrointestinal tract and liver: an update. Hepatology 9:126–138
Martin DF, Montgomery E, Dobek AS, Patrissi GA, Peura DA (1989) *Campylobacter pylori*, NSAIDs, and smoking: risk factors for peptic ulcer disease. Am J Gastroenterol 84:1268–1272
McCallum RW, Singh D, Wollman J (1979) Endoscopic and histologic correlations of the duodenal bulb. Arch Pathol Lab Med 103:169–172

McCarthy DM (1989) Nonsteroidal antiinflammatory drug-induced ulcers: management by traditional therapy. Gastroenterology [Suppl] 96:662–674
Meikle DD, Taylor KB, Truelove SC, Whitehead R (1976) Gastritis, duodenitis and circulating levels of gastrin in duodenal ulcer before and after vagotomy. Gut 17:719–728
Menguy R, Masters YF (1963) Effect of cortisone on mucoprotein secretion by gastric antrum of dogs: pathogenesis of steroid ulcer. Surgery 54:19–27
Merki HS, Fimmel CJ, Walt RP, Harre K, Rohmel J, Witzel L (1988) Patterns of 24-hour intragastric acidity in active duodenal ulcer disease and in healthy controls. Gut 29:1583–1587
Mersereau WA, Hinchey EJ (1982) Role of gastric mucosal folds in formation of focal ulcers in the rat. Surgery 91:150–155
Messer J, Reitman D, Sacks HS, Smith H, Chalmers TC (1983) Association of adrenocorticosteroid therapy and peptic-ulcer disease. N. Engl J Med 309: 21–24
Miller TA (1987) Mechanisms of stress-related mucosal damage. Am J Med [suppl 6A] 83:8–14
Miller TA (1988) Gastroduodenal mucosal defense: factors responsible for the ability of the stomach and duodenum to resist injury. Surgery 103:389–396
Miranda M, Defilippi C, Valenzuela JE (1985) Abnormalities of interdigestive motility complex and increased duodenogastric reflux in gastric ulcer patients. Dig Dis Sci 30:16–21
Mogard MH, Maxwell V, Reedy TJ, Walsh JH (1987) Gastric acidification inhibits meal-stimulated gastric acid secretion after prostaglandin synthesis inhibition by indomethacin in humans. Gastroenterology 93:63–68
Moore SC, Malagelada J-R, Shorter RG, Zinsmeister AR (1986) Interrelationships among gastric mucosal morphology, secretion and motility in peptic ulcer disease. Dig Dis Sci 31:673–684
Morris A, Nicholson G (1987) Ingestion of *Campylobacter pyloridis* causes gastritis and raises fasting gastric pH. Am J Gastroenterol 82:192–197
O'Brien P, Schultz C, Gannon B, Browning J (1986) Protective effects of the synthetic prostaglandin enprostil on the gastric microvasculature after ethanol injury in the rat. Am J Med [Suppl 2A] 81:12–17
O'Conner HJ, Wyatt JI, Ward DC, Dixon MF, Axon ATR, Dewar EP, Johnston D (1986) Effect of duodenal ulcer surgery and enterogastric reflux on *Campylobacter pyloridis*. Lancet 2:1178–1180
O'Conner HJ, Dixon MF, Wyatt JI, Axon ATR, Dewar EP, Johnston D (1987) *Campylobacter pylori* and peptic ulcer disease (Letter). Lancet 2:633–634
Oates PJ, Hakkinen JP (1988) Studies on the mechanism of ethanol-induced gastric damage in rats. Gastroenterology 94:10–21
Oi M, Oshida K, Sugimura S (1959) The location of gastric ulcer. Gastroenterology 86:45–56
Oi M, Ito Y, Kumagai F, Yoshida K, Tanaka Y, Yoshikawa K, Miko O, Kijima M (1969) A possible dual control mechanism in the origin of peptic ulcer. A study on ulcer location as affected by mucosa and musculature. Gastroenterology 57:280–293
Okada M, Fuchigama T, Lida M, Omae T, Kimihiro A, Onoyama K (1985) Adrenocorticosteroid therapy and gastroduodenal lesions. Gastrointest Endosc 31:188–190
Ottenjan R (1970) Chronische Gastritis. Dtsch Med Wochenschr 95:1235–1240
Parks DA (1989) Oxygen free radicals: mediators of gastrointestinal pathophysiology. Gut 30:293–298
Parl FF, Lev R, Thomas E, Pitchumoni CS (1979) Histologic and morphometric study of chronic gastritis in alcoholic patients. Hum Pathol 10:45–56
Pearson J, Allen A, Venables C (1980) Gastric mucus. Isolation and polymeric structure of the undegraded glycoprotein: its breakdown by pepsin. Gastroenterology 78:709–715

Perez-Perez GI, Dworkin BM, Chodos JE, Blaser MJ (1988) *Campylobacter pylori* antibodies in humans. Ann Intern Med 109:11–17
Perrault J, Fleming R, Dozois RR (1988) Surreptitious use of salicylates: a cause of chronic recurrent ulcers. Mayo Clin Proc 63:337–342
Peterson GM, Lam SK, Samloff IM, Jing J, Rotter JI (1985) Genetic factors predict duodenal ulcer healing (abstract). Gastroenterology 88:1538A
Peterson WJ, Lee E, Feldman M (1988) Relationship between *Campylobacter pylori* and gastritis in healthy humans after administration of placebo or indomethacin. Gastroenterology 95:1185–1197
Pounder R (1989) Silent peptic ulceration: deadly silence or golden silence. Gastroenterology [Suppl] 96:626–631
Price AB, Levi J, Dolby JM, Dunscomb PL, Smith A, Clark J, Stephenson ML (1985) *Campylobacter pyloridis* in peptic ulcer disease: microbiology, pathology and scanning electron microscopy. Gut 26:1183–1188
Quimby GF, Bonnice CA, Burstein SH, Eastwood GL (1986) Active smoking depresses prostaglandin synthesis in human gastric mucosa. Ann Intern Med 104:616–619
Ramsey EJ, Carey KV, Peterson WL, Jackson JJ, Murphy FK, Read NW, Taylor KB, Trier JS, Fordtran JS (1979) Epidemic gastritis with hypochlorhydria. Gastroenterology 76:1449–1457
Rathbone BJ, Wyatt JI, Worsley BW, Shires SE, Trejdosiewicz LK, Heatley RV, Losowsky MS (1986) Systemic and local antibody response to gastric *Campylobacter pyloridis* in nonulcer dyspepsia. Gut 27:642–647
Rauws EAJ, Langenberg W, Houthoff HJ, Zanen HC, Tytgat GNJ (1988) *Campylobacter pyloridis*-associated chronic active antral gastritis. Gastroenterology 94:33–40
Redfern JS, Blair AJ, Lee E, Feldman M (1987) Gastrointestinal ulcer formation in rabbits immunized with prostaglandin E_2 Gastroenterology 93:744–752
Reynolds JC (1989) Famotidine for active duodenal ulcers. Ann Intern Med 111:7–14
Rhodes J (1964) Experimental production of gastric epithelium in the duodenum. Gut 5:454
Richardson CT (1989) Gastric ulcer. In: Sleisinger MH, Fordtran JS (eds) Gastrointestinal disease 4th ed. Saunders, Philadelphia, pp 879–909
Robert A, Nezamis JE, Lancaster C, Janchar AJ (1979) Cytoprotection by prostaglandin in rats. Prevention of gastric necrosis produced by alcohol, HCl, NaOH, hypertonic NaCl, and thermal injury. Gastroenterology 77:433–443
Rotter JI, Sones JW, Samloff IM, Richardson CT, Gursky JM, Walsh JH, Rimoin DL (1979) Duodenal ulcer disease associated with elevated serum pepsinogen I: an inherited autosomal dominant disorder. N Engl J Med 300:63–65
Rume SJ (1973) pH in the human duodenum. Digestion 8:261–268
Rutten MJ, Ito S (1983) Morphology and electrophysiology of guinea pig gastric mucosal repair in vitro. Am J Physiol 244:G171–G182
Samloff IM (1989) Peptic ulcer: the many proteinases of aggression. Gastroenterology [Suppl] 96:586–595
Samloff IM, Liebman WM (1973) Cellular localization of the group II pepsinogens in human stomach and duodenum by immunofluorescence. Gastroenterology 65:36–42
Sarosiek J, Slomiany A, Slomiany BL (1988) Evidence for weakening of gastric mucus integrity by *Campylobacter pylori*. Scand J Gastroenterol 23:585–590
Sarosiek J, Bilski J, Murty VLN, Slomiany A, Slomiany BL (1989) Colloidal bismuth subcitrate (De Nol) inhibits degradation of gastric mucus by *Campylobacter pylori* protease. Am J Gastroenterol 84:506–510
Schlegel W, Wenk K, Dollinger HC (1977) Concentrations of prostaglandins A-, E- and F-like substances in gastric mucosa of normal subjects and of patients with various gastric diseases. Clin Sci Mol Med 52:255–258
Schoen RT, Vender RJ (1989) Mechanisms of nonsteroidal anti-inflammatory drug-induced gastric damage. Am J Med 86:449–458

Schrager J, Spink R, Mitra S (1967) The antrum in patients with duodenal and gastric ulcers. Gut 8:497–508
Schwarz K (1910) Über penetrierende Magen- und Jejunalgeschwüre. Beitr Klin Chir 67:96–128
Selling JA, Hogan DL, Koss MA (1985) Human proximal versus distal duodenal bicarbonate secretion: effect of endogenous prostaglandin synthesis (Abstr). Gastroenterology 88:A1580
Semble EL, Turner RA, Wu WC (1987) Clinical and genetic characteristics of upper gastrointestinal diseases in rheumatoid arthritis. J Rheumatol 14:692–699
Shimoda SS, Saunders DR, Rubin CE (1968) The Zollinger-Ellison syndrome with steatorrhea. Gastroenterology 55:705–723
Shorrock CJ, Rees WDW (1988) Overview of gastroduodenal mucosal protection. Am J Med [Suppl 2A] 84:25–34
Shousha S, Spiller RC, Parkins RA (1983) The endoscopically abnormal duodenum in patients with dyspepsia: biopsy findings in 60 cases. Histopathology 7:23–34
Silen W (1985) Pathogenic factors in erosive gastritis. Am J Med [Suppl 2C] 79:45–48
Silen W, Ito S (1985) Mechanisms for rapid re-epithelialization of the gastric mucosal surface. Annu Rev Physiol 47:217–229
Silen W, Merhaw A, Simson JNL (1981) The pathophysiology of stress ulcer disease. World J Surg 5:165–174
Silvoso GR, Ivey KJ, Butt JH, Lockard OO, Holt SD, Sisk C, Baskin WN, Mackercher PA, Hewett J (1979) Incidence of gastric lesions in patients with rheumatic disease on chronic aspirin therapy. Ann Intern Med 91:517–520
Skillman JJ, Lisbon A, Long PC, Silen W (1984) 15[R]-15-methyl prostaglandin E_2 does not prevent gastrointestinal bleeding in seriously ill patients. Am J Surg 147:451–455
Slomiany BL, Kasinathan C, Slomiany A (1989) Lipolytic activity of *Campylobacter pylori*: effect of colloidal bismuth subcitrate (DeNol). Am J Gastroenterol 84:1273–1277
Smith CL, Hillier K (1985) Duodenal mucosal synthesis of prostaglandins in duodenal ulcer disease. Gut 26:237–240
Smith SM, Grisham MB, Manci EA, Granger DN, Kvietys PR, Russell JM (1987) Gastric mucosal injury in the rat: role of iron and xanthine oxidase. Gastroenterology 92:950–956
Soll AH (1980) Specific inhibitions by prostaglandin E_2 and I_2 of histamine-stimulated [^{14}C] aminopyrine accumulation and cyclic adenosine monophosphate generation by isolated canine parietal cells. J Clin Invest 65:1222–1229
Soll AH, Kurata J, McGuigan JE (1989) Ulcers, nonsteroidal anti-inflammatory drugs and related matters. Gastroenterology [Suppl] 96:561–568
Sontag SJ (1988) Current status of maintenance therapy in peptic ulcer disease. Am J Gastroenterol 83:607–617
Sontag SJ, ACG Committee on FDA-Related Matters (1986) Prostaglandins and acid peptic disease. Am J Gastroenterol 81:1021–1028
Spiro H (1983) Is the steroid ulcer a myth? (Editorial). N Engl J Med 309:45–47
Stadelmann O, Elster K, Stolte M, Miederer SE, Deyhle P, Demling L, Siegenthaler W (1971) The peptic gastric ulcer – histotopographic and functional investigations. Scand J Gastroenterol 6:613–623
Strickland RG, Mackay IR (1973) A reappraisal of the nature and significance of chronic atrophic gastritis. Dig Dis 18:426–440
Szabo S, Frankel PW, Trier JS (1981) Sulphydryl compounds may mediate gastric cytoprotection. Science 214:200–202
Taha AS, Boothman P, Holland P, McKinlay A, Upadhyay R, Kelly RW, Lee F, Russell RI (1990) Gastric mucosal prostaglandin synthesis in the presence of *Campylobacter pylori* in patients with gastric ulcers and non-ulcer dyspepsia. Am J Gastroenterol 85:47–50
Tatsuta M, Okuda S (1975) Location, healing and recurrence of gastric ulcer in relation on fundal gastritis. Gastroenterology 69:897–902

Tatsuta M, Iishi H, Makoto I, Noguchi S, Okuda S, Taniguchi H (1985) Chromoendoscopic observations on extension and development of fundal gastritis and intestinal metaplasia. Gastroenterology 88:70–74
Tatsuta M, Iishi H, Okuda S (1986) Location of peptic ulcers in relation to antral and fundal gastritis by chromoendoscopic follow-up examinations. Dig Dis Sci 31:7–11
Thomas WEG (1984) The possible role of duodenogastric reflux in the pathogenesis of both gastric and duodenal ulcers. Scand J Gastroenterol [Suppl 92] 19:151–155
Thompson GN, Barr GA, Collier N, Spencer J, Bush A, Cope L, Gribble R, Baron J (1985) Basal, sham-feed, and pentagastrin-stimulated gastric acid, pepsin and electrolytes after omeprazole 20 mg and 40 mg daily. Gut 26:1018–1024
Turnberg LA, Ross IN (1984) Studies of the pH gradient across gastric mucus. Scand J Gastroenterol [Suppl 92] 19:48–50
Vaira D, Holton J, Londei M, Beltrandi E, Salmon PR, d'Anastasio C, Dowsett JF, Bertoni F, Grauenfels P, Gandolfi L (1988). *Campylobacter pylori* in abattoir workers: is it a zoonosis? Lancet 2:725–726
Van Deventer GM, Elashoff JD, Reedy TJ, Schneidman D, Walsh JH (1989) A randomized study of maintenance therapy with ranitidine to prevent the recurrence of duodenal ulcer. N Engl J Med 320:1113–1119
Varis K (1988) Gastritis – a misused term in clinical gastroenterology. Scand J Gastroenterol [Suppl 155] 23:53–59
Venables CW (1985) Duodenitis. Scand J Gastroenterol [Suppl 109] 20:91–97
Wagner BM (1985) Gastric morphology in ulcer patients receiving misoprostol. Dig Dis Sci [Suppl] 30:129s–132s
Walker V, Taylor WH (1980) Pepsin 1 secretion in chronic peptic ulceration. Gut 21:766–771
Wallace JL, Whittle BJ (1986) Role of mucus in the repair of gastric epithelial damage in the rat. Inhibition of epithelial recovery by mucolytic agents. Gastroenterology 91:603–611
Warren JR, Marshall BJ (1983) Unidentified curved bacilli on gastric epithelium in active chronic gastritis. Lancet 1:1273
Weiss A, Pittman ER, Graham EC (1961) Aspirin and gastric bleeding. Am J Med 31:266–278
Whitehead R, Truelove SC, Gear MWL (1972) The histologic diagnosis of chronic gastritis in fiberoptic gastroscope biopsy specimens. J Clin Pathol 25:1–11
Wilcox CM, Spenney JG (1988) Stress ulcer prophylaxis in medical patients: who, what and how much? Am J Gastroenterol 83:1199–1211
Wilson DE, Levendoglu H, Adams A, Ramsamooj E (1984) A new PGE_1 analogue (CL115, 574) 111. Effects on gastric acid and mucus secretion in man. Prostaglandins 28:5–11
Woolfe MM, Soll AH (1988) The physiology of gastric acid secretion. N Engl J Med 319:1707–1715
Wright JP, Young GO, Klaff LJ, Weeks LA, Price SK, Marks IN (1982) Gastric mucosal prostaglandin E levels in patients with gastric ulcer disease and carcinoma. Gastroenterology 82:263–267
Wyatt JI (1989) The role of *Campylobacter pylori* in the pathogenesis of peptic ulcer disease. Scand J Gastroenterol [Suppl 157] 24:7–11
Wyatt JI, Rathbone BJ (1988) Immune response of the gastric mucosa to *Campylobacter pylori*. Scand J Gastroenterol [Suppl 142] 23:44–49
Wyatt JI, Rathbone BJ, Dixon MF, Heatley RV (1987) *Campylobacter pyloridis* and acid induced gastric metaplasia in the pathogenesis of duodenitis. J Clin Pathol 40:841–848

CHAPTER 9

Nonulcer Dyspepsia

D.A. Johnson

A. Introduction

> How are we to explain this . . . disease that is not; this wealth of balsams for sufferings which can not be named? Is there no distress to lull, no pain to lenify?
>
> T.C. Allbutt, 1884, *Neuroses of the Viscera*

Dyspepsia defies definition yet has been part of our language for centuries. In fact the term "nonulcer dyspepsia" may be a term in search of a disease. In addition to being an epiphenomenon of organic lesions of the digestive tract at various levels (peptic ulcers, hepatobiliary disease, pancreatic disease, neoplasia, etc.), the symptom complex of dyspepsia is a dysfunctional condition for which, to date, no organic basis can be found. If physicians all agreed on the definition of nonulcer dyspepsia the nosology of epigastric distress would be much simpler and we would be a long way towards appropriate therapy and indications for diagnosis. The problem lies in the term itself, which defines a disorder by the absence of the characteristics of another disorder. Nonulcer dyspepsia therefore is not a homogeneous disorder, but one which has many diseases and processes hidden within the confines of the clinical diagnosis.

B. Definition

> The abdomen is such a temple of mystery that attempts at too great specificity are unwise.
>
> Howard Spiro. 1985

Multiple definitions have been proposed for dyspepsia although many are mutually incompatible and a few even diametrically opposed (DeDombal 1981). A random survey of publications on dyspepsia showed that more than two-thirds contained no definition (DeDombal and Hall 1979). As a working definition, patients with nonulcer dyspepsia have symptoms that prompt a physician to believe an ulcer may be present, but no ulcer is found on evaluation. More recently, assistance with the definition was offered by a consensus of a symposium directed towards the management of dyspepsia. Nonulcer dyspepsia was defined as upper abdominal or retrosternal pain, discomfort, heartburn, nausea, vomiting, or other symptom considered to be referable to the proximal alimentary tract. The symptom complex, as defined, persisted for a minimum of 4 weeks, was unrelated to exercise, and a focal lesion or systemic disease could not be implicated in the genesis of the complaints (HANSEN 1832). In contrast, "organic dyspepsia" was defined as dyspepsia due to specific lesions – such as peptic ulcer, esophagitis, and cholelithiasis – which was identified on routine investigation.

There are a variety of synonyms for nonulcer dyspepsia, which is a relatively recent term and supercedes several synonyms popularized in the literature. The term "pseudo-ulcer syndrome" was introduced in 1932 by Hansen and popularized by BOCKUS (1963), who also described "pyloroduodenal instability." Other terms for nonulcer dyspepsia have included "epigastric distress syndrome" (NYREN et al. 1987), "essential dyspepsia" (TALLEY and PIPER 1985), "functional dyspepsia" (ALVARE 1917), and "nervous dyspepsia" (ALVARE 1943). The nomenclature becomes even more confusing when pathologic concepts are introduced. Some authors have related nonulcer dyspepsia to "gastritis" (GUSTAVSSON et al. 1985) – at best a tenuous relation inasmuch as more than 50% of these patients have no histologic evidence of gastritis (NYREN et al. 1987; VILLAKO et al. 1984).

C. Epidemiology

Epidemiologic data on nonulcer dyspepsia have been gathered by a number of investigators but the imprecise definition of dyspepsia makes extrapolation of valid prevalence and incidence data hazardous. As cited, however, the prevalence ranges from 20% to 55% (URAG 1982; THOMPSON and HEATON 1980; MOLLMAN et al. 1975) and annual incidence is over 1% (BONNEVIE 1982). In fact, it is at least twice as common as peptic ulcer disease (KRAG 1982; THOMPSON 1984). One must recognize the prevalence in order to appreciate the fact that dyspepsia has considerable implications for individual suffering, medical work load, and financial cost. Nearly half of a gastroenterological practice involves the management of patients in whom no organic basis for the complaints is found, and many of whom have dyspepsia (HARVEY et al. 1983; VILLAKO et al. 1984). The approach to such patients in general involves expensive diagnostic testing and consequent time lost from work, as well as the drug costs of empiric treatment (NYREN et al. 1986b). A study from Sweden estimated that the cost of outpatient care and drugs for dyspepsia was 47 million dollars for a population of approximately 8 million. When the cost of lost earnings and sick leave was considered the annual cost was about 506 million dollars (NYREN et al. 1985).

D. Categories of Nonulcer Dyspepsia

> How do I feel today? I feel as unfit as an unfiddle and it is the result of a certain turbulence in the mind and an uncertain turbulence in the middle.
>
> OGDEN NASH

It is possible to divide patients with nonulcer dyspeptic symptoms into subsets based on the specific symptoms which suggest, albeit imperfectly, causative factors (COLIN-JONES 1988).

I. Gastroesophageal Reflux-Like Dyspepsia

Gastroesophageal reflux is a common medical problem and is usually diagnosed by the history. There may be no difference in the symptom type, frequency, or severity between patients with and without macroscopic evidence of disease. The symptomatology of substernal or burning epigastric discomfort with or without regurgitation is classic. In one study, however, belching was the leading symptom in patients with microscopic and severe esophagitis while heartburn was most common in mind esophagitis (WEINBECK and BERGES 1985). Upper abdominal pain, nausea, and vomiting were present in 31%, 24% and 22% of patients respectively. Clearly, gastroesophageal reflux-like dyspepsia is not infrequently accompanied by symptoms which resemble those of other causes of dyspepsia. As we have seen with other disorders of the upper gastrointestinal tract, sole reliance on symptoms to localize the disease process is potentially fraught with hazard.

II. Dysmotility-Like Dyspepsia

This subject overlaps with the irritable bowel syndrome. These patients complain of flatulence, bloating, distention, and meteorism. Surprisingly, although profound postprandial satiety may be seen, emesis is relatively infrequent. Patients may complain of multiple or poorly localized abdominal pains which are rarely nocturnal. Pain events tend to be continuous and not episodic and patients may give a history of variable and multiple food intolerance. The criteria as set forth by MANNING et al. (1978) are helpful in distinguishing dysmotility-like dyspepsia from true irritable bowel syndrome. The four symptoms which are most closely associated with irritable bowel syndrome are: abdominal distention, pain eased after bowel movement, and more frequent and loose stools at the onset of pain. Nearly two-thirds of patients with irritable bowel syndrome have at least three of these four symptoms. Additional features include alternating diarrhea and constipation, mucous-like stools, and a sensation of incomplete evacuation (KRUIS et al. 1984).

III. Ulcer-Like Dyspepsia

Symptoms in patients with ulcer-like dyspepsia – i.e., nocturnal awakening, postprandial relief of pain, or relief with antacids – are suggestive of an ulcer yet no ulcer is found. It has been suggested that these patients represent a stage in the spectrum of peptic ulcer disease and similar physiologic characteristics are demonstrated regardless of whether they possess an ulcer at the time of evaluation (SPIRO 1974).

IV. Aerophagia

Aerophagia has been defined as "deglutition of air in hysterics" (JONES 1967). There has been, however, no objective evidence of major psychopathology in patients with aerophagia (TALLEY and PIPER 1986; TALLEY et al. 1986). The typical features of aerophagia include repetitive belching or bloating, frequent dry swallows and gulping, and a characteristic forward movement of the neck when swallowing (COLIN-JONES 1988). This symptom complex is most frequently postprandial and may be exacerbated by stress. Relief of symptoms is rarely obtained by belching although such efforts are invariably repetitive.

V. Idiopathic/Essential Dyspepsia

This subgroup accounts for approximately 20% of nonulcer dyspeptic patients who have no specific features on history or examination which could allow categorization in the previously discussed groups. For want of a better name, these patients are classified as having essential dyspepsia (TALLEY et al. 1986).

E. Pathophysiology

> If the physician is to understand the correct meaning of health he must know that there are more than a hundred indeed more than a thousand kinds of stomach, consequently if you gather a thousand persons, each of them will have a different kind of digestion, each unlike the others.
>
> PARACELSUS, 1500, *Three Books of Surgery*

The causes of nonulcer dyspepsia remain poorly understood but several pathophysiologic factors have been proposed. A discussion of these factors is important not only for better understanding of the disease but also to prepare a better framework to structure the approach to therapy of this chronic disorder.

I. Gastric Acid

In that gastric acid secretion is well accepted in the pathogenesis of peptic ulcer disease, it is logical that the role of acid in nonulcer dyspepsia has been well studied. Several studies have failed to show a consistent difference between acid secretion in nonulcer dyspeptic patients and normal controls (NYREN et al. 1987; KRAG 1969; BONNEVIE et al. 1971). In another study of two groups of patients with functional dyspepsia, one with and one without ulcer-like pain, the results showed that even in these two clinical variants of dyspepsia, objective differences could not be demonstrated in either gastric secretion or serum gastrin response to physiologic stimulation (BONNEVIE et al. 1971). Similarly, a study of basal and stimulated levels of gastrin and pancreatic polypeptide showed that nonulcer dyspeptic patients lacked the exaggerated responses demonstrated in ulcer patients and the pattern response was similar instead to that in healthy controls (ROTOLO et al. 1988). In one study, a group of patients with nonulcer dyspepsia and acid hypersecretion were subjected to a vagotomy and drainage procedure (NYREN et al. 1986). Although, as expected, the postoperative acid outputs decreased, dyspeptic complaints remained prominent in many of these patients (NYREN et al. 1986). Similarly, a controlled trial in which gastric acid was neutralized or suppressed supports the concept that acid is not of major pathogenetic importance (CHRISHANSEN et al. 1973).

The mucosal injury effected by acid, i.e., gastritis and/or duodenitis, has also been studied in regard to nonulcer dyspepsia. Studies of representative samples of the population have defined prevalence rates similar to those reported in dyspeptics (TALLEY and PHILLIPS 1988; SIURALA et al. 1968; VILLAKO et al. 1976). Erosive duodenitis may be a cause of nonulcer dyspepsia (CHEI et al. 1983) but it more likely represents a component of duodenal ulcer disease (GREENLAW et al. 1980; JOFFE 1981). In fact, gastric acid secretion in some studies in patients with symptomatic duodenitis is higher than normal and comparable to that in patients with duodenal ulcer disease (SIRCUS 1985; MYREN 1981). In contrast, patients with nonulcer dyspepsia have basal and stimulated gastric secretion and gastrin responses that are no different than those in healthy controls (NYREN et al. 1986a; ROTOLO et al. 1988). A more recent study of nonulcer dyspepstic patients – both with and without duodenitis – demonstrated normal basal acid output in both groups (COLLEN and LOWENBERG 1989). The acid profiles from this study do not support the view that nonulcer dyspepsia with or without duodenitis is a spectrum of the same acid peptide process as duodenal ulcer disease (COLLEN and LOWENBERG 1989).

Some investigators have suggested that 30%–70% of patients with nonulcer dyspepsia have histologic evidence of chronic type B antral gastritis independent of the endoscopic appearance of the mucosa (THOMPSON 1984; COLLEN and LOWENBERG 1989; GREENLAW et al. 1980). A similar prevalence of chronic antral gastritis, however, may be seen in a healthy asymptomatic patient population (GREENLAW et al. 1980). The prevalence of chronic antral gastritis clearly increases with age, at least 50% of patients being affected by the fifth decade (GREENLAW et al. 1980; TOUKAN et al. 1985; KRUENING et al. 1978; CHELI et al. 1980). Similarly, although one study demonstrated that

53% of nonulcer dyspeptic patients had antral gastritis, the investigators found a 57% prevalence when studying a matched control population (CHELI et al. 1980).

II. *Helicobacter pylori*

During the last few years there has been a plethora of articles centering on this newly recognized enteric pathogen. This organism has been implicated in an incredible catalogue of conditions involving the stomach and duodenum – including gastritis, duodenal ulcer, gastric ulcer, gastric cancer, epidemic achlorhyria, and nonulcer dyspepsia (BARTLETT 1988; DOOLEY 1988).

Helicobacter pylori (formerly *Campylobacter pylori*) infection has been detected in approximately 50% of patients presenting for diagnostic evaluation of nonulcer dyspepsia (DOOLEY 1988; GRAHAM and KLEIN 1987; ROKKAS et al. 1987a). There is both direct and indirect evidence of such an association. *H. pylori* has been cultured from patients with nonulcer dyspepsia (ROKKAS 1987) although the strength of the association is less convincing than that with gastritis or peptic ulcer. The nonulcer dyspepsia story is complicated by the relatively high incidence of *H. pylori* in the community at large. Studies have shown a steady increase with age in the Morris population with *H. pylori* infections (ROKKAS et al. 1987a; GRAHAM et al. 1986; MORRIS et al. 1986). Additionally, active *H. pylori* infection and gastritis are frequent in asymptomatic people (PEREZ-PEREZ et al. 1988; LANGENBERG et al. 1984; BARTHEL et al. 1988). Since about half of 50-year-old individuals may have *H. pylori*-associated gastritis and many of those investigated for nonulcer dyspepsia are within this age range, it is difficult to establish an absolute etiologic significance for the fact that some nonulcer dyspeptic patients have infections with *H. pylori* (GRAHAM and KLEIN 1987). Furthermore adding to the confusion are the observations that there are no discernible differences in the symptomatology of *H. pylori*-positive and *H. pylori*-negative dyspeptics (M.L. LANGENBERG et al. 1984) and, secondly, that some patients with *H. pylori* and nonulcer dyspepsia have no histologic evidence of gastritis (BARTHEL et al. 1988). That the dyspeptic symptoms attributed to *H. pylori*-associated gastritis might be attributed to a consequent delay in gastric emptying has recently been studied and appears not to be the case (WEGNER et al. 1988).

Confirmation of a causal relationship between *H. pylori* infection and nonulcer dyspepsia will require large well-controlled blinded trials using specific and effective agents to eradicate the organism. There is some preliminary support provided by a few trials to date. One controlled trial assigned nonulcer dyspeptic patients to receive antacid, erythromycin, or bismuth salicylate (RATHBONE et al. 1988). Treatment with bismuth was associated with clearance of the organism and resolution of the gastritis. Improvement in symptomatology was seen in the patients who were cleared of *H. pylori* but this improvement was not statistically significant in the small number of patients studied. Preliminary results from other clinical trials show similar effects of bismuth agents on *H. pylori*-associated gastritis and improvement in symptoms in those cleared of the organism (HCNULTY et al. 1986; BRODY et al. 1987a,b; LAMBERT et al. 1987; ROKKAS et al. 1987b). These data suggest that *H. pylori* may be causally related to nonulcer dyspepsia at best in a proportion of these patients. The topic for the moment remains an area of heated debate and continued investigation.

There is a paucity of data to define the natural history of untreated dyspeptic patients with *H. pylori*-associated gastritis. One recent study provided longitudinal follow-up for 12–33 months of both individuals with untreated *H. pylori*-associated gastritis and noninfected patients who also had nonulcer dyspepsia (W. LANGENBERG et al. 1988). In this study, patients underwent serial reexamination with endoscopy (including biopsy and culture) as well as serologic testing for *H. pylori*. Of interest is that there was no spontaneous disappearance of *H. pylori* infection or the associated gastritis in any of the nine patients followed. Twelve nonulcer dyspeptic patients who were negative for *H. pylori* gastritis remained negative through the follow-up period. One patient developed a positive culture with gastritis but this was attributed to contamination of the biopsy specimen during sampling. No patient in either the *H. pylori*-positive or the *H. pylori*-negative group developed ulceration. This result contrasts with the considerable rate of recurrent ulceration observed in patients who present with a duodenal ulcer (BARDHAM et al. 1982) and emphasizes the idea that if *H. pylori* infection is a risk factor for peptic ulceration, other patient- or microorganism-related factors are also implicated.

III. Motility

> Behold my belly is as wine which hath no vent, it is ready to burst like new bottles.
>
> *Bible*, Job 32:19

Disordered motility of the upper gastrointestinal tract has been implicated in the genesis of nonulcer dyspepsia (CAMILLERI et al. 1986; REES et al. 1980; PETERSEN 1982). A complex of symptoms such as postprandial fullness, abdominal distention, bloating, and flatulence is compatible with an underlying disorder of motility. Under stress, normal antral motility may change to hypomotility in some patients (CAMILLERI et al. 1986). Motility studies have shown that approximately 50% of patients with dyspeptic symptoms of unknown origin have some delay in gastric emptying, with antral hypomotility (MALAGELADA and STANGHELLINI 1985). A criticism of the cited study is that many of the patients studied had associated metabolic and neurologic diseases which likely influenced the results of the manometric studies. Somewhat surprisingly, the symptoms were not well correlated with the manometric findings (MALAGELADA and STANGHELLINI 1985). The relationship between gastric dysrhythmias and the findings and symptoms of nonulcer dyspepsia at present is unclear. Clearly, major gastric dysrhythmias can precipitate severe gastroparesis (YOU and CHEY 1984; ABELL et al. 1985a; STODDARD et al. 1981). Transient dysrhythmias, however, have been seen in entirely asymptomatic patients after vagotomy or cholecystectomy (STODDARD et al. 1987). Antral tachygastria has been described in some patients with postprandial upper gastrointestinal distress (STODDARD et al. 1981). An increased frequency of antral slow waves (6–10/min compound with normal 3–4/min) has been indicted as the cause of the dyspeptic complaints in these patients (ABELL et al. 1985b). Most dyspeptic patients, however, are not as ill as those reported to have antral tachygastria.

Reflux of duodenal contents (especially bile) has been implicated in some patients with nonulcer dyspepsia (NIEMELA 1985). Although this may reflect a motility disorder, duodenogastric reflux occurs commonly in healthy asymptomatic persons (HUGHES et al. 1982). Comparative studies of nonulcer dyspeptic patients show a prevalence of duodenogastric reflux comparable to that in a control population (HUGHES et al. 1982; WATSON and LORE 1987). The evidence for duodenogastric reflux as having a major role in the pathogenesis of nonulcer dyspepsia is obviously lacking.

Another hypothesis linking motility disturbances to nonulcer dyspepsia is that functional disturbances of the upper gastrointestinal tract may be mediated by a disrupted circulating concentration of gut hormones (SMITH 1983). Cholecystokinin can elicit postprandial satiety (SMITH 1983) and other peptides have been shown to alter both fundic and antral motility, although the physiologic roles are yet to be established (BLACKBURN et al. 1980; WALSH 1987). There have been a few studies which have specifically evaluated the role of gut hormones in patients with nonulcer dyspepsia. In one study, circulating levels of insulin, gastrin, gastric inhibitory polypeptide, pancreatic polypeptide, and neurotensin were measured (WATSON et al. 1986). No differences were found between controls and symptomatic patients with flatulent dyspepsia. Another group of investigators found that release of motilin (the levels of which fluctuate with the migrating motor complex) was impaired in 22 patients with nonulcer dyspepsia who also had an idiopathic marked delay in gastric emptying (LABO et al. 1986).

The role of endogenous opiates and functional dyspepsia has also been studied (NARDUCCI et al. 1986). It is known that morphine and related opioid substances may inhibit gastric emptying (TAMHI and SULLIVAN 1983; SULLIVAN et al. 1981). Studies have demonstrated the presence of endogenous opiate-like substances (enkephalinis) in the myenteric plexus of the gastrointestinal tract, with particularly high concentrations in the stomach and upper small intestine (POLAK et al. 1977; GEISHON and ERDE 1987; BITAR and MAKHLOUF 1982). Furthermore, specific opioid receptors in the smooth-muscle cells of the stomach (BITAR and MAKHLOUF 1982) and small bowel (BITAR and MAKHLOUF 1983) have been demonstrated. The hypothesis that increased endogenous opiate-like activity might be responsible for idiopathic gastric stasis was evaluated by NARDUCCI et al. (1986). A selective opioid antagonist (naloxone hydrochloride) was administered and improvement in gastric emptying was seen in patients with gastric hypomotility. In contrast, the subset of patients who had gastric stasis due to duodenal dyskinesia had normalization of gastric emptying effected by naloxone. This suggests that endogenous opiates may participate in the pathogenesis of gastric stasis in this subgroup of nonulcer dyspeptic patients.

There is some evidence that dysmotility of the biliary tree may be responsible for abdominal discomfort (GOFF et al. 1988; DODDS et al. 1988). Dyskinetic function of the sphincter of Oddi has been characterized by one or more of the following: episodic severe upper abdominal pain, an elevated amylase, alkaline phosphatase, or bilirubin level, dilatation of the common bile duct, and delayed drainage during endoscopic retrograde cholangiopancreatography (HOGAN et al. 1983; MESHKINPOUR and MALLOT 1987). Overall this disorder is probably uncommon (HOGAN et al. 1983; MESHKINPOUR and MALLOT 1987) and dyspepsia as the sole manifestation of biliary dyskinesia is distinctly unusual.

IV. Psychosocial Factors

> Deep sorrow occasionally produces dyspepsia.
>
> CALEB PERRY, 1815, *Elements of Pathology and Therapeutics*

The gastrointestinal physiologic effects of stress are known to include alteration of secretion, motility, and vascularity (TALLEY et al. 1986). In that nonulcer dyspepsia is considered to be a functional disorder and that emotional factors are presumed to influence such disorders through the above physiologic effects, psychosocial factors and stress have been implicated in the pathogenesis of nonulcer dyspepsia – hence the synonym nervous dyspepsia (TALLEY et al. 1996; ALVAREZ 1943). There does not appear to be a personality profile, however, that is unique to nonulcer dyspepsia (NYREN et al. 1988).

Similarly, it does not appear that psychosocial factors (socioeconomic class, marital status, family structure, migration) or childhood factors (parental separation, number of siblings, birth order, country of birth) have a discriminant causal role in essential dyspepsia (TALLEY et al. 1988). From case control studies it appears that major life events are not strikingly more common in dyspeptic patients than in controls but that these patients are slightly more neurotic. Furthermore, in response to acute stress, the autonomic response may be suppressed (TALLEY et al. 1986).

Unlike ulcer patients, whose absence from work is, for the most part, due to abdominal complaints, patients with nonulcer dyspepsia report a variety of symptoms dominated by musculoskeletal pains (Nyren et al. 1988). These patients have a heightened perception of physiologic function, although this aspect is difficult to evaluate in that there may be uncontrolled factors (such as ethnic and cultural differences) which may distort a comparative analysis of all patients with nonulcer dyspepsia (Nyren et al. 1985).

V. Environmental Factors

When belly with bad pains doth swell, it matters nought what else goes well.

Saadi (Muslia-ud-Din), ca. 1250, *In Gulistaug*

Patients with nonulcer dyspepsia are usually advised to avoid exposure to cigarettes, alcohol, analgesics, or coffee substances, which have been implicated in causing or exacerbating dyspepsia (Dal Monte 1983; Hecrei 1983). Talley et al. (1988) studied the patterns of ingestion of analgesic drugs (aspirin, acetaminophen, dextropropoxyphene, non-steroidal anti-inflammatory drugs), alcohol, coffee, and tea and smoking in patients with essential dyspepsia. These investigators were able to define that only acetaminophen use was associated with essential dyspepsia. Such usage, in fact, was present both before the onset of the essential dyspepsia and before the diagnosis. Although this suggested association is a novel concept, the authors did not consider the possibility that dyspeptic patients may have a bias against aspirin and therefore prefer acetaminophen.

Constituents of the diet including essential oils may have effects on gastrointestinal motility (Evans et al. 1975). Clearly, long chain fatty acids delay gastric emptying and fat-stimulated cholecystokinin release influences motility at various levels of the gut (Hunt and Unox 1968; Harvey and Read 1973). Furthermore, many patients report that their symptoms are meal related (Horrocks and DeDombal 1978) and that certain foods, in particular fatty foods, precipitate dyspepsia (Oal Monk 1983; Taggart and Billington 1966). Taggart and Billington (1966) showed, however, in a double-blind study, that despite the alleged fatty food exacerbation, patients did not have dyspepsia when they ate disguised meals. Other uncontrolled studies have also shown that dyspeptic complaints cannot be attributed to particular (G.Friedman 1948; Koch and Donaldson 1964). The relationship between foods and dyspepsia therefore remains unestablished.

Various drugs can affect the gastrointestinal tract and cause dyspepsia. Most attention has focused on the effects of non-steroidal anti-inflammatory agents (Tarkai et al. 1987; Collins et al. 1986) although a large variety of drugs, e.g., digoxin, antibiotics, or corticosteroids, may cause various dyspeptic symptoms. With the exception of the previously cited incrimination of acetaminophen (Talley et al. 1988), no clear association of a specific drug or drug class has been linked with essential dyspepsia.

F. Diagnostic Approach

> Disease is very old and nothing about it has changed. It is we who change as we learn to recognize what was formerly imperceptible.
>
> J.M. Charcot

Traditional teaching and practice suggest that a diagnosis of nonulcer or nonorganic dyspepsia can be made only after organic disease has been excluded by investigation. The limits of this investigation are in general governed by several considerations: the availability, acceptability, and cost of various procedures as well as the fear of "missing something" and the consequent fear of litigation. Indeed, a positive diagnosis of nonulcer dyspepsia is usually possible on clinical grounds alone (Loof et al. 1985), although clearly there have been diagnostic refinements allowing better recognition of formerly imperceptible disease.

The diagnostic approach begins with the history. Symptom markers that are helpful in suggesting the diagnosis of nonorganic dyspepsia are listed in Table 1. In the history it is important to define what drugs the patient is taking, particularly if the patient is taking nonsteroidal anti-inflammatory agents. Daily dyspepsia is evident in approximately 5% of patients taking these agents chronically (Committee on the Savety of Medicine 1986).

Physical examination in patients with nonulcer dyspepsia will demonstrate no masses or organomegaly. These patients are well nourished although many surgical scars may be evident (Chaudhary and Truelove 1962; Goulston 1972; Fielding 1977). The presence or absence of tenderness in the epigas-

Table 1. Markers which are useful in the symptomatic diagnosis of nonulcer dyspepsia

Symptoms are not described convincingly; emphasis or priorities of symptoms as described may shift during interview or follow-up
Symptoms are disproportionate to clinical well-being
Symptoms patterns not conforming to distinctly recognizable disease conditions
Poorly localized or multicentric abdominal pains
Dramatic description of pain
Daily, continuous unremittent pain
Pain on awakening – not cause for awakening
Nausea, retching, or early morning preprandial emesis
Belching, burping, and flatulence are generally not related to organic disease – beware of occult presentation for cardiac disease (infarction)
Anorexia without weight loss
Behavioral characteristics of anxiety or lowered affect
Previous psychiatric history
Longstanding symptoms extending to childhood
Stress factors worsening or precipitating symptoms
Young age at time of diagnosis

trium is not a reliable indicator of peptic ulcer disease (Priebe et al. 1982). Furthermore, the results of routine hematologic and biochemical investigations, including serum chemistries, electrolytes, amylase, and lipase, are normal.

The diagnostic possibilities for evaluating the patient with dyspepsia include immediate study with a upper gastrointestinal barium x-ray series or study with esophagoduodenoscopy. An alternative, however, is empiric treatment, reserving diagnostic evaluation for those patients with complications or persistence of symptoms despite therapy. In an effort to maximize the cost-effectiveness of the diagnostic evaluation, adopting the strategy of treating all dyspeptic patients (Who do not have clinical evidence of serious disease) by withdrawal of offending agents (i.e. alcohol, ulcerogenic medications, cigarettes) and by prescribing antacids or H_2 blockers appears efficacious (Heath and Public Policy Committee, American College of Physicians; Kahn and Greenfield 1986). Adoption of this recommendation, however, must be modified in light of each patient's clinical presentation and relative risks. Patients with weight loss, systemic illness, multisystemic disease, evidence of bleeding, obstruction, or perforation, suspicion of neoplasia, or other suspect atypical symptoms should undergo prompt diagnostic evaluation. This strategy, which provides empiric therapy as the initial approach to dyspeptic patients meeting the above criteria, reserves further diagnostic evaluation for two subsets of patients. One is those patients who have no or minimal response to 7–10 days of active therapy. The other is the approximately 30% of patients whose symptoms persist (albeit partially improved) after 6–8 weeks of therapy.

There is not absolute uniformity of opinion on empiric therapy for dyspeptic patients (Talley and Phillips 1988; Sampliner 1986). Although the prevalence of gastric cancer is low in primary practice (Kahn and Greenfield 1986; Sampliner 1986), H_2 antagonists may mask symptoms and heal even malignant ulcers (Tragardh and Haglund 1985). Conceivably the use of H_2 antagonists may also weaken the value of subsequent endoscopy. Duodenitis or superficial erosions may be the primary diagnosis or indicate partially healed ulceration (Cotton and Shorvon 1984). Furthermore, the positive yield from early endoscopy may vary with age, being reported as 30% for patients over 40 years but nearly 60% for patients over 65 years of age (Fjosne et al. 1986). Empiric use of H_2 antagonists may also lead to inappropriate long-term therapy (Cocco and Cocco 1981) and to serious side-effects. Such concerns have led some authors (Talley and Phillips 1988) to recommend. Investigation of patients over the age of 40 with new onset of dyspepsia, chronic symptoms that have not previously been investigated, or clinical evidence of organic disease (e.g., bleeding, vomiting, weight loss, dysphagia, jaundice, biliary pain, abdominal mass, anemia, or a strong family history of peptic ulceration). Other authors have proposed screening questionnaires employing a standardized data sheet which is analyzed by computer. A relative risk score is generated by which the need for further investigation is determined. Overall, it must be recognized, however, that despite the numerous recommendations discussed in this text, an optimal management/diagnostic approach to patients with nonulcer dyspepsia has yet to be rigorously tested.

After selecting the group of patients whose symptoms warrant further investigation, the question must be asked whether the usual pattern of upper gastrointestinal barium x-ray followed by esophagogastroduodenoscopy is still the appropriate sequence. It can be argued that the higher false-negative rate of 18%–40% and the false-positive rate of 13%–35% for the upper gastrointestinal series are unacceptable, relative to the yield by endoscopy (KNUTSON et al. 1978; MARTTN et al. 1980; SCHUOIANN 1972). Furthermore, the use of the double contrast technique reduces the false-negative rate only to 9%–17% and the false-positive rate to 8%–10% (MONTAGNE et al. 1978; HERLINGER et al. 1977). In addition, barium studies do not allow the opportunity for biopsy or cytologic examination, which is indicated in patients with radiographically suspicious lesions. Furthermore, biopsies for *H. pylori* can be obtained if this is of diagnostic concern. Overall, to detect cancer or to decide on long-term or modified therapy, the more accurate diagnostic modality of upper endoscopy is preferable.

If no evidence of mucosal disease is found on endoscopic examination, additional tests are of little value (DAL MONTE 1983). Clearly, an ultrasonogram of the biliary tract (including the pancreas, bile ducts, and gallbladder) would be required if the symptoms were suggestive of cholelithiasis. Upper abdominal ultrasonography is recommended by some as a routine test for dyspeptic patients although other investigators have shown a low yield in screening nonselected dyspeptic patients in such a fashion (NYREN et al. 1987; TALLEY and PIPER 1985). Screening for giardiasis should be considered in that the prevalence of this infection in dyspeptic patients in one study was 15.5% (CARR et al. 1988). Surprisingly, however, this was not different than a control population of nondyspeptic patients undergoing endoscopy. Additionally, if the patients had vomiting and diarrhea as part of their symptom complex, the prevalence of giardiasis was 38.5%. The role of endoscopic retrograde cholangiopancreatography was evaluated in another study of patients with atypical dyspepsia and there was no evidence of pancreatic disease in any of the patients evaluated by this technique (VATN et al. 1985). Intraesophageal acid perfusion (Bernstein test) and/or 24-h esophageal pH monitoring may be helpful, particularly if reflux-like dyspepsia is suspect. There is no role (outside of an investigational protocol) for analysis of gastric secretion in patients with nonulcer dyspepsia. Gastric emptying studies using radioisotopic markers are noninvasive and may be useful in documenting aberrant emptying. Gastrointestinal motility studies clearly provide valuable data in selected patients but these tests are not widely available.

In patients with lower abdominal symptoms present, diagnostic testing should also be focused to exclude small intestinal and colonic pathology. A proposed diagnostic schema for excluding major diseases is shown in

Table 2. Diagnostic tests to exclude diseases associated with dyspepsia

Exclusion concern	Diagnostic tests of choice
Peptic ulcer disease	Endoscopy
Esophagogastric neoplasia	Endoscopy
Gastroesophageal reflux	Bernstein test Twenty-four hour pH monitoring Endoscopy
Biliary tract disease	Ultrasonography Oral cholecystography Endoscopic retrograde cholangiopan-creatography ± biliary manometry
Pancreatitis (chronic)	Ultrasonography Computed tomography Endoscopic retrograde cholangiopan-creatography "Pancreatic function" tests
Irritable bowel syndrome	Bood count with differential and ESR Serum chemistries Stool occult blood tests Colonoscopy or combination flexible sigmoidoscopy and barium enema (especially if ≥40 years) Hydrogen breath test Stool examination for ova and parasites

Table 2. Other causes of dyspepsia should also be considered before ascribing the symptoms to functional disease. A list of diseases and disorders reportedly associated with dyspepsia (KRAG 1987) is provided in Table 3.

G. Treatment

> What comfort can the vortices of Descartes give to a man who has a whirlwind in his bowels?
>
> BENJAMIN FRANKLIN

Given the uncertainty of what constitutes nonulcer or nonorganic dyspepsia, coupled with its widely different symptomatic presentation, it is not surprising that there is no universal strategy for treatment. The high placebo response noted in treatment of this disorder makes it difficult to interpret the results of the clinical trials that have been carried out. No specific medication or class thereof appears effective in treating all patients with dyspepsia. A therapeutic approach that directs therapy to the category of the dyspeptic complaints seems most prudent. A proposed management plan is shown in Table 4. A major criticism of most of the therapeutic trials evaluating various medications in nonulcer dyspeptic patients is that a subcategorization of the dyspeptic complaints was not considered in the selection of patients entered. Accordingly, it would be unlikely that a patient with ulcer-like dyspepsia

Table 3. Differential diagnosis of diseases and disorders reported to cause dyspepsia

A. *Gastrointestinal diseases*
Irritable bowel syndrome
Gastroesophageal reflux
Biliary tract disease
Peptic ulcer
Esophagogastric neoplasia
Chronic pancreatitis
Malabsorptive syndromes
Infection (esp. giardiasis)
Adhesions (intra-abdominal)
Liver disease
Vascular diseases
Intestinal angina
Ischemic colitis
B. *Disorders of other abdominal organs*
Urinary tract
Nephrolithiasis
Hydronephrosis
Pyelonephritis
Genital organs
Menstruation
Pregnancy
Salpingitis
Ovarian cyst/tumor
Uterine myoma/carcinoma
Endometriosis
C. *Diseases or disorders of other systems*
Metabolic disorders
Uremia
Diabetes mellitus
Porphyria
Electrolyte abnormalities
Endocrine disorders
Thyroid (hyper/hypo)
Parathyroid (hyper/hypo)
Adrenal
Cardiac
Congestive heart failure
Coronary artery disease (ischemia/infarction)
Pericarditis
Collagen diseases
Systemic lupus
Periarteritis nodosa
Dermatomyositis
Amyloidosis
Psychiatric diseases
Neurologic diseases
Orthopedic diseases
Facet syndrome
Costochondritis
Intercostal neuralgia
Spindle reflux pain syndrome

Table 4. Proposed management plan for nonulcer dyspepsia

Dyspepsia group	Initial treatment
Reflux-like	Dietary/mechanical antireflux precautions H_2 receptor antagonist (b.i.d. dose)
Ulcer-like	H_2 receptor antagonist (nocturnal dose)
Aerophagia-like	Modification of diet and dietary habits Correct any denture problems Exclude psychiatric illness
Dysmotility-like	Cisapride Domperidone Metoclopramide
Essential/idiopathic type	Counselling/reassurance Treatment of *C. pylori* if present with gastritis (bismuth and antibiotics)

would benefit from a prokinetic motility agent or that conversely a patient with a dysmotility-like dyspepsia would benefit from an H_2 antagonist or antacid.

The rationale for treatment of nonulcer dyspepsia directed at neutralization or suppression of gastric acid has not been substantiated. Despite the continued widespread use of such agents in such patients, placebo-controlled studies have failed to consistently demonstrate efficacy (Evberi et al. 1988). The results of these clinical trials are provided in Table 5. Subgroups of patients with reflux-like dyspepsia or ulcer-like dyspepsia are those most likely to respond to this treatment approach (Johannessen et al. 1988; Horrocks and De Dombal 1978).

The prokinetic class of drugs may have a particular role in treatment of patients known or suspected to have gastroduodenal dysmotility. The potential side-effects of metoclopramide (particularly extrapyramidal reactions) argue against its use (especially in elderly patients) even in patients with an established visceral dysmotility (McCallum and Albibi 1983). The newer agents such as domperidone and cisapride may have a broader therapeutic index and thus be the drugs of choice in long-term management of the visceral stasis syndromes (Friedman 1948; McCallum 1985). A comparative summary of the pharmacology of these agents is provided in Table 6. These drugs have not been extensively studied in patients with nonulcer dyspepsia. Some trials, however, appear promising, especially those investigating domperidone and cisapride in patients with gastroduodenal dysmotility. A summary of the literature is provided in Table 7.

The specific therapies available for *H. pylori*-related infection are discussed elsewhere in this text, but a summary of the relative paucity of literature concerning treatment of infected patients with nonulcer dyspepsia is shown in Table 8. Clearly, there may be a subgroup of patients with nonulcer dyspepsia whose symptoms are related to *H. pylori* (Berstad et al.

Table 5. Controlled trials of neutralization or suppression of gastric acid in patients with nonulcer dyspepsia

Pts. (*n*)	Entry criteria	Study medication	Control medication	Study design	Results	Ref.
123	Peptic ulcer-like symptoms ⩾6 mo	Cimetidine	Placebo	Double-blind Multi-crossover	Cimetidine group had less symptoms than placebo overall Subgroup of cimetidine responders with reflux-like dyspepsia Endoscopic/histologic examination showed no differences in responders/nonresponders	Johannessen et al. 1988
159	Epigastric pain ⩾2 mo	Cimetidine	Placebo	Double-blind	No difference, including no difference in patients with endoscopic or histologic evidence of gastritis or duodenitis	Nyren et al. 1986c
30	Upper abdominal pain and normal upper endoscopy	Cimetidine	Placebo	Not stated	No difference	Zuberi et al. 1988
220	Dyspepsia of unknown origin	Cimetidine or antacid	Placebo	Double-blind	Cimetidine superior to antacids and placebo in relieving pain and nausea but not bloating	Gotthard et al. 1988
62	Dyspepsia pain or nausea ⩾1 mo	Cimetidine or pirenzipine	Placebo	Double-blind Crossover	Cimetidine superior to placebo in decreasing abdominal pain episodes and number; absolute improvement small No difference between pirenzipine and placebo	Talley et al. 1986
60	Peptic ulcer-like epigastric pain ⩾3 mo	Cimetidine	Placebo	Double-blind	No difference	Lance et al. 1986

Table 5 (continued)

Pts. (*n*)	Entry criteria	Study medication	Control medication	Study design	Results	Ref.
50	Epigastric pain ≥1 mo	Cimetidine	Placebo	Double-blind	No difference	Velbaek et al. 1985
414	Dyspepsia ≥3 mo	Cimetidine	Placebo	Double-blind	Cimetidine more effective in relieving pain severity/frequency	Delattre et al. 1985
251	Dyspepsia ≥2 wks	Ranitidine	Placebo	Double-blind	Ranitidine more effective than placebo in resolution of dyspeptic symptoms	Saunders et al. 1986
90	Dyspeptic symptoms ≥3 mo	Antacid and/or pirenzipine	Placebo	Double-blind	Neither pirenzipine nor low dose antacid (120 mmol/day acid neutralizing capacity) superior to placebo	Webergand Berstad 1988
15	Peptic ulcer-like dyspepsia	Antacids	None	Prospective Longitudinal	Antacids 30 cc taken 1 and 3 h postprandially improved symptom and histologic scores although the improvements in symptom scores and histologic scores did not correlate	Kerkar et al. 1988

Table 6. Pharmacologic profile of prokinetic therapies for nonulcer dyspepsia

	Metoclopramide	Domperidone	Cisapride
Mechanism of action	Cholinergic agonist Dopamine antagonist ? Smooth muscle effect	Dopamine antagonist	Cholinergic agonist Increased acetylcholine release at myenteric plexus without effects on secretory gland
Therapeutic effects	Esophagus to small bowel	Esophagus to small bowel	Esophagus to colon
Dosage	5–20 mg q.i.d.	20–30 mg q.i.d.	10 mg t.i.d. 10–20 mg t.i.d.
Administration	p.o., i.v., s.c.	p.o., i.v., rectal suppository	i.v., p.o.
Side-effects	Overall: 20% Drowsiness, restlessness, akathisia, lightheadedness Extrapyramidal: 1% Oculogyric crises, opisthotonos trismus, torticollis Elevates prolactin levels Breast enlargement/tenderness, galactorrhea, menstrual irregularity	Elevates prolactin levels Breast enlargement/tenderness, galactorrhea, menstrual irregularity/amenorrhea Rare extrapyramidal/dystonic reactions	Negligible side-effects Negligible side-effects
Comments	Subcutaneous route makes drug more bioavailable; may increase incidence of side-effects. Contraindicated in: mechanical obstruction, pheochromocytoma, parkinsonism	Does not cross blood–brain barrier ? Associated with cardiac arrhythmias when given parenterally	Antagonist of serotonin in animal models ? Role in diarrheal states

Table 7. Published trials of prokinetic agents in patients with nonulcer dyspepsia

Pts. (*n*)	Entry criteria	Study medication	Control medication	Study design	Results	Ref.
42	Flatulent dyspepsia	Metoclopramide	Placebo	Double-blind Crossover	Significant improvement with metoclopramide although drowsiness was a prominent side-effect (caused withdrawal from trial in four patients)	Johnson 1971
18	Flatulent dyspepsia	Metoclopramide	Placebo	Double-blind	Postprandial fullness relieved with metoclopramide	Selxar 1977
20	Dysmotility-like dyspepsia	Domperidone or metoclopramide	Placebo	Double-blind Crossover	In an open pilot trial of 40 pts, significant improvement was noted in dyspepsia while taking domperidone. In the crossover study, both domperidone and metoclopramide were statistically better than placebo; domperidone was also better than metoclopramide in 7/9 target symptoms.	De Loose 1979
16	Dyspepsia with known gastric or duodenal dysmotility	Domperidone	Placebo	Double-blind	Domperidone effective in treatment of some symptoms (abdominal pain, early satiety), although no effect on nausea, emesis, or bloating. Effect on gastric emptying in patients with idiopathic gastric stasis and gastroduodenal motor dysfunction was equivocal.	Davis et al. 1988
32	Chronic post-prandial dyspepsia	Domperidone	Placebo	Double-blind	Excellent or global improvement in 71% of domperidone-treated pts compared to only 13% of placebo-treated pts	Van de Mierop et al. 1979

44	Chronic dyspepsia	Domperidone	Placebo	Double-blind Crossover	Compared with placebo, treatment with domperidone achieved symptomatic improvement in 84% of patients, with regard to belching, postprandial fullness, abdominal distention, and heartburn.	Sarin et al. 1986
11	Chronic post-prandial dyspepsia	Domperidone	Placebo	Double-blind Crossover	No difference	Vagler and Miskovitz 1981
40	Chronic dyspepsia and delayed gastric emptying	Domperidone	Placebo	Double-blind	Symptomatic improvement, gastric emptying response not studied	Bekhti and Rutgeerts 1979
48	Chronic post-prandial dyspepsia	Domperidone	Placebo	Double-blind Crossover	Significant improvement on active drug although placebo-related improvement was not infrequent	Englet and Schlich 1979
8	Idiopathic dyspepsia with delayed gastric emptying	Cisapride	None	Unblinded	Acute intravenous or chronic oral administration of cisapride improved gastric emptying. Symptomatic response not addressed	Urbain et al. 1988
118	Nonulcer dyspepsia	Cisapride	Placebo	Double-blind	Significant improvement with cisapride over placebo (81% vs 31%), especially in postprandial discomfort and gastroesophageal reflux-type symptoms	Rosch 1987
12	Nonulcer dyspepsia with idiopathic gastroparesis	Cisapride	Placebo	Double-blind Crossover	Cisapride was more effective than placebo in improving delayed gastric emptying but no significant difference was observed in total symptoms score	Corinaldesi et al. 1987

Table 8. Published trials involving treatment of *H. pylori* in nonulcer dyspepsia

Pts. (*n*)	Entry criteria	Study medications	Control medications	Study design	Results	Ref.
50	NUD with HP	De-Nol Erythromycin Ethylsuccinate	Placebo	Double-blind	Significant improvement in gastritis in patients who cleared HP (14/18 De-Nol, 1/15 erythromycin, 0/17 placebo). No statistically significant association between severity of symptoms and gastritis before or after treatment. Symptoms improvement: 87% De-Nol group, 64% erythromycin, 67% placebo.	McNulty et al. 1986
43	NUD and HP positive	De-Nol	Placebo	Double-blind	Significant improvement in symptoms correlated with improvement in chronic gastritis and HP disappearance.	Brody et al. 1987a
33	NUD	De-Nol	Placebo	Not stated	Eradication of bacteria in 73% De-Nol treated (vs 6% placebo) resulted in relief of pain but not nausea/vomiting, fullness, or flatulence. HP found in 66% of initial 54 patients with NUD.	Lambert et al. 1987
40	NUD	De-Nol	Placebo	Not stated	HP was present in 10/20 De-Nol-treatment patients and 6/20 placebo group. Symptomatic improvement with De-Nol correlated with eradication of HP and improvement in gastritis.	Brody et al. 1987b
89	NUD >3 months	Antacids Pirenzipine	Placebo	Double-blind	28% patients had HP; 10 patients with HP received antacid – density of colonization decreased in all and HP disappeared in five. Neither pirenzipine nor placebo affected HP. Antacids reduced or eliminated HP without healing gastritis or relieving symptoms.	Morgan et al. 1988

51	NUD	De-Nol	Placebo	Double-blind	Overall, no difference between groups in respect of symptom relief, reduction of gastritis, or HP. If, however, gastritis was present De-Nol improved symptoms, gastritis, and reduced HP.	RAWWS et al. 1988
106	NUD with antral gastritis and HP	Nitrofurantoin Furazolidine	Placebo	Double-blind	Resolution of gastritis paralleled clearance of HP with antibiotics but significant relief of symptoms was not evident.	GREGORY et al. 1972
164	NUD	Cimetidine Sucralfate De-Nol Amoxicillin De-Nol and amoxicillin	No treatment	Prospective Longitudinal	164/200 patients with NUD screened had CP. De-Nol and/or amoxicillin were effective in eliminating CP but recurrence occurred within 1 month following eradication in 60%. No clearance of CP with cimetidine or sucralfate. Symptoms in response to therapy not addressed.	BRUMMER and HALKINEN 1959

Abbreviations: NUD, nonulcerative dyspepsia; HP, *Helicobacter pylori*.

1988; Kang et al. 1988). To bolster a causal association of pain in nonulcer dyspepsia with *H. pylori* infection, it will be necessary to prove that eradication of the infection brings relief of dyspepsia. Until such data are released from the large prospective ongoing studies, caution should temper our zeal for interpreting the role of *H. pylori* in symptomatic nonulcer dyspepsia. Such caution in judgment is heralded by the following quote:

> I have no data yet. It is a capital mistake to theorize before one has the data. Insensibly one begins to twist facts to suit theories instead of theories to suit facts.
>
> Sherlock Holmes, *A Scandal in Bohemia*

There is no single dietary manipulation which effects a favorable response in the majority of dyspeptic patients. For those dyspeptic patients with symptoms suggesting an acid-related pathogenesis, some dietary modification such as avoidance of tobacco and aspirin may be helpful. It is clear that certain foods may exacerbate symptoms – as detailed by the patient. Common offenders include citrus juice and carbonated sodas. It is important to listen to the patient, taking into account the related symptoms and exacerbating factors. Coupling this information to working knowledge of gastric physiology, the physician should be able to come up with a workable dietary guide with which the patient can live.

A key part of the therapeutic strategy is the psychological support and understanding in managing these often distressing problems (Johannessen et al. 1988), especially in patients with the idiopathic or essential subtype of nonulcer dyspepsia. Reassurance is the cornerstone of this approach in asmuchas many patients have an inordinate fear of cancer that reinforces and magnifies these symptoms. The role of psychotherapy in patients with nonulcer dyspepsia has not been well studied (Almy 1977). A trained psychotherapist may well help to alleviate certain stresses and tensions which can in turn alter gastric acid output, but there is no reason as a general principle to recommend costly psychotherapy for most dyspeptic patients. In my practice, I believe that achieving reasonable expectations in any patient with chronic functional symptoms is important. I tell them early in the course of the evaluation that their symptoms may not be relieved entirely with dietary and pharmacologic modifications, although I believe that we can improve them somewhat. Furthermore, we will exclude diseases (neoplastic and other diseases) for which we have a more directed treatment. Patients can seemingly adapt to and live with a variety of chronic symptoms, relieved that the mere persistence of any symptoms does not mean that they have a disease that is being missed or perhaps they are on the wrong medication – or worse – have selected the wrong physician!

H. Prognosis

The art of medicine is entertaining the patient until nature heals the disease.

VOLTAIRE

Although the prognosis of nonulcer dyspepsia is excellent in terms of life expectancy, symptoms left to nature's healing continue in 25%–66% over several years of follow-up (GREGORY et al. 1972; POUNDER 1989). In one study with a follow-up of 17 months (BRUMMER and HALKINEN 1959), the authors found that the best predictor of the course of upper abdominal pain in patients with chronic dyspepsia was the number of days of pain in the 6 months prior to diagnosis. Furthermore, the taking of medications for dyspepsia and the development of gastroesophageal reflux were also associated with more days of pain over the follow-up period. Demographic and environmental factors, length of dyspepsia history, and past history of ulcer were of no significant predictive value. Surprisingly, there was no evidence of a "burn-out" of abdominal dyspeptic pain symptoms, in contrast to the symptoms of peptic ulcer disease (FRY 1964). Patients with a history of dyspepsia of more than 1–5 years did exhibit a burn-out although this was transient and if the first two data periods following endoscopy were excluded this effect disappeared. This effect may have occurred because of a placebo effect of endoscopy with the reassurance that serious organic disease had been excluded. These findings are also consistent with another previous study (GRIEBE et al. 1974).

Four studies have demonstrated that some patients with nonulcer dyspepsia will develop demonstrable peptic ulcer in follow-up of 5–27 years (GREGORY et al. 1972; POUNDER 1989; BONNEVIE 1982; KRAG 1965). It is likely, however, that the techniques used in the earlier studies were inaccurate in excluding demonstrable peptic ulcer disease. The more recent of these series had only 3% of patients developing an ulcer after 6 years of follow-up (BONNEVIE 1982). It seems logical that at least a percentage of these patients, especially those with the "Moynihan's disease" variant of nonulcer dyspepsia, will at some point have peptic ulcer disease. A criticism of these studies, however, is the reliance on radiographic rather than endoscopic evaluation and, therefore, the sensitivity for detection is compromised. Furthermore, in that recurrent peptic ulcer disease is not infrequently asymptomatic (165), a regimen of endoscopic surveillance would have to be ensured to establish the true prevalence of ulcer disease in the follow-up of these patients.

J. Conclusions

> The abdomen is the reason why man does not easily mistake himself for a god.
>
> FREDERICK WITZCHE, *Beyond Good and Evil*

Nonulcer dyspepsia is a commonly encountered clinical problem, the pathophysiology of which remains poorly understood. It almost certainly represents a "wastebasket" of various physiological and psychological observations. Numerous investigative tools are available for the diagnosis and treatment of these patients although it is possible that with judicious avoidance we may minimize the discomfort of an extensive evaluation at least in some patients. The newer therapeutic modalities such as the prokinetic agents and treatment of *C. pylori* infection await larger prospective studies to establish clear efficacy. Another possibility for treatment in the future is electrical pacing of portions of the gastrointestinal tract. If abnormal myoelectric activity is causing dysmotility in some dyspeptic patients, we may be able to override the abnormal gastrointestinal pacemaker in the same way the cardiologists treat cardiac arrhythmias. The future will be determined by the extent of our knowledge. If we can identify what is causing these symptoms, conceivably we can develop therapies for them.

References

Abell TL, Lucas AR, Brown ML, Malagelada JR (1985a) Gastric electrical dysrhythmias in anorexia nervosa. Gastroenterology 88:1300 (abstr)

Abell TL, Camilleri M, Malagelada JR (1985b) High prevalence of gastric electrical dysrhythmias in diabetic gastroparesis. Gastroenterology 88:1299 (abstr)

Almy TP (1977) Therapeutic strategy in stress-related digestive disorders. Gastroenterol 6(3):709–721

Alvarez WC (1917) The syndrome of mild reverse peristalsis. JAMA 69:2018–2024

Alvarez WC (1943) Nervousness, indigestion and pain. Hoeber, New York

Bardham K, Cole DS, Hawkins BW, Franks CR (1982) Does treatment with cimitidine extended beyond initial healing of duodenal ulcer reduce the subsequent relapse rate? Br Med J 284:621–623

Barthel JS, Westbloom TU, Harvey AD, Gonzalez F, Evertt D (1988) Gastritis and *Campylobacter pylori* in healthy asymptomatic controls. Arch Intern Med 148:1149–1151

Bartlett JG (1988) *Campylobacter pylori*: fact or fancy? Gastroenterology 94:229–238

Bekhti AA, Rutgeerts L (1979) Domperidone in the treatment of functional dyspepsia in patients with delayed gastric emptying. Postgrad Med J [Suppl 1] 55:28–29

Berstad A, Alexander B, Weberg R, Serck-Hanssen A, Holland S, Hurschowitz BI (1988) Antacids reduce *Campylobacter pylori* colonization without healing the gastritis in patients with non-ulcer dyspepsia and erosive prepyloric changes. Gastroenterology 95:619–624

Bitar KN, Makhlouf GM (1982) Specific opiate receptors on isolated mammalian gastric smooth muscle cells. Nature 297:72–74

Bitar KN, Makhlouf GM (1983) Opiate receptors are present on circular and selectively absent from longitudinal muscle cells of the intestine. Gastroenterology 84:1107 (abstr)

Blackburn AM, Fletcher DR, Bloom SR et al. (1980) Effect of neurotensin on gastric function in man. Lancet i:987–989
Bockus HL (1963) Gastroenterology, vol 1. Saunders, Philadelphia, p 521
Bonnevie O (1982) Outcome of non-ulcer dyspepsia. Scand J Gastroenterol [Suppl 79] 17:135–138
Bonnevie OH, Kallehauge HE, Wulff HR, Wulff MR (1971) Prognostic value of the augmented histamine test in ulcer disease and x-ray negative dyspepsia. Scand J Gastroenterol 6:723–729
Brody T, Hennissy W, Daskaalopoulos G, Carrick J, Hazell S (1987a) Double blind trial of De-Nol in non-ulcer dyspepsia associated with *Campylobacter pyloridis* gastritis. Gastroenterology 92:1324 (abstr)
Brody T, Daskalpoulos G, Brandl S, Carrick J, Hazell S (1987b) Dyspeptic symptoms improve following eradication of gastric *Campylobacter pyloridis*. Gastroenterology 92:1324 (abstr)
Brummer P, Halkinen I (1959) x-ray negative dyspepsia: a follow-up study. Acta Med Scand 165:329–332
Camilleri M, Malagelada JR, Kao PC, Zinsmeister AR (1986) Gastric and autonomic responses to stress in functional dyspepsia. Dig Dis Sci 31:1169–1177
Carr MF, Ma J, Green PHR (1988) *Giardia lamblia* in patients undergoing endoscopy: lack of evidence for a role in non-ulcer dyspepsia. Gastroenterology 95:972–974
Chaudhary NA, Truelove SC (1962) The irritable colon syndrome. A study of the clinical features, predisposing causes, and prognosis in 130 cases. Q J Med 31:307–322
Chei R, Perasso A, Giacosa A (1983) Dyspepsia and chronic gastritis. Hepatogastroenterology 30:21–23
Cheli R, Simon L, Aste H et al. (1980) Atrophic gastritis and intestinal metaplasia in asymptomatic Hungarian and Italian populations. Endoscopy 12:105–108
Christiansen J, Aagaard P, Koudahl G (1973) Truncal vagotomy and drainage in the treatment of ulcer-like dyspepsia without ulcer. Acta Chir Scand 139:173–175
Cocco AE, Cocco DV (1981) A survey of cimetidine prescribing. N Engl J Med 304:1281
Colin-Jones DG (1988) Management of dyspepsia: report of a working party. Lancet i:576–579
Collen MJ, Lowenberg MJ (1989) Basal gastric acid secretion in non-ulcer dyspepsia with or without duodenitis. Dig Dis Sci 34(2):246–250
Collins AJ, Davies J, Dixon ASJ (1986) Contrasting presentation and findings between patients with rheumatic complaints taking non-steroidal anti-inflammatory drugs and a general population referred for endoscopy. Br J Rheumatol 25:50–53
Committee on the Safety of Medicine (1986) Update 1. Non-steroidal anti-inflammatory drugs and serious gastrointestinal adverse reactions. Br Med J 292:614
Corinaldesi R, Stanghellini V, Racti C, Rea E, Salgemini R, Barbara L (1987) Effect of chronic administration of cisapride on gastric emptying of a solid meal and on dyspeptic symptoms in patients with idiopathic gastroparesis. Gut 28:300–305
Cotton PB, Shorvon PJ (1984) Analysis of endoscopy and radiography in the diagnosis, follow-up and treatment of peptic ulcer disease. Clin Gastroenterol 13:383–403
Dal Monte PR (1983) Treatment of non-ulcerative dyspepsia (editorial). Hepatogastroenterology 30:1–2
Davis RH, Clench MH, Mathias JR (1988) Effects of domperidone in patients with chronic unexplained upper gastrointestinal symptoms: a double-blind placebo-controlled study. Dig Dis Sci 33(12):1505–1511
DeDombal FT (1981) Analysis of foregut symptom. In: Baron JH, Moody FC (eds) Gastroenterology, vol 1. Foregut. Butterworth, London, pp 49–66 (Butterworth's international medical reviews)

DeDombal FT, Hall R (1979) The evaluation of medical care from the clinician's point of view: what should we measure and can we trust our measurements? In: Alperovitch A, DeDombal FT, Gremuy F (eds) Evaluation of efficacy of medication action. North Holland, Amsterdam, pp 13–22
Delattre M, Malesky MA, Prinzie A (1985) Symptomatic treatment of non-ulcer dyspepsia. Curr Ther Res 37:980–991
De Loose F (1979) Domperidone in chronic dyspepsia: a pilot open study and a multicentre general practice crossover comparison with metoclopramide and placebo. Pharmatherapeutica 2:140–146
Dodds WJ, Hogan WJ, Geenen JE (1988) Perspectives about function of the sphincter of Oddi. Viewpoint. Dig Dis 20(3):9–12
Dooley CP (1988) The clinical significance of *Campylobacter pylori*. Ann Intern Med 108:70–79
Englert W, Schlich D (1979) A double-blind crossover trial of domperidone in chronic postprandial dyspepsia. Postgrad Med J [Suppl 1] 55:28–29
Evans BK, Heatley RV, James KC, Luscombe DK (1975) Further studies on the correlation between biological activity and solubility of some carminatives. J Pharma Pharmacol [Suppl 66] 27
Fielding JF (1977) The irritable bowel syndrome, pt I: clinical spectrum. Clin Gastroenterol 6:607–622
Fjosne U, Kleveland PM, Waldum H, Halvorsen T, Petersen H (1986) The clinical benefit of routine upper gastrointestinal endoscopy. Scand J Gastroenterol 21:433–440
Friedman G (1983) Domperidone. Am J Gastroenterol 78(1):47–48
Friedman MH (1948) Peptic ulcer and functional dyspepsia in the armed forces. Gastroenterology 10:586–605
Fry J (1964) Peptic ulcer: a profile. Br Med J 2:809–812
Geishon D, Erde SM (1981) The nervous system of the gut. Gastroenterology 80:1571–1594
Goff JS (1988) The human sphincter of Oddi: physiology and pathophysiology. Arch Intern Med 148(12):2673–2677
Gotthard R, Bodemar G, Brokin V, Jonsson KA (1988) Treatment with cimetidine, antacid or placebo in patients with dyspepsia of unknown origin. Scand J Gastroenterol 23:7–18
Goulston K (1972) Clinical diagnosis of the irritable colon syndrome. Med J Aust 1:1122–1125
Graham DY, Klein PD (1987) *Campylobacter pyloridis* gastritis: the past, the present and speculations about the future. Am J Gastroenterol 82:283–286
Graham DY, Klein PD, Evans DG et al. (1986) Rapid noninvasive diagnosis of the presence of gastric campylobacter: the ^{13}C urea breath test. Gastroenterology 90:1435
Greenlaw R, Sheahan DG, DeLuca V, Miller D, Myerson P (1980) Gastroduodenitis. A broader concept of peptic ulcer disease. Dig Dis Sci 25:660–672
Gregory DW, Davies GT, Evans KT, Rhodes J (1972) Natural history of patients with x-ray negative dyspepsia in general practice. Br Med J 4:519–520
Griebe J, Bugge P, Gyorup T, Lauretzen T, Bonnevie O, Wulff HR (1977) Long-term prognosis of duodenal ulcer: follow-up study and survey of doctor's estimates. Br Med J 2:1572–1574
Gustavsson S, Bates S, Adami HO, Loof L, Nyren O (1985) Definition and discussion of nomenclature. Scand J Gastroenterol [Suppl] 109:11–13
Hansen H (1932) Pseudoulcera ventriculi mit besonderer Berucksichtigung der benignen Tuberkulose. Levin and Munksgaard. Copenhagen, pp 21, 69
Harvey RF, Read AE (1973) Effect of cholecystokinin on colonic motility and symptoms in patients with irritable bowel syndrome. Lancet i:1–3
Harvey RF, Salih SY, Read AE (1983) Organic and functional disorders in 2000 outpatients attending a gastroenterology clinic. Lancet i:632–634

Health and Public Policy Committee, American College of Physicians (1985) Endoscopy in the evaluation of dyspepsia. Ann Intern Med 102:266–269

Hecker R (1983) Indigestion and flatulence. Aust Fam Physician 1983; 10:447–451

Herlinger H, Glamville JN, Kreel L (1977) An evaluation of the double contrast meal (DCBM) against endoscopy. Br Med J 28:307–314

Hogan WJ, Geenen JE, Toouli J, Dodds EJ, Arndorfer RC (1983) Motility and biliary dyskinesia. In: Chey WY (ed) Functional disorders of the digestive tract. Raven, New York, pp 267–275

Horrocks JC, DeDombal FT (1978) Clinical presentation of patients with "dyspepsia": detailed symptomatic study of 360 patients. Gut 19:19–26

Hughes K, Robertson DA, James WB (1982) Duodenogastric reflux in normal and dyspeptic subjects. Clin Radiol 33:461–466

Hunt JN, Knox MT (1968) A relation between chain length of fatty acids and the slowing of gastric emptying. J Physiol (Lond) 194:327–326

Joffe SN (1981) Relevence of duodenitis to nonulcer dyspepsia and peptic ulceration. Scand J Gastroenterol 17(79):88–97

Johannessen T, Fjosne V, Kleveland PM et al. (1988) Cimetidine responders in non-ulcer dyspepsia. Scand J Gastroenterol 23:327–336

Johnson AG (1971) Controlled trial of metoclopramide in the treatment of flatulent dyspepsia. Br Med J 2:25–26

Jones FA (1967) Burbulence. A fresh look at flatulent dyspepsia. Practitioner 198:367–370

Kahn KL, Greenfield S (1986) The efficacy of endoscopy in the evaluation of dyspepsia. A review of the literature and development of a sound strategy. J Clin Gastroenterol 8(3):346–358

Kang JY, Tay HH, Guan R, Math MV, Yap I (1988) The effect of colloidal bismuth subcitrate on symptoms and gastric histology in non-ulcer dyspepsia – a double-blind placebo-controlled trial. Gut 29[10]:A1440 (abstr)

Kelbaek H, Linde J, Eucksen J, Munkgaard S, Moesgaard F, Bonnevie O (1985) Controlled clinical trial of treatment with cimetidine for non-ulcer dyspepsia. Acta Med Scand 217:281–287

Kerkar PG, Naik SR, Dalvi HG, Vora IM (1988) Effect of high dose liquid antacids on symptoms and endoscopic and histological changes in gastroduodenal mucosa in non-ulcer dyspepsia. Indian J Gastroenterol 7:81–83

Knutson CO, Max MH, Ahmad W, Polk HC Jr (1978) Should flexible fiberoptic endoscopy replace barium contrast study of the upper gastrointestinal tract? Surgery 84:609–615

Koch JP, Donaldson RM (1964) Survey of food intolerance in hospitalized patients. N Engl J Med 271:657–660

Krag E (1965) Pseudo-ulcer and true peptic ulcer: a clinical, radiographic and statistical follow-up study. Acta Med Scand 178:713–728

Krag E (1969) The pseudo-ulcer syndrome. A clinical radiographic and statistical follow-up study of patients with ulcer symptoms but no demonstrable ulcer in the stomach or duodenum. Dan Med Bull 16:6–9

Krag E (1982) Non-ulcer dyspepsia introduction: epidemiological data. Scand J Gastroenterol [Suppl] 79:6–8

Krag E (1987) Other causes of dyspepsia. Scand J Med [Suppl 79] 17:32–34

Kruening J, Bossman FT, Kuper G, Wal AM, Lindeman J (1978) Gastric and duodenal mucosa in "healthy" individuals. An endoscopic and histopathological study of 50 volunteers. J Clin Pathol 31:69–77

Kruis W, Thieme CH, Weinzierl M, Schussler P, Holl J (1984) A diagnostic score for the irritable bowel syndrome. Its value in the exclusion of organic disease. Gastroenterology 87:1–7

Labo G, Bortolotti M, Vezzadini P, Bonora G, Bersani G (1986) Interdigestive gastroduodenal motility and serum motilin levels in patients with idiopathic delay in gastric emptying. Gastroenterology 90:20–26

Lambert JR, Borromeo M, Korman MG, Hansky J (1987) Role of *Campylobacter pyloridis* in non-ulcer dyspepsia – a randomized controlled trial. Gastroenterology 92:1488 (abstr)

Lance P, Wastell C, Schiller KFR (1986) A controlled trial of cimetidine for the treatment of non-ulcer dyspepsia. J Clin Gastroenterol 8(4):414–418

Langenberg ML, Tytgat GNJ, Schipper MEI et al. (1984) Campylobacter-like organisms in the stomach of patients and healthy individuals. Lancet i:1348

Langenberg W, Rouns EAJ, Houthoff HJ et al. (1988) Follow-up study of individuals with untreated *Campylobacter pylori*-associated gastritis and of noninfected persons with non-ulcer dyspepsia. J Infect Dis 157(6):1245–1249

Loof L, Hans-Olov A, Agenas I, Gustavsson S, Nyberg A, Nyren O (1985) Symposium on Dyspepsia. Scand J Gastroenterol [Suppl] 109:35–39

Malagelada JR, Stanghellini V (1985) Manometric evaluation of functional upper gut symptoms. Gastroenterology 88:1223–1231

Manning AP, Thompson DG, Heaton KW, Morris AF (1978) Towards positive diagnosis of the irritable bowel syndrome. Br Med J ii:653–656

Martin TR, Vennes JA, Silvis SG, Ansel HI (1980) Upper gastrointestinal endoscopy versus radiography: Is radiography obsolete? J Clin Gastroenterol 2:27–30

McCallum RW (1985) Review of the current status of prokinetic agents in gastroenterology. Am J Gastroenterol 80:1008–1016

McCallum RW, Albibi R (1983) Metoclopramide: pharmacology and clinical application. Ann Intern Med 98:86–95

McNulty CA, Gearity JC, Crump B et al. (1986) *Campylobacter pyloridis* and associated gastritis: investigator blind, placebo controlled trial of bismuth salicylate and erythromycin ethylsuccinate. Br Med J 293:645–649

Meshkinpour H, Mallot M (1987) Bile duct dyskinesia and unexplained abdominal pain. A clinical and manometric study. Gastroenterology 92:1533 (abstr)

Mollman KM, Bonnevie O, Gudmanel-Hoyer E, Wulff HR (1975) A diagnostic study of patients with upper abdominal pain. Scand J Gastroenterol 10:805–809

Montagne J, Moss AA, Margulis AR (1978) Double-blind study of single and double contrast upper gastrointestinal examinations using endoscopy as a control. Am J Roentgenol 130:1041–1045

Morgan D, Kraft W, Bender M, Pearson A (1988) Nitrofurans in the treatment of gastritis associated with *Campylobacter pylori*. Gastroenterology 95:1178–1184

Morris A, Micholson G, Lloyd G et al. (1986) Seroepidemiology of *Campylobacter pyloridis*. NZ Med J 99:657–659

Myren J (1981) Gastric secretion in duodenitis. Scand J Gastroenterol 17(79):98–101

Narducci F, Bassotti G, Granata MT et al. (1986) Functional dyspepsia and chronic idiopathic gastric stress – role of endogenous opiates. Arch Intern Med 146:716–720

Niemela S (1985) Duodenogastric reflux in patients with upper abdominal complaints with particular reference to reflux-associated gastritis. Scand J Gastroenterol [Suppl] 115:1–56

Nyren O, Adam HO, Gustavsson S, Loof L, Nyberg A (1985) Social and economic effects of non-ulcer dyspepsia. Scand J Gastroenterol [Suppl 109] 20:41–47

Nyren O, Adami HO, Bergstrom R, Gustavsson S, Loof L, Lundquist G (1986a) Basal and food stimulated levels of gastrin and pancreatic polypeptide in non-ulcer dyspepsia and duodenal ulcer. Scand J Gastroenterol 21:471–477

Nyren O, Adami HO, Gustavsson S, Loof L (1986b) Excess sick listing in social and economic non-ulcer dyspepsia. J Clin Gastroenterol 8:339–345

Nyren O, Adami HO, Bates S et al. (1986c) Absence of therapeutic benefit from antacids or cimetidine in non-ulcer dyspepsia. N Engl J Med 314:339–343

Nyren O, Adami HO, Gustavsson S, Lindgren PG, Loof L, Nyberg A (1987) The epigastric distress syndrome: a possible disease entity identified by history and endoscopy in patients with non-ulcer dyspepsia. J Clin Gastroenterol 9:303–309

Nyren O, Adami HO, Gustavsson S, Loof L (1988) Excess sicklisting in non-ulcer dyspepsia. J Clin Gastroenterol 8(3):339–345

Perez-Perez GI, Dworkin BM, Chodos JE, Blaser MJ (1988) *Campylobacter pylori* antibodies in humans. Ann Intern Med 109:11–17

Petersen H (1982) Further investigations and treatment of non-ulcer dyspepsia. Scand J Gastroenterol [Suppl] 79:130–134

Polak JM, Sullivan SN, Bloom SR et al. (1977) Enkephalin-like immunoactivity in the human gastrointestinal tract. Lancet i:972–974

Pounder R (1989) Silent peptic ulceration: deadly silence or golden silence? Gastroenterology 96:626–631

Priebe WM, Da Costa LR, Beck IT (1982) Is epigastric tenderness a sign of peptic ulcer disease? Gastroenterology 82:16–19

Rathbone BJ, Wyatt J, Healthy RV (1988) Symptomatology in *C.pylori*-positive and -negative non-ulcer dyspepsia. Gut 24:A1473 (abstr)

Raw EAJ, Langenberg W, Houthoff HJ, Zanen HC, Tytgat GNJ (1988) *Campylobacter pyloridis*-associated chronic active antral gastritis: a prospective study of its prevalence and the effects of antibacterial and antiulcer treatment. Gastroenterology 94:33–40

Rees WD, Miller LJ, Malagelada JR (1980) Dyspepsia, antral motor dysfunction, and gastric stasis of solids. Gastroenterology 78:360–365

Rokkas T, Pursey C, Uzoechina E et al. (1987a) *Campylobacter pylori* and non-ulcer dyspepsia. Am J Gastroenterol 82:1149–1152

Rokkas T, Pursey C, Simmons NA, Filipe MI, Slader GE (1987b) Non-ulcer dyspepsia and colloidal bismuth subcitrate therapy: the role of *Campylobacter pyloridis*. Gastroenterology 92:1599 (abstr)

Rosch W (1987) Cisapride in non-ulcer dyspepsia: results of a placebo controlled trial. Scand J Gastroenterol 22:161–164

Rotolo G, DiFede G, Mascellin MR, Rizzo G, Scardavi M, Rini GB (1988) Pattern of gastric acidity and gastrin blood level in basic conditions and following the administration of food in subjects with ulcer-like and non-ulcer like dyspepsia. Panminerva Med 30:37–41

Sampliner RE (1986) Are H_2 blockers for symptom relief (editoral)? J Clin Gastroenterol 8:8–9

Sarin SK, Sharma P, Chawla YK, Gopinath P, Nundy S (1986) Clinical trial on the effect of domperidone on non-ulcer dyspepsia. Indian J Med Res 83:623–628

Saunders JHB, Oliver RJ, Higson DL (1986) Dyspepsia: incidence of non-ulcer disease in a controlled trial of ranitidine in general practice. Br Med J 292:665–668

Schuman BM (1972) The gastroscopic yield from the negative upper gastrointestinal series. Gastrointest Endosc 19:79–82

Sekar ASC (1977) Metoclopramide treatment of non-ulcer dyspepsia. Ann R Coll Physicians Surg Can 10:52 (abstr)

Sircus W (1985) Duodenitis: a clinical, endoscopic and histopathologic study. Q J Med 56:593–600

Siurala M, Isokoski M, Vares K, Kakki M (1968) Prevalence of gastritis in a rural population. Bioptic study of subjects selected at random. Scand J Gastroenterol 3:211–223

Smith GP (1983) Gut hormones and postprandial satiety. In: Chey WY (ed) Functional disorders of the digestive tract. Raven New York, pp 29–33

Spiro HM (1974) Moynihan's disease? The diagnosis of duodenal ulcer. N Engl J Med 291:567–569

Stoddard CJ, Smallwood RH, Duthie HL (1981) Electrical arrhythmias in the human stomach. Gut 22:705–712

Sullivan SN, Tamki L, Corcoran P (1981) Inhibition of gastric emptying by enkephalin analogue. Lancet ii:86–87

Taggart D, Billington BP (1966) Fatty foods and dyspepsia. Lancet ii:465–466

Talley NJ, Phillips SF (1988) Non-ulcer dyspepsia: potential causes and pathophysiology. Gastroenterology 108:865–879
Talley NJ, Piper DW (1985) The association between non-ulcer dyspepsia and other gastrointestinal disorders. Scand J Gastroenterol 20:896–900
Talley NJ, Piper OW (1986a) Major life event stress and dyspepsia of unknown cause. A case control study. Gut 27:127–134
Talley NJ, Piper DW (1986b) Comparison of the clinical features and illness behavior of patients presenting with dyspepsia of unknown cause (essential dyspepsia) and organic disease. Aust NZ J Med 16:352–359
Talley NJ, Fung LH, Gilligan IG, NcNeil D, Piper DW (1986a) Association of anxiety, neuroticism, and depression with dyspepsia of unknown cause. A case control study. Gastroenterology 90:886–892
Talley NJ, McNeil D, Hayden A, Piper DW (1986b) Randomized double-blind, placebo controlled crossover trial of cimetidine and pirenzepine in non-ulcer dyspepsia. Gastroenterology 91:149–156
Talley NJ, NcNeil D, Piper DW (1988a) Environmental factors and chronic unexplained dyspepsia – association with acetaminophen but not other analgesics, alcohol, coffee, tea or smoking. Dig Dis Sci 33(6):641–648
Talley NJ, Jones M, Piper DW (1988b) Psychosocial and childhood factors in essential dyspepsia. A case control study. Scand J Gastroenterol 23:341–346
Tamki L, Sullivan S (1983) A study of gastrointestinal opiate receptors: the role of the mu receptor on gastric emptying: concise communication. J Nucl Med 24:689–692
Tarkai EN, Smith JL, Lidsky MD, Graham DY (1987) Gastroduodenal mucosa and dyspeptic symptoms in arthritic patients during chronic nonsteroidal anti-inflammatory drug use. Am J Gastroenterol 82:1153–1157
Thompson WG (1980) Non-ulcer dyspepsia. Can Med Assoc J 130:565–569
Thompson WG, Heaton KW (1980) Functional bowel disorders in apparently healthy people. Gastroenterology 79:283–288
Toukan AV, Kamel MF, Amr SS, Arnaout MA, Abu-Romiyeh AS (1985) Gastroduodenal inflammation in patients with non-ulcer dyspepsia: a controlled endoscopic and morphometric study. Dig Dis Sci 30:313–320
Tragardh B, Haglund U (1985) Endoscopic diagnosis of gastric ulcer. Evaluation of the benefits of endoscopic follow-up observation for malignancy. Acta Chir Scand 151:37–41
Urbain JLC, Siegel JA, Debie NC, Pauwels SP (1988) Effect of cisapride on gastric emptying in dyspeptic patients. Dig Dis Sci 33(7):779–783
Vagler J, Miskovitz P (1981) Clinical evaluation of domperidone in the treatment of chronic postprandial idiopathic upper gastrointestinal distress. Am J Gastroenterol 76:495–499
Van de Mierop L, Rutgeerts L, Van den Langenbergh B, Staessen A (1979) Oral domperidone in chronic postprandial dyspepsia. Digestion 19:244–250
Vatn MH, Favsa O, Gjone E (1985) Diagnostic value of gastrointestinal endoscopy in patients with uncharacteristic abdominal disorders. Scand J Gastroenterol 20:636–640
Villako K, Tamm A, Savisaar E, Ruttas M (1976) Prevalence of antral and fundic gastritis in a randomly selected group of an Estonian rural population. Scand J Gastroenterol 11:817–822
Villako, K, Ihamaki T, Tamm A, Tammur R (1984) Upper abdominal complaints and gastritis. Ann Clin Res 16:192–194
Walsh JH (1987) Gastrointestinal hormones. In: Johnson LR (ed) Physiology of the gastrointestinal tract, 2nd edn. Raven New York, pp 181–253
Watson RG, Love AH (1987) Intragastric bile acid concentration is unrelated to symptoms of flatulent dyspepsia in patients with and without gallbladder disease and postcholecystectomy. Gut 28:131–136

Watson RG, Shaw C, Buchanan KD, Love AH (1986) Circulating gastrointestinal hormones in patients with flatulent dyspepsia, with and without gallbladder disease. Digestion 35:211–216
Weberg R, Berstad A (1988) Low dose antacids and pirenzipime in the treatment of patients with non-ulcer dyspepsia and erosive prepyloric changes: a randomized, double-blind, placebo controlled trial. Scand J Gastroenterol 23:237–243
Wegner M, Borsch G, Schaffstein J, Schultz-Flake C, Mai U, Leverkus F (1988) Are dyspeptic symptoms in patients with *Campylobacter pylori* associated type B gastritis linked to delayed gastric emptying? Am J Gastroenterol 83(7):737–740
Weinbeck M, Berges W (1985) Esophageal disorders in the etiology and pathophysiology of dyspepsia. Scand J Gastroenterol [Suppl 109] 20:133–137
You CH, Chey WY (1984) Study of electromechanical activity of the stomach in humans and in dogs with particular attention to tachygastria. Gastroenterology 86:1460–1468
Zuberi SJ, Qureshi H, Najmuddin S et al. (1988) Lack of therapeutic benefit of cimetidine in non-ulcer dyspepsia. JAMA 38(1):168–169

CHAPTER 10

The Natural History of Duodenal Ulcer Disease: Has It Been Altered by Drug Therapy?

J.H. LEWIS

A. Introduction

> If one cannot free the patient from the disease it should be helpful to discover how best to fit him to it.
>
> EMERY and MONROE, 1935

Duodenal ulcer (DU) disease has been largely defined by aphorisms such as "once an ulcer, always an ulcer" (SPIRO 1977). While there is general agreement that DU is a chronically relapsing disease characterized by recurrent exacerbations and remissions, our knowledge and understanding of this common disorder remain incomplete. Only a few studies have attempted to rigorously define the long-term natural history of DU, nearly all of which were conducted prior to endoscopy and the availability of H_2 receptor antagonists and other new ulcer-healing drugs and the recognition of epidemiologic factors such as *Helicobacter pylori* (formerly *Campylobacter pylori*) as will be discussed.

In the past three decades, more than 60 compounds with the ability to heal DU have been developed (BOYD et al. 1983a), although relatively few are currently available for use in the United States. As BONFILS et al. (1984) have recently opined, "progress in ulcer therapy has advanced the treatment only of the ulcer lesion. No drug has been shown to affect the natural history of ulcer disease." On what evidence are these authors basing such a statement? Surely there are many who believe that with all of the new pharmacologic weapons and modern diagnostic tools at our disposal, we are winning what some have termed the "battle" against ulcer disease. The following chapter will examine this question; to find out just how far we have come and how far we have to go in understanding the natural course of DU and formulating a rational approach to the medical treatment of the disorder.

B. Incidence of Duodenal Ulcer – Historical Perspectives

Although DU is presently one of the most commonly diagnosed disorders, with a lifetime prevalence estimated to be 5%–12% for the United States and other Western populations (IVY 1946; KURATA and HAILE 1984; MONROE and MACMAHON 1969), it appears to have grown into medical prominence from truly humble beginnings. Whereas accurate pathologic descriptions of gastric ulcer (GU) date as far back as 1586 (WILBUR 1935), it was not until the early eighteenth century that DU was first recognized as a distinct clinicopathologic entity (CRAIG 1948; JORDAN 1985, WILBUR 1935). According to MOYNIHAN (1910), one of the earliest mentions of DU in the medical literature is found in the London *Medico-Chirurgical Transactions* of 1817. This and other seminal reports emanated from Europe; SARGENT in 1854 and O'HARA in 1875 are credited with being among the first to describe cases of DU in the United States. All of these early reports came from postmortem examinations of fatal DUs that had perforated acutely, as the disorder was largely unrecognized during life. Chvostek has been cited as the first clinician to diagnose a perforated DU prior to death (MOYNIHAN 1910).

While symptoms compatible with peptic ulcer disease were mentioned in antiquity, not until 1828 were the symptoms we commonly associate with DU and GU carefully described, first by John Abercrombie and later by Cruveilhier (JORDAN 1985; MOYNIHAN 1910). MOYNIHAN's classic description of the pain–food–relief sequence in DU was not published until after the turn of this century (MOYNIHAN 1910).

Throughout the eighteenth and nineteenth centuries, DU was considered extremely rare based on its prevalence in autopsy series. For example, in a study published by BRINTON in 1857, DU is not mentioned as being present among more than 7000 cases. Autopsy records amassed from 17652 individuals from the years 1826–1892 by PERRY and SHAW (1893) at Guy's Hospital in London gave the prevalence of active or healed DU as only 0.4%, compared to 5% for GU. A similar DU prevalence (0.26%) was reported by FENWICK and FENWICK (1900) in their monograph detailing more than 13000 postmortem examinations. By the turn of this century, the ratio of GU to DU in the United States and Great Britain was conservatively estimated to be 20–40:1 (HURST and STEWART 1929; JORDAN 1985).

Duodenal ulcer became more commonly recognized after 1900, largely through the efforts of MOYNIHAN in England (MENDELOFF 1974; MOYNIHAN 1910; WILBUR 1935) and the MAYO brothers (1906) and Julius FRIEDENWALD (1912) in the United States. On both sides of the Atlantic, DU quickly assumed increasing clinical importance and its frequency rapidly outstripped that of GU. By 1946, the autopsy prevalence of the two entities was equal, prompting IVY (1946) to suggest that since the overall frequency of peptic ulcer disease had not changed, "It would then appear that during the past hundred years the location of about half the peptic ulcers which occur has shifted from the stomach to the duodenum." Accompanying this shift in frequency was a reversal in the sex ratio from a female to a male predominance (IVY 1946; KURATA et al. 1985). These changes in DU frequency were recorded in both the autopsy records and the mortality statistics for the first half of this century and conformed to the clinical experience being recorded by physicians of that time (BLUMENTHAL 1968; BONNEVIE 1985; CRAIG 1948; IVY 1946; IVY et al. 1950; JENNINGS 1940).

Just why DU seemingly went from being a wallflower who hardly anyone noticed prior to 1900 to the belle of the ball after 1900 is a question still being debated. Moynihan is said to have referred to DU as a "new disease" (JORDAN 1985), but was it in fact "new"? MAYO (1906) was convinced that as many as 90% of DUs were misdiagnosed as GUs, and that DU constituted at least 40% of all ulcer disease. IVY, GROSSMAN, and BACHRACH (1950), in an exhaustive review of the early clinical and autopsy evidence, describe the attempts by some more "modern-day" pathologists to discredit much of the early autopsy data by suggesting that the duodenum was either incompletely examined or overlooked entirely. Similarly, JORDAN (1985) has suggested that some DUs, especially those located at the pylorus, were probably misdiagnosed as GUs in early autopsy studies. Just how prevalent DU actually was prior to 1900 remains open to speculation.

In writing about the changing incidence of perforated peptic ulcers in 1940, JENNINGS emphasized that unlike uncomplicated ulcers, which are subject to various diagnostic influences, "the diagnosis of acute perforations . . . is not a matter of [diagnostic] fashion, either there is an operation or the patient dies." In arguing that the perceived increase in DU incidence after 1900 was indeed real, based on the rising number of perforated ulcers being encountered, JENNINGS appropriately asked, "How did the many fine 18th-century physicians miss such a striking clinical picture, if [perforated ulcer] was as common then as it afterwards became in the 19th century?" The answer is: they probably didn't and it probably wasn't, as will be discussed below.

I. Cohort Phenomena

In 1946, IVY suggested that some unidentified etiologic factor must have been responsible for the increasing frequency and male predominance of DU. The incidence of DU in the United States and Great Britain continued to increase until the 1950s, when, according to several reports, it began to fall (KURATA 1983; MENDELOFF 1974; PULVERTAFT 1968; STURDEVANT 1976; SUSSER and STEIN 1962). This apparent "recession" was seen primarily in younger men and women as the incidence of DU continued to rise in individuals over the age of 65 years. In order to explain these divergent and seemingly incongruent changes in incidence among the different age groups, SUSSER and STEIN (1962) suggested that "each generation has carried its own particular risk of bearing ulcers throughout adult life." It was calculated that the generation born in Great Britain circa 1890 carried the highest risk of developing DU based on a cohort analysis (i.e., following the same group over time). They postulated that individuals born in that particular time period suffered experiences that increased their ulcer risk to a greater extent than did experiences in subsequent generations.

Labeling DU a "disease of civilization," they suggested that these "experiences" related to the physical and emotional stresses common to a developing industrialized society. Such stresses could be expected to increase as society grew more complex, and would ultimately affect an increasing number of individuals as more and more people were caught up in the urban life-style. They further suggested that it was the "early phase" of industrialization and urbanization that was most likely responsible for the highest risk of DU. As subsequent generations learned how to adapt to the increasing demands of industrialized society and as older individuals with the highest risk gradually died out, the risk, and therefore the incidence, of DU would eventually fall. The unequal response of the sexes to societal upheavals and other events exerting an impact on urban life was offered as the explanation for the change from a female to a male predominance of DU.

C. Recent Time Trends in the Incidence of Duodenal Ulcer

Twenty years after the cohort hypothesis was first put forth, SUSSER (1967, 1982) remained convinced that it had accurately predicted the decline in ulcer mortality recorded in England and Wales from 1900 through 1977. Corroborating reports were published by SONNENBERG, who analyzed the age-and sex-specific deaths rates from GU and DU disease in Germany (SONNENBERG and FRITSCH 1983) and Switzerland (SONNENBERG 1984), and concluded that the cohort phenonomen existed, but was not unique to Great Britian. Indeed, in a subsequent analysis, SONNENBERG and his colleagues (1985) demonstrated that the temporal changes in peptic ulcer mortality in all of the remaining European nations also could be attributed to birth-cohort determinants.

The cohort analysis seemed to satisfy the clinical impression that the incidence of DU had changed dramatically over the preceding 150 years. However, as SUSSER (1967, 1982), BONNEVIE (1985), DONALDSON (1975), STURDEVANT (1976), and KURATA and his co-workers (KURATA 1983, 1989; KURATA and CORBOY 1988; KURATA and HAILE 1984; KURATA et al. 1983, 1985) have since acknowledged, incidence studies are subject to a great many limitations. To complicate the matter still further, DU rates seem to be declining for some populations but not for others. For example, while the incidence of DU in the United States and Great Britain is reported to have dropped steadily since the 1950s (KURATA 1989; KURATA and HAILE 1984; KURATA et al. 1983; MEADE et al. 1968; MENDELOFF 1974; MONSON and MACMAHON 1969; PULVERTAFT 1968; STURDEVANT 1976; SUSSER and STEIN 1962; VOGT and JOHNSON 1980), epidemiologic studies from Denmark (BONNEVIE 1985) and Iceland (Jonasson et al. 1983) show a stable incidence over this period and recent studies from Hong Kong (Koo et al. 1983) and Norway (Ostensen et al. 1983b) suggest an actual rise in DU incidence.

Several possible explanations have been cited for these divergent incidence curves, including more accurate means of diagnosis and various environmental influences. MENDELOFF wondered in 1974 whether the United States "was really witnessing the decline of a disease which has been one of the great endemics of the twentieth century" or if peptic ulcer was just as common as in the past but was taking on a "different form." By this he was referring to the increasing number of diagnoses of gastritis, duodenitis, and esophagitis made possible by the introduction of endoscopy, which undoubtedly reduced the number of actual "duodenal ulcers" being diagnosed in dyspeptic patients. Reflecting, in part, on the potential inaccuracies of pre-endoscopic diagnoses, and on the implications this held for determining incidence figures, MENDELOFF suggested that "it is thus impossible to construct a reasonable idea as to the time trend for the frequency of occurrence of this disease before 1940, and it is better not to try." A similar sentiment had been voiced by JENNINGS (1940) more than three decades earlier based on what he referred to as changes in "diagnostic fashions." A decline in DU incidence based on a reduction in the number of ulcers diagnosed at endoscopy continues to be cited as a plausible explanation, along with changes in hospitalization criteria and coding practices (KURATA 1983, 1989; KURATA and HAILE 1984; KURATA et al. 1983). KURATA (1989) notes that data from the National Health Interview Survey show an *increase* in self-reported ulcer disease, although most patients reporting dyspepsia which they attribute to ulcer disease may not have undergone confirmatory studies. Interestingly, the fall in the rate of DU in women has been less than that for men, a circumstance attributed to the rising number of women who smoke and the pressures experienced by the increasing number of women who have entered the work place (BONNEVIE 1985; COGGON et al. 1981).

A novel (though uncorroborated) hypothesis recently put forth by HOLLANDER and TARNAWSKI (1986) to explain the decline in peptic ucler disease in this country deserves special mention. They note that the dietary availability of vegetable oils containing E class prostaglandin precursors has increased 200% since 1909 in both the United States and the United Kingdom. As a result, they propose that this steady rise in the consumption of essential fatty acids might be responsible for enhanced gastroduodenal mucosal protection through the increased production of endogenous prostaglandins. While no definite cause and effect relationship to peptic ulcer incidence or virulence has been established, this diet-related cytoprotection theory remains provocative. So, too, are the theories dealing with eradication of *H. pylori*, as will be discussed below.

D. Geographic Influences

Perhaps no less important in attempting to explain and understand the differences in DU incidence being recorded for various populations are the geographic, ethnic, and racial variations (even within national borders) that are evident for DU (BONNEVIE 1985; IVY et al. 1950; MOSHAL et al. 1981; SASAKI et al. 1984; SONNENBERG 1985; SUSSER 1961). Included among these environmental influences are the various occupational and dietary factors said to convey an increased risk of DU, such as for fishermen in Norway and Scotland (Ostensen et al. 1985a), low fiber diets in Scandinavia (Rydning and Berstad 1985), and night shift workers in Japan (Segawa et al. 1987). A recent study by Moshal et al. (1981), however, points out the potential problems inherent in the interpretation of such incidence data. These authors observed a decline in the incidence of new DUs diagnosed endoscopically for certain African and Indian populations living in Durban, South Africa, during the late 1970s, after an initial rise in incidence had been detected during the early 1970s for the same groups. However, as the number of endoscopic procedures performed also rose during the first half of the decade, the apparent increase in the number of new DU cases was discounted by the authors. In contrast, the decline in DU incidence after 1976 was considered real since the number of endoscopies performed held steady during the second half of the decade.

Highlighting the geographic influences is a report from Ostensen et al. (1985b), who found that the increasing incidence of DU (as well as GU) correlated, in part, with increasing age of the population. Interestingly, younger patients displayed an incidence pattern very different from the elderly and similar to non-Scandinavian regions, suggesting a possible cohort phenomenon. In Finland, the DU to GU ratio is 1:1, which is significantly lower than for most Western countries but higher than in Japan and similar to that in Alaska and Norway. The phenomenon of "Arctic behavior" of peptic ulcer disease has been mentioned to explain the lower DU to GU ratio in these northernmost countries (Tilvis et al. 1987).

E. Recent Trends in Hospitalization and Surgery for Duodenal Ulcer

Whether or not the incidence of DU in the United States is actually falling, there is general agreement that hospitalization rates for DU in this country and several Western European nations have been declining for the past two to three decades (Christensen et al. 1988; Coggon et al. 1981; Elashoff and Grossman 1980; Gustavasson et al. 1988; Kurata 1989; Kurata and Corboy 1988; Kurata and Haile 1984; Kurata et al. 1983; Schmidt et al. 1984; Sonnenberg 1987). Sonnenberg (1987) reviewed physician visits for DU during the period 1958–1984 and found a 20-year decline, with a steeper decline for men than for women. Gustavsson et al. (1988) notes that these trends started well before the introduction of H_2 blockers. At the Mayo Clinic, a more than eightfold decrease in elective surgery during the years 1956–1985 was observed in previously unoperated patients. Again, the decline was greater for men than women, and it was felt that the decline in surgical therapy was related to improvements in the diagnosis of ulcer disease as fewer elective operative procedures were required to make a diagnosis of benign as well as malignant disorders.

Paralleling this trend in hospitalization, the death rate for DU in the United States also has been decreasing steadily since 1962 (COGGON et al. 1981; ELASHOFF and GROSSMAN 1980; KURATA and HAILE 1984; WYLLIE et al. 1981), although KURATA (KURATA 1983; KURATA and CORBOY 1988) mentions that figures from the United States Office of Vital Statistics showed a reversal in this trend with a slight increase in ulcer mortality from 1978 to 1979 and an increase for 1982. The fall in hospitalization rates was observed largely for uncomplicated DUs as little recent change in the incidence of ulcer perforations or hemorrhage had been recorded for the United States or Western Europe (CHRISTENSEN et al. 1988; ELASHOFF and GROSSMAN 1980; KURATA 1983). For example, CHRISTENSEN et al. (1988) found that H_2 blockers have not changed the incidence of severe ulcer complications requiring emergency surgery in Denmark. Similarly, GUSTAVSSON et al. (1988) found that the incidence of emergency operations at the Mayo Clinic has remained steady over the past 30 years.

Several groups have suggested that H_2 blockers also have contributed directly to the recent decline in the number of elective surgical procedures for DU (BARDHON and HINCHLIFFE 1981; FINEBERG and PEARLMAN 1981; WYLLIE et al. 1981). However, as mentioned by GUSTAVASSON et al. and others, this decline preceded the marketing of these drugs as dramatically demonstrated by the fact that in the mid-1970s, the Veterans Administration was forced to cancel two large cooperative studies (one dealing with the treatment of bleeding ulcers and the other comparing parietal cell vagotomy to truncal vagotomy and antrectomy) because of a lack of patients (MENDELOFF 1974; POSTLETHWAIT 1979). GILLEN et al. (1986) also concluded that the introduction of the H_2 blockers has not altered the reoperation rate for patients with chronic ulcer perforation managed initially by an oversew procedure in England. A report by SMITH (1977) is one of the few that has chronicled a decrease in ulcer perforations coincident with a decline in ulcer surgery. What ultimate effect the available H_2 receptor antagonists and newer ulcer-healing drugs will have on the future need for hospitalization and surgery for DU has yet to be determined.

Any study attempting to examine the effect of H_2 blockers on ulcer disease must take into account whether or not patients were taking these medications. I think it is fair to conclude that patients who developed complications were not receiving drug therapy at the time. For example, in the study by GILLEN et al. (1986), after their initial oversew procedure, patients received cimetidine for 8 weeks followed by a maintenance dose for 3 months, after which the treatment was stopped. Since the mean time at which a reoperation was required was 17.5–27.4 months, it must be assumed that these patients were not receiving the medication at the time of their next perforation. In contrast, as will be discussed, the complication rate can be shown to decline in patients who continue to receive maintenance therapy.

As with DU incidence rates, hospitalization rates and ulcer complications also appear to be subject to geographic and environmental influences. For example, in Hong Kong, KOO et al. (1983) observed a 21% *increase* in hospital admissions for DU and a 71% *rise* in perforations during the 1970s. Both increases were most prominent in the elderly, although the overall mortality for DU actually fell by 26%, a circumstance attributed to improvements in hospital care. Retrospective studies from the United Kingdom and Western Europe also have shown an increase in the incidence of bleeding and perforated peptic ulcers among patients over age 65 during the past 25 years (TILVIS et al. 1987; WALT et al. 1986). While the reason or reasons for this increase in perforations are often not specifically stated, one of the most important factors cited for patients in Great Britain and elsewhere is the frequent ingestion of nonsteroidal anti-inflammatory drugs (NSAIDs) (COLLIER and PAIN 1985; TILVIS et al. 1987), a factor that also appears to contribute to the risk of bleeding from peptic ulcers (MATTHEWSON et al. 1988; SOMMERVILLE et al. 1986).

In Germany, hospitalization rates remained constant from 1956 to 1980, with ulcer mortality falling slightly during this period but with significant gender differences (SONNENBERG and FRITSCH 1983). As reported by SONNENBERG and FRITSCH (1983), mortality from GU and DU for women actually increased, but this increase was offset by a decline in mortality from GU for men (male mortality from DU remained constant). These differences were due largely to deaths among elderly patients and corroborated the observations made by BONNEVIE (1977, 1978) and others (PERMUTT and CELLO 1982) that ulcer mortality increases with age. In Japan, LEE et al. (1989b) found no excess mortality due to DU compared to age-matched controls in patients followed for up to 23 years. In addition, survival rates for surgically treated patients did not differ from the general population, a finding in agreement with the observations of KRAUSE from Scandinavia more than 25 years earlier (KRAUSE 1963).

F. Seasonal Variations in Duodenal Ulcer

In temperate climates, a distinct spring and fall seasonality for DU has been mentioned for more than 50 years (GIBINSKI 1983). EINHORN (1930) remarked that most recurrences in his 800 patients occurred in the fall (42%) and spring (35%), compared to the winter (19%) and summer (4%). He noted that this pattern was nearly identical to his patients' past recurrences, and speculated that the low incidence seen in the summer correlated with ulcer patients going on vacation and leaving their urban life-styles and stresses behind. The autumn increase was related to a return to the city and a resumption of their employment. The spring rise was thought to be secondary to frequent changes in the weather that predisposed to colds and other respiratory ailments. Indeed, colds were present in more than half of all observed ulcer recurrences. External and psychic stresses accounted for one-third, diet for nearly one-tenth, and unknown causes for one-quarter of recurrences. IVY (1946) also wondered whether the tradition of taking a summer vacation might be associated with a transient decrease in acid secretion, as had been demonstrated in animals.

Writing in 1935, EUSTERMAN and BALFOUR observed that about half of their ulcer patients experienced a spring or fall exacerbation, regardless of whether they lived in a rural or urban environment. They postulated that the cause for this seasonal increase in ulcer activity was due to "nutritional factors" or possibly "increased bacterial activity in ulcerated tissues." FLOOD (1948) observed DU peaks in March and November among his patients in a 1948 analysis. Similarly, SMITH and RIVERS (1953) wrote that "it is well known that duodenal ulcer seems to have a tendency to become reactivated during the spring and again in the fall of the year." They go on to say that this tendency is often lost when ulcer complications supervene. The reason for the seasonal occurrence was thought to be respiratory or other intercurrent infections in some cases and nervous tension in others.

WELSH and WOLF (1960) reviewed the available clinical evidence for this apparent seasonal variation in 1960 and concluded that there were indeed clusterings of cases in the spring and fall in many studies, but not in all. Reasons they cited to explain the phenomenon included an increase in volume and acidity of gastric juice in the autumn and spring and seasonal effects on the cardiovascular system and chemical composition of the blood. Environmental factors, including changes in barometric pressure, ambient air temperature, ionizing radiation, and rainfall, were additional factors being suggested by others (BINGHAM 1960).

In keeping with the seasonal appearance of ulcer symptoms, an increased frequency of DU complications in the spring and fall also has been observed by several groups (AHMED et al. 1963; BOLES and WESTERMAN 1954; GARDINER et al. 1966; WILLIAM BEAUMONT SOCIETY 1966). For example, among nearly 2200 individuals studied in five different geographic areas by the William Beaumont Society (1966), fewer instances of bleeding from both DU and GU were reported during the summer months. Similar observations were made by BOLES and WESTERMAN (1954) and GARDINER et al. (1966), although other investigators did not find any seasonal trend for ulcer bleeding (DOLL et al. 1951; TIDY 1945).

With regard to ulcer deaths, IVY (1946) cited mortality data from the first half of this century that confirmed the general impression that deaths due to DU peaked in April and November. Nearly 40 years later, KURATA and HAILE (1984) found that deaths from ulcer disease remained highest in the winter and lowest in the summer during the 1970s, although they pointed out that deaths from *all* causes were highest during the winter months.

Among patients studied prospectively, OSTENSEN et al. (1985c) followed 87 DU, 100 GU, and 1749 nonulcer dyspepsia patients in northern Norway with monthly upper gastrointestinal series. They found a significant increase in the radiologic diagnosis of DU in October and November and a decrease in DU during August. Symptoms most often developed during September and October. Corresponding months with the highest incidence of GU were January and September with the fewest number of GUs being diagnosed in April, June, and July. GU symptoms were most prominent during November and January. Similar findings were recorded for nonulcer dyspepsia patients, with the most symptomatic months being September, October, and November. This apparent autumnal increase in peptic ulcer disease was attributed, in part, to the extreme climatic conditions that exist in northern Norway, where winters last 10 months of the year (so-called Arctic behavior).

I. Seasonal Variations Studied Endoscopically

All of the studies cited above relied on either symptoms or radiographic findings to diagnose DU. However, even studies evaluating seasonal variations with the aid of endoscopy have yielded conflicting results. For example, Palmas and his colleagues (1984) in Italy observed a significant drop in DU incidence during August, with the disease exhibiting peaks in July and in the fall months among 1668 individuals. Hospitalization rates for complicated DU (e.g., perforations) followed a similar seasonal pattern, although neither GU nor gastric cancer followed a seasonal trend. Gibinski and co-workers (1982) from Poland examined 41 DU patients endoscopically an average of 5.6 times per year for 1–5 years. They found that complaints of ulcer pain were most frequent in the fall and least frequent during the spring and late summer. The only positive correlation they observed, however, was for ulcer pain and DU niches during the autumn months, and this association was less than perfect.

In a study of 882 DU and GU patients from Germany, Safrany et al. (1982) were unable to document any statistically significant seasonal clustering of ulcer disease. However, this study has been criticized by Gibinski (1983), who suggests that the investigators counted the number of patient visits rather than the true occurrence of new ulcers. In Israel, Fich et al. (1988) found an increased DU incidence in winter with a nadir during the summer months based on their endoscopic analysis of nearly 1700 DUs. Although this study was conducted in the Middle East, where winters are relatively mild compared to more temporate or arctic areas, their findings were corroborated by a higher death rate from peptic ulcer disease in winter compared to other seasons (Slater 1989) as described for peptic ulcer disease in the United States (Kurata and Haile 1984). What can we conclude from these studies that purport a seasonal trend for DU? I think it is fair to say that a fall–winter rise in incidence with a decline during the summer months appears to be present in many individuals, although the optimal study to definitely prove or disprove this observation has yet to be conducted.

G. Natural History of Duodenal Ulcer – Pre-H_2 Blocker Studies

With this background of changing incidence, hospitalization, and surgery rates, and geographic and seasonal variations, it should not be hard to imagine the problems that must be overcome in order to record a meaningful and accurate natural history of DU. Add to these difficulties the problems inherent in following a large group of DU patients over a period of time long enough that the emerging trends carry clinical significance, and it is not surprising that only a few investigators have attempted to chronicle the natural course of the disorder. The following section summarizes the work of those hearty souls who were willing to try.

In 1930 BROWN published a review of the course of 923 DU patients treated from 1912 to 1927 with the Sippy regimen. He found that nearly half of the patients remained "cured" over this period of time. However, he was careful to point out that "In applying the term 'cured' to a certain group of cases it must be understood that the word is used to describe the present status of the patient, with complete understanding of the fact that during the next five years probably more than a few individuals in the present cured group will again be suffering from peptic ulcer." This sentiment was echoed by several investigators, including EMERY and MONROE, who had stated in 1929 that "all evidence points to the fact that ulcer is a chronic disease and that all present methods of treatment are merely palliative. Cure is probably rare." To prove their point, 6 years later they presented the results of an evaluation of 1435 patients with peptic ulcer disease (gastric and duodenal) followed at the Peter Bent Brigham Hospital in Boston (EMERY and MONROE 1935). In this long-term analysis, they observed that untreated ulcer disease follows an up and down course for many years with symptoms fluctuating between spontaneous remissions and relapses. The interval between ulcer attacks was found to be quite variable. Among 131 patients who experienced a spontaneous remission, 95 (72.5%) remained in remission for up to 3 years and 35 (27%) for up to 6 years. Sustained remissions beyond 6 years were uncommon, although two patients went 9 years and three others went 20 years between symptomatic relapses. BOCKUS (1974) mentioned that in his practice, symptomatic relapses were separated by as many as 45 years for some patients.

EMERY and MONROE (1935) remarked that the longer they followed their ulcer patients, the fewer the number of medical "cures" they observed. Only 7.4% of patients were described as being "cured" (i.e., totally without symptoms) after 11–15 years. However, they also observed that medical failures became fewer over this period of time. Ulcer disease was rarely fatal among their patients and it did not appear to shorten the life expectancy of the group as a whole; only 6% of patients died as a result of ulcer-related complications. While the percentage of patients who experienced nonfatal complications rose from approximately 40% at the time of initial treatment to nearly 60% after two or three decades of disease, the authors concluded that, in general, "The ulcer has little tendency to become worse as time goes on." In contrast, EUSTERMAN and BALFOUR (1935) wrote that "in about half of the cases the symptoms become progressively more severe as the condition continues. The chronic nature of the disease is evidenced by the fact that the majority of the patients who have duodenal ulcer, as seen in the clinic, do not undergo an operation until the disease has existed an average period of 10 years."

In 1955, FLOOD (1955) reported his 20-year experience with 233 DU patients followed at Columbia Presbyterian Hospital in New York. His results suggested that the majority of DU patients experienced one or more relapses within a 5-year period. Recurrences were recorded for 78% of patients, a rate that was in keeping with that compiled by ALTHAUSEN (1949) for nearly all series published in the first half of this century. FLOOD observed that recurrences were unpredictable, often occurring without any precipitating event. The average relapse occurred once every 2.1 years after initial therapy. Diet did not appear to protect against relapse and medical management in general was not thought to have influenced the natural course of the disease. A subgroup of patients with a better than average course (one relapse every 4 years) was identified by having a short history of ulcer symptoms prior to therapy, the absence of complications, and the lack of the need for hospitalization. Conversely, among patients with a slow response to initial medical therapy or who suffered multiple episodes of hemorrhage, relapses occurred once every 1.2 years, a rate nearly twice that of the group in general.

I. Scandinavian Studies

Several long-term follow-up studies from Scandinavia were published between 1943 and 1966 (KRAG 1966; KRARUP 1946; KRAUSE 1963; MALMROS and HIERTONN 1949; NATVIG et al. 1943; QUIGSTAD and ROMCKE 1946; ROMCKE and HIERTONN 1949). What makes these studies particularly unique is the fact that large numbers of DU patients were seen at regular intervals for up to 25 years, often by the same physician in the same community. In addition, the absence of the external pressures and societal upheavals that were encountered by patients from war-ravaged European nations contributed to a relatively static population of DU patients available for study.

ROMCKE and his colleagues (NATVIG et al. 1943; QUIGSTAD and ROMCKE 1946; ROMCKE and LOKEN 1956) followed 230 medically treated patients for up to 9½ years and noted that 34% were symptom-free after 3 years but only 11% remained in complete remission at the end of the observation period. Patients with a long ulcer history (>5 years) and younger patients (<25 years old) had the poorest prognosis and surgery was recommended for those individuals who relapsed after initial treatment and whose symptoms could not be controlled by diet. KRARUP (1946) followed 297 DU patients diagnosed by barium meal for 5–11 years and observed that 20% remained healed but only 3% healed after a relapse. A poor result from medical therapy was recorded for nearly one-third of the group, a less favorable prognosis correlating with a longer ulcer history.

MALMROS and HIERTONN (1949) followed 495 DU patients after an initial 3-week course of bed rest, bland diet, and treatment with what they referred to as "pulvis antacidus" (a combination of magnesium subcarbonate, bismuth subsalicylate, and extract of belladonna) given between meals along with phenobarbital. More than 90% of ulcers healed as judged by their complete resolution on barium meal. Patients were subsequently observed over the next 7–10 years. A "favorable" course was enjoyed by 29% of the group (12.7% of whom were completely symptom-free); 22% had a "less favorable" course; and 41% had a "serious" course (with 3.9% dying from DU-related complications). No differences were seen with regard to gender, but those patients with shorter ulcer histories (<5 year duration) had a more favorable course (37%) compared to 12.5% in those with a history greater than 5 years. In addition, patients who had not received any ulcer therapy prior to that given at the outset of the study also fared better. These authors concluded that "in the long run the course of the disease is very little influenced by a single course of treatment or by repeated courses." They also stated that medical therapy appeared to be nearly a complete failure against preventing a relapse, adding that for many patients "the ulcer certainly heals but troubles recur."

A fourth large long-term Scandinavian study was reported by KRAUSE in 1963. In voicing his opinion that assumptions about ulcer disease based on the results of only 5 or 10 years of follow-up might not be entirely valid, he followed 371 DU patients at 5-year intervals beginning in 1925, most of whom were observed for a period of at least 25 years or until their deaths. As in all of the pre-endoscopic studies, the ulcers were diagnosed by barium meal. Symptomatic relapses were systematically recorded following an initial 4- to 6-week course of medical therapy. He observed that nearly 38% of men and 46% of women relapsed within 12 months, and 70% of both groups had relapsed within 5 years. After 25 years, 11% of men and 18% of women remained ulcer-free on x-ray but only 6.5% and 10.9% were asymptomatic. When "fresh case" DU patients (i.e., those with an ulcer history less than 5 years in duration and no prior treatment) were analyzed, the relapse figures were similar.

This "life prognosis" of DU disease provided KRAUSE with the opportunity to examine factors predictive of relapse and to determine the proper indications for surgical treatment. He found that male sex, younger age, previous medical therapy, and a long (>5 year) history of DU portended a less favorable prognosis and a higher relapse rate. Seventy percent of males and 66% of females with DU required surgical intervention during the observation period. The percentage was the same for "fresh cases" as for patients with a long ulcer history. Among those who did not undergo surgery, there was no excess mortality from ulcer disease; deaths due to perforation were rare. A few DU patients died of gastric carcinoma, an association that is now regarded as being unusual (LEWIS and WOODS 1982), but certainly not unexpected in the pre-endoscopic era.

Recognizing that medical treatment of ulcer disease would invariably change in the future, KRAUSE (1963) summarized the importance of the medical regimen available to his patients as being "rather small, on the whole, so that it will probably not have any great effect [on long-term prognosis]." Nevertheless, it was his impression that DU disease stabilized after 20 years, as few additional relapses occurred after that length of time.

Krag (1966) reported on the 17- to 26-year follow-up of 347 patients with DU or GU. A favorable course was reported for 28% of DU patients, a less favorable course requiring rehospitalization for bleeding or pain in 16%, and a serious course with two or more readmissions for bleeding or surgery in 56%. Overall, 39% of DU patients required surgery and 25% had bleeding. Krag did note, however, that for most patients, there was little or no change in their course of disease over a 25-year span.

II. European Studies

In 1964, Fry published the outcome of 212 DU patients diagnosed by barium meal who were followed in his general practice in a London suburb during the years 1948–1963. He observed that once symptoms began, they generally caused increasing disability and recurrent exacerbations over a 5- to 10-year period, with a peak in severity occurring 8.1 years for men and 7.1 years for women from the onset of symptoms. Afterwards, a steady and progressive remission in symptoms occurred, culminating in the ulcer tending to "burn itself out."

Elective surgical treatment among Fry's patients was reserved for those individuals (16% of the group) with severe or disabling symptoms. He remarked that this "tendency toward natural remissions" in the majority of DU patients seen in his office was quite different from what he had encountered while in training at Guy's Hospital. In discussing the possible influence of medical treatment on the course of ulcer disease, Fry, like those before him, concluded that it "very likely had no bearing on the final outcome." Interestingly, he noted that as a group, surgically treated patients fared better than those who were treated medically. A potential problem with Fry's analysis, however, can be found in the fact that most of his patients were lost to follow-up over the years and their ulcer histories were not included. This stands in contrast to the very high percentage of patients who were continuously followed after initial healing in the various studies from Scandinavia.

Levrat et al. (1968) chronicled the course of 421 ulcer patients over a 10-year span in Lyon, France, during 1943–1956. They observed that 35% of the nonoperated group (217 patients) continued to "suffer regularly" and that only 38% considered themselves "cured completely." The proportion of ulcer patients "cured" without surgical intervention dropped to 20% when all 421 individuals were considered, prompting the authors to conclude that their findings "could lead to the adoption of a more surgical attitude to treatment of gastro-duodenal ulcer."

In an earlier report, Levrat and his co-workers (1966) reported on their experience with 287 elderly ulcer patients over that age of 60 seen during an

11-year period and diagnosed by x-ray or at surgery. More than half the group had the onset of their ulcer disease after age 60 and only 20% had symptoms prior to age 50. The authors remarked that it was unusual for an ulcer originating at an early age to remain continuously or intermittently active after the age of 60. Indeed, they observed that the majority of ulcers in young individuals became asymptomatic prior to the seventh decade. This was in keeping with the results of a study conducted from 1930 to 1958 at the Mayo Clinic (MICHENER et al. 1960) in which ulcers beginning in childhood (prior to age 15) had a 50% chance of persisting or recurring into adolescence or adulthood. In contrast, the rate of ulcer complications in the older age group was very high (50%) and increased steadily with increasing age. In the endoscopic era, bleeding episodes have been found to be more prevalent amoung elderly DU patients, but pain is less often reported as a major symptom (SCAPA et al. 1989).

In 1977, GREIBE et al. summarized their experience with a group of 227 Danish DU patients who had been diagnosed in 1963, 154 of whom were available for follow-up interviews in 1976. The authors found that 37% of medically treated patients were asymptomatic, 29% were having mild symptoms, 12% were having moderate to severe symptoms, and 22% had undergone surgery for severe symptoms or ulcer complications over this 13-year period. Echoing the conclusions of previous investigators, their findings also suggested that medical therapy had little or no influence on the natural course of the disorder, although for many patients, DU disease did not appear to worsen appreciably over time.

III. CURE Study

In contrast to the celebrated conclusion reached by FRY (1964) that DU may, in fact, ultimately "burn itself out," ELASHOFF and her colleagues (1983) at the Center for Ulcer Research and Education (CURE) in Los Angeles offered a dissenting view. They analyzed the course of 190 male patients with an average DU history of 13 years on entry to the CURE Center, who were followed for up to 6 additional years. Although medical therapy was not specifically identified, since their report was published in 1983 it can be assumed that cimetidine was available to some, if not most patients during the latter part of the follow-up period. A complication rate of 2.7% per year was observed for those individuals with no prior history of ulcer complications, but the rate nearly doubled to 5% per year for patients who had previous ulcer-related problems. A long history of ulcer disease and a history of frequent hospitalizations prior to the observation period were both predictive of a more severe course later on. Patient age, age at onset of DU, smoking status, and family history of ulcer disease all failed to show a statistically significant relationship to the severity of the disorder.

A subset of DU patients (16%) were classified as having disease of low severity (i.e., they did not require hospitalization or the use of cimetidine, did not experience nighttime pain, and reported only mild–moderate ulcer systems over time). These patients notwithstanding, the majority of patients with a long ulcer history and more past problems due to ulcer disease continued to have ulcer-related disability or complications during the follow-up period, leading these investigators to conclude that their findings were "inconsistent with the idea that ulcer disease tends to burn itself out." Although nearly two-thirds of DU patients showed a reduction in ulcer pain scores during the follow-up period, the authors suggested that this tendency for ulcer pain to decrease might well have been due to the benefits of close medical attention rather than to spontaneous "burnout" of the ulcer.

What can be concluded about the natural history of DU from these early studies, all of which (except the latter part of the CURE study) were conducted prior to the introduction of the H_2 blockers? Notwithstanding the fact that the diagnosis of DU in these studies was made on the basis of symptoms and a barium meal examination, neither of which is as accurate as endoscopy (DOOLEY et al. 1984; DUNN and ETTER 1962), few would argue with the fact that DU is a chronic relapsing disorder with most patients experiencing periodic exacerbations and remissions. Just how long the disease remains active, however, cannot be completely ascertained from the data available. From the 25-year follow-up study by MALMROS and HIERTONN (1949), it can be reasonably inferred that sustained remissions are possible after initial medical therapy. FRY's (1964) observations made without the benefit of endoscopy or modern-day healing agents have continued to be widely quoted as defining the natural history of DU (DEW 1987; SONTAG 1988; WALAN and STROM 1985). However, whether or not DU disease ever truly "burns itself out" (i.e., *never* to recur again) is still not known, since relapses after 40–50 years of quiescent disease have been described (BOCKUS 1974), and the longest period of controlled observation has been only 25 years.

H. Duodenal Ulcer Disease in the H_2 Blocker Era

The medical therapy available to peptic ulcer disease patients prior to the introduction of cimetidine in 1978 consisted largely of combinations of a bland diet, antacid preparations, anticholinergic–antispasmodic compounds, gastric irradiation, sedation, reassurance, and stress reduction (BOCKUS 1974; IVY et al. 1950; PALMAS et al. 1984; PALMER 1974; SMITH and RIVERS 1953). The sentiment of MALMROS and HIERTONN (1949) that medical therapy was "almost a complete failure against preventing a relapse," was echoed by nearly all of the authors of the early studies examining the natural history of DU (BONNEVIE 1987). IVY (1946) was prescient is his 1946 prediction that "since the mechanism for the formation of hydrochloric acid by the parietal cell is so specific for the parietal cell, some substance which blocks the mechanism should be found in the course of time." Indeed, the introduction of the first H_2 receptor antagonists in the late 1970s was greeted with emotional fanfare by many patients and physicians faced with the prospect of treating severe ulcer disease without surgery. But have the H_2 blockers and other potent antisecretory drugs made a substantial difference? With over a decade of widespread use behind us, it is time to stop and reflect.

I. How Long Does a Duodenal Ulcer Stay Healed After Treatment?

The advent of endoscopically controlled healing trials has done much to advance our knowledge about ulcer relapse.[1] The first placebo-controlled endoscopic healing trial for DU was published by BROWN et al. in 1972. Literally hundreds of similar trials have followed and the results of the various agents that have been compared in short-term healing efficacy studies are summarized in a number of recent reviews (SONTAG 1988; THOMAS and MISIEWICZ 1984; TYTGAT et al. 1984; WALAN 1984). What emerges from a perusal of all these healing trials is that on average, 60%–80% of DUs heal within 4 weeks. Continuing therapy for an additional 2–4 weeks can be expected to increase the healing rates to 90%–95%. No single agent emerges as being truly superior to any other in terms of acute uncomplicated DU healing, although in Europe, very rapid 2- and 4-week healing rates (up to 100% in a few trials) (GUSTAVSSON et al. 1983; NAESDAL et al. 1985) were achieved with omeprazole. In general, however, greater antisecretory potency has not been equated with greater ulcer healing efficacy. Indeed, omeprazole was not recommended for the treatment of uncomplicated DU at its initial FDA Advisory Committee hearing (STERN 1989), as no superiority over the H_2 blockers in terms of efficacy or safety was demonstrated in several North American studies. As a result, the choice of ulcer therapy has grown to depend more on the issues of safety, side-effects, cost, and compliance than on the ability to simply heal the ulcer and relieve symptoms (LEWIS 1991).

As capable as all these drugs are in their ability to heal ulcers, most seem equally incapable of keeping ulcers healed after therapy is withdrawn. The majority of endoscopic studies have demonstrated a 12-month relapse rate that approaches 80% and more, regardless of the agent used to initially heal the DU (BOYD et al. 1983a; LANE and LEE 1988; LEWIS 1989a; SONTAG 1988; STRUM 1986). This high rate of relapse does not appear to be influenced by the duration of acute therapy. Even extending full-dose treatment for up to 1 year has not altered the relapse rate after therapy is stopped, as demonstrated by CARGILL et al. (1978) and DRONFIELD et al. (1979), who extended cimetidine therapy for 6 months, and by BARDHAN et al. (1984) and KORMAN et al. (1980), who extended cimetidine therapy for up to 12 months. After the drug was discontinued, the observed rate of relapse in each of these studies was the

1. The term "relapse" connotes the reappearance of the same or a different ulcer after medical therapy; "recurrence" is preferred when the ulcer reoccurs after surgery, but the terms are used interchangeably.

same as that seen following the usual 4- to 8-week treatment period for H_2 blockers and other agents (THOMAS and MISIEWITZ 1984; TYTGAT et al. 1984; WALAN 1984). Many studies indicate that most DUs tend to recur at the same site or in an adjacent quadrant of the duodenum (FULLMAN et al. 1985; MOSHAL et al. 1981; SOLHAUG et al. 1987).

J. Role of *Helicobacter pylori*

A number of reports from the late 1970s and early 1980s suggested that DU relapse was less likely to occur after short-term therapy with colloidal bismuth preparations compared to H_2 blockers and other agents (DOBRILLA et al. 1988; HAMILTON et al. 1986; LEE et al. 1985; MARTIN et al. 1981). For example, in a study by MARTIN et al. (1981), relapse rates following 4–8 weeks of therapy with tripotassium dicitrato bismuthate (5 ml q.i.d.) or cimetidine (1 g daily) were 13% and 70% at 6 months and 39% and 85% at 12 months, respectively. At the end of 18 months, the percentage of ulcers that had relapsed endoscopically was 52% for bismuth and 89% for cimetidine. These differences were statistically significant, although the study has been criticized because not all of the asymptomatic bismuth-treated patients had follow-up endoscopies. Furthermore, the results of other bismuth studies have been conflicting. KANG and PIPER (1982), SHREEVE et al. (1983), and BIANCHI PORRO et al. (1986) all failed to show a significantly lower relapse rate with colloidal bismuth compared to cimetidine. And in a recent report by LANE and LEE (1988), the apparent early protective effects of bismuth treatment were shown not to extend beyond the first 12 months.

Nevertheless, these studies subsequently served as an important link in the discovery of the association of *H. pylori* with ulcer disease (COGHLAN et al. 1987; MARSHALL 1988; MARSHALL et al. 1988; SHREEVE et al. 1983) (as is discussed in more detail elsewhere in this monograph). The theory that DU disease is declining because of the increasing use of antibiotics since the 1950s leading to the serendipitous eradication of the organism (MARSHALL 1988), is provocative but remains unproven. It is still too early to assess the long-term consequences of eradicating *H. pylori* and its associated gastritis on the long-term natural history of DU.

K. Natural History of Untreated Ulcers

Only a few studies have attempted to determine the endoscopic healing rate of DU using a true placebo or by means of simple passive observation. In a study by COLLEN et al. (1980), a placebo cimetidine tablet was compared to the actual drug and no p.r.n. antacids were allowed. The healing rate for cimetidine was slightly greater at 2 weeks, but the rates at 4 weeks (67% vs 72%) were not significantly different.

FREDERIKSEN et al. (1984) studied 91 DU subjects (mostly out patients) and found that 29 (32%) showed complete endoscopic healing at 2 weeks and a total of 52 (57%) healed within 6 weeks on "passive observation" combined with avoidance of aspirin and the use of p.r.n. antacids. "Spontaneous" healing was most frequently observed in women and in men with lower acid outputs. The 52 patients who healed "spontaneously" were then entered into a 2-year follow-up study utilizing the same "nontherapy" with endoscopic examinations scheduled every 3 months. Thirteen patients (25%) remained in complete remission; 19 suffered one or two relapses that healed "spontaneously"; 11 developed symptomatic relapses that necessitated active drug therapy; and nine individuals failed to complete the study for various reasons. In sum, 69% relapsed (or otherwise failed) during this 2-year observation period, a figure not dissimilar from relapse rates recorded for patients who come off active maintenance therapy or who receive placebo in clinical trials (LANE and LEE 1988; SONTAG 1988).

An interesting observation made by FREDERIKSEN et al. (1984) was the fact that spontaneous relapses may heal spontaneously. This phenomenon had been alluded to (LEWIS 1985), but was never actually documented during continuous maintenance therapy with an active agent until BOYD et al. (1989) performed monthly endoscopies in 34 healed DU patients for 1–13 months and found that DUs could indeed relapse and reheal spontaneously while on continuous low-dose H_2 blocker therapy (ranitidine 150 mg h.s.). Identifying individuals who do not require active DU drug treatment would seem to be difficult at best. From a practical standpoint, as concluded by FREDERIKSEN and his colleagues (1984), it is probably best to simply prescribe an active therapeutic agent for all DU patients at the time of diagnosis. If factors can be uncovered that accurately predict who will heal *without* an active agent, then this approach can be altered.

L. Natural History of Unhealed Ulcers

At the conclusion of nearly every published short-term (4–8 week) DU healing trial, 10%–25% of patients' ulcers remain unhealed on active therapy as assessed by endoscopy (HOWDEN et al. 1985; THOMAS and MISIEWICZ 1984; TYTGAT et al. 1984; WALAN 1984). Just why these ulcers do not heal has been attributed to multiple factors, including noncompliance (BOYD et al. 1983b), active smoking (BOYD et al. 1983c; KIKENDALL et al. 1984; KORMAN et al. 1983), continued use of NSAIDs (LANGMAN 1989), hypersecretion of acid (COLLEN et al. 1989), large ulcer diameter (BARDHAN 1984; LAM et al. 1985), male gender (SOUNENBERG et al. 1981), long duration of ulcer symptoms (BARDHAN 1984), invasion of the ulcer by fungi (THOMAS and REDDY 1983), lower socioeconomic status (HASAN and SIRCUS 1981), spice-filled diet (KUMAR et al. 1984), alcohol ingestion (REYNOLDS 1989), poor initial pain relief (REYNOLDS 1989), and a positive family history of DU (BARDHAN 1984; HASAN and SIRCUS 1981). However, there is far from a complete consensus of opinion regarding the importance of these individual factors (IPPOLITI 1985). For example, in several reports, smoking (KORMAN et al. 1983), alcohol (SONNENBERG et al. 1981), male gender (KORMAN et al. 1983), and lower socioeconomic status (SONNENBERG et al. 1981) were not associated with impaired DU healing.

"Resistance" to cimetidine is the reason cited for healing failures in several reports (DANILEWITZ et al. 1982; GALMICHE et al. 1982; MAZZACCA et al. 1982; WITZEL and WOLBERGS 1982), as healing was subsequently accomplished with ranitidine. However, true "resistance" to an active agent is considered to be exceedingly rare (LAM et al. 1985; STEINBERG et al. 1984), and it has been suggested that simply prolonging therapy with the same drug would be equally as effective as switching to another agent. In support of this contention is a study by QUATRINI et al. (1984) in which patients who failed to heal on cimetidine 1 g/day for 6 weeks were randomized to receive ranitidine 300 mg/day or to continue to receive cimetidine 1 g/day for an additional 6 weeks. Nearly identical rates of healing were observed for both groups at the end of the trial, suggesting that some patients are simply "slow healers," as defined by BARDHAN (1981), and require more than the traditional 4–8 weeks of acute therapy or increased doses of medication.

M. Can Drug Therapy Prevent Duodenal Ulcer Relapse?

As previously mentioned, once a DU has healed on short-term therapy, the risk of an endoscopically documented relapse within the next 12–24 months approaches 90%, regardless of the agent (SONTAG 1988; LANE and LEE 1988). The real problem then with DU therapy, as stated by WORMSLEY (1982) and others, is not so much being able to heal the ulcer as being able to keep it healed. Physicians in the pre-H_2 blocker era were uniformly unsuccessful in sustaining a remission, which prompted the following remark by EMERY and MONROE in 1935: "If one cannot free the patient from the [ulcer] disease it should be helpful to discover how best to fit him to it."

The use of continuous low-dose H_2 blocker therapy reduces ulcer relapse rate from approximately 80% down to 20%–30% during the 1st year of therapy (SONTAG 1988). Scores of trials have confirmed the efficacy of various agents in low-dose regimens in the prevention of DU relapse (LEWIS 1989a; SONTAG 1988; STRUM 1986; THOMAS and MISIEWICZ 1984; TYTGAT et al. 1984; VAN DEVENTER 1984; WALAN 1984). On the surface it would appear that for the first time we can control DU disease. Or can we?

"Low-dose" H_2 blocker therapy for relapse prevention is a somewhat arbitrarily defined concept, with the recommended dose generally being one-half that used for acute healing. The H_2 receptor blocking agents are usually given at bedtime, based on the observations of DRAGSTED (1969) and others nearly 50 years ago, recently reconfirmed (DE GARA et al. 1986; JONES et al. 1987), that nocturnal acid secretion appears to be the most important in terms of ulcer pathogenesis. This knowledge served as the impetus for subsequent studies that demonstrated the ability of a single nocturnal dose of H_2 blocker to heal a DU acutely (CAPURSO et al. 1984; DYCK et al. 1982; GITLIN et al. 1987; HOWDEN et al. 1985; IRELAND et al. 1984).

The half-strength doses that are currently used to prevent relapses (e.g., cimetidine 400 mg h.s., ranitidine 150 mg h.s., famotidine 20 mg h.s., nizatidine 150 mg h.s.) may not be effective in all patients, especially those with one or more of the factors that predict ulcer recurrence as described below. For example, FITZPATRICK et al. (1982) observed a 59% relapse rate at 6 months in patients receiving cimetidine 400 mg h.s. (vs 63% among placebo recipients), but only a 30% relapse rate when those patients still in remission were given 800 mg h.s. over the next 6 months. Similarly, WALAN and STROM (1985) intimated that higher doses of cimetidine are often necessary to prevent relapse, and followed up on that statement with a study that demonstrated the best dose to be 400 mg b.i.d. for any DU patient who fails to heal completely after 6 weeks of initial treatment with 1 g/day (STROM et al. 1986). They observed that such "slow healers" had the highest relapse rates on 400 mg h.s. and that even 400 mg b.i.d. was successful in establishing a remission in only about half of these individuals. The relapse rate for slowly healing prepyloric ulcers was even higher on 400 mg h.s. and the remission rate lower (31%) compared to DU, even with the 400 mg b.i.d. regimen.

Prolonging *full-dose* cimetidine (BARDHAN et al. 1984; KORMAN et al. 1983) or ranitidine (LEE et al. 1989a) for up to 12 months will prevent DU relapse in most patients during the time the drug is taken. Although it has been suggested that such a regimen may expose the patient to unnecessary medication with its attendant compliance and cost issues and the potential for unwanted side-effects (ANDERSEN 1985), adverse effects during therapy for up to 9 years have been very rare to date (LEWIS 1989b; PENSTON 1990; PENSTON and WORMSLEY 1988; WALAN et al. 1987).

Predicting DU relapse: On average, 25%–35% of patients receiving continuous low-dose maintenance therapy with H_2 blockers will suffer a "breakthrough" relapse (SONTAG 1988; STRUM 1986; THOMAS and MISIEWICZ 1984; TYTGAT et al. 1984; WALAN 1984). In head-to-head comparisons with the two most widely used agents, ranitidine maintenance treatment has led to statistically fewer DU relapses than cimetidine both in large multicenter trials (GOUGH et al. 1984; SILVIS et al. 1985) and in meta-analyses of multiple studies (CHAMBERS et al. 1987; KURATA et al. 1987). This difference may not be too surprising given the fact that ranitidine has also been shown to heal slightly more acute duodenal ulcers in short-term healing trials (MCISAAC et al. 1987). Its superiority in preventing DU relapse is probably the result of its greater nocturnal acid suppression at the maintenance doses used (JONES et al. 1987).

Several other factors have been suggested to explain why duodenal ulcers relapse. The first is compliance, or more strictly speaking the lack of compliance. The failure to adhere to a drug treatment schedule has been cited as one of the most important reasons why maintenance treatment fails (BOYD et al. 1983b). DIAZ-RUBIO (1988) found that informing the patient of the need and rationale for maintenance therapy had a positive influence on compliance, as only about one-third of patients permanently stopped their therapy compared to 100% who did not receive such information. Similarly, JENSSEN et al. (1989) recently reported that among patients being followed after treatment for an acutely bleeding DU, many stopped maintenance therapy despite the recommendation not to do so. Of these, 26% suffered the consequences of ulcer rebleeding compared to only 3.5% who complied with the treatment regimen. In a study by PENSTON and WORMSLEY (1988), only 1% of DU patients followed for up to 9 years developed breakthrough ulcer rebleeding on maintenance. There is no evidence to support the possibility that any of the H_2 blockers lose efficacy over time. Although transient resistance to an active agent (DANILEWITZ et al. 1982; GALMICHE et al. 1982; MAZZACCA et al. 1982; WITZEL and WOLBERGS 1982) and marked individual variations in the sensitivity to cimetidine have been observed (LEWIS et al. 1982), true resistance remains more of a theoretical than a factual possibility.

Several investigators have cited hyperacidity as an important reason why ulcers relapse (BATTAGLIN et al. 1984; COLLEN et al. 1989; KRAG 1966). Active smoking (BOYD et al. 1983c; KORMAN et al. 1983; SONTAG et al. 1984), continued used of NSAIDs (MELLEM et al. 1985), and alcohol (VAN DEVENTER et al. 1989) also may interfere with the ability of a maintenance drug regimen to prevent relapses. Whether or not smokeless tobacco or substances used to help patients quit smoking (e.g., Nicorette) have an adverse effect on ulcer healing or relapse is a question that has not been adequately studied.

Another important reason why ulcers may relapse is that they may not have been completely healed at the start of maintenance therapy (PAOLUZI et al. 1985). Other factors, such as long duration of ulcer disease (BATTAGLIA et al. 1984), early onset of ulcer disease (BATTAGLIA et al. 1984), positive family history (SILVIS et al. 1985), male gender (IPPOLITI 1985), and blood group A (BTTAGLIA et al. 1984), all have been cited as predictors of DU relapse. However, just as with the factors that may impair initial ulcer healing, not all studies find that these relapse risk factors listed above can be substantiated. Emotional stress, for example, while long cited as an important reason for recrudescence of ulcer disease (WOLF 1981), has in fact been difficult to consistently prove in a cause and effect relationship (PETERS and RICHARDSON 1983). A case in point, LOOF et al. (1987) found no benefit to psychological counseling compared to maintenance drug therapy, while COLGAN (1988) observed hypnotherapy to be beneficial in his study, in keeping with the findings of KLEIN and SPIEGEL (1989) that hypnosis can modulate acid secretion. In a recent report from Australia (NASIRY et al. 1987), marriage breakup and divorce adversely affected ulcer disease, but alcohol, smoking, and male gender did not. In contrast, no correlation between DU relapse and marital status or other psychological stresses was apparent in a Swedish study (ADAMI et al. 1987).

N. Other Agents for "Short-Term" Maintenance Therapy

I. Antacids

Until recently, little information was available on the efficacy of antacids in the prevention of DU relapse, despite their undoubtedly widespread uncontrolled use for this purpose. In an early double-blind comparison published in 1957 by CAYER et al., 144 patients with DU diagnosed by barium meal were given either dihydroxy aluminum aminoacetate (four tablets 2 after meals and at bedtime) or placebo and were instructed to maintain a bland diet. After 8.5 months the relapse rate, as judged by a return of ulcer symptoms, was 50% for the antacid group and 88% for the placebo group. This is obviously an unacceptable rate of relapse by today's standards even in the absence of endoscopically verified relapses, but antacids did appear to have some beneficial effect as 74% of antacid recipients reported "good to excellent" results compared to only 24% in the placebo group.

Only a few endoscopically controlled trials have been reported using antacids for the prevention of DU relapse. In a preliminary report, BARDHAN and co-workers (1986) found that Maalox TC (three tablets each morning and at bedtime) was as effective as cimetidine 400 mg h.s. in reducing cumulative relapse rates (25% vs 27% at 12 months) and both treatment regimens were superior to placebo (53% at 12 months) and to Maalox three tablets h.s. (43% at 12 months). BYTZER et al. (1986) also reported that after 1 year, relapse rates were similar among patients receiving ranitidine 150 mg b.i.d. or high dose antacid (Novaluzid 10 ml seven times daily). BRESCI et al. (1986) compared maintenance doses of cimetidine (400 mg h.s.), ranitidine (150 mg h.s.), and pirenzipine (50 mg h.s.) to antacids taken only as needed for pain and recorded 1-year relapse rates of 17.5%, 21%, 21.7%, and 49.8% respectively, suggesting that intermittent antacid therapy is ineffective as prophylaxis.

The results of a recent international multicenter study found tablet antacids (3 Maalox tablets after breakfast and at bedtime) to be as effective as climetidine (400 mg h.s.) at 12 months. Antacid tablets taken only at night had intermediate efficacy (MILLER 1990).

II. Anticholinergics

Anticholinergics were not found to be successful in preventing DU relapse in the pre-endoscopic era and are still not regarded as being useful for this purpose (WALAN 1984). The one exception might be pirenzepine, a tricyclic compound with anticholinergic properties which has been better than placebo in a few long-term maintenance studies but which has generally led to higher relapse rates compared to H_2 blockers (SONNENBERG et al. 1981; TYTGAT et al. 1984; WALAN 1984). More recent reports, however, have shown similar efficacy (FONTANA et al. 1986).

III. Tricyclic Antidepressants

Trimipramine has maintained DU remission in 36%–66% of patients given 25 mg nocturnally for periods of up to 12 months, but has been numerically inferior to H2 blockers (BECKER et al. 1984; RIES et al. 1984; VALNES et al. 1982). Thus, it may not be appropriate as maintenance therapy, but may serve an adjunctive role.

IV. Sucralfate

Forty years ago IVY (1946) suggested that if it was possible to increase the resistance of the gastroduodenal mucosa or to increase its healing potential then ulcer recurrence might be prevented. Results with sucralfate and other "cytoprotective" agents appear to support IVY's contention. The results of studies utilizing a maintenance dose of 1 g b.i.d. show a 20% 6-month relapse rate and a 12-month relapse rate of approximately 30% (figures comparable to H_2 blockers) (BEHAR et al. 1986; CLASSEN et al. 1983; LEWIS 1986). The 12-month relapse rate of a single nocturnal 1 g dose of sucralfate for maintenance, however, has been considerably higher (47%) and the dose approved for a DU maintenance indication in the United States was 1 g b.i.d.

The combination of sucralfate 2 g/day plus cimetidine 400 mg/day was compared to both agents given alone in a maintenance study by TAKEMOTO et al. (1986). Their results suggested that no additional benefit was conferred by the use of both drugs simultaneously in preventing DU relapse.

V. Bismuth

As previously mentioned, a number of studies have suggested that DU relapse might be delayed following initial healing with bismuth compounds, possibly because of their ability to eradicate *H. pylori* (DOBRILLA et al. 1988; MARSHALL 1988; MARSHALL et al. 1988). However, the results of long-term follow-up studies do not show any extended benefit of an initial course of bismuth therapy (LANE and LEE 1988) and there are no long-term continuous low-dose bismuth treatment studies that have been published to date, although such trials are reportedly ongoing BIANCHI PORRO 1986). As mentioned previously, just how the successful eradication of *H. pylori* will influence the natural history of DU remains to be determined.

VI. Omeprazole

No extended maintenance studies in DU patients are currently available for review with omeprazole and, at present, it is not indicated for maintenance treatment of DU pending the results of long-term safety data in non-Zollinger-Ellison syndrome ulcer patients (STERN 1980). Six-month duodenal ulcer relapse rates off of therapy have been no different from those with placebo in several studies, indicating that in spite of its potent antisecretory abilities, acute treatment with this agent does not change the natural history of DU (BROOK et al. 1987; WALAN et al. 1985).

O. How Long Should Maintenance Therapy Be Continued?

In 1978, FORDTRAN asked "whether prolonged maintenance therapy [for DU] will reduce the frequency of complications and need for surgical treatment? Even if it does, will it be worth the cost, possible risks and effort?" From the data available thus far, extended maintenance therapy with H_2 blockers has been shown to be both safe and effective over an extended period of several years. For example, in a 4-year trial conducted by the Anglo-Irish Study Group (WALAN et al. 1987), patients received cimetidine 40 mg h.s. with endoscopy performed every 6–12 months or as needed for the assessment of symptoms. Cumulative DU relapse rates were 33% at the end of the 1st year and subsequently rose to 62% at the end of 4 years. While this cumulative relapse rate seems unacceptably high at first glance, the percentage of patients with ulcer relapses was only 12% between the 1st and 2nd years, 13% between the 2nd and 3rd years, and just 4% between the 3rd and 4th years.

A nearly identical reduction in cumulative DU relapse has been observed by BIANCHI PORRO and PETRILLO (1986). Among their patients whose DUs remained healed on cimetidine 400 mg h.s. at the end of 1 year, 17% relapsed after 2 years and the relapse rate at the end of the 3rd year was only 10%, both figures being significantly less than the average rate of relapse observed in most 1-year studies. Similarly, BOYD et al. (1984a) observed an 18% relapse rate during the 2nd year of maintenance therapy with ranitidine 150 mg h.s. compared to 38% during the 1st year of therapy and PENSTON and WORMSLEY (1988) showed a decline in the annual relapse rates during a 6-year trial using ranitidine or cimetidine, with annual relapse rates between years falling to only 3%–5% by the end of the study. In patients receiving ranitidine in maintenance as well as full treatment doses for up to 9 years, PENSTON and WORMSLEY have reported no serious side-effects, and no instances of gastric carcinoids or carcinoma (PENSTON 1990; PENSTON and WORMSLEY 1988; SONTAG 1988; WORMSLEY 1984).

In 1978, an Editorial in the *British Medical Journal* entitled "Cimetidine for ever (and ever and ever ...)?," first raised the possibility of truly "long-term" therapy. Just how long maintenance therapy should be continued, however, is a question that still cannot be answered since the longest studies employing periodic endoscopy to determine the course of DU have been conducted for fewer than 10 years, a fraction of the time that ultimately may be required to define the true natural history.

Some authorities have suggested that maintenance therapy might have to be continued lifelong, especially in patients who, by virtue of an increased risk of DU relapse, remain at increased risk of ulcer morbidity and complications (SONTAG 1988; WORMSLEY 1984, 1988). However, pending the results of truly long-term studies, others have suggested that continuous therapy may be inappropriate given the as yet unresolved issues of continued cost of therapy, long-term compliance, possible untoward side-effects, and potential for drug interactions from some agents during prolonged daily therapy (ANDERSEN 1985; EDITORIAL 1978). As a result, a number of alternative medical approaches to relapse prevention have been proposed: "on demand," "intermittent," and "seasonal" forms of therapy.

I. On-Demand Versus Intermittent Therapy

POUNDER (1981) defined "on-demand" therapy as the self-administration of full-dose ulcer medication by the patient at the time that symptoms reappear. Therapy is continued for at least 2 weeks after symptoms have abated (usually 3–4 weeks' total). This form of therapy relies on the patient's assessment of his or her own symptoms and is unmonitored (SONTAG 1988). In contrast, "intermittent" therapy is initiated by the physician for a documented ulcer relapse (either by clinical assessment, upper gastrointestinal series, or endoscopic findings). Full-dose therapy is also continued for at least 2 weeks after symptoms resolve. Utilizing these two forms of therapy, it has been estimated that the average DU patient will take only 4–6 weeks of medication annually (BARDHAN 1988; POUNDER 1981). In a recent analysis, VAN DEVENTER et al. (1989) concluded that intermittent therapy was successful in preventing relapses in many patients although the direct medical and indirect costs of ulcer disease (absenteeism and death) were somewhat lower with a continuous regimen of daily maintenance therapy compared to the traditional (intermittent) treatment approach. Even when compared to surgical therapy, continuous daily maintenance therapy remains cost-effective for periods of 15–32 years (SONNENBERG 1989).

The observation that ulcer disease has a seasonal periodicity gave rise to a third treatment option, "seasonal prophylaxis." PALMAS et al. (1984) employed low-dose treatment with ranitidine in a dose of 300 mg daily for the first 3 weeks of April followed by 150 mg until the end of June. An identical cycle of ranitidine prophylaxis was repeated during October and November. When compared to treatment with 150 mg daily for the entire year, no difference in ulcer relapse was observed. Similarly, preliminary results with pirenzepine in a seasonal type of maintenance therapy show it to be as effective in preventing relapses as continuous maintenance therapy (GIBINSKI et al. 1986).

All three of these alternative maintenance regimens have the advantage of requiring less medication and are therefore less costly to the patient. Since on-demand therapy is initiated by the patient, treatment of symptomatic relapses is often started sooner than with physician-initiated intermittent therapy. While an attractive approach to long-term maintenance therapy for some patients, these alternative forms of therapy nevertheless have their detractors. One disadvantage of on-demand therapy is that it tends to miss asymptomatic relapses, which may place the patient at risk for future ulcer complications (BARDHAN 1988). As reported by BOYD et al. (1984b), ulcer relapses in patients receiving placebo during the 2nd year of maintenance therapy tended to cause symptoms and were more likely to be associated with hemorrhage than were those in whom patients continued to receive ranitidine 150 mg h.s. Breakthrough relapses on active therapy were often clinically silent, even though they seldom healed despite continuation of maintenance therapy. Therefore, it was these authors' recommendation that continuous ranitidine therapy was safer than no maintenance treatment, even for patients with asymptomatic ulcers, a point corroborated by more long-term studies (JONES et al. 1987; PENSTON and WORMSLEY 1988; WALAN et al. 1987).

Intermittent forms of therapy have been considered unsuitable for individuals with a history of frequent recurrences, prior complications, or the presence of additional factors that portend a high risk of DU relapse (BARDHAN 1988; SONTAG 1988; VAN DEVENTER 1984). Under those circumstances, most authorities would recommend continuous daily maintenance therapy to prevent further ulcer morbidity (SONNENBERG 1985; WORMSLEY 1988). A patient with a first-time uncomplicated ulcer may not suffer a relapse for years, if ever, and the on-demand or intermittent therapy approach would seem most appropriate (BARDHAN 1988; LEWIS 1989a).

P. Summary

It seems apparent that while we can heal most, if not all, DUs with the agents at hand, short-term drug therapy does not alter the long-term natural history of the disease, given the high rate of relapse observed when therapy is stopped. As mentioned by WORMSLEY (1982), any drug capable of reducing DU recurrence would make an important contribution to our armentarium, but "merely deferring recurrence for a few months is not likely to be very valuable." Although the incidence, mortality, and the need for hospitalization for DU have steadily declined in the United States in recent years, medical, social, and economic costs of peptic ulcer disease remain high, suggesting that we must consider altering our present approach to ulcer management. Maintenance therapy using H_2 blockers (and sucralfate and possibly other agents for which there are controlled data) is effective in preventing ulcer relapse in most individuals at the doses recommended, but once discontinued does not provide any long-term prevention against relapse. Continuing therapy beyond 1 year (and possibly at full ulcer-healing doses) has been shown to further reduce the cumulative rate of relapse, but the optimal duration (and dose) of chronic therapy has not been defined. Additional studies on the role of short-term therapy of *H. pylori* (with bismuth and antibiotic combination) on long-term DU relapse rates will be eagerly awaited.

In some patients, treatment is likely to be recommended for many years or even decades, but treatment recommendations are constrained by current limitations on our knowledge of the natural history of a disease that has not been fully defined endoscopically, and for which we have only relatively limited experience using ulcer medications monitored continuously for "extended" periods of time (i.e., <10 years). If such studies continue to show that the H_2 blockers (and sucralfate and other agents) remain safe and effective at the currently recommended doses when given for more than 5–10 years, then we will continue to be justified in recommending such "long-term" treatment. In the meantime, alternative forms of maintenance therapy, such as on-demand, intermittent, or seasonal prophylaxis, may be appropriate for individuals not wishing to continue continuous treatment beyond 1 or 2 years. For some patients who develop breakthrough relapses or who suffer from frequent relapses whenever therapy is discontinued (because of compliance difficulties or other reasons), surgical intervention may be appropriate, although the optimal surgical procedure to prevent ulcer disease has not been defined and operative and postoperative morbidity and mortality should be taken into account before considering this approach.

Until such time as the true (i.e., the endoscopic), life-long natural history of DU is defined, we must realize that our present approach to the medical therapy and prevention of DU is, if not still in its infancy, then certainly not beyond its adolescent years. Perhaps someone updating this topic 20 or 30 years from now will be in a better position to comment on the impact that "long-term" therapy has had on the natural history of duodenal ulcer disease.

References

Adami H-O, Bergstrom R, Nyren O et al. (1987) Is duodenal ulcer really a psychosomatic disease? A population-based case-control study. Scand J Gastroenterol 22:889–896

Ahmed SZ, Levine M, Finkbiner R (1963) The seasonal incidence of complications of peptic ulcer. Ann Intern Med 59:165–171

Althausen TL (1949) Prevention of recurrence in peptic ulcer. Ann Intern Med 30:544–599

Andersen D (1985) Prevention of ulcer recurrence – medical vs. surgical treatment. The surgeon's view. Scand J Gastroenterol [Suppl 110] 10:89–92

Bardhan KD (1981) Non-responders to cimetidine treatment, part 2. In: Baron JH (ed) Cimetidine in the 80's. Churchill Livingstone, Edinburgh, pp 42–57

Bardhan KD (1984) Refractory duodenal ulcer. Gut 25:697–702

Bardhan KD (1986) Are antacids as effective as cimetidine in preventing duodenal ulcer relapse? A multi-center study. Gastroenterology 90:1336

Bardhan KD (1988) Intermittent treatment of duodenal ulcer for long-term medical management. Postgrad Med J [Suppl 1] 64:40–46

Bardhan KD, Hinchliffe RFC (1981) Effect of cimetidine on surgery for duodenal ulcer. Lancet II:38
Bardhan K, Cole DS, Hawkins BW, Franks CR (1984) Does treatment with cimetidine extended beyond initial healing of duodenal ulcer reduce the subsequent relapse rate? Br Med J 284:621–623
Battaglia G, Farini R, Di Mario F et al. (1984) Recurrence of duodenal ulcer under continuous antisecretory treatment: an approach to the detection of predictive markers. Am J Gastroenterol 1984; 79:831–834
Becker U, Faurschou V, Jensen J et al. (1984) Relapse prevention of duodenal ulcers with trimipramine, cimetidine or placebo. Scand J Gastroenterol 19:405–410
Behar J, Roufail W, Thomas E et al. (1986) Efficacy of sucralfate in the prevention of recurrence of duodenal ulcer. Gastroenterology 90:1343
Bianchi Porro G (1986) Maintenance therapy with De-Nol in peptic ulcer disease. De-Nol symposium: mucosal protection and peptic ulcer disease; World Congress of Gastroenterology, Sao Paulo, September 8, 1986
Bianchi Porro G, Petrillo M (1986) The natural history of peptic ulcer disease: the influence of H_2-antagonist treatment. Scand J Gastroenterol [Suppl 121] 21:46–52
Bingham JR (1960) Relation between climate and hemorrhage from duodenal ulcer. Gastroenterology 38:959
Blumenthal IS (1968) Digestive disease as a national problem. III. Social cost of peptic ulcer. Gastroenterology 54:86–92
Bockus HL (1974) The therapy of peptic ulcer, part I. Management of uncomplicated peptic ulcer. Gastroenterology 1 (30):674–710
Boles RS Jr, Westerman MP (1954) Seasonal incidence and precipitating causes of hemorrhage from peptic ulcer. JAMA 156:1379–1383
Bonfils S, Baron JH, Blum A (1984) Uncontrolled factors in controlled trials of peptic ulcer. Dig Dis Sci 29:858–861
Bonnevie O (1975) The incidence of duodenal ulcer in Copenhagen County. Scand J Gastroenterol 10:385–393
Bonnevie O (1977) Causes of death in duodenal and gastric ulcer. Gastroenterology 73:1000–1004
Bonnevie O (1978) Survival in peptic ulcer. Gastroenterology 75:1055–1060
Bonnevie O (1985) Changing demographics of peptic ulcer disease. Dig Dis Sci 30 (Suppl):8s–14s
Bonnevie O (1987) Developments in the treatment of peptic ulcer. Scand J Gastroenterol [Suppl 127] 22:51–54
Boyd EJS, Wilson JA, Wormsley KG (1983a) Review of ulcer treatment; role of ranitidine. J Clin Gastroenterol [Suppl 1] 5:133–141
Boyd EJS, Wilson JA, Wormsely KG (1983b) Effects of treatment compliance and overnight gastric secretion on outcome of maintenance therapy of duodenal ulcer with ranitidine. Scand J Gastroenterol 18:193–200
Boyd EJS, Wilson JA, Wormsley KG (1983c) Smoking impairs therapeutic gastric inhibition. Lancet I:95–97
Boyd EJS, Wilson JA, Wormsley KG (1984a) Safety of ranitidine maintenance treatment of duodenal ulcer. Scand J Gastroenterol 19:394–400
Boyd EJS, Wilson JA, Wormsley KG (1984b) The fate of asymptomatic recurrences of duodenal ulcer. Scand J Gastroenterol 19:808–812
Boyd EJS, Penston JG, Johnston DA, Wormsley KG (1989) Does maintenance therapy keep duodenal ulcers healed? Lancet I:1324–1327
Bresci G, Capria A, Federici G, Rindi G, Geloni M, Corsini G (1986) Prevention of relapse with various antiulcer drugs. Scand J Gastroenterol [Suppl 121] 21:58–62
Brinton W (1857) On the pathology symptoms and treatment of ulcer of the stomach. Churchill, London, p 155
Brook CW, Yeomans ND, McCarthy PG, Dudley FJ, Smallwood RA (1987) Relapse of duodenal ulceration after healing with omeprazole. Med J Aust 147:595–597

Brown P, Salmon PR, Thien-Htut, Read AE (1972) Double-blind trial of carbenoxolone sodium capsules in duodenal ulcer therapy, based on endoscopic diagnosis and follow-up. Br Med J iii:661–664
Brown RC (1930) The results of medical treatment of peptic ulcer. JAMA 95:1144–1148
Bytzer P, Lauritsen K, Rask-Madsen J (1986) Symptomatic recurrence of healed duodenal and prepyloric ulcers after treatment with ranitidine or high-dose antacid. A 1-year follow-up study. Scand J Gastroenterol 21:765–768
Capurso L, Dal Monte PR, Mazzeo F et al. (1984) Comparison of cimetidine 800 mg once daily and 400 mg twice daily in acute duodenal ulceration. Br Med J 289:1418–1420
Cargill JM, Peden N, Saunders JHB, Wormsley KG (1978) Very long-term treatment of peptic ulcer with cimetidine. Lancet II:1113–1115
Cayer D, Sohmer MF, Ruffin JM (1957) The effect of prolonged continuous therapy on the course of chronic recurring peptic ulcer. Antacid therapy with dihydroxy aluminum aminoacetate (Alglyn). NC J 18:315–317
Chambers JB, Pryce D, Bland JM, Northfield TC (1987) Effect of bedtime ranitidine on overnight gastric acid output and intragastric pH: dose/response study and comparison with cimetidine. Gut 28:294–299
Christensen A, Bousfield R, Christiansen J (1988) Incidence of perforated and bleeding peptic ulcers before and after the introduction of H_2-receptor antagonists. Ann Surg 207:4–6
Classen M, Bethge H, Brunner G et al. (1983) Effect of sucralfate on peptic ulcer recurrence: a controlled double-blind multicenter study. Scand J Gastroenterol [Suppl] 18:61–68
Coggon D, Lambert P, Langman MJS (1981) 20 years of hospital admissions for peptic ulcer in England and Wales. Lancet I:1302–1304
Coghlan JG, Gilligan D, Humphries H et al. (1987) *Campylobacter pylori* and recurrence of duodenal ulcers – a 12 month follow-up study. Lancet II:1109–1111
Colgan SM, Faragher EB, Whorwell PJ (1988) Controlled trial of hypnotherapy in relapse prevention of duodenal ulceration. Lancet I:1299–1300
Collen MJ, Hanan MR, Maher JA et al. (1980) Cimetidine vs. placebo in duodenal ulcer therapy: six-week controlled double-blind investigation without any antacid therapy. Dig Dis Sci 25:744–749
Collen MJ, Stanczak VJ, Ciarleglio CA (1989) Refractory duodenal ulcers (nonhealing duodenal ulcers with standard doses of antisecretory medication). Dig Dis Sci 34:233–237
Collier DStJ, Pain JA (1985) Anti-inflammatory drugs and upper gastrointestinal ulcer perforation. Clin Rheumatol 4:389–391
Craig JD (1948) The evolution of gastric and duodenal ulceration. Br Med J 2:330–334
Danilewitz M, Tim LO, Hirschowitz B (1982) Ranitidine suppression of gastric hypersecretion resistant to cimetidine. N Engl J Med 306:20–22
De Gara CJ, Gledhill T, Hunt RH (1986) Nocturnal gastric acid secretion: its importance in the pathophysiology and rational therapy of duodenal ulcer. Scand J Gastroenterol [Suppl 121] 21:17–24
Dew MJ (1987) Asymptomatic peptic ulcer disease. Br Med J 295:401
Diaz-Rubio M (1988) Obstacles to maintenance therapy in peptic ulcer. Res Clin Forums 10(2):63–70
Dobrilla G, Vallaperta P, Amplatz S (1988) Influence of ulcer healing agents on ulcer relapse after discontinuation of acute treatment: a pooled estimate of controlled clinical trials. Gut 29:181–187
Doll R, Jones FA, Bukatzsch MM (1951) Occupational factors in the etiology of gastric and duodenal ulcers with an estimate of their incidence in the general population. Medical Research Cancelled Special Report Series, no 276, p 96. HRM Stationery Office

Donaldson RM (1975) Factors complicating observed associations between peptic ulcer and other diseases. Gastroenterology 68:1608–1614
Dooley CP, Larson AW, Stace NH et al. (1984) Double-contrast barium meal and upper gastrointestinal endoscopy: a comparative study. Ann Intern Med 101:538–545
Dragstedt LR (1969) Peptic ulcer, an abnormality in gastric secretion. Am J Surg 117:143–156
Dronfield MW, Batchelor AJ, Larkworthy W, Langman MJS (1979) Controlled trial of maintenance cimetidine treatment in healed duodenal ulcer: short and long-term effects. Gut 20:526–530
Dunn JP, Etter LE (1962) Inaccuracy of the medical history in the diagnosis of duodenal ulcer. N Engl J Med 266:68–72
Dyck WP, Cloud ML, Offen WW et al. (1987) Treatment of duodenal ulceration in the United States. Scand J Gastroenterol [Suppl 136] 22:47–55
Editorial (1978) Cimetidine for ever (and ever and ever . . .)? Br Med J I:1435–1436
Einhorn M (1930) Seasonal incidence and study of factors influencing the production of one thousand recurrences in eight hundred patients. Am J Med Sci 179:259–264
Elashoff JD, Grossman MI (1980) Trends in hospital admissions and death rates for peptic ulcer in the United States from 1970 to 1978. Gastroenterology 78:280–285
Elashoff JD, Van Deventer G, Reedy TJ et al. (1983) Long-term follow-up of duodenal ulcer patients. J Clin Gastroenterol 5:509–515
Emery ES Jr, Monroe RT (1979) Peptic ulcer: a study of five hundred and fifty six cases. Arch Intern Med 43:846–873
Emery ES Jr, Monroe RT (1935) Peptic ulcer: nature and treatment based on a study of one thousand, four hundred and thirty five cases. Arch Intern Med 55:271–292
Eusterman GB, Balfour DC (eds) (1935) The stomach and duodenum. Saunders, Philadelphia
Fenwick S, Fenwick WS (1900) Ulcer of the stomach and duodenum. Churchill, London
Fich A, Goldin E, Zimmerman J, Rachmilewitz D (1988) Seasonal variations in the frequency of endoscopically diagnosed duodenal ulcer in Israel. J Clin Gastroenterol 10:380–382
Fineberg HV, Pearlman LA (1981) Surgical treatment of peptic ulcer in the United States: trends before and after the introduction of cimetidine. Lancet I:1305–1307
Fitzpatrick WJF, Blackwood WS, Northfield JC (1982) Bedtime cimetidine maintenance treatment: optimum dose and effect on subsequent natural history of duodenal ulcer. Gut 23:239–242
Flood CA (1948) Recurrence in duodenal ulcer under medical management. Gastroenterology 10:184–185
Flood CA (1955) The results of medical treatment of peptic ulcer. J Chronic Dis 1:43–50
Fontana G, Nizzoli N, Da Broi GL et al. (1986) Pirenzepine for long-term treatment of duodenal ulcer: a controlled multicenter trial. Dig Dis Sci [Suppl 10] 31:208s
Fordtran JS (1978) Placebo, antacids and cimetidine for duodenal ulcer. N Engl J Med 298:1081–1083
Frederiksen JHB, Matzen P, Madsen P et al. (1984) Spontaneous healing of duodenal ulcers. Scand J Gastroenterol 19:417–421
Friedenwald J (1912) A clinical study of a thousand cases of ulcers of the stomach and duodenum. Am J Med Sci 144:157–170
Fry J (1964) Peptic ulcer: a profile. Br Med J II:809–812
Fullman H, Van Deventer G, Schneidman D, Walsh J, Elashoff J, Weinstein W (1985) "Healed" duodenal ulcers are histologically ill. Gastroenterology 88:1390
Galmiche JP, Desechalliers JP, Denis P et al. (1982) Ranitidine treatment of cimetidine resistant peptic ulcers: preliminary clinical and 24-hour intragastric

acidity results. In: Misiewicz JJ, Wormsley KG (eds) Clinical use of ranitidine. 2nd international symposium on ranitidine London, October 1981. Oxford, Medicine Publishing Foundation, pp 243–250

Gardiner GC, Pinsky W, Myerson RM (1966) The seasonal incidence of peptic ulcer activity – fact or fancy? With special reference to gastrointestinal hemorrhage. Am J Gastroenterol 45:22–28

Gibinski K (1983) Step by step towards the natural history of peptic ulcer disease. J Clin Gastroenterol 5:299–302

Gibinski K, Rybicka J, Nowak A, Czarneck A (1982) Seasonal occurrence of abdominal pain and endoscopic findings in patients with gastric and duodenal ulcer disease. Scand J Gastroenterol 17:481–485

Gibinski K, Nowak A, Butruk E et al. (1986) Seasonal prevention of duodenal ulcer recurrence with pirenzepine. Dig Dis Sci [Suppl 10] 31:200s

Gillen P, Ryan W, Peel ALG, Devlin HB (1986) Duodenal ulcer perforation: the effect of H_2 antagonists? Ann R Coll Surg Engl 68:240–242

Gitlin N, McCullough AJ, Smith JL et al. (1987) A multicenter, double-blind, randomized, placebo-controlled comparison of nocturnal and twice-a-day famotidine in the treatment of active duodenal ulcer disease. Gastroenterology 92:48–53

Gough KR, Korman MG, Bardhand KD et al. (1984) Ranitidine and cimetidine in prevention of duodenal ulcer relapse. Lancet II:659–662

Greibe J, Bugge P, Gjorup T, Lauritzen T, Bonnevie O, Wulff HR (1977) Long-term prognosis of duodenal ulcers; follow-up study in survey of doctor's estimates. Br Med J 2:1572–1574

Gustavsson S, Adami H-O, Loof L, Nyberg A, Nyren O (1983) Rapid healing of duodenal ulcers with omeprazole: double-blind dosecomparative trial. Lancet II:124–125

Gustavsson S, Kelly KA, Melton LJ III, Zinsmeister AR (1988) Trends in peptic ulcer surgery. A population-based study in Rochester, Minnesota, 1956–1985. Gastroenterology 94:688–694

Hamilton I, O'Conner JH, Wood NC, Bradbury I, Axon ATR (1986) Healing and recurrence of duodenal ulcer after treatment with tripotassium dicitrato bismuthate (TDB) tablets or cimetidine. Gut 27:106–110

Hasan M, Sircus W (1981) Factors determining success or failure of cimetidine treatment of peptic ulcer. J Clin Gastroenterol 3:225–229

Hollander D, Tarnawski A (1986) Dietary essential fatty acids and the decline in peptic ulcer disease – a hypohesis. Gut 27:239–242

Howden CW, Jones DB, Hunt RH (1985) Nocturnal doses of H_2 receptor antagonists for duodenal ulcer. Lancet I:647–648

Hurst AF, Stewart MJ (1929) Gastric and duodenal ulcer. Oxford University Press, New York, p 544

Ippoliti AF (1985) Prognostic factors in ulcer disease: are they real, are they relevant? J Clin Gastroenterol 7:445–446

Ireland A, Colin-Jones DG, Gear P et al. (1984) Ranitidine 150 mg twice daily vs 300 mg nightly in treatment of duodenal ulcers. Lancet II:274–276

Ivy AC (1946) The problem of peptic ulcer. JAMA 132:1053–1059

Ivy AC, Grossman MI, Bachrach WH (1950) Peptic ulcer. Blakiston, Philadelphia

Jennings D (1940) Perforated peptic ulcer. Changes in age-incidence and sex-distribution in the last 150 years. Lancet I:395–398; 444–447

Jensen DM, Machicado GA, Kovacs TOG et al. (1989) Long-term recurrence rates of peptic ulceration and rebleeding with H_2 maintenance, surgery or no maintenance therapy. Gastroenterology 96:A239

Jonasson TA, Brekkan A, Jonmundsson E, Bjarnason T, Bonnevie O (1983) Epidemiologic study of peptic ulcer in Iceland. Scand J Gastroenterol [Suppl 86] 18:32

Jones DB, Howden CW, Burget DW, Kerr GD, Hunt RH (1987) Acid suppression in duodenal ulcer: a meta-analysis to define optimal dosing with antisecretory drugs. Gut 28:1120–1127

Jordan PH Jr. (1985) Duodenal ulcers and their surgical treatment: where did they come from. Am J Surg 149:2–14

Kang JY, Piper DW (1982) Cimetidine and colloidal bismuth in treatment of chronic duodenal ulcer. Comparison of initial healing and recurrence after healing. Digestion 23:73–79

Kikendall JW, Evaul J, Johnson LF (1984) Effect of cigarette smoking on gastrointestinal physiology and non-neoplastic digestive disease. J Clin Gastroenterol 6:65–79

Klein KB, Spiegel D (1989) Modulation of gastric acid secretion by hypnosis. Gastroenterology 96:1383–1387

Koo J, Ngany K, Lam SK (1983) Trends in hospital admissions, perforation, and mortality of peptic ulcer in Hong Kong from 1970 to 1980. Gastroenterology 84:1558–1562

Korman MG, Hetzel DJ, Hansky J, Shearman DJC, Don G (1980) Relapse rate of duodenal ulcer after cessation of long-term cimetidine treatment. A double-blind controlled study. Dig Dis Sci 25:88–91

Korman MG, Hansky J, Eaves ER, Schmidt GT (1983) Influence of cigarette smoking on healing and relapse in duodenal ulcer disease. Gastroenterology 85:871–874

Krag E (1966) Long-term prognosis in medically treated peptic ulcer. A clinical, radiographical and statistical follow-up study. Acta Med Scand 180:657–670

Krarup NB (1946) On the results of the medical treatment of peptic ulcer. Acta Med Scand 123:181–207

Krause U (1963) Long-term results of medical and surgical treatment of peptic ulcer. A follow-up investigation of patients initially treated conservatively between 1925–34. Acta Chir Scand [Suppl 310] 125:1–111

Kumar N, Vij JC, Sorin SK et al. (1984) DO chillies influence healing of duodenal ulcer? Br Med J 288:1803–1804

Kurata JH (1983) What in the world is happening to ulcers? Gastroenterology 84:1623–1625

Kurata JH (1989) Ulcer epidemiology: an overview and proposed research framework. Gastroenterology [2,2 Suppl] 96:569–580

Kurata JH, Corboy ED (1988) Current peptic ulcer time trends. An epidemological profile. J Clin Gastroenterol 10:259–268

Kurata JH, Haile DM (1984) Epidemiology of peptic ulcer disease. Clin Gastroenterol 13:289–307

Kurata JH, Elashoff JD, Haile BM et al. (1983) A reappraisal of time trends in ulcer disease: factors related to changes in ulcer hospitalization and mortality rates. Am J Public Health 73:1066–1072

Kurata JH, Haile BM, Elashoff JD (1985) Sex differences in peptic ulcer disease. Gastroenterology 88:96–100

Kurata JH, Koch GG, Nogawa AN (1987) Comparison of ranitidine and cimetidine ulcer maintenance therapy. J Clin Gastroenterol 9:644–650

Lam S-K, Lai C-L, Lee LNW et al. (1985) Factors influencing healing of duodenal ulcer. Control of nocturnal secretion by H_2 blockade and characteristics of patients who fail to heal. Dig Dis Sci 30:45–51

Lane MR, Lee SP (1988) Recurrence of duodenal ulcer after medical treatment. Lancet I:1147–1149

Langman MJ (1989) Epidemologic evidence on the association between peptic ulceration and antiinflammatory drug use. Gastroenterology [2, 2 Suppl] 96:640–646

Lee FI, Samloff IM, Hardman M (1985) Comparison of tri-potassium di-citrato bismuthate tablets with ranitidine in healing and relapse of duodenal ulcers. Lancet I:1299–1302

Lee FI, Hardman M, Jaderberg M (1989a) Maintenance treatment of duodenal ulceration: comparison of ranitidine 300 mg and 150 mg at night. Am J Gastroenterol 84:1165

Lee S, Iida M, Yao T, Shindo S, Fujishima M, Okabe H (1989b) Long-term follow-up of 2529 patients with gastric and duodenal ulcer: survival rate and causes of death. Gastroenterology 96:381–386

Levrat M, Pasquier J, Lambert R, Tissot A (1966) Peptic ulcer in patients over 60. Experience in 287 cases. Am J Dig Dis 11:279–285

Levrat M, Descos L, Pasquier J et al. (1968) Evolution a long terme des ulceres gastro-duodenaux. Statistique de 421 malades avec un recurl de plus de 10 ans. Arch Fr Mal App Dig 57:141–152

Lewis JH (1985) Summary of the Gastrointestinal Drugs Advisory Committee Meeting-March 21 and 22, 1985. Am J Gastroenterol 80:581–583

Lewis JH. Summary of the 20th meeting of the Food and Drug Administration Gastrointestinal Drugs Advisory Committee January 16–17, 1986. Am J Gastroenterol 1986; 81:495–498.

Lewis JH (1989a) Long-term management of peptic ulcer disease. Compr Ther 15:55–61

Lewis JH (1989b) Safety profile of long-term H_2-antagonist therapy. Transatlantic Converence on acid/peptic disorders. AV/MD Group, New York, pp 22–25

Lewis JH (1991) Peptic ulcer. In: Rakel RE (ed) Conn's current therapy, 1991 edn. Saunders, Philadelphia, pp 474–481

Lewis JH, Woods M (1982) Gastric carcinoma occurring in patients with unoperated duodenal ulcer disease. Am J Gastroenterol 77:368–373

Lewis JH, Steinberg WS, Katz DM (1982) Variable pH response to cimetidine. Gastroenterology 82:1114

Loof L, Adami H-O, Bates S et al. (1987) Psychological group counseling for the prevention of ulcer relapses. J Clin Gastroenterol 9:400–407

Malmros H, Hiertonn T (1949) A post-investigation of 687 medically treated cases of peptic ulcer. Acta Med Scand 133:229–252

Marshall BJ (1988) *The Campylobacter pylori* story. Scand J Gastroenterol [Suppl 146] 23:58–66

Marshall BJ, Goodwin CS, Warren JR et al. (1988) Prospective double-blind trial of duodenal ulcer relapse after eradication of *Campylobacter pylori*. Lancet II:1437–1442

Martin DF, Hollanders D, May SJ, Ravenscroft MM, Tweedle DEF, Miller JP (1981) Difference in relapse rates of duodenal ulcer after healing with cimetidine or tripotassium dicitrato bismuthate. Lancet 1:7–10

Matthewson K, Pugh S, Northfield TC (1988) Which peptic ulcer patients bleed? Gut 29:70–74

Mayo WJ (1906) Ulcers of the duodenum from a surgical standpoint. Br Med J 2:1299–1302

Mazzacca G, D'Agostino L, D'Arienzo A et al. (1982) Cimetidine or ranitidine non-responder patients. Treatment of duodenal ulcers resistant to one H_2 blocker with the other. Scand J Gastroenterol [Suppl 78] 17:103

McIsaac RL, McCanless I, Summers K, Wood JR (1987) Ranitidine and cimetidine and the healing of duodenal ulcer: meta-analysis of comparative clinical trials. Aliment Pharmacol Ther 1:369–381

Meade TW, Arie THD, Brewis M et al. (1968) Recent history of ischemic heart disease and duodenal ulcer in deaths. Br Med J 3:701–704

Mellem H, Stave R, Myren J et al. (1985) Symptoms in patients with peptic ulcer and hematemesis and/or melena related to the use of non-steroid anti-inflammatory drugs. Scand J Gastroenterol 20:1246–1248

Mendeloff AI (1974) What has been happening to duodenal ulcer? Gastroenterology 67:1020–1022

Michener WM, Kennedy RLJ, DuShane JW (1960) Duodenal ulcer in childhood: ninety-two cases with follow-up. Am J Dis Child 100:814–817
Miller JP (1990) Maintenance of duodenal ulcer healing by antacids. Scand J Gastroenterol 25 (Suppl 174):54–59
Monson RR, MacMahon B (1969) Peptic ulcer in Massachusetts physicians. N Engl J Med 281:11–15
Moshal MG, Spitaels JM, Robbs JV, MacLeod IN, Good CJ (1981) Eight-year experience with 3392 endoscopically proven duodenal ulcers in Durban, 1972–79. Rise and fall of duodenal ulcers and a theory of changing dietary and social factors. Gut 22:327–331
Moshal MG, Spitaels JM, Khan F (1981) Short- and long-term studies of duodenal ulcer with sucralfate. J Clin Gastroenterol [Suppl 2] 3:159–161
Moynihan BGA (1910) Duodenal ulcer. Saunders, Philadelphia
Naesdal J, Lind T, Bergsaker-Aspoy J et al. (1985) The rate of healing of duodenal ulcers during omeprazole treatment. Scand J Gastroenterol 20:691–695
Nasiry RW, McIntosh JH, Byth K, Piper DU (1987) Prognosis of chronic duodenal ulcer: a prospective study of the effects of demographic and environmental factors and ulcer healing. Gut 28:533–540
Natvig P, Romcke O, Svaar-Seljesaeter O (1943) Results of medical treatment of gastric and duodenal ulcer. Acta Med Scand 113:444–458
O'Hara H (1875) Perforating or corrosive ulcer of the duodenum. Trans Pathol Soc Phil 6:37
Ostensen H, Burhol PG, Stormer J, Bonnevie O (1985a) The incidence of peptic ulcer disease related to occupation in the northern part of Norway. A prospective epidemiological and radiological study. Scand J Gastroenterol 20:79–82
Ostensen H, Gudmundsen TE, Bolz KD, Burhol PG, Bonnevie O (1985b) The incidence of gastric ulcer and duodenal ulcer in north Norway. A prospective epidemiological study. Scand J Gastroenterol 20:189–192
Ostensen H, Gudmundsen TE, Burhol PG, Bonnevie O (1985c) Seasonal periodicity of peptic ulcer disease. A prospective radiologic study. Scand J Gastroenterol 20:1281–1284
Palmas F, Andriulli A, Canepa G et al. (1984) Monthly fluctuations of active duodenal ulcers. Dig Dis Sci 29:983–987
Palmas F, Andriulli A, Verme G (1984) Seasonal treatment with ranitidine. Lancet II:698–699
Palmer WL (1974) The therapy of peptic ulcer. II. Radiation therapy. Gastroenterology 1 (30):710–719
Paoluzi P, Ricotta G, Ripoli F et al. (1985) Incompletely and completely healed duodenal ulcers' outcome in maintenance treatment: a double blind controlled study. Gut 26:1080
Penston JG (1990) The efficacy and safety of long-term maintenance treatment of duodenal ulcers with ranitidine. Scand J Gastroenterol 25 (Suppl) 177:1–104
Penston JG, Wormsley KG (1988) Long-term treatment of duodenal ulcers. Gastroenterology 94:A349
Permutt RP, Cello JP (1982) Duodenal ulcer disease in the hospitalized elderly patient. Dig Dis Sci 27:1–6
Perry EA, Shaw LE (1893) On disease of the duodenum. Guys Hosp Rep 50:171–176
Peters MN, Richardson CT (1983) Stressful life events, acid hypersecretion, and ulcer disease. Gastroenterology 84:114–119
Postlethwait RW (1979) Retrospective study of operations for peptic ulcer. Surg Gynecol Obstet 149:703–708
Pounder RE (1981) Model of medical treatment for duodenal ulcer. Lancet I:29–30
Pulvertaft CN (1968) Comments on the incidence and natural history of gastric duodenal ulcer. Postgrad Med J 44:597–602

Quatrini M, Basilisco G, Bianchi PA (1984) Treatment of "cimetidine-resistant" chronic duodenal ulcers with ranitidine or cimetidine: a randomized multicentre study. Gut 25:1113–1117

Quigstad I, Romcke O (1946) Post-investigation of medically treated gastric and duodenal ulcers. II. Acta Med Scand 126:34–39

Reynolds JC (1989) Famotidine therapy for active duodenal ulcers. A multivariate analysis factors affecting early healing. Ann Intern Med 111:7–14

Ries RK, Gilbert DA, Katon W (1984) Tricyclic antidepressant therapy for peptic ulcer disease. Arch Intern Med 144:566–569

Romcke O, Loken E (1956) Prognosis of peptic ulcer in young patients. Acta Med Scand 155:373–375

Rydning A, Berstad A (1985) Dietary aspects of peptic ulcer disease. Scand J Gastroenterol [Suppl 110] 20:29–33

Safrany L, Schott B, Portocarrero G, Krause S, Neuhaus B (1982) Spring and autumn disposition to gastroduodenal ulcer. Dtsch Med Wochenschr 107:685–687

Sargent J (1954) Fatal peritonitis from perforation of the duodenum. Am J Med Sci 28:116–117

Sasaki H, Nagulesparan M, Samloff IM, Straus E, Sievers ML, Dubois A (1984) Low acid output in Pima Indians. A possible cause for the rarity of duodenal ulcer in this population. Dig Dis Sci 29:785–789

Scapa E, Horowitz M, Waron M, Eshchar J (1989) Duodenal ulcer in the elderly. J Clin Gastroenterol 11:502–506

Schmidt K, Mosbech J, Banke L (1984) Morbidity of peptic ulcer. Registration of hospital discharges in Denmark 1978–1980. Scand J Gastroenterol 19:849–852

Segawa K, Nakazawa S, Tsukamoto Y et al. (1987) Peptic ulcer is prevalent among shift workers. Dig Dis Sci 32:449–453

Shreeve DR, Klass HJ, Jones PE (1983) Comparison of cimetidine and tripotassium discitrato bismuthate in healing and relapse of duodenal ulcers. Digestion 28:96–101

Silvis SE et al. (1985) Final report on the United States multicenter trial comparing rantidine to cimetidine as maintenance therapy following healing of duodenal ulcer. J Clin Gastroenterol 7:482–487

Slater PE (1989) High winter incidence of duodenal ulcer in Israel. J Clin Gastroenterol 11:587–588

Smith LA, Rivers AB (1953) Peptic ulcer; pain patterns, diagnosis and medical treatment. Appleton-Century Crofts, New York

Smith MP (1977) Decline in duodenal ulcer surgery. JAMA 237:987–988

Solhaug JH, Carling L, Glise H et al. (1987) Ulcer recurrences following initial ulcer healing with sucralfate or cimetidine. Scand J Gastroenterol [Suppl 127] 22:77–80

Somerville K, Faulkner G, Langman M (1986) Non-steroidal anti-inflammatory drugs and bleeding peptic ulcer. Lancet I:462–464

Sonnenberg A (1984) The occurrence of a cohort phenomenon in peptic ulcer mortality from Switzerland. Gastroenterology 86:398–401

Sonnenberg A (1985) Geographic and temporal variations in the occurrence of peptic ulcer disease. Scand J Gastroenterol [Suppl 110] 20:11–24

Sonnenberg A (1985) Decision analysis of different strategies for long-term treatment of duodenal ulcer. Gastroenterology 88:1593

Sonnenberg A (1989) Costs of medical and surgical treatment of duodenal ulcer. Gastroenterology 96:1445–1452

Sonnenberg A (1987) Changes in physician visits for gastric and duodenal ulcer in the United States during 1958–1984 as shown by National Disease and Therapeutic Index (NDTI). Dig Dis Sci 32:1–7

Sonnenberg A, Fritsch A (1983) Changing mortality of peptic ulcer disease in Germany. Gastroenterology 84:1553–1557

Sonnenberg A, Muller-Lissner SA, Vogel E et al. (1981) Predictors of duodenal ulcer healing and relapse. Gastroenterology 81:1061–1067

Sonnenberg A, Muller H, Pace F (1985) Birth-cohort analysis of peptic ulcer mortality in Europe. J Chronic Dis 38:309–317
Sontag SJ (and the ACG Committee on FDA-Related Matters) (1988) Current status of maintenance therapy in peptic ulcer disease. Am J Gastroenterol 93:607–617
Sontag S, Graham DY, Belsito A et al. (1984) Cimetidine, cigarette smoking, and recurrence of duodenal ulcer. N Engl J Med 311:689–693
Spiro HM (1977) Clinical gastroenterology, 2nd edn. Macmillan, New York, p 270
Steinberg WM, Lewis JH, Katz DM (1984) Transient cimetidine resistance. J Clin Gastroenterol 6:355–359
Stern WR (1989) Summary of the 34th meeting of the Food and Drug Administration Gastrointestinal Drugs Advisory Committee March 15 and 16, 1989 (omeprazole and domperidone). Am J Gastroenterol 84:1351–1355
Strom M, Berstad A, Bodemar G, Walan A (1986) Results of short- and long-term cimetidine treatment in patients with juxtapyloric ulcers, with special reference to gastric acid and pepsin secretion. Scand J Gastroenterol 21:521–530
Strum WB (1986) Prevention of duodenal ulcer recurrence. Ann Intern Med 105:757–761
Sturdevant RAL (1976) Epidemiology of peptic ulcer. Am J Epidemiol 104:9–14
Susser M (1961) Environmental factors and peptic ulcer. Practitioner 186:302–311
Susser M (1967) Causes of peptic ulcer. A selective epidemiologic review. J Chronic Dis 20:435–456
Susser M (1982) Period effects, generation effects and age effects in peptic ulcer mortality. J Chronic Dis 35:29–40
Susser M, Stein A (1962) Civilisation and peptic ulcer. Lancet I:115–119
Takemoto T, Okita K, Kimura K (1986) Efficacy of sucralfate, cimetidine and their combination in the prevention of peptic ulcer recurrence. A double-blind multicenter study. The 4th international sucralfate symposium, Sao Paulo, Brazil, September 8, 1986. Abstract no 9
Thomas JM, Misiewicz G (1984) Histamine H_2-receptor antagonist in the short- and long-term treatment of duodenal ulcer. Clinics Gastroenterol 13:501–541
Thomas E, Reddy KR (1983) Nonhealing duodenal ulceration due to *Candida*. J Clin Gastroenterol 5:55–58
Tidy H (1945) The incidence of peptic ulcer at St. Thomas Hospital 1910–1937. Br Med J II:319
Tilvis RS, Vuoristo M, Varis K (1987) Changed profile of peptic ulcer disease in hospital patients during 1969–1984 in Finland. Scand J Gastroenterol 22:1238–1244
Tytgat GNJ, Hameeteman W, Van Olffer GH (1984) Sucralfate, bismuth compounds, substituted benzimidazoles, trimipramine and pirenzepine in the short- and long-term treatment of duodenal ulcer. Clin Gastroenterol 13:543–568
Valnes K, Myren J, Witterhus S et al. (1982) Long-term treatment of duodenal ulcer with trimipramine. Scand J Gastroenterol 17:1003–1007
Van Deventer GM (1984) Approaches to the long-term treatment of duodenal ulcer disease. Am J Med [Suppl 5b] 77:15–22
Van Deventer GM, Elashoff JD, Reedy TJ, Schneidman D, Walsh JH (1989) A randomized study of maintenance therapy with ranitidine to prevent the recurrence of duodenal ulcer. N Engl J Med 320:1113–1119
Vogt TM, Johnson RE (1980) Recent changes in the incidence of duodenal and gastric ulcer. Am J Epidemiol 111:713–720
Walan A (1984) Antacids and anticholinergics in the treatment of duodenal ulcer. Clin Gastroenterol 13:473–449
Walan A, Strom M (1985) Prevention of ulcer recurrence – medical vs. surgical treatment. The physician's view. Scand J Gastroenterol [Suppl 110] 20:83–88

Walan A, Bardhan KD, Bianchi Porro G et al. (1985) A comparison of two different doses of omeprazole versus ranitidine in duodenal ulcer (DU) healing. Gastroenterology 88:1625
Walan A, Bianchi-Porro G, Hentschel E, Bardhan KD, Delattre M (1987) Maintenance treatment with cimetidine in peptic ulcer disease for up to 4 years. Scand J Gastroenterol 22:397–405
Walt R, Katschinski B, Logan R, Ashley J, Langman M (1986) Rising frequency of ulcer perforation in elderly people in the United Kingdom. Lancet I:489–491
Welsh JD, Wolf S (1960) Geographical and environmental aspect of peptic ulcer. Am J Med 29:754–760
Wilbur DL (1935) The history of diseases of the stomach and duodenum with reference also to their etiology. In: Eusterman GB, Balfour DC (eds) The stomach and duodenum. Saunders, Philadelphia, pp 1–21
William Beaumont Society (1966) U.S. Army Report. Seasonal incidence of upper gastrointestinal tract bleeding; report of the standing committee on upper gastrointestinal bleeding. JAMA 198:184–185
Witzel L, Wolbergs E (1982) Peptic ulcer healing with ranitidine in cimetidine resistance. Lancet II:1224
Wolf S (1981) The psyche and the stomach. A historical vignette. Gastroenterology 80:605–614
Wormsley KG (1982) Problems in the treatment of peptic ulcer. Scand J Gastroenterol [Suppl 80] 17:43–48
Wormsley KG (1984) Assessing the safety of drugs for the long-term treatment of peptic ulcers. Gut 25:1416–1423
Wormsley KG (1988) Long-term treatment of duodenal ulcer. Postgrad Med J [Suppl 1] 64:47–53
Wylie CM (1981) The complex wane of peptic ulcer. I. Recent national trends in deaths and hospital care in the United States. J Clin Gastroenterol 3:327–332
Wyllie JH, Clark CG, Alexander-Williams J et al. (1981) Effect of cimetidine on surgery for duodenal ulcer. Lancet I:1307–1308

CHAPTER 11

Refractory Duodenal Ulcer

J.W. RADEMAKER and R.H. HUNT

A. Introduction

The term "refractory duodenal ulcer" has been used since the introduction of the H_2 receptor antagonist cimetidine and represents the more severe end of a disease spectrum for which the underlying pathophysiological mechanisms remain complex and poorly understood.

Studies of this difficult and now relatively rare group of ulcer patients are complicated by the arbitrary and inconsistent definitions given in both the reviews (BARDHAN 1982, 1989; PIPER 1987; POUNDER 1987; WALT and DANESHMEND 1988; DOMSCHKE et al. 1989) (Table 1) and the medical (BARDHAN 1984; QUATRINI et al. 1984; AMOURETTI et al. 1985; DAL MONTE et al. 1985; BARDHAN et al. 1987; 1988; LAM et al. 1984; BIANCHI-PORRO et al. 1987; GUSLANDI et al. 1983; NEWMAN et al. 1987; TYTGAT et al. 1987; BRUNNER et al. 1988; DELCHIER et al. 1989) (Table 2) and surgical (HANSEN and KNIGGE 1984; PICKARD and MACKAY 1984; WEAVER and TEMPLE 1985; PRIMROSE et al. 1988; ANDERSEN et al. 1990) (Table 3) literature.

I. Definition

For the purposes of this chapter a refractory duodenal ulcer is defined as a duodenal ulcer which either fails to heal following 3 months of full-dose treatment with an H_2 receptor antagonist or recurs within 1 year of healing despite maintenance treatment.

A review of treatment trials confirms that current medical treatment heals approximately 90%–95% of duodenal ulcers following an 8-week course of an H_2 receptor antagonist (HUNT et al. 1986; JONES et al. 1987). After initial healing and continued maintenance therapy with any of the available H_2 receptor antagonists, approximately 25%–35% of duodenal ulcers recur annually (THOMAS and MISENWICZ 1984; FRESTON 1987a). This figure varies considerably and often underestimates the true rate because asymptomatic recurrence commonly occurs and detection is dependent on the time interval between endoscopies. Asymptomatic ulcers are more often detected in studies where regular and more frequent endoscopies have been undertaken (BOYD et al. 1988).

Table 1. Definition of refractory duodenal ulcer from reviews

BARDHAN (1982): Incomplete healing of ulcer following treatment with cimetidine 1 g per day for 3 months or symptomatic recurrence despite full maintenance dose.
PIPER (1987): Ulcer that fails to heal despite 3 months of active treatment or recurs within 1 year despite maintenance therapy with H_2 receptor antagonist or frequent/persistent symptomatic relapse.
POUNDER (1987): Failure of ulcer healing after 8 weeks full-dose treatment with modern antiulcer drug.
WALT and DANESHMEND (1988): Failure of ulcer healing after 2 months of full-dose treatment with H_2 receptor antagonist.
DOMSCHKE et al. (1989): Incomplete healing after 2–3 months of H_2 receptor antagonist treatment or recurrence despite low dose maintenance therapy with H_2 receptor antagonist.
BARDHAN (1989): A symptomatic endoscopically proven ulcer that does not heal after at least 2 months of treatment with 1 g or more of cimetidine per day.

The important questions for the patient and gastroenterologist are:

1. Why has the ulcer failed to heal?
2. Why has the ulcer relapsed despite maintenance treatment with an H_2 receptor antagonist?
3. What further management options are available?

These issues and the possible underlying pathophysiological mechanisms which may be involved will be discussed.

II. Adequate Treatment and Compliance

Adequate antisecretory treatment requires that both the correct dose and the correct regimen of an H_2 receptor antagonist be prescribed. Initial therapeutic regimens aimed to suppress gastric acid to as great a degree and for as much of the 24-h period as possible. This seems logical since the majority of patients with duodenal ulcer show acid hypersecretion throughout the 24-h period (FELDMAN and RICHARDSON 1986). Also the recent meta-analysis to explore the relationship of acid suppression to ulcer healing by antisecretory drugs has demonstrated that a clear correlation exists between nocturnal acid suppression with the H_2 receptor antagonists and duodenal ulcer healing (JONES et al. 1987). This study confirms that targeting treatment to the nighttime period optimizes the pharmacological action of H_2 receptor antagonists, which suppress basal acid secretion more effectively than daytime food-stimulated acid secretion. The nocturnal period is a prolonged period of basal acid secretion during which hyperacidity is not buffered by food.

Compliance has often been raised as a major concern in the management of chronic peptic ulcer disease, especially in patients who are refractory, and has recently been reviewed (BADER and STANESCU 1989). Although the differences in definition and measurement in clinical trials did not permit

Table 2. Medical treatment trials for refractory duodenal ulcer

Reference	No. of patients	Definition of refractory	Treatment	Duration	Number healed (%)
BARDHAN (1984)	66	Cimetidine 1 g (3 months)	Cimetidine 1 g Cimetidine 2 g Cimetidine 3 g	>6 months >6 months >6 months	8/57 (14) 25/41 (61) 4/8 (50)
QUATRINI et al. (1984)	40	Cimetidine 1 g (6 weeks)	Cimetidine 1 g Ranitidine 0.3 g	6 weeks 6 weeks	12/19 (63) 13/21 (62), NS
AMOURETTI et al. (1985)	285	Cimetidine 1 g	Cimetidine 1 g Ranitidine 0.3 g	6 weeks 6 weeks	(60) (71)*
DAL MONTE et al. (1985)	11	Cimetidine 1 g (>2 months)	Cimetidine 0.8 g Pirenzipine 0.1 g or combined	1–6 months 1–6 months 1–6 months	0/25 (0)– 8/23 (35) 0/25 (0)– 9/22 (41), NS 20/25 (83)–17/20 (84)*
BARDHAN et al. (1987)	131	Cimetidine or ranitidine (8 weeks)	Cimetidine 0.8 g Cimetidine 1 g Pirenzipine 0.15 g	6 weeks	39/59 (66) 39/65 (57), NS
LAM et al. (1984)	25	Cimetidine 1 g (4 weeks)	Cimetidine 1.6 g Bismuth subcitrate	8 weeks 8 weeks	15/25 (40) 17/25 (85)**
BIANCHI-PORRO et al. (1987)	52	Various H_2RAs (8 weeks)	Cimetidine 1.2 g Cimetidine 2.0 g Bismuth subcitrate	4–8 weeks 4–8 weeks 4–8 weeks	7 (39) –11 (65) 7 (44) –12 (75) 14 (82)*–16 (94)*
GUSLANDI (1987)	20	Cimetidine 1 g Ranitidine 0.3 g (8 weeks)	Sucralfate 3 g	6 weeks	26 (81)
NEWMAN et al. (1987)	225	Cimetidine or ranitidine (4 weeks)	Misoprostol 0.8 g or placebo	4–8 weeks 4–8 weeks	37/101 (37)* 20/92 (22)
TYTGAT et al. (1987)	11	Various H_2RAs and other treatments	Omeprazole 0.4 g	2–4 weeks	9/11 (82)–11/11 (100)

Table 2 (continued)

Reference	No. of patients	Definition of refractory	Treatment	Duration	Number healed (%)
Brunner et al. (1988)	11	Ranitidine 0.45–0.6 g (3 months)	Omeprazole 0.4 g	2–4 weeks	4/11 (37)–11/11 (100)
Bardhan et al. (1988)	107	Cimetidine 1 g Ranitidine 0.3 g (8 weeks)	Omeprazole 0.4 g continue H_2RA	4–8 weeks 4–8 weeks	45/52 (87)–50/52 (98)* 18/47 (39)–28/47 (60)
Delchier et al. (1989)	151	Cimetidine 0.8 g Ranitidine 0.3 g	Omeprazole 0.2 g or Ranitidine 0.3 g	2–4 weeks 2–4 weeks	33/68 (47)–53/66 (71), NS 33/41 (43)–52/73 (68)

NS, not significant; * $P < 0.05$; ** $P < 0.01$.
H_2RA, H_2 receptor antagonist.

Table 3. Surgical treatment trials for refractory duodenal ulcer

Reference	No. of patients	Definition or refractory	Surgical treatment	Recurrence (%)
Hansen and Knigge (1984)	45	Cimetidine 1 g 1–2 months	Proximal gastric vagotomy	44% 2–5 yr
Pickard and Mackay (1984)	52	Cimetidine 2 months	Truncal vagotomy	5% 2 yr
Weaver and Temple (1985)	57	Cimetidine 1 g or maintenance 0.4 g	Proximal gastric vagotomy	5% 1–2 yr
Primrose et al. (1988)	57	Various H_2 receptor antagonists	Proximal gastric vagotomy	18% 2 yr and 34% 5 yr
Andersen et al. (1990)	86	Cimetidine	Vagotomy	16% 5 yr

direct comparison for psychological and treatment factors to be made between studies, the compliance rates between randomized groups within studies were similar and apparently did not introduce bias into the analysis. However, in the real world situation outside of clinical studies compliance must always be considered for patients who fit the criteria of nonresponse, especially when they are taking maintenance therapy.

III. Hypersecretory Disorders and Nonpeptic Ulcer Disease

Acid hypersecretion is associated with rare conditions such as Zollinger-Ellison syndrome (Mignon and Bonfils 1988), antral G cell hyperplasia or G cell hyperfunction (Lewin et al. 1984), retained gastric antrum, and systemic mastocytosis (Cherner et al. 1988), all of which must be excluded in the refractory patient. Fasting serum gastrin levels, basal and peak acid output to pentagastrin stimulation, and 24-h intragastric pH measurements should be considered, and if abnormal lead to further confirmatory investigations.

The widespread availability of endoscopy readily allows for accurate diagnosis and follow-up to confirm healing, and multiple biopsies may be taken from any suspicious or atypical lesions. This enables the rare nonpeptic causes for duodenal ulcer to be excluded, such as Crohn's disease, tuberculosis, lymphoma, carcinoma, or cytomegalovirus infections in the immunocompromised patient. However, in the majority of patients no cause is found and these represent one extreme of the spectrum of duodenal ulcer disease with either impaired healing or a persistent imbalance between luminal aggressive and mucosal defensive factors, thus inhibiting healing or promoting recurrent injury. Possible pathophysiological mechanisms which may be involved include: increased acid secretion, impaired mucosal defense, and environmental factors such as smoking, nonsteroidal anti-inflammatory drugs (NSAIDs), or *Helicobacter pylori* infection either alone or in combination and occurring in a genetically susceptible individual.

B. Factors Which Affect Healing and Recurrence

Analysis of ulcer treatment trials to determine the factors related to impaired healing are complicated by the geographical variation observed in spontaneous healing rates (Sonnenberg 1985) and the change in the incidence of duodenal ulcer disease which has occurred since the mid-1960s and appears independent of the introduction of effective medical therapies (Kurata 1989).

Factors which are considered to influence healing have received much attention (Bardhan 1982; Lam and Koo 1983; Sonnenberg et al. 1981) and, although there is not necessarily consistency between studies, include the following which are considered to be of definite importance: long duration of history, large ulcer size, increased acid secretion, and somking. In addition, factors possibly involved are: elderly age, male sex, and NSAID ingestion.

The factors which affect recurrence have also been reviewed (FRESTON 1987b; ORLANDO 1987) and include genetic susceptibility, acid hypersecretion, impaired mucosal defense, environmental factors including smoking, NSAIDs, and *H. pylori.*

Furthermore the effect of initial therapy may be important since several meta-analyses of the effect of initial therapy on recurrence have been performed (McLEAN et al. 1985; MILLER and FARAGHER 1986; DOBRILLA et al. 1988; CHIVERTON and HUNT 1989), all of which show a significantly increased relapse following H_2 receptor antagonist therapy when compared to all other drugs. In one study (DOBRILLA et al. 1988) this difference was due solely to the beneficial effect of bismuth subcitrate. The bactericidal effect of bismuth against *H. pylori* has been acclaimed as one reason for its impact, although bismuth probably has additional, as yet undefined effects.

Refractory duodenal ulcer treatment trials to date have explored many of these factors to determine any possible association which might help to identify the patient who would develop a refractory ulcer. The findings show no consistent trend apart from smoking and the use of NSAIDs; therefore appropriate early advice should be given to all patients.

I. Acid Hypersecretion

The consideration of acid hypersecretion in refractory duodenal ulcer disease has two main components: namely the differences in acid secretory capacity, which includes the basal and stimulated response when acidity and acid output are measured, and the evidence for differences in response to conventional therapy.

The evidence that patients with refractory duodenal ulcer have increased acid secretory capacity is conflicting, with studies reporting both increased (GLEDHILL et al. 1984; COLLEN et al. 1989) and unchanged (BARDHAN 1984; QUATRINI et al. 1984; LAM et al. 1984; BIANCHI-PORRO et al. 1987) basal and stimulated acid secretion. The differences in results have been attributed to male sex, variability of measurements, and the overlap seen between healthy volunteers and duodenal ulcer patients (LAM 1985). No obvious relationship to previous treatment with an H_2 receptor antagonist was shown by COLLEN et al. (1989), who found that patients with nonhealing duodenal ulcer have a basal acid output greater than 10 mEq/h. However, considerable overlap occurred between the healing and the nonhealing groups, with the latter group containing extreme results which might have affected the statistical analysis. Basal acid output of greater than 10 mEq/h probably should not be used as an absolute marker for nonhealing. Furthermore the patients appeared to have been studied soon after stopping long-term H_2 receptor antagonist therapy, and therefore may have been studied during a period of rebound hypersecretion (FULLARTON et al. 1989); NWOKOLO et al. 1989a (vide infra).

The term "cimetidine nonresponders" originally employed by HUNT (1981) applied to patients who failed to suppress basal nocturnal acid secretion with standard doses of cimetidine. This abnormality was corrected by either performing a proximal gastric vagotomy (GLEDHILL et al. 1983) or the addition of the anticholinergic atropine to cimetidine (GLEDHILL et al. 1984). The cimetidine blood levels measured in these patients were not different from those in historical controls, suggesting that a pharmacodynamic rather than pharmacokinetic abnormality was responsible, although in subsequent studies this pharmacodynamic failure of response did not appear to correlate with healing. Possible mechanisms which might account for these observed differences in response include altered parietal cell sensitivity, altered receptor regulation, tolerance or tachyphylaxis, and hypergastrinemia.

1. Parietal Cell Sensitivity

An increased parietal cell sensitivity when measured by dose–response stimulation of acid secretion to pentagastrin was originally reported by ISENBERG et al. (1975) in duodenal ulcer patients compared to matched controls. The authors proposed several possible mechanisms, including increased vagal tone, decreased inhibition of gastrin release, and decreased metabolism of pentagastrin. These observations of an increased parietal sensitivity have been confirmed by some workers (HALTER et al. 1982; LAM and JARLEY 1985) but disputed by others (ALY and EMAS 1982; FELDMAN et al. 1983; HIRSCHOWITZ 1984); the latter attributed the differences to male gender, body weight, and the analytic methods used to transform the dose–response data. The effect of duodenal ulcer disease activity on pentagastrin-stimulated acid secretion, which ACHORD (1981) demonstrated to increase during active ulceration and subsequently decrease with healing, was not considered and may have confounded these results. Moreover, a recent study (YANAKA and MUTO 1988) examining factors related to early ulcer relapse suggests that parietal cell sensitivity may be increased by smoking, which was not standardized for in many of these studies.

Increased parietal cell sensitivity following treatment with an H_2 receptor antagonist has also been reported in controlled studies with pentagastrin (AADLAND et al. 1977), pentagastrin and histamine (AADLAND and BERSTAD 1979; MARKS et al. 1989), and the specific H_2 receptor agonist impromidine (JONES et al. 1988). Studies with both cimetidine (SEWING et al. 1978) and ranitidine (PRICHARD et al. 1986) showed a decreased effectiveness of intravenous H_2 receptor antagonist in reducing pentagastrin-stimulated acid secretion in patients on long-term therapy. These studies can be criticized for several aspects of their design and analysis because: (a) H_2 receptor antagonist inhibition of pentagastrin-stimulated acid secretion is noncompetitive (Aadland et al. 1977; Konturek et al. 1981); (b) there was failure to correct for basal acid secretion (Aadland and Berstad 1979; Jones et al. 1988); (c) a possible carry-over effect of the H_2 receptor antagonist may have occurred (Prichard et al. 1986); and (d) most of the studies failed to confirm healing endoscopically (Sewing et al. 1978; Aadland and Berstad 1979; Jones et al. 1988).

In conclusion, the increased parietal cell sensitivity seen following duodenal ulcer healing with an H_2 receptor antagonist may be a concomitant effect of the increased sensitivity seen with H_2 receptor antagonist therapy (Aadland et al. 1977; Aadland and Berstad 1979; Marks et al. 1989; Jones et al. 1988) and the decreased sensitivity occurring with healing (Isenberg et al. 1975; Achord 1981; Halter et al. 1982; Aly and Emas 1982), which would predispose to failed healing or early ulcer recurrence. The mechanisms which have been proposed include receptor up-regulation, originally observed in healthy individuals with cimetidine (Sewing et al. 1978) and subsequently in duodenal ulcer patients in remission with ranitidine (Aadland and Berstad 1979), and altered parietal cell sensitivity following treatment with an H_2 receptor antagonist, which was less marked following treatment with the site-protective agent sucralfate than with ranitidine (Marks et al. 1989).

2. Tolerance

Tolerance or tachyphylaxis to an H_2 receptor antagonist reflects a decrease in the antisecretory response seen with repeated doses of the drug. This phenomenon has been reported in children (Hyman et al. 1985) and in adults (Smith et al. 1989; Nwokolo et al. 1989b); Wilder-Smith et al. 1989).

The study reporting tolerance to intravenous ranitidine in children requiring nutritional supplementation following bowel surgery (Hyman et al. 1985) can be criticized for the small numbers and the effect of short bowel syndrome.

The adult studies were carried out in volunteers with various oral H_2 receptor antagonists. The results showed that following both short- and long-term treatment an increase in the intragastric acidity occurs and correlates with an increase in gastrin. Furthermore, a short-term study with pharmacological doses of pentagastrin demonstrated a similar loss of effect of H_2 receptor antagonist therapy, suggesting that hypergastrinemia might be one factor responsible for this phenomenon (Nwokolo et al. 1989c). All of these studies have only been reported in abstract and have inconsistencies which cannot be resolved without fuller details. The studies involved small numbers and for the different ranitidine dosage regimens the increase in acidity observed with time was not paralleled by equivalent changes in gastrin levels (Nwokolo et al. 1989b; Smith et al. 1989). Also H_2 receptor blockade is known to be overcome by pharmacological doses of pentagastrin as well as peptone- or food-stimulated gastrin release.

It is clear from these studies that tolerance occurs rapidly, within 1–2 weeks, but the mechanisms involved are not well understood. Further in vitro studies will be required to examine the response to histamine and gastrin in order to determine receptor numbers and sensitivity before we are able to clarify the gastrin link.

3. Rebound Hypersecretion

Rebound hypersecretion following cessation of H_2 receptor antagonist therapy was not seen in the original basal or pentagastrin-stimulated acid secretory studies. More recent studies have shown evidence for rebound hypersecretion on cessation of therapy when nocturnal acid output was measured in duodenal ulcer patients (Fullarton et al. 1989) and 24-h intragastric acidity was measured in healthy volunteers (Nwokolo et al. 1989a). The lack of change in the basal and pentagastrin-stimulated response in the original studies is probably explained by their study designs, which did not take into account (a) the possible carry-over effect of treatment with cimetidine or ranitidine, (b) their noncompetitive kinetics with pentagastrin-stimulated acid secretion (Aadland et al. 1977; Konturek et al. 1981), or (c) any possible effect of healing on acid secretion (Achord 1981).

The duodenal ulcer patient study (Fullerton et al. 1989) using nizatidine 300 mg h.s. showed a marked increase of 77% in nocturnal acid output following cessation of therapy but no difference in daytime acidity. This study has been criticized for the small number of patients studied and the statistical methods used.

In healthy normal volunteers significant increases in nocturnal (21%) and 24-h acidity (9%) were seen only when the cimetidine 800 mg h.s., nizatidine 300 mg h.s., and famotidine 40 mg h.s.groups were combined (Nwokolo et al. 1989a).

4. Gastrin

Studies which only measured fasting plasma gastrin levels have been conflicting, with both increased (Sewing et al. 1978; Richardson 1978) and unchanged (Bank et al. 1977; Vantini et al. 1978) levels reported. When 24-h gastrin profiles are measured, all drugs which suppress gastric acid secretion show an inverse relationship between acid suppression and gastrin levels (Lanzon-Miller et al. 1987a). The increase in gastrin levels which occurs is temporary even with omeprazole (Sharma et al. 1987). The possible trophic effect of gastrin on the parietal cell mass has not yet been demonstrated following antisecretory therapy but is unlikely to be of the same clinical significance as in the Zollinger-Ellison syndrome. The slight increase in plasma gastrin levels which are seen with the H_2 receptor antagonists has been suggested as one possible cause for tachyphylaxis (vide supra) (Nwokolo et al. 1989b).

Meal-stimulated gastrin response also increases following treatment with H_2 receptor antagonists (RICHARDSON 1978) as a result of the decreased intragastric acidity altering the autoregulation of gastrin release (FRISLID et al. 1986). This could also lead to an increase in meal-related acid secretion following H_2 receptor antagonist therapy (BLAIR et al. 1987) but the duration of effect and the relationship to healing or recurrence have not been determined.

5. Clinical Significance

Despite a better understanding of the pharmacological mechanisms of altered parietal cell sensitivity, tolerance, receptor up-regulation, and hypergastrinemia, which may act alone or in combination to alter acid secretion, their clinical significance in relationship to refractory ulcer healing or early relapse with H_2 receptor antagonists remains unclear. The duration of these observed effects on acid output rather than acidity needs further investigation. Current medical therapy is able to effectively suppress acid but the degree and duration of acid suppression needed to initially heal a duodenal ulcer and prevent recurrence are not known (HUNT 1988).

II. Smoking

Smoking has been shown consistently to correlate with delayed healing and recurrence of duodenal ulcer (KORMAN et al. 1983; SONTAG et al. 1984), with a threshold of ten or more cigarettes per day (KORMAN et al. 1983; MACCARTHY 1984). A recent meta-analysis of smoking in duodenal ulcer treatment trials (CHIVERTON et al. 1988) has confirmed that smoking impairs healing in patients while on placebo and all classes of drugs by about 10%. When the therapeutic gain above placebo was calculated, there was no difference in healing between smokers (33%) and nonsmokers (32%). Thus ulcer-healing drugs are equally effective in smokers and nonsmokers and no individual drug class showed superior healing or appeared to have an impaired therapeutic response.

The pathophysiological effects of smoking on gastroduodenal physiology are complex and controversial (WORMSLEY 1978; GUSLANDI 1988) and the mechanisms include the impairment of mucosal defense and an increase in acid secretion (WHITFIELD and HOBSLEY 1987). Smoking reduces prostaglandin E_2 levels in gastric secretions (MCCREADY et al. 1985) and in the gastric but apparently not the duodenal mucosa (QUINBY et al. 1986). Decreases in bicarbonate secretion by the duodenal mucosa (BOCHNENEK and KORONCZEWSKI 1973) and the pancreas (BYNUM et al. 1972) are reported. Chronic smokers also appear to have increased basal and pentagastrin-stimulated acid secretion (PARENTE et al. 1985; WHITFIELD and HOBSLEY 1987). Furthermore, smoking inhibits salivary, pancreatic, and duodenal epidermal growth factor secretion, which appears to play an important role in both mucosal protection and wound healing (Konturek et al. 1989).

III. Nonsteroidal Anti-Inflammatory Drugs

Epidemiological evidence supports the association of NSAIDs with gastric and duodenal mucosal damage and peptic ulceration, although the relative risk of gastric ulceration is about five times higher than that of duodenal ulceration (Langman 1989). Our understanding of the underlying mechanisms involved has increased from animal studies (Szabo 1987; Kauffman 1989) but little is known with respect to the adverse effects on healing (Lam and Koo 1983).

The proposed mechanisms include (a) impairment of mucosal defense mechanisms by inhibition of the cyclooxygenase pathway, leading to a reduction in local and systemic prostaglandin synthesis with a subsequent decrease in mucus and bicarbonate secretion, (b) a reduction in mucosal blood flow, (c) decreased cell turnover, (d) impaired platelet aggregation (Kauffman 1989), and (e) increased acid secretion (Feldman and Colturi 1984; Levine and Schwartzel 1984). The effects of decreasing prostaglandin synthesis may potentiate arachidonic acid metabolism by the lipooxygenase pathways to increase production of leukotrienes, which in animal studies act as potent vasoconstrictors and stimulate acid secretion (Halter 1988). The net effect would be to impair mucosal defense and predispose the mucosa to recurrent damage by acid and pepsin, which would result in delayed healing or early recurrence.

IV. *Helicobacter pylori*

Helicobacter pylori is considered important because of the significant association with peptic ulcer disease and is now widely accepted as the cause of type B gastritis (Marshall and Warren 1984). The organism is highly adapted for the ecological niche which it occupies below the mucus layer overlying the gastric epithelium and areas of gastric metaplasia in the duodenal cap.

The mechanisms by which this organism or specific virulent strains cause mucosal damage are unknown (Goodwin et al. 1986; Graham 1989) but may include mucus depletion, cellular invasion and cytotoxicity, the associated inflammatory response, and ammonia production by the potent urease activity. It remains unclear whether gastric metaplasia in the duodenal cap results from mucosal adaptation to an excess acid load or from direct damage by *H. pylori*. Furthermore, controversy exists as to whether the organism is associated with altered acid secretion although recent evidence suggests that there is an inappropriate gastrin response which may result from antral alkalinization by ammonia secretion, producing hypergastrinemia (Levi et al. 1989). Chronic inflammation may be associated with decreased mucosal prostaglandins (GOREN 1989), and in isolated animal parietal cell preparations *H. pylori* may cause direct inhibition of acid secretion (CAVE and VARGAS 1989; DEFIZE et al. 1989).

Treatment trials show that antisecretory agents do not clear or eradicate *H. pylori*, but bismuth compounds (colloidal bismuth subcitrate or bismuth subsalicylate) result in clearance in about 45%–50% of cases and to a greater extent when combined with a variety of antibiotics including amoxycillin, tetracycline, metronidazole, and tinidazole (COGHLAN et al. 1987; MARSHALL et al. 1988; MCNULTY et al. 1986). Duodenal ulcer healing rates for bismuth and antibiotic combinations are similar to those for H_2 receptor antagonists alone but significantly lower recurrence rates of 30%–40% are seen after eradication of the organism (COGHLAN et al. 1987; HUMPHREYS et al. 1986; MARSHALL et al. 1988). Bismuth may be acting by eradication of the organisms or as a site-protective agent resulting in better healing of the associated duodenitis (GOODWIN 1988; PRICHARD and KERR 1985). It may thus have a dual role in preventing the synergistic action of *H. pylori* and acid, thereby preventing recurrent ulceration.

The relationship between *H. pylori* and refractory duodenal ulcer has not been discussed in any trial to date and this must be considered in future trials in view of the significantly improved 4-week healing rates with bismuth subcitrate (80%) compared with cimetidine (40%) in refractory duodenal ulcer studies (LAM et al. 1984; BIANCHO-PORRO et al. 1987).

V. Ulcer Morphology

The relationship of different morphological characteristics of duodenal ulcer to healing and relapse have been extensively studied (KOHN et al. 1972; SONNENBERG et al. 1981; LAM and KOO 1983; NAVA et al. 1979); these characteristics include ulcer size, shape, number, and location. Healing rates appear to correlate exponentially with ulcer size (SCHEURER et al. 1977) but the measurement techniques used are difficult to apply to irregular ulcers and the depth of the ulcer crater has not been considered in vivo. Refractory duodenal ulcers are usually irregular, linear, multiple, located near the pylorus, and associated with scar deformity and erosive pathology. Associated *Candida* infection has been reported in case series more commonly for gastric ulcer (KATZENSTEIN and MAKSEN 1974) than duodenal ulcer (THOMAS and REDDY 1983). The finding of *Candida* probably only reflects poor nutritional or immunological status since patients were often immunocompromised or malnourished alcoholics (PETERS et al. 1980).

C. Outcome of Refractory Duodenal Ulcer Treatment Trials

The majority of refractory duodenal ulcer studies involve assessment of the effect of different treatments on healing and have included an attempt to increase acid suppression by changing the dose or class of the antisecretory drug or switching to a mucosal protective agent. More recently the potent H^+,K^+-ATPase or "proton pump" blocker omeprazole (TYTGAT et al. 1987; BRUNNER et al. 1988; BARDMAN et al. 1988; DELCHIER et al. 1989) and the role of surgery (HANSEN and KNIGGE 1984; PICKARD and MACKAY 1984; WEAVER and TEMPLE 1985; PRIMROSE et al. 1988; ANDERSEN et al. 1990) have been assessed with respect to acid suppression and healing.

All studies which have increased the dose of the initial drug or changed the agent clearly increase the duration of treatment, which is considered one of the more important factors in ulcer healing (BARDMAN 1982; HUNT et al. 1986; JONES et al. 1987). Both the degree and the duration of acid suppression produced by different antisecretory agents correlate with duodenal ulcer healing (HUNT et al. 1986; JONES et al. 1987).

I. Acid Suppression

In an early report BARDMAN (1984) attempted to increase acid suppression by increasing the dose of cimetidine from 1 g to 2 g per day but this only increased healing to 56% after an average 9 months' treatment. This result is probably explained by the fact that standard doses of cimetidine already produce peak whole blood concentrations towards the top of the dose–response curve and are unlikely to further inhibit acid secretion. Changing to a more potent H_2 receptor antagonist such as ranitidine or famotidine has the added advantage of increasing the degree and to some extent the duration of acid suppression. Published trials have only compared ranitidine with cimetidine and have shown no significant advantage (QUATRINI et al. 1984) or only a minor improvement of 11% (AMOURETTI et al. 1985).

Medical regimens using H_2 receptor antagonists currently aim to suppress the nocturnal unbuffered acid secretion. In early studies with cimetidine, a subgroup of pharmacological nonresponders achieved successful acid suppression following either vagotomy (GLEDHILL et al. 1983) or the addition of atropine (GLEDHILL et al. 1984), thus supporting GLEDHILL and co-workers' suggestion of an excessive vagal drive in these patients. However, in clinical trials which combined cimetidine with the M_1 anticholinergic pirenzipine, which has fewer severe side-effects than atropine, there was no advantage compared to cimetidine alone (DAL MONTE et al. 1985; BARDMAN et al. 1987).

Changing to omeprazole produces the most profound and sustained inhibition of acid secretion by irreversible blockade of the H^+,K^+-ATPase proton pump of the parietal cell. Dose–responses studies with omeprazole have shown considerable variation in response at 20 mg daily, but at higher doses of 30 or 40 mg daily omeprazole produces almost 100% inhibition of 24-h intragastric acidity (SHARMA et al. 1984). Initial uncontrolled studies of duodenal ulcer patients resistant to H_2 receptor antagonists (TYTGAT et al. 1987; BRUNNER et al. 1988) using omeprazole 40 mg daily produced 100%

healing rates at 4 weeks. A more recent controlled study comparing omeprazole 40 mg daily and continued H_2 receptor antagonist therapy reported significantly increased healing rates at both 4 and 8 weeks (BARDHAN et al. 1988) while another study comparing omeprazole 20 mg daily and ranitidine 150 mg b.i.d. found no significant difference in healing (DELCHIER et al. 1989). The latter study probably did not use a high enough dose of either omeprazole or ranitidine to adequately suppress acid secretion, which was not measured, and the ranitidine group also appeared to have smaller ulcers.

Recent 24-h intragastric acidity studies have shown that ranitidine 300 mg four times daily (LANZON-MILLER et al. 1987b) and famotidine 20–40 mg daily (SANTANA et al. 1986) produce similar degrees of acid suppression to omeprazole but neither drug regimen has been tested in refractory ulcer trials. A simple single-dose regimen of omeprazole is probably preferable in nonresponders to enhance compliance and avoid the potential adverse pharmacological effects of increased parietal cell sensitivity, tolerance, and receptor up-regulation which may occur following H_2 receptor antagonist therapy.

II. Mucosal Protective Agents

Mucosal protective agents have been studied in nonresponders with promising results. Improved healing has been observed with tripotassium dicitrato bismuthate (LAM et al. 1984; BIANCH-PORRO et al. 1987), sucralfate (GUSLANDI et al. 1983), and misoprostol (NEWMAN et al. 1987). However, all these studies have used inconsistent definitions of refractory duodenal ulcer and the quality of the trials has varied widely with problems of blinding and duration of treatment making comparison and generalization difficult.

The two studies using tripotassium dicitrato bismuthate (LAM et al. 1984; BIANCH-PORRO et al. 1987) have shown significantly improved healing rate at 4 weeks of 85% compared to 40% when treatment with higher doses of cimetidine was continued. The mechanism of ulcer healing with bismuth is not fully understood but mainly involves mucosal protective properties of coating the ulcer base (KOO et al. 1982), increasing local prostaglandin production (KONTUREK et al. 1986), accumulating epidermal growth factor (KONTUREK et al. 1988), and perhaps the more specific bacteriostatic action against *H. pylori* infection.

The open sucralfate study for refractory ulcer, which was defined as a duodenal ulcer that failed to heal after 8 weeks of cimetidine or ranitidine, demonstrated 80% healing; however, this study was only reported in abstract, which limits further comment.

The study using the prostaglandin E_1 analogue misoprostol (NEWMAN et al. 1987), which defined refractory ulcers as those which failed to heal after only 4 weeks' treatment with cimetidine or ranitidine, showed improved healing when compared to placebo. Misoprostol was prescribed at a dose of

200 μg four times daily, which produces a measurable antisecretory effect rather than a mucosal protective action. Although a statistical difference was seen in the healing rates for the misoprostol and placebo groups (37% vs 22% respectively), the difference at 4 weeks was too small to be of clinical value.

III. Surgery

Gastric surgery has been traditionally used to reduce gastric acid secretion but more specifically to manage the complications of peptic ulcer disease, in particular bleeding, perforation, and severe obstructive deformity of the duodenum. Surgical techniques are now extremely sophisticated, with proximal gastric vagotomy and drainage the preferred procedure. When performed by an experienced surgeon, this procedure effectively reduces acid secretion and is associated with a low morbidity and mortality (AMDRUP 1988). The results of surgery for refractory duodenal ulcer have been variable, with differences in study design and outcome measures. Clinical improvement following surgery has been shown in only one study (PICKARD and MACKAY 1984) and disputed by others (BARDHAN 1982; HANSEN and KNIGGE 1984; PRIMROSE et al. 1988) who all reported high recurrence rates and complications. A more recent large controlled study (ANDERSEN et al. 1990) found no difference in cumulative recurrence or Visick gradings after 5 years for duodenal ulcers sensitive and resistant to cimetidine.

The important issues involved are not only whether surgery will heal the refractory duodenal ulcer, which it appears to do successfully, but also whether it will improve the quality of life for patients who would otherwise be committed to long-term maintenance therapy with the inevitable cost-benefit issues. More radical surgical procedures such as antrectomy and gastrectomy reduce the acid secretory capacity to a greater degree but at the cost of increasing the risks of long-term complications.

D. Management

The management of refractory duodenal ulcer depends on several factors, including a satisfactory and widely accepted definition. Assuming that adequate H_2 receptor antagonist therapy has been prescribed with good patient compliance, and if endoscopically confirmed ulcer healing has not occurred after at least 3 months of medical treatment, further investigations are required to exclude acid hypersecretory states and nonpeptic causes for duodenal ulceration. Fasting serum gastrin levels should be measured; endoscopy and biopsies should be repeated, and if necessary gastric secretory function tests performed. These should include basal and stimulated secretory tests, and in addition 24-h intragastric pH monitoring might also be considered to assess the degree of response to a particular antisecretory drug or dose.

I. General Advice

All patients with refractory duodenal ulcer must be advised to stop smoking, to avoid NSAIDs, to eat a well-balanced diet which includes three regular meals a day, and particularly to avoid bedtime snacks or drinks.

II. Specific Treatment

The specific therapeutic options available to heal the refractory ulcer are dependent on both the general health of the individual patient and the severity of the ulcer disease; hence each case must be considered individually. The choice of treatment includes either changing to a more potent antisecretory regimen or changing to a mucosal protective agent. Omeprazole is a logical first choice because of the high degree of efficacy seen in clinical trials in general and the refractory ulcer patient in particular. Once healing is achieved the choice of maintenance therapy is not clear since experience of maintenance treatment with omeprazole is limited and currently not approved. Furthermore there remains a significant concern over the long-term issues of safety with omeprazole although no serious adverse effects have been reported. An alternative would be to revert to full-dose H_2 receptor antagonists which are well established and safe.

In patients who are unable to comply with long-term maintenance therapy, proximal gastric vagotomy and a drainage procedure should be considered. Limited data are available for postvagotomy failures but the results are usually independent of the earlier response to medical treatment and recurrent ulcers usually heal with a standard dose of an H_2 receptor antagonist (Berstad et al. 1981).

The outcome of the refractory ulcer trials reconfirms Schwarz's often misquoted dictum "no acid – no ulcer," which, when correctly translated, states that "peptic ulcer disease is a product of self-digestion; it results from an excess of autopeptic power of gastric juice over the defensive power of the gastric and intestinal mucosa" (Schwarz 1910). Duodenal ulcer healing appears to be dependent on the degree and duration of acid suppression (Hunt et al. 1986; Jones et al. 1987) produced by the antisecretory agents used. Whether a short but marked decrease in acidity as against a prolonged and more moderate decrease in acidity, or the total acid load secreted, is important needs further investigation (Hunt 1988). The role of surgery is controversial and it remains to be seen whether it will be necessary for the duodenal ulcers "refractory to omeprazole." Further well-designed long-term trials comparing optimal medical and surgical treatment are required and must include an assessment of all known factors – specifically acid secretory function, *H. pylori* status, and measures which assess not only healing but also the quality of life.

References

Aadland E, Berstad A (1979) Parietal and chief cell sensitivity to histamine and pentagastrin stimulation before and after ranitidine treatment in healthy subjects. Scand J Gastroenterol 14:933–938

Aadland E, Berstad A, Semb LS (1977) Effect of cimetidine on pentagastrin stimulated gastric secretion in healthy man. Scand J Gastroenterol 12:501–506

Achord JL (1981) Gastric pepsin and acid secretion in patients with acute and healed duodenal ulcer. Gastroenterology 81:15–18

Aly A, Emas S (1982) Sensitivity of the oxyntic and peptic cells to pentagastrin in duodenal ulcer patients and healthy subjects with similar secretory capacity. Digestion 25:88–95

Amdrup E (1988) Surgery and its sequelae. In: Piper DW (ed) Balliere's clinical gastroenterology. Balliere Tindall, London, pp 699–710

Amouretti M, Ansenay M, Bader JP, Baillet J, Bel A, Belaiche J, Benzenou A, Bertrand G, Bonfils S, Boncekknie J (1985) A multicentre controlled trial of ranitidine and cimetidine-resistant peptic ulcer disease. Gastroenterol Clin Biol 9:147–152

Andersen D, Amdrup E, Hanberg Sorensek F (1990) Parietal cell vagotomy in patients resistant to cimetidine. (in press).

Bader JP, Stanescu L (1989) Problems with patients' compliance in peptic ulcer therapy. J Clin Gastroenterol [Suppl 1] 11:S25–S28

Bank S, Barbezat GO, Vinik AI, Helman C (1977) Serum gastrin levels before and after 6 weeks of cimetidine therapy in patients with duodenal ulcer. Digestion 15:157–161

Bardhan KD (1982) Non-responders to cimetidine treatment. In: Baron JH (ed) Cimetidine in the 80's. Livingston, Edinburgh, pp 42–57

Bardhan KD (1984) Refractory duodenal ulcer. Gut 25:711–717

Bardhan KD (1989) Omeprazole in the management of refractory duodenal ulcer disease. Scand J Gastroenterol [Suppl 166] 24:63–73

Bardhan KD, Thompson M, Bose K, Hincliffe RFC, Crowe J, Weir DG McCarthy C, Walters J, Thompson TJ, Thompson MH, Gait JE, King C, Prudham D (1987) Combined anti-muscarinic and H_2 receptor blockade in the healing of refractory duodenal ulcer. A double blind study. Gut 28:1505–1509

Bardhan KD, Naesdal J, Bianchi-Porro G, Lazzorini M, Hincliffe RFC, Thompson M, Morris P, Daly MJ, Carroll NJH, Walan A (1988) Treatment of refractory peptic ulcer with omeprazole (Abstr) Gut 29:A724

Berstad A, Aadland E, Bjerke K (1981) Cimetidine treatment of recurrent ulcer after proximal gastric vagotomy. Scand J Gastroenterol 16:981–986

Bianchi-Porro G, Parente F, Lazzaroni M (1987) Tripotassium dicitrato bismuthate (TDB) versus two different dosages of cimetidine in the treatment of resistant duodenal ulcers. Gut 28:907–911

Blair AJ, Richardson CT, Walsh JH, Feldman M (1987) Variable contribution of gastrin to gastric acid secretion after a meal in humans. Gastroenterology 92:944–949

Bochnenek WJ, Koronczewski R (1973) Effect of cigarette smoking on bicarbonate and volume of the duodenal contents. Am J Dig Dis 18:729–733

Boyd EJS, Penston JG, Johnston KA, Wormsley KG (1988) Does maintenance therapy keep duodenal ulcer healed? Lancet 2:134–137

Brunner G, Creutzfeldt W, Harke U, Lamberts R (1988) Therapy with omeprazole with peptic ulcerations resistant to extended high-dose ranitidine treatment. Digestion 39:80–90

Bynum TE, Solomon TE, Johnson LR, Jacobson ED (1972) Inhibition of pancreatic function in man by cigarette smoking. Gut 13:361–365

Cave DR, Vargas M (1989) Effect of a *Campylobacter pylori* protein on acid secretion by parietal cell. Lancet 2:187–189

Cherner JA, Jensen RT, Dubois A, O'Dorisio TM, Gardner JD, Metcalfe DD (1988) Gastrointestinal dysfunction in systemic mastocytosis. A prospective study. Gastroenterology 95:657–667
Chiverton SG, Burget D, Hunt RH (1988) Smoking does not impair the response to therapy in duodenal ulcer healing. (Abstr). Gastroenterology 94:A69
Chiverton SG, Hunt RH (1989) Initial therapy and relapse of duodenal ulcer: possible acid secretory mechanisms. Gastroenterology 96:632–639
Coghlan JG, Humphries H, Dooley C, Keane C, Gilligan, McKenna D, Sweeney E, O'Morain C (1987) *Campylobacter pylori* and recurrence of duodenal ulcers – a 12 month follow up study. Lancet 2:1109–1111
Collen MJ, Stanczak VJ, Ciarleglio CA (1989) Refractory duodenal ulcers (non healing duodenal ulcers with standard doses of antisecretory medication). Dig Dis Sci 34:233–237
Dal Monte PR, D'Imperio M, Ferri M, Fratucello F, del Soladato P (1985) A combination of pirenzipine and cimetidine: a new approach to treatment of duodenal ulcer in "non-responders". Hepatogastroenterology 32:126–128
Defize J, Goldie J, Hunt RH (1989) Inhibition of acid production by *Campylobacter pylori* in isolated guinea pig parietal cells. (Abstr). Gastroenterology 96:A114
Delchier JC, Isal JP, Eriksson S, Soule JC (1989) Double blind multicentre comparison of omeprazole 20 mg once daily versus ranitidine 150 mg twice daily in the treatment of cimetidine or ranitidine resistant duodenal ulcers. Gut 30:1173–1178
Dobrilla G, Vallaperta P, Amplatz S (1988) Influence of ulcer healing agents on ulcer relapse after discontinuation of acute treatment: a pooled estimate of controlled clinical trials. Gut 27:106–110
Domschke W, Lam SK, Pounder RE, Anderson D (1989) H_2-blocker resistant duodenal ulceration. Gastroenterol Int 2:85–91
Feldman M, Colturi TJ (1984) Effect of indomethacin on gastric acid and bicarbonate secretion in humans. Gastroenterology 87:1339–1343
Feldman M, Richardson CT (1986) Total 24-hour gastric acid secretion in patients with duodenal ulcer. Comparison with normal subjects and effects of cimetidine and parietal cell vagotomy. Gastroenterology 90:540–544
Feldman M, Richardson CT, Walsh JH (1983) Sex related differences in gastrin release and parietal cell sensitivity to gastrin in healthy human beings. J Clin Invest 71:715–720
Freston JW (1987a) H_2-receptor antagonist and duodenal ulcer recurrence: analysis of efficacy and commentary on safety, costs, and patient selection. Am J Gastroenterol 82:1242–1249
Freston JW (1987b) Mechanisms of relapse in peptic ulcer disease. J Clin Gastroenterol [Suppl 1] 11:S34–S38
Frislid K, Aadland E, Berstad A (1986) Augmented postprandial gastric acid secretion due to exposure to ranitidine in healthy subjects. Scand J Gastroenterol 21:119–122
Fullarton AM, McLaughlin G, MacDonald A, Crean GP, McColl KEL (1989) Rebound nocturnal hypersecretion after four weeks treatment with an H_2 receptor antagonist. Gut 30:449–454
Gledhill T, Buck M, Hunt RH (1983) Cimetidine or vagotomy? Comparison of the effects of proximal gastric vagotomy, cimetidine and placebo on nocturnal intragastric acidity and acid secretion in patients with cimetidine resistant duodenal ulcer. Br J Surg 70:704–706
Gledhill T, Buck M, Hunt RH (1984) Effect of no treatment, cimetidine 1 g/day, cimetidine 2 g/day and cimetidine combined with atropine on nocturnal gastric secretion in cimetidine non-responders. Gut 25:1211–1216
Goodwin CS (1988) Duodenal ulcer, *Campylobacter pylori* leaking and the "roof" concept. Lancet 2:1467–1469
Goodwin CS, Armstrong JA, Marshall BJ (1986) *Campylobacter pyloridis*, gastritis, and peptic ulceration. J Clin Pathol 39:353–365
Goren A (1989) *Campylobacter pylori* and acid secretion (Letter). Lancet 2:212–213

Graham DY (1989) *Campylobacter pylori* and peptic ulcer disease. Gastroenterology 96:70–90
Guslandi M (1988) How does smoking harm the duodenum? Br J Med 296:311–312
Guslandi M, Ballarin E, Tittobello A (1983) Sucralfate in refractory duodenal ulcers. (Abstr). Gut 24:A498
Halter F (1988) Mechanism of gastrointestinal toxicity of NSAIDs. Scand J Rheumatol [Suppl] 73:16–21
Halter F, Bangerter U, Häcki WH, Schlup M, Varga L, Wyder S, Rotzer A, Galeazzi R (1982) Sensitivity of the parietal cell to pentagastrin in health and duodenal ulcer disease: A reappraisal. Scand J Gastroenterol 17:539–544
Hansen JH, Knigge U (1984) Failure of proximal gastric vagotomy for duodenal ulcer resistant to cimetidine. Lancet 2:84–85
Hirschowitz BI (1984) Apparent and intrinsic sensitivity to pentagastrin of acid and pepsin secretion in peptic ulcer. Gastroenterology 86:843–851
Humphreys H, Bourke S, Dooley C, McKenna D, Power B, Keane CT, Sweeney EC, O'Morain C (1988) Effect of treatment on *Campylobacter pylori* in peptic disease: a randomized prospective trial. Gut 29:279–283
Hunt RH (1981) Non-responders to cimetidine treatment. In: Baron JH (ed) Cimetidine in the 80's. Livingstone, Edinburgh, pp 331–341
Hunt RH (1988) Acid suppression and ulcer healing: dichotomy, degree, and dilemma. Am J Gastroenterol 83:964–966
Hunt RH, Howden CW, Jones DB, Burgett DW, Kerr GD (1986) The correlation between acid suppression and peptic ulcer healing. Scand J Gastroenterol [Suppl 125] 21:22–29
Hyman PE, Abrams C, Garvey TQ (1985) Ranitidine tachyphylaxis (Abstr). Gastroenterology 88:1426
Isenberg JI, Grossman MI, Maxwell V, Walsh JH (1975) Increased sensitivity to stimulation of acid secretion by pentagastrin in duodenal ulcer. J Clin Invest 55:330–337
Jones DB, Howden CW, Burget DW, Kerr GD, Hunt RH (1987) Acid suppression in duodenal ulcer: a meta-analysis to define optimal dosing with antisecretory drugs. Gut 28:1120–1127
Jones DB, Howden CW, Burget DW, Siletti C, Hunt RH (1988) Alteration of H_2 receptor sensitivity in duodenal ulcer patients following maintenance treatment with an H_2 receptor antagonist. Gut 29:890–893
Katzenstein ALA, Maksen J (1974) *Candida* infection of gastric ulcer. Histology, incidence and clinical significance. Am J Clin Pathol 71:137
Kauffman G (1989) Aspirin-induced gastric injury: lessons learned from animal models. Gastroenterology 96:606–614
Kohn Y, Misahi F, Kawai K (1972) Endoscopic follow-up observation of duodenal ulcer. Endoscopy 4:202–208
Konturek SJ, Obtulowicz W, Kweicien N, Kopp B, Oleksy J (1981) Dynamics of gastric acid inhibition by ranitidine in duodenal ulcer patients. Digestion 22:119–125
Konturek SJ, Radecki T, Piastucki I, Drozdowicz D (1986) Advances in the understanding of the mechanism of cytoprotective action of colloidal bismuth subcitrate. Scand J Gastroenterol [Suppl 122] 21:6–10
Konturek SJ, Dembinski A, Warzecha Z, Bielanski W, Brzorowski T, Dorozdowilz D (1988) Epidermal growth factor in the gastroprotection and ulcer healing action of colloidal bismuth subcitrate. Gut 29:894
Konturek JW, Bielanski W, Konturek SJ, Bogdal J, Oleksy J (1989) Distribution and release of epidermal growth factor in man. Gut 30:1194–1200
Koo J, Ho J, Lam SK, Wong J, Ong GB (1982) Selective coating of gastric ulcer by tripotassium dicitrato bismuthate in the rat. Gastroenterology 82:864–870
Korman MG, Hansky J, Eaves ER, Schmidt GT (1983) Influence of cigarette smoking on healing and relapse in duodenal ulcer disease. Gastroenterology 85: 871–874

Kurata JH (1989) Ulcer epidemiology: an overview and proposed research framework. Gastroenterology [Suppl 2] 96:569–580

Lam SK (1985) Heterogeneous nature of hyperacidity in duodenal ulcer Krevning J, Samloff, Rotter J, Eriksson AW (eds). In: Pepsinogens in man: clinical and genetic advances. Arliss, New York, pp 255–271

Lam SK, Koo J (1985) Gastrin sensitivity in duodenal ulcer. Gut 26:485–490

Lam SK, Koo J (1983) Accurate prediction of duodenal-ulcer healing rate by discriminant analysis. Gastroenterology 85:403–412

Lam SK, Lee NW, Koo J, Hui WM, Fok KH, Ng M (1984) Randomized crossover trial of tripotassium dicitrato bisumthate versus high dose cimetidine for duodenal ulcers resistant to standard dose of cimetidine. Gut 25:703–706

Langman MJS (1989) Epidemiological evidence on the association between peptic ulceration and anti-inflammatory drug use. Gastroenterology 96:640–646

Lanzon-Miller S, Pounder RE, Hamilton MR, Ball S, Chronos NAF, Raymond F, Olausson M, Cedeberg C (1987a) Twenty-four hour intragastric acidity and plasma gastrin concentration before and during treatment with either ranitidine or omeprazole. Aliment Pharmacol Ther 1:239–251

Lanzon-Miller S, Pounder RE, Chronos NAF, Hamilton M, Ball S, Raymond F (1987b) Can high dose ranitidine eliminate intragastric acid and what does it do to plasma gastrin? (Abstr). Gastroenterology 92:1491

Levi S, Beardshall K, Haddad G, Playford R, Ghosh P, Calam J (1989) *Campylobacter pylori* and duodenal ulcers: the gastrin link. Lancet 2:1467–1469

Levine RA, Schwartzel EH (1984) Effect of indomethacin on basal and histamine stimulated gastric acid secretion. Gut 25:718–722

Lewin KJ, Yang K, Ulich T, Glashoff, Walsh J (1984) Primary gastrin cell hyperplasia: a report of five cases and review of the literature. Am J Surg Pathol 8:821–832

MacCarthy DM (1984) Smoking and ulcers – time to quit. N Engl J Med 311:726–728

Marks IN, Young GO, Tigler-Wybrandi NA, Bridger S, Newton KA (1989) Acid secretory response and parietal cell sensitivity in patients with duodenal ulcer before and after healing with sucralfate or ranitidine. Am J Med [Suppl 6A] 86:145–147

Marshall BJ, Warren JR (1984) Unidentified curved bacilli in the stomach of patients with gastritis and peptic ulceration. Lancet 1:1312–1315

Marshall BJ, Goodwin CS, Warren JE, Murray R, Blincow ED, Blackbourn SJ, Phillips M, Waters TE, Sanderson CR (1988) Prospective double-blind trial of duodenal ulcer relapse after eradication of *Campylobacter pylori*. Lancet 2:1437–1442

McCready DR, Clark L, Cohen MM (1985) Cigarette smoking reduces human gastric luminal prostaglandin E_2. Gut 26:1192–1196

McLean AJ, Harrison PM, Ionnides-Demos L, Byrne AJ, McCarthy P, Dudley FJ (1985) The choice of ulcer healing agent influences ulcer healing rate and long term clinical outcome. Aust N Z J Med 15:367–374

McNulty CAM, Gearty JC, Crump B, Davis M, Donovan IA, Melikan V, Lister DM, Wise R (1986) *Campylobacter pyloridis* and associated gastritis: investigator blind, placebo controlled trial of bismuth salicylate and erythromycin ethylsuccinate. Br Med J 293:645–649

Mignon M, Bonfils S (1988) Diagnosis and treatment of Zollinger-Ellison syndrome. In: Piper DW (ed) Bailliere's clinical gastroenterology. Balliere Tindall, London, pp 677–689

Miller JP, Faragher EB (1986) Relapse of duodenal ulcer: does it matter which drug is used in initial treatment? Br Med J 293:1117–1118

Nava G, Pippa G, Ballanti R, Papi C, Nava G Jr (1979) Role of ulcer morphology in evaluating prognosis and therapeutic outcome in duodenal ulcer. Scand J Gastroenterol [Suppl 54] 124:41–43

Newman RD, Gitlin N, Lacayo EJ, Safdi AV, Ramsey EJ, Engel SL, Rubin A, Nissen CH, Swabb EA (1987) Misoprostol in the treatment of duodenal ulcer refractory to H_2-blocker therapy. Am J Med [Suppl 1A] 83:27–31

Nwokolo CU, Smith JTL, Pounder RE (1989a) Rebound intragastric hyperacidity following dosing with cimetidine, nizatidine and famotidine. (Abstr). Gastroenterology 96:A369
Nwokolo CU, Gavey CJ, Smith JLT, Gavey C, Sawyerr A, Pounder RE (1989b) Tolerance during 29 days of conventional dosing with cimetidine, nizatidine, famotidine, or ranitidine. (Abstr). Gut 30:A1487
Nwokolo CU, Smith JLT, Sawyerr A, Pounder RE (1989c) Intravenous pentagastrin can overcome H_2 blockade in man: a possible mechanism for tolerance. (Abstr). Gut 30:A1487
Orlando RC (1987) Peptic ulcer: factors influencing recurrence. Clin J Gastroenterol [Suppl 1] 9:2–7
Parente F, Lazzaroni M, Sangaletti O, Baroni S, Bianchi Porro G (1985) Cigarette smoking, gastric acid secretions and serum pepsinogen I concentrations in duodenal ulcer patients. Gut 26:1327–1332
Peters M, Weiner J, Whelan G (1980) Fungal infection associated with gastroduodenal ulceration: Endoscopic and pathologic appearances. Gastroenterology 78:350–354
Pickard WR, MacKay C (1984) Early results of surgery in patients considered cimetidine failures. Br J Surg 71:67–68
Piper DW (1987) The refractory ulcer. World J Surg 11:268–273
Pounder RE (1987) What is an intractable duodenal ulcer and how should it be managed? Aliment Pharmacol Therap 1:4395–4465
Prichard PJ, Kerr GD (1985) Duodenitis and ulcer relapse. Lancet 2:102
Prichard PJ, Jones DB, Yeomans ND, Mikaly GW, Smallwood RA, Louis WJ (1986) The effectiveness of ranitidine in reducing gastric acid secretion decreases with continued therapy. Br J Clin Pharmacol 22:663–668
Primrose JN, Axon ATR, Johnston D (1988) Highly selective vagotomy and duodenal ulcers that fail to respond to H_2 receptor antagonists. Br Med J 296:1031–1035
Quatrini M, Basilico G, Bianchi PA (1984) Treatment of 'cimetidine-resistant' chronic duodenal ulcers with ranitidine or cimetidine: a randomised multicentre study. Gut 25:1113–1117
Quinby GF, Avundk-Bonnice AC, Burstein SH, Eastwood GL (1986) Active smoking depresses prostaglandin synthesis in human gastric mucosa. Ann Intern Med 104:616–619
Rack J, Sonnenberg A (1983) The influence of smoking and intravenous nicotine on gastric mucus. Hepatogastroenterology 30:258–260
Richardson CT (1978) Effect of H_2-receptor antagonists on gastric acid secretion and serum gastrin concentration: a review. Gastroenterology 74:366–370
Santana IA, Lanzon-Miller S, Pounder RE (1986) Effect of oral famotidine on 24-hour intragastric acidity. Postgrad Med J [Suppl 2] 62:39–42
Scheurer U, Witzel L, Halter F, Keller HM, Huber R, Caleazzi R (1977) Gastric and duodenal ulcer healing under placebo treatment. Gastroenterology 72:838–841
Schwarz K (1910) Ueber penetrierende Magen-und Jejunalgeschwüre. Beitr Z Klin Chir 67:69–128
Sewing KF, Hagie L, Ippoliti AF, Isenberg JI, Samloff IM, Sturderant RAL (1978) Effect of one month treatment with cimetidine on gastric secretion and serum gastrin and pepsinogen levels. Gastroenterology 74:376–379
Sharma BK, Walt RP, Pounder RE, Gomes EFA, Wood EC, Logan LH (1984) Optimal dose of oral omeprazole for maximal 24 hour decrease of intragastric acidity. Gut 25:957–964
Sharma B, Alexson M, Pounder RE, Lundberg P, Öman M, Sanatana A, Talbot M, Cederberg C (1987) Acid secretory capacity and plasma gastrin concentration after administration of omeprazole to normal subjects. Aliment Pharmacol Therap 1:67–76
Smith JLT, Gavey CJ, Nwokolo CU, Pounder RE (1989) Tolerance during eight days of high dose H_2 blockade: placebo controlled studies of 24 hour acidity and gastrin. (Abstr). Gut 30:A1487

Sonnenberg A (1985) Geographic and temporal variations in the occurrence of peptic ulcer disease. (Suppl 10). Scand J Gastroenterol 20:11–24

Sonnenberg A, Müller-Lissner SA, Vogel E, Schmid P, Gonvers JJ, Peter P, Strohmeyer G, Blum AL (1981) Predictors of duodenal ulcer healing and relapse. Gastroenterology 81:1061–1067

Sontag S, Graham DY, Belisto A, Belsito A, Weiss J, Farley A, Grunt R, Coben N, Kinnear D, Davis W, Archambault A, Achord J, Thayer W, Gillies R, Sidorov J, Sabesin SM, Dyck W, Fleshler B, Cheator I, Wengen J, Opekun A (1984) Cimetidine, cigarette smoking, and recurrence of duodenal ulcer. N Engl J Med 311:689–693

Szabo S (1987) Mechanisms of mucosal injury in the stomach and duodenum: time-sequence analysis of morphologic, functional, biochemical and histological studies. Scand J Gastroenterol [Suppl 121] 22:21–28

Thomas JM, Misenwicz JJ (1984) Histamine H_2 receptor antagonists in short and long term treatment of duodenal ulcer. Clin Gastroenterol 13:501–505

Thomas E, Reddy KR (1983) Non-healing duodenal ulceration to *Candida*. J Clin Gastroenterol 5:55

Tytgat GNJ, Lamers CBHW, Hameeteman W, Jansen JMBJ, Wilson JA (1987) Omeprazole in peptic ulcers resistant to histamine H_2-receptor antagonists. Aliment Pharmacol Therap 1:31–38

Vantini I, Ederlene A, Bovo P, Voama B, Biubello W, Benini L, Carabellini G, Scuoro LA (1987) Serum fasting gastrin levels after short term treatment with cimetidine in patients with duodenal ulcer. Acta Hepato-Gastroenterol (Study) 25:376–379

Walt RP, Daneshmend TK (1988) Resistant duodenal ulcer: when, why, and what to do? Post Grad Med J 64:369–372

Weaver RM, Temple JG (1985) Proximal gastric vagotomy in patients resistant to cimetidine. Br J Surg 72:177–178

Whitfield PF, Hobsley M (1987) Comparison of maximal gastric secretion in smokers and non-smokers with and without duodenal ulcer. Gut 28:557–560

Wilder-Smith CH, Ernst T, Gennoni M, Zeyen B, Varga L, Röehmel J, Halter F, Merki HS (1989) Acute tolerance to H_2 receptor antagonists. Gut 30:A1489

Wormsley KG (1978) Smoking and duodenal ulcer. Gastroenterology 75:139–142

Yanaka A, Muto H (1988) Increased parietal cell responsiveness to tetragastrin in patients with recurrent duodenal ulcer disease. Dig Dis Sci 33:1459–1465

CHAPTER 12

Idiopathic Gastric Acid Hypersecretion

M.J. COLLEN

A. Introduction

Clearly, hypersecretion of gastric acid exists in the clinical setting and at times is the reason why many acid-peptic disorders do not respond to standard antisecretory medication (COLLEN et al. 1987a,b, 1988a,b, 1989a,b, 1991; COLLEN and GALLAGHER 1990; COLLEN and JOHNSON 1991; COLLEN and LOEBENBERG 1989; COLLEN 1989, 1990; JENSEN et al. 1983). It is recommended that patients with refractory acid-peptic symptoms and/or mucosal disease (i.e., duodenal ulcer) be evaluated for gastric acid hypersecretion, namely, Zollinger-Ellison syndrome (JENSEN et al. 1983; COLLEN et al. 1989d, 1991; SPINDEL et al. 1986; BARON 1981). Patients with Zollinger-Ellison syndrome can be identified by noting gastric acid hypersecretion and an elevated serum gastrin concentration and by demonstrating a positive provocative secretin test (JENSEN et al. 1983). However, it is estimated that less than 1% of patients with gastric acid hypersecretion actually have Zollinger-Ellison syndrome, and almost all other patients except for less than 1% with other specific causes for gastric acid hypersecretion have no apparent etiology for their gastric acid hypersecretory states (JENSEN et al. 1983; COLLEN 1989; MCCARTHY 1982) (Table 1). The patients with no apparent etiology for their gastric acid hypersecretory states are classified as having idiopathic gastric acid hypersecretion.

Since very few patients with gastric acid hypersecretion have Zollinger-Ellison syndrome, a condition in which a serum gastrin concentration can be used to identify these patients with gastric acid hypersecretion, most of the time the presence of a gastric acid hypersecretory state can only be diagnosed by gastric analysis which determines gastric acid secretion either in the basal state (basal acid output) or the stimulated state (maximal acid output) (JENSEN et al. 1983; COLLEN et al. 1989; MCCARTHY 1982). Most define gastric acid hypersecretion including Zollinger-Ellison syndrome, in the face of no previous gastric surgery, to be a basal acid output of greater than 15 mEq/h (JENSEN et al. 1983; MCCARTHY 1982; KIRKPATRICK and HIRSCHOWITZ 1980). However, some consider patients with basal acid outputs of greater than 10 mEq/h to have gastric acid hypersecretion (COLLEN 1989; BARON 1981). BARON (1981) recommended that patients with refractory duodenal ulcers be evaluated with gastric analysis and that those with basal acid outputs of

Table 1. Conditions associated with gastric acid hypersecretion

Associated with increased gastrin
Zollinger-Ellison syndrome
Retained gastric antrum
Gastric outlet obstruction
Renal failure
Antral G cell hyperfunction
Antral G cell hyperplasia
Short bowel syndrome
Associated with increased histamine
Systemic mastocytosis
Basophilic granulocytic leukemia
Unknown etiology
Idiopathic
Associated with the immediate postoperative period
Associated with pancreatic tumors (nongastrinoma)
Associated with intracranial lesions

greater than 10 mEq/h have fasting serum gastrin concentrations determined to rule out Zollinger-Ellison syndrome. His recommendations are probably correct in light of the fact that as many as 3%–32% of patients with Zollinger-Ellison syndrome have basal acid outputs of less than 15 mEq/h and some patients with Zollinger-Ellison syndrome may have basal acid outputs of less than 10 mEq/h (JENSEN et al. 1983).

Many feel that the only way to define gastric acid hypersecretion is by the determination of basal acid output (JENSEN et al. 1983; MCCARTHY 1982; KIRKPATRICK and HIRSCHOWITZ 1980). However, others have tried to utilize maximal acid output to define gastric acid hypersecretion (JENSEN et al. 1983). They have found that as many as 40% of patients with Zollinger-Ellison syndrome with basal acid outputs of greater than 15 mEq/h (basal gastric acid hypersecretion) have maximal acid outputs in the normal range (JENSEN et al. 1983; COLLEN et al. 1988c). Therefore, maximal acid output does not reliably identify many patients with basal gastric acid hypersecretion with or without Zollinger-Ellison syndrome.

It is quite easy to clearly determine the level for basal acid output for patients with Zollinger-Ellison syndrome that defines gastric acid hypersecretion, since serum gastrin concentration is a "marker" that identifies patients with Zollinger-Ellison syndrome (JENSEN et al. 1983; SPINDEL et al. 1986; MCCARTHY 1982). Therefore, it is well accepted that a basal acid output of greater than 15 mEq/h is the definition for gastric acid hypersecretion in patients with Zollinger-Ellison syndrome (JENSEN et al. 1983; MCCARTHY 1982). A basal acid output of greater than 15 mEq/h identifies 68%–97% of patients with Zollinger-Ellison syndrome (JENSEN et al. 1983). Furthermore, a basal acid output of greater than 10 mEq/h identifies 99% of patients with Zollinger-Ellison syndrome (JENSEN et al. 1983). However, it may be wrong to accept basal acid output of greater than 15 mEq/h as the definition for idiopathic gastric acid hypersecretion in that the level for basal acid output that defines idiopathic gastric acid hypersecretion may be either higher or lower than 15 mEq/h. Since there is no "marker" (such as serum gastrin concentration as in Zollinger-Ellison syndrome) for idiopathic gastric acid hypersecretion, it is difficult to identify these patients, thereby making it difficult to determine the level for basal acid output that defines idiopathic gastric hypersecretion. Therefore, other means are required to determine the level for basal acid output that defines idiopathic gastric acid hypersecretion.

The level for basal acid output that defines idiopathic gastric acid hypersecretion may be determined on a statistical basis and a functional basis. If it is defined on a statistical basis, then it should be defined relative to the normal population. If it is defined on a functional basis then it should be defined as that level of basal acid output which causes refractory acid-peptic mucosal disease (i.e., duodenal ulcer) in patients being treated with standard doses of antisecretory medication.

In the present chapter, idiopathic gastric acid hypersecretion will be defined both statistically and functionally. Data will be presented that clearly show that idiopathic gastric acid hypersecretion should be defined as a basal acid output of greater than 10 mEq/h. This is in contrast to Zollinger-Ellison syndrome and other gastric acid hypersecretory states where a specific etiology is identified, in which a basal acid output of greater than 15 mEq/h defines gastric acid hypersecretion. Also, data will be shown from over 90 patients with idiopathic gastric acid hypersecretion identified during 4 years of gastric analysis.

B. Method of Doing Gastric Analysis

There are many ways to do a gastric analysis in order to determine basal acid output and/or maximal acid output. This can be done by either intragastric titration (Fordtran and Walsh 1973; Malagelada et al. 1976) or gastric aspiration (Feldman 1979; Raufman et al. 1983). The data from gastric analysis presented in this chapter were determined by gastric aspiration which utilized the nasogastric tube. Basal acid output was determined in the basal state in the absence of any antisecretory medication for at least 72 h and maximum acid output was determined in the stimulated state after giving pentagastrin 6 μg/kg subcutaneously, and both were measured as previously described (Raufman et al. 1983). In brief, a nasogastric tube is inserted into the gastric antrum; the accurate position of the tube is confirmed by recovery of greater than 80% of a 30 ml water load in lieu of fluoroscopy. After the gastric residual is emptied by aspiration, four consecutive 15-min samples of gastric fluid are collected by continuous aspiration. Samples are titrated to pH 7.0 with 0.01 NaOH. All results are expressed in milliequivalents of acid per hour (mEq/h).

In the present chapter, idiopathic gastric acid hypersecretion is defined as a basal acid output of greater than 10 mEq/h and all patients with basal acid outputs of greater than 10 mEq/h had serum gastrin concentrations determined. The patients with elevated serum gastrin concentrations of greater than 100 pg/ml had secretin tests (2 units/kg of secretin, Kabi-Ferring Laboratories, Suffern, New York) (FRUCHT et al. 1989). The criterion for the diagnosis of Zollinger-Ellison syndrome was an elevated fasting serum gastrin concentration of greater than 100 pg/ml with a positive secretin test defined as an increase above baseline fasting serum gastrin concentration of greater than 200 pg/ml after intravenous injection of the secretin (FRUCHT et al. 1989).

C. Definition of Idiopathic Gastric Acid Hypersecretion

I. Statistical Definition

Basal acid output was determined in 65 normal subjects, both males and females (Fig. 1) (COLLEN and SHERIDAN 1991). Even though the mean basal acid output for the group of male normal subjects was higher than for the group of female normal subjects, they were not significantly different (Table 2) (COLLEN and SHERIDAN 1991). The 95% confidence intervals for the mean basal acid outputs for all 65 normal subjects, the 28 males and 37 females, are in a narrow range which statistically verifies that the 65 normal subjects are representative of the general population (COCHRAN and SNEDECOR 1980). Statistically, the ranges for the upper limits of basal acid output for all 65 normal subjects, the 28 male normal subjects, and the 37 female normal subjects are similar, with values for the mean basal acid output plus two standard deviations and the mean basal acid output plus three standard deviations for the 65 normal subjects being 8.4 and 11.1 mEq/h respectively. Therefore, 95% to greater than 99% of the normal population have basal acid outputs of less than 8.4 mEq/h and 11.1 mEq/h respectively, and the upper limits for basal acid output for the normal population would be in the range between 8.4 and 11.1 mEq/h. Consequently, statistically the level for basal acid output which should be used to define idiopathic gastric acid hypersecretion is between 8.4 and 11.1 mEq/h.

II. Functional Definition

The functional definition for idiopathic gastric acid hypersecretion was determined in studies that were previously reported (COLLEN et al. 1987b, 1989d, 1991) in which the following questions were asked: Are basal acid outputs of patients whose duodenal ulcers do not heal during 8 weeks of treatment with standard doses of antisecretory medication higher than the basal acid outputs of patients whose duodenal ulcers do heal during 8 weeks of standard antisecretory medication? And, if the basal acid outputs are higher, is there a threshold for the basal acid output of those patients with the refractory duodenal ulcers? In that, do patients with nonhealed duodenal

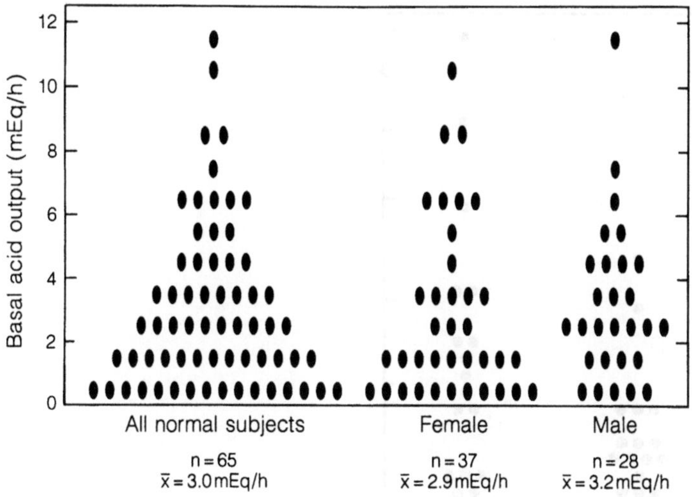

Fig. 1. Distribution of basal acid outputs from normal subjects, both female and male (COLLEN and SHERIDAN 1991)

Table 2. Characteristics of normal subjects (COLLEN and SHERIDAN 1991)

Groups	No.	Age (years)	BAO (mEq/h)			Mean BAO (mEq/h)
		x ± SD	x ± SD	x + 2SD	x + 3SD	95% CI
All	65	36 ± 12	3.0 ± 2.7	8.4	11.1	2.4–3.7
Male	28	35 ± 15	3.2 ± 2.6	8.4	11.0	2.2–4.1
Female	37	37 ± 11	2.9 ± 2.8	8.5	11.3	2.0–3.8

BAO, basal acid output; 95% CI, 95% confidence interval; x ± SD, mean ± 1 standard deviation; x + 2SD, mean + 2 standard deviations; x + 3SD, mean + 3 standard deviations.

ulcers after 8 weeks of standard antisecretory therapy have their basal acid outputs greater than a certain level? If there is a threshold for basal acid output for duodenal ulcers which are refractory to standard treatment, then that threshold could be utilized as the functional definition for idiopathic gastric acid hypersecretion. Also, would that threshold level for basal acid output fall between the range of 8.4 and 11.1 mEq/h, which is the statistical definition for idiopathic gastric acid hypersecretion?

The reason that standard doses of antisecretory medication were used was that it appears that refractoriness of a duodenal ulcer is a function of potency and the amount of antisecretory medication used during therapy. When more potent doses of antisecretory medication (i.e., omeprazole) are utilized, then very little refractory duodenal ulcer disease is found (GUSTAVSSON et al. 1983).

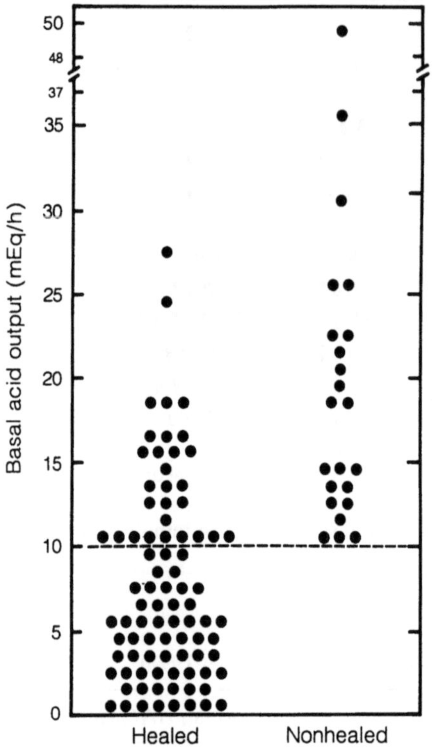

Fig. 2. Distribution of basal acid outputs from patients with active duodenal ulcers treated with standard doses of antisecretory medications (COLLEN and SHERIDAN 1991)

The data presented in Fig. 2 are an expansion of a previously published paper in which 75 patients were reported (COLLEN et al. 1989d). In the present study (COLLEN et al. 1991) 110 patients with active duodenal ulcers were investigated and basal acid outputs were determined. Each of the 110 patients received 8 weeks of standard antisecretory medication: 9–cimetidine 1200 mg/day, 95–ranitidine 300 mg/day, 6–famotidine 40 mg/day. In 23 patients the duodenal ulcers did not heal during 8 weeks of standard antisecretory therapy. The mean basal acid output for the 23 patients with nonhealed duodenal ulcers was 19.4 mEq/h (range 10.1–49.1 mEq/h) while for the 87 patients with healed duodenal ulcers it was 7.5 mEq/h (range 0.0–27.9 mEq/h); this difference was statistically significant ($P < 0.001$). Even though there was an overlap of basal acid outputs between the patients with healed duodenal ulcers and those with nonhealed duodenal ulcers during 8 weeks of therapy, all patients with nonhealed duodenal ulcers had basal acid outputs of greater than 10 mEq/h (Fig. 2). Therefore, the threshold for basal acid output found in patients with refractory duodenal ulcers, which is utilized here to determine the functional definition for idiopathic gastric acid hypersecretion, is a basal acid output of greater than 10 mEq/h.

The functional definition for idiopathic gastric acid hypersecretion, i.e., a basal acid output of greater than 10 mEq/h, is in the range of the statistical

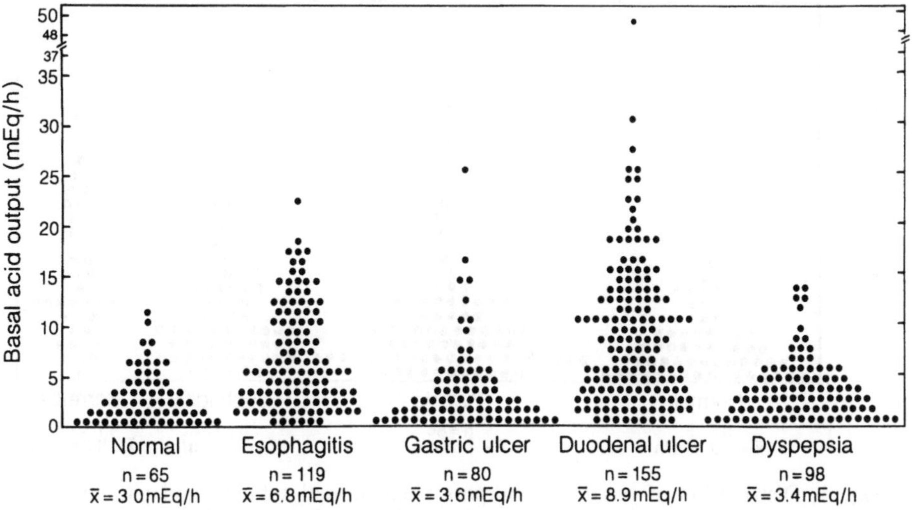

Fig. 3. Distribution of basal acid outputs from normal subjects and patients with erosive esophagitis, gastric ulcers, duodenal ulcers, and nonulcer dyspepsia

definition for idiopathic gastric acid hypersecretion, which is a basal acid output between 8.4 and 11.1 mEq/h.

It may be that a basal acid output of greater than 10 mEq/h is too low for the definition of gastric acid hypersecretion for Zollinger-Ellison syndrome and other gastric acid hypersecretory states in which there is a "marker" for the disease; however, since there is no "marker" for idiopathic gastric acid hypersecretion and since the statistical definition and the functional definition coincide, I feel that idiopathic gastric acid hypersecretion should be defined as a basal acid output of greater than 10 mEq/h. As will be pointed out later in this chapter, that definition for idiopathic gastric acid hypersecretion has tremendous clinical application in that a basal acid output of greater than 10 mEq/h clearly identifies all patients who will have refractory duodenal ulcers (Collen et al. 1987b, 1989d, 1991) when treated with standard doses of antisecretory medication and will also identify many patients with gastroesophageal reflux disease (Collen et al. 1990) who will be refractory to standard doses of antisecretory medication.

D. Diseases Associated with Idiopathic Gastric Acid Hypersecretion

A basal acid output of greater than 10 mEq/h is found in all aspects of acid-peptic disease irrespective of the degree of symptoms and/or mucosal disease (Fig. 3). The highest basal acid outputs and the highest percent of

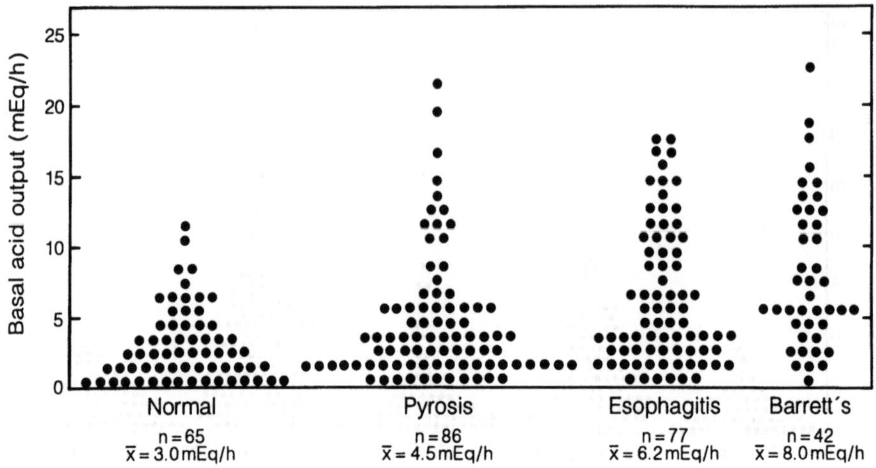

Fig. 4. Distribution of basal acid outputs from normal subjects and patients with pyrosis, erosive esophagitis, and Barrett's esophagus (COLLEN and GALLAGHER 1990)

hypersecretion are found in patients with duodenal ulcers; however, elevated basal acid outputs and hypersecretion are quite common in patients with gastroesophageal reflux disease (mainly esophagitis with or without Barrett's esophagus). There is very little hypersecretion found in patients with gastric ulcers, and patients with nonulcer dyspepsia have basal acid outputs similar to those of normal subjects.

I. Gastroesophageal Reflux Disease

The distribution of basal acid outputs from patients with gastroesophageal reflux disease are shown in Fig. 4. Basal acid outputs and the amount of hypersecretion increase with the severity of the gastroesophageal reflux disease (COLLEN and GALLAGHER 1990). Esophagitis and Barrett's esophagus have the highest basal acid outputs and the most gastric acid hypersecretion, and that accounts for the poor response of more severe esophagitis to treatment with standard antisecretory medication (COLLEN et al. 1990).

II. Duodenal Ulcer Disease

The highest basal acid outputs and most gastric acid hypersecretion (41%) are found in patients with duodenal ulcer disease (Fig. 3). Patients with bleeding duodenal ulcers have higher basal acid outputs and more hypersecretion than nonbleeding ulcers (63% and 39% hypersecretion respectively, $P < 0.002$) (COLLEN et al. 1991). The amount of gastric acid hypersecretion found in patients with bleeding duodenal ulcers accounts for the refractoriness to standard antisecretory medication.

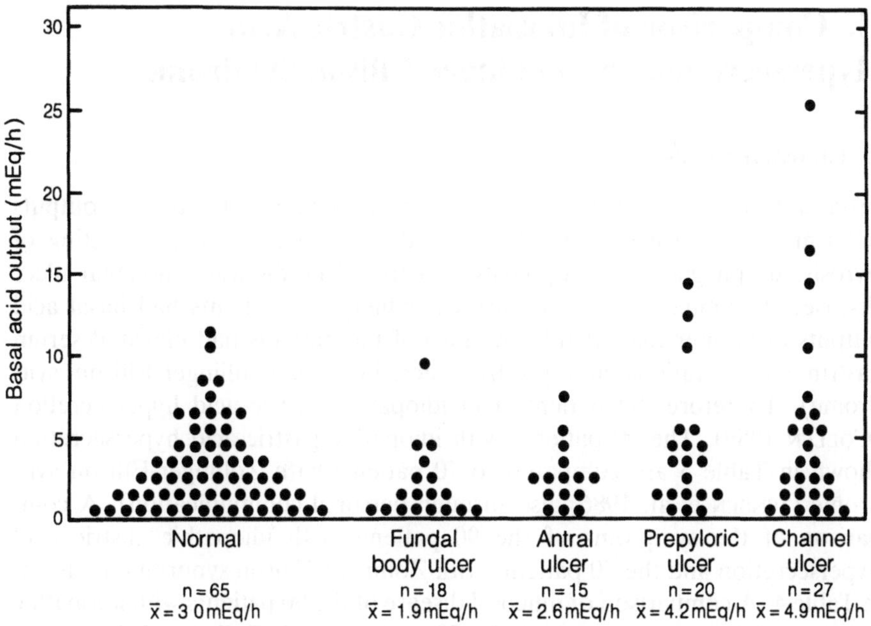

Fig. 5. Distribution of basal acid outputs from normal subjects and patients with gastric ulcers located in the body/fundus, antrum, prepyloric area, or gastric channel

III. Gastric Ulcer Disease

Basal acid outputs for all patients with gastric ulcers are similar to those for normal subjects (Fig. 3). As the gastric ulcer is located nearer the pyloris, basal acid outputs tend to be higher and more hypersecretion is found; however, basal acid outputs are never in the range for patients with duodenal ulcers (Figs. 5) (Collen et al. 1987b). From the acid secretory profiles, it appears that prepyloric gastric ulcers and channel gastric ulcers are different from duodenal ulcers (Figs. 3, 5). Many studies in the literature have previously included prepyloric and channel ulcers with duodenal ulcers, but from the acid secretory profiles it appears that they should be evaluated separately.

IV. Nonulcer Dyspepsia

Patients with nonulcer dyspepsia have basal acid outputs similar to normal subjects (Fig. 3) (Collen and Loebenberg 1989; Collen 1990). Also the distribution of basal acid outputs for patients with nonulcer dyspepsia with and without duodenitis is similar (Collen and Loebenberg 1989). Previously, duodenitis was considered to be a spectrum of duodenal ulcer disease; however, according to the acid secretory profiles, it does not appear that nonulcer dyspepsia with or without duodenitis and duodenal ulcer disease are a spectrum of the same acid-peptic process.

E. Comparison of Idiopathic Gastric Acid Hypersecretion and Zollinger-Ellison Syndrome

I. Characteristics

From January 1985 to January 1989, there were 619 basal acid outputs determined for problems which included esophageal disease consisting of pyrosis, dysphagia, and esophagitis, gastric ulcer disease, duodenal ulcer disease, abdominal pain, and diarrhea. Ninety-two patients had basal acid outputs of greater than 10 mEq/h. Two of the patients had elevated serum gastrin concentrations and positive secretin tests (Zollinger-Ellison syndrome). Therefore, 90 patients had idiopathic gastric acid hypersecretion (COLLEN 1989). The 90 patients with idiopathic gastric acid hypersecretion shown in Table 3 are compared to 70 patients with Zollinger-Ellison syndrome (JENSEN et al. 1986, also through personal communication). A comparison of the symptoms of the 90 patients with idiopathic gastric acid hypersecretion and the 70 patients with Zollinger-Ellison syndrome is shown in Table 4. A comparison of mucosal disease of the 90 patients with idiopathic gastric acid hypersecretion and the 70 patients with Zollinger-Ellison syndrome is shown in Table 5. It appears from the data that the major difference between patients with idiopathic gastric acid hypersecretion and patients with Zollinger-Ellison syndrome is the significant elevation of basal acid outputs found in patients with Zollinger-Ellison syndrome (Table 3). That most likely accounts for the significant amount of diarrhea found in Zollinger-Ellison syndrome patients (Table 4).

Of the 90 patients with idiopathic gastric acid hypersecretion, 42 (47%) required standard doses of ranitidine 300 mg/day for adequate treatment. The mean basal acid output for that group was 14.0 mEq/h (range 10.1–27.9 mEq/h). Patients who did not respond were given increased doses of ranitidine

Table 3. Characteristics of the 90 patients with idiopathic gastric acid hypersecretion and the 70 patients with Zollinger-Ellison syndrome (COLLEN 1989; JENSEN et al. 1986)

Characteristics	Idiopathic gastric acid hypersecretion	Zollinger-Ellison syndrome
Sex (M/F)	74/16	45/25
(% males)	82	64
Age at diagnosis (years)	45	45
(range)	(19–77)	(19–68)
Family history of acid-peptic disease (%)	21	21
Basal acid output (mEq/h)[a]	15.3	53
(range)	(10.1–49.1)	(9–150)

[a] Significantly different ($P < 0.001$).

Table 4. Comparison of symptoms of the 90 patients with idiopathic gastric acid hypersecretion and the 70 patients with Zollinger-Ellison syndrome (COLLEN 1989; JENSEN et al. 1986)

Characteristics	Idiopathic gastric acid hypersecretion	Zollinger-Ellison syndrome
Age at onset (years)	32	41
(range)	(11–77)	(15–64)
Duration before diagnosis (years)	13	4
(range)	(0–45)	(0–19)
Initial (%)		
Abdominal pain	66	–
Diarrhea (alone)	8 (2)	–
Esophageal disease (alone)	49 (19)	–
At some time (%)		
Abdominal pain	69	72
Diarrhea (alone)[a]	13	64 (35)
Esophageal disease	52	45

[a] Significantly different ($P < 0.001$).

Table 5. Comparison of muscosal disease in the 90 patients with idiopathic gastric acid hypersecretion and the 70 patients with Zollinger-Ellison syndrome (COLLEN 1989; JENSEN et al. 1986)

Characteristics	Idiopathic gastric acid hypersecretion	Zollinger-Ellison syndrome
Age at onset (years)	38	–
(range)	(16–77)	
Duration before diagnosis (years)	7	–
(range)	(0–41)	
Initial (%)		
Duodenal ulcer	57	–
Gastric ulcer	3	–
Esophageal disease (alone)	24 (20)	–
At some time (%)		
Duodenal ulcer	59	76
Gastric ulcer	6	2
Esophageal disease	31	43

every 12 h. Gastric analysis by nasogastric suction was determined the hour before the next dose of ranitidine, which was the 12th hour post drug. When only symptoms were present, each patient was given enough ranitidine to treat symptoms. With duodenal or gastric ulcer disease, each was given enough ranitidine to reduce gastric acid secretion to less than 10 mEq/h for the hour before the next dose. That level of inhibition of gastric acid secretion was selected because previous studies in patients with Zollinger-Ellison syndrome and other gastric acid hypersecretory states with basal acid outputs of greater than 10 mEq/h have shown that reduction of gastric acid secretion to less than 10 mEq/h allows healing of acid-peptic disease and prevents further acid-peptic complications (RAUFMAN et al. 1983; COLLEN et al. 1984). With esophageal disease, each patient was given enough ranitidine to reduce gastric acid secretion to less than 1 mEq/h for the hour before the next dose. That level of inhibition of gastric acid secretion was selected because in patients with Zollinger-Ellison syndrome and other gastric acid hypersecretory states with basal acid outputs of greater than 10 mEq/h it has previously been shown that reduction of gastric acid secretion to less than 1 mEq/h appears crucial to the successful treatment of gastroesophageal reflux disease (COLLEN et al. 1990, MILLER et al. 1990). Of the 90 patients with idiopathic gastric acid hypersecretion, 48 (53%) required increased doses of ranitidine. Mean ranitidine dose was 925 mg/day (range 600–1800 mg/day). Mean basal acid output was 16.4 mEq/h (range 10.1–49.1 mEq/h). There was no significant difference in mean basal acid output between the patients with idiopathic gastric acid hypersecretion who responded to standard therapy and those who required increased doses of ranitidine. There were no side-effects or biochemical toxicity with any of the patients who were taking increased doses of ranitidine. Some of the patients have been treated with large doses of ranitidine for as long as 4 years.

The above data show that 15% of patients with acid-peptic related diseases have gastric acid hypersecretion defined as a basal acid output of greater than 10 mEq/h. Also, symptoms and/or mucosal disease are similar between idiopathic gastric acid hypersecretion and Zollinger-Ellison syndrome except for diarrhea, which is more common in patients with Zollinger-Ellison syndrome. Furthermore, 53% of patients with idiopathic gastric acid hypersecretion required increased doses of standard medication to treat symptoms and/or mucosal disease. On the basis of these data I would like to reiterate that since Zollinger-Ellison syndrome is an infrequent cause of gastric acid hypersecretion (less than 1%), and since patients with idiopathic gastric acid hypersecretion can have symptoms and/or mucosal disease similar to Zollinger-Ellison syndrome, gastric analysis which determines basal acid output and not serum gastrin concentration is the test of choice when evaluating patients with refractory acid-peptic disease.

II. Basal Acid Output, Maximal Acid Output, and Basal Acid Output/Maximal Acid Output Ratio

Basal and maximal gastric acid hypersecretion in Zollinger-Ellison syndrome are caused by a gastrin-secreting tumor. The increased maximal acid output is attributed to increased parietal cell mass and the increased basal acid output/maximal acid output ratio of greater than 0.6 is attributed to increased basal stimulation.

Table 6. Basal acid output (BAO), maximal acid output (MAO), and basal acid output/maximal acid output (BAO/MAO) ratio in normal subjects (NS) and patients with idiopathic gastric acid hypersecretion (IGAH) or Zollinger-Ellison syndrome (ZES) (COLLEN et al. 1988c)

	BAO (mEq/h)		MAO (mEq/h)		BAO/MAO ratio	
Group	Mean ± SD	Range	Mean ± SD	Range	Mean ± SD	Range
NS	3.4 ± 3.0	0.0–10.4	19.3 ± 10.3	0.2–43.3	0.16 ± 0.14	0.00–0.51
IGAH[a]	16.6 ± 7.5	10.1–49.1	39.9 ± 14.7	14.2–96.4	0.44 ± 0.18	0.20–0.99
ZES	62.4 ± 36.0	13.0–150.0	75.5 ± 39.4	19.0–150.0	0.84 ± 0.14	0.54–1.00

[a] There was a significant difference in BAO, MAO, and BAO/MAO ratio between the patients with IGAH and both the NS ($P < 0.001$) and the patients with ZES ($P < 0.001$).

Maximal acid output and basal acid output/maximal acid output ratio in patients with idiopathic gastric acid hypersecretion were compared to those in 22 normal subjects and 12 patients with Zollinger-Ellison syndrome who were previously reported (COLLEN et al. 1984, 1988c). Table 6 shows basal acid outputs, maximal acid outputs, and basal acid output/maximal acid output ratios in all subjects. Of the 38 patients with idiopathic gastric acid hypersecretion, 24 (63%) had their maximal acid outputs in the range of the normal subjects. There was a significant correlation between basal acid output and maximal acid output in the 38 patients with idiopathic gastric acid hypersecretion ($r = 0.62$, $P < 0.001$).

The interesting finding is that mean maximal acid output and mean basal acid output/maximal acid output ratio of the patients with idiopathic gastric acid hypersecretion were significantly higher than in the normal subjects. The interpretation is that like Zollinger-Ellison syndrome, idiopathic gastric acid hypersecretion is associated with increased parietal cell mass and increased basal stimulation. Previously, idiopathic gastric acid hypersecretion was attributed to increased vagal tone (FELDMAN et al. 1980); however, if there is an increased parietal cell mass in patients with idiopathic gastric acid hypersecretion, as alluded to by the data, then there must be some growth factor (i.e., gastrin-like) that is causing an increased parietal cell mass and increased basal stimulation.

F. *Helicobacter pylori* Associated with Idiopathic Gastric Acid Hypersecretion

Helicobacter pylori has been found in the gastric antrum in 80%–90% of most patients with duodenal ulcers (RAUWS et al. 1988) but in less than 50% of patients with Zollinger-Ellison syndrome with duodenal ulcers (FICH et al. 1989). In contrast, *H. pylori* has been found in less than 40% of many patients with nonduodenal ulcer acid-peptic disease such as gastroesophageal reflux disease (PAULL and YARDLEY 1988). The difference between patients with Zollinger-Ellison syndrome with duodenal ulcers and other groups of patients with duodenal ulcers has been attributed to the high level of gastric acid hypersecretion in patients with Zollinger-Ellison syndrome, in that patients with Zollinger-Ellison syndrome almost always have basal acid outputs of greater than 15 mEq/h (JENSEN et al. 1983). If the decrease in *H. pylori* found in Zollinger-Ellison syndrome is due to gastric acid hypersecretion, then there should be less *H. pylori* found in other gastric acid hypersecretory states.

Twenty-nine patients with idiopathic gastric acid hypersecretion were investigated for *H. pylori* (COLLEN et al. 1989a). Fourteen patients had duodenal ulcer disease and 15 patients had nonduodenal ulcer acid-peptic disease, including five patients with Barrett's esophagus with esophagitis, four patients with esophagitis, two patients with pyrosis, two patients with diarrhea, one patient with nausea and vomiting, and one patient with

Table 7. Characteristics of 29 patients with idiopathic gastric acid hypersecretion with either positive or negative CLO tests (COLLEN et al. 1989a)

Characteristics	Duodenal ulcer disease	Nonduodenal ulcer acid-peptic disease
Sex (M/F)	12/2	10/5
Age (years)	41 ± 14	48 ± 15
Mean ranitidine dose (mg/day)*	643	1592
(range)	(300–1500)	(300–2700)
Basal acid output (mEq/h)	16.9 ± 6.1[a]	14.3 ± 2.8[a]
(range)	(10.1–30.3)	(10.1–19.9)
Positive CLO test**	12 (86%)	2 (13%)

* Significantly different ($P < 0.001$); ** significantly different ($P < 0.0001$).
[a] Mean ± 1 standard deviation.

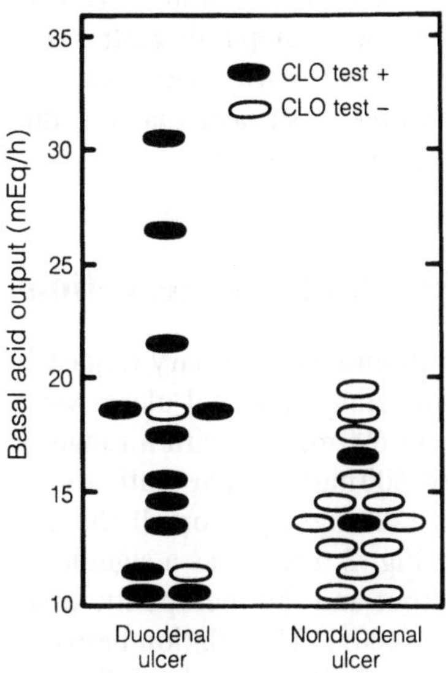

Fig. 6. Distribution of basal acid outputs from the 14 patients with duodenal ulcer disease and the 15 patients with nonduodenal ulcer acid-peptic disease (COLLEN et al. 1989a)

dyspepsia. The CLO test was used to determine the presence of *H. pylori*. The CLO test detects the presence of urease produced by *H. pylori*. It has been shown to have a sensitivity and specificity of about 90% (SCHNELL and SCHUBERT 1989). A comparison of the two groups is shown in Table 7. Fig. 6 illustrates the distribution of basal acid outputs for the patients with duodenal ulcer disease and nonduodenal ulcer acid-peptic disease. The distribution of basal acid outputs for the patients with duodenal ulcer disease and nonduodenal ulcer acid-peptic disease are similar. Eight patients with duodenal ulcer disease and five patients with nonduodenal ulcer acid-peptic disease had basal acid outputs of greater than 15 mEq/h, which is the level of basal acid output found in patients with Zollinger-Ellison syndrome. Seven of the eight patients with duodenal ulcer disease with basal acid outputs of greater than 15 mEq/h had positive CLO tests, while only one of the five patients with nonduodenal ulcer acid-peptic disease with basal acid outputs of greater than 15 mEq/h had a positive CLO test. Furthermore, the three patients with the highest basal acid outputs, which were all greater than 20 mEq/h, had duodenal ulcer disease with positive CLO tests. In addition, there was no significant difference in mean basal acid outputs when comparing all patients with positive CLO tests and all patients with negative CLO tests.

From the following data, it was found that 86% of patients with idiopathic gastric acid hypersecretion with duodenal ulcers had *H. pylori* in the gastric antrum, which is similar to other groups of patients with duodenal ulcers. This was in marked contrast to patients with Zollinger-Ellison syndrome with duodenal ulcers, who have been reported to have a significantly lower percent of *H. pylori* in the gastric antrum. The difference might be attributed to the higher level of gastric acid hypersecretion in patients with Zollinger-Ellison syndrome. However, because many of the patients with idiopathic gastric acid hypersecretion with duodenal ulcers had levels of gastric acid secretion similar to patients with Zollinger-Ellison syndrome, I suspect that the difference is secondary to other factors such as hypergastrinemia.

G. Therapy for Idiopathic Gastric Acid Hypersecretion

As shown in Fig. 2, refractory duodenal ulcer disease is secondary to gastric acid hypersecretion. The 23 patients with nonhealing duodenal ulcers were treated with increased doses of ranitidine, mean 690 mg/day with a range of 600–1200 mg/day. Seventeen patients required 600 mg/day, five patients required 900 mg/day, and one patient required 1200 mg/day. For all the 110 patients with duodenal ulcer disease shown in Fig. 2, there was a significant correlation between the level of basal acid output and the therapeutic daily dose of antisecretory medication ($r = 0.68$, $P < 0.001$). The relation between basal acid output and daily ranitidine dose was best fit by the following equation: daily ranitidine dose = 67 + 33 × basal acid output. The criterion used to treat refractory duodenal ulcer disease is the same criterion that was established for treating Zollinger-Ellison syndrome (Raufman et al. 1983). That criterion consists of giving patients with gastric acid hypersecretion enough antisecretory medication to reduce postdrug gastric acid secretion to a level of less than 10 mEq/h for the hour before the next dose of medication. That level of inhibition of gastric acid secretion was selected because previous studies in patients with Zollinger-Ellison syndrome and other gastric acid hypersecretory states with basal acid outputs of greater than 10 mEq/h have shown that reduction of gastric acid secretion to less than 10 mEq/h allows healing of acid-peptic disease and prevents further acid-peptic complications (Raufman et al. 1983; Collen et al. 1984). For all duodenal ulcers treated that criterion was utilized.

As previously mentioned, patients with bleeding duodenal ulcers have signficantly more gastric acid hypersecretion (63% vs 39%) than nonbleeders. This is probably the reason why patients with bleeding duodenal ulcers have significantly more refractory disease and often rebleed when treated with standard doses of antisecretory medication (COLLEN et al. 1991).

Not only are the acid secretory data different for gastric ulcer disease compared to duodenal ulcer disease, but it appears that there is no difference in basal acid outputs between patients with refractory gastric ulcers and those with gastric ulcers that heal in 8 weeks during treatment with standard doses of antisecretory medication (COLLEN et al. 1988c). Also, it was found that not all gastric ulcers healed after increasing the dose of antisecretory medication for an additional 8 weeks. This was in marked contrast to duodenal ulcer disease, in that when patients with refractory duodenal ulcers were given enough antisecretory medication to reduce gastric acid secretion to less than 10 mEq/h for the hour before the next dose of medication, all duodenal ulcers healed during an additional 8 weeks of increased doses of antisecretory medication (COLLEN et al. 1987c, 1989d, 1991). These data are supported by reports of others (HUNT et al. 1986; JONES et al. 1987) that the rate and degree of healing of duodenal ulcers are proportionate to the potency of antisecretory medication. They also found that in contrast, with gastric ulcer disease, there was no correlation between potency of antisecretory medication and healing of gastric ulcers (HUNT et al. 1986; HOWDEN et al. 1988). However, from the present data (COLLEN et al. 1991) it was found that in patients with prepyloric gastric ulcers or channel gastric ulcers who had gastric acid hypersecretion, gastric ulcers often healed with an additional 8 weeks of antisecretory medication after increasing the dose. Possibly, those patients had refractory gastric ulcers secondary to gastric acid hypersecretion.

Gastroesophageal reflux disease is another acid-peptic condition that responds to increasing the dose of antisecretory medication. As shown in Fig. 4, there is significant gastric acid hypersecretion in all degrees of gastroesophageal reflux disease (i.e., pyrosis, esophagitis, Barrett's esophagus). However, in marked contrast to duodenal ulcer disease, when treating gastroesophageal reflux disease, gastric acid secretion has to be significantly reduced. In a study (COLLEN et al. 1990) in which 23 patients with gastroesophageal reflux disease were treated with standard doses of ranitidine (300 mg/day), 12 of the patients had refractory reflux disease. In order to achieve complete disappearance of symptoms and heal esophagitis, doses had to be increased to as much as 1800 mg/day. The mean dose of the 12 patients was 1280 mg/day: two patients responded to doubling the dose (600 mg/day) while the remaining ten patients required three to six times the usual ulcer healing dose (300 mg/day). Nine of the 12 patients (75%) had gastric acid hypersecretion accounting for the refractory gastroesophageal reflux disease (Fig. 7). Of the 23 patients treated, 11 had underlying columnar epithelium (Barrett's esophagus). Ten of the 11 patients did not respond to standard doses of ranitidine (300 mg/day), which supports other studies in

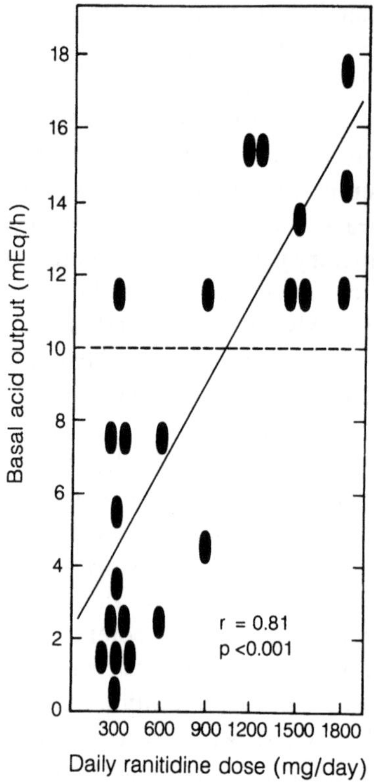

Fig. 7. Basal acid output versus daily ranitidine dose in 23 patients treated for gastroesophageal reflux disease (Collen et al. 1990)

that patients with more severe esophageal disease secondary to gastroesophageal reflux do not respond to standard doses of antisecretory medication (Hetzel et al. 1988; Koelz et al. 1986). There was a significant correlation between daily ranitidine dose required to eliminate gastroesophageal reflux symptoms and basal acid output (Fig. 7). The relation between basal acid output and daily ranitidine dose was best fit by the following equation: daily ranitidine dose = −221 + 100 × basal acid output. Based on the results of that study, when acid hypersecretion was identified, doses of ranitidine often had to be increased by two fold to six fold for clinical and statistically significant healing and symptomatic relief of gastroesophageal reflux disease to be attained. The degree of acid suppression was directly correlated with symptomatic and endoscopic response in that study. In most patients, gastric acid secretion had to be reduced to less than 1 mEq/h the hour before the next dose of medication in order to achieve complete disappearance of all symptoms and healing of all mucosal disease (Fig. 8). That significant reduction was irrespective of the initial basal acid output and the degree of esophagitis. Reduction of gastric acid secretion to less than 1 mEq/h in patients with gastroesophageal reflux disease is crucial in order to have successful treatment, not only because of the near elimination of gastric acid in the refluxate but also because of the concomitant inactivation of pepsin at the higher pH values achieved. When present in the

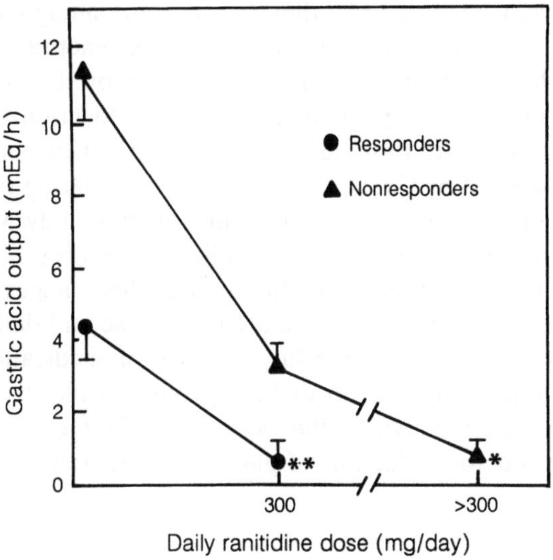

Fig. 8. Gastric acid output from 23 patients treated for gastroesophageal reflux disease showing the responders and nonresponders during no ranitidine therapy (basal state) and during therapy with ranitidine. Significantly different from no ranitidine therapy: $^{*}P < 0.001$; $^{**}P < 0.01$ (COLLEN et al. 1990)

refluxate, pepsin caused necrosis of esophageal mucosa only when the pH remained less than 4. Because near-total suppression of gastric acid is required in patients with gastroesophageal reflux disease compared to patients with duodenal ulcer disease, it is not surprising that a drug such as omeprazole that can completely abolish gastric acid secretion through the inhibition of H^+,K^+-ATPase has been shown to be superior to standard doses of H_2 receptor antagonists in the treatment of gastroesophageal reflux disease (VANTRAPPEN et al. 1988; SANDMARK et al. 1988).

Even though gastric acid secretory profiles in nonulcer dyspepsia are similar to normal (Fig. 3), basal acid output does identify the patients with nonulcer dyspepsia with or without duodenitis who have gastric acid hypersecretion and whose nonulcer dyspepsia symptoms may respond to increased doses of antisecretory medication (COLLEN 1990). Nonulcer dyspepsia in general is most likely not an acid-peptic condition; however, patients with nonulcer dyspepsia with concomitant gastric acid hypersecretion often respond to increased doses of H_2 receptor antagonists (COLLEN 1990).

With most of the data from patients with idiopathic gastric acid hypersecretion presented in this chapter, ranitidine was used either in standard doses or increased doses; however, from previous experience I suspect that similiar results would have been attained with other H_2 receptor antagonists (COLLEN et al. 1984; HOWARD et al. 1985). In patients with gastric acid hypersecretion, including Zollinger-Ellison syndrome, irrespective of the H_2 receptor antagonists used for treatment (i.e., cimetidine, ranitidine, famotidine), those who required increased doses of one H_2 receptor antagonist also required increased doses of other H_2 receptor antagonists to reduce gastric acid secretion. This is in contrast to doses of omeprazole required to treat patients with idiopathic gastric acid hypersecretion. Unlike H_2 receptor antagonists, the dose of omeprazole required for reduction of gastric acid secretion does not correlate with the dose of ranitidine (COLLEN et al. 1989b). The dose ranges studied by COLLEN et al. were up to 1800 mg ranitidine daily and up to 60 mg omeprazole daily. The results of that study were similar to the findings in a group of patients with Zollinger-Ellison syndrome treated with omeprazole (MATON et al. 1989). In the same dose ranges, there was no correlation between daily ranitidine maintenance dose and daily omeprazole maintenance dose. However, when larger doses of medication were used (up to 10 g ranitidine daily and up to 120 mg omeprazole daily), there was a significant correlation between the dose of ranitidine and the dose of omeprazole required for reduction of gastric acid secretion (MATON et al. 1989).

H. Other Data on Idiopathic Gastric Acid Hypersecretion

I. Basal Acid Output in Children

Basal acid outputs in children, aged 2–18 years, are similar to those in adult subjects (COLLEN et al. 1988b). When 28 pediatric patients with atypical recurrent abdominal pain were compared to a group of adult patients with nonulcer dyspepsia, basal acid outputs were similar. There was no significant correlation between basal acid output and body weight. Of the 28 children studied, there were seven with acid-peptic mucosal disease who were treated with ranitidine. Gastric acid hypersecretion was found in an 11-year-old child with erosive esophagitis and a basal acid output of 14.1 mEq/h who did not respond to standard H_2 antagonist therapy. Children with hypersecretion who do not respond to standard doses of H_2 receptor antagonists often respond when the doses are increased. The above-mentioned child became asymptomatic with complete healing of the esophagitis when treated with increased doses.

II. Basal Acid Output in Other Disorders

Gastric acid hypersecretion has been found in other disorders such as hereditary angioedema (COLLEN et al. 1989c). When 21 patients were investigated, five were found to have gastric acid hypersecretion, of whom three had refractory abdominal pain to standard treatment for angioedema that was subsequently found to be caused by acid-peptic disease. When the three patients were treated with increased doses of ranitidine, all symptoms disappeared and mucosal disease healed.

I feel that any disease that has an acid-peptic component can be associated with idiopathic gastric acid hypersecretion. Zollinger-Ellison syndrome, which is a disease associated with basal acid hypersecretion, has symptoms and mucosal disease secondary to gastric acid hypersecretion. Interestingly, the main mucosal diseases associated with Zollinger-Ellison syndrome are gastroesphageal reflux disease with erosive esophagitis and duodenal ulcer (Table 5). Both gastroesophageal reflux disease and duodenal ulcer disease are associated with idiopathic gastric acid hypersecretion (Table 5); however, a disease such as gastric ulcer disease which has much less idiopathic gastric acid hypersecretion is very rarely found in Zollinger-Ellison syndrome. Even prepyloric gastric ulcers and channel gastric ulcers are rarely found in Zollinger-Ellison syndrome.

J. Conclusions

Idiopathic gastric acid hypersecretion is quite common in the acid-peptic disorders in which acid appears to be the primary component of injury, i.e., gastroesophageal reflux disease and duodenal ulcer disease. This is substantiated by the fact that patients with Zollinger-Ellison syndrome get primarily esophageal disease and duodenal ulcer disease. Gastric ulcer disease and nonulcer dyspepsia are associated with much less gastric acid hypersecretion.

The disorders that are associated with gastric acid hypersecretion respond consistently to increased doses of antisecretory medication, and if they are associated with refractory symptoms and/or mucosal disease when treated with standard doses of antisecretory medication, then gastric acid hypersecretion appears to be the reason for the refractoriness. This has been shown in essentially all patients with duodenal ulcer disease and most patients with gastroesophageal reflux disease. These patients respond to increased doses of antisecretory medication (i.e., H_2 receptor antagonists) and more potent antisecretory medication such as the H^+,K^+-ATPase inhibitors (e.g., omeprazole). That is the reason a disorder such as gastric ulcer disease that is not associated with gastric acid hypersecretion is much less affected by more potent antisecretory medication.

It can be seen that idiopathic gastric acid hypersecretion is a much more common disorder than Zollinger-Ellison syndrome. And from the previous discussion, it is quite apparent that when one wishes to evaluate a patient for gastric acid hypersecretion, gastric analysis which evaluates basal acid output and not serum gastrin concentration is the test of choice.

References

Baron JH (1981) When should a clinician perform gastric analysis? J Clin Gastroenterol 3:87–89

Cochran WG, Snedecor GW (1980) Statistical methods, 7th edn. Iowa State University Press, Ames

Collen MJ (1989) Idiopathic gastric acid hypersecretory states (Abstr). Gastroenterology 96:93

Collen MJ (1990) Gastric analysis (basal acid output) in nonulcer dyspepsia (Letter). Dig Dis Sci 35:540–541

Collen MJ, Gallagher JE (1990) Basal acid output and gastric acid hypersecretion in patients with gastroesophageal reflux disease (Abstr). Gastroenterology 98:32

Collen MJ, Loebenberg MJ (1989) Basal gastric acid secretion in nonulcer dyspepsia with or without duodenitis. Dig Dis Sci 34:246–250

Collen MJ, Sheridan MJ (1991) Definition for idiopathic gastric acid hypersecretion: A statistical and functional evaluation. Dig Dis Sci (in press)

Collen MJ, Johnson DA (1991) Correlation between basal acid output and daily ranitidine dose required for therapy in Barrett's esophagus. Dis Sci (in press)

Collen MJ, Howard JM, McArthur KE, Raufman J-P, Cornelius MJ, Ciarleglio CA, Gardner JD, Jensen RT (1984) Comparison of ranitidine and cimetidine in the treatment of gastric acid hypersecretion. Ann Intern Med 100:52–58

Collen MJ, Stanczak VJ, Ciarleglio CA (1987a) Duodenal ulcer disease and gastric acid hypersecretion (Abstr). Gastroenterology 92:1351

Collen MJ, Stanczak VJ, Ciarleglio CA (1987b) Basal acid output in patients with gastric ulcer disease (Abstr). Gastroenterology 92:135

Collen MJ, Stanczak VJ, Ciarleglio CA (1987c) Basal acid output in patients with refractory duodenal ulcer disease (Abstr). Gastroenterology 92:135

Collen MJ, Ciarleglio CA, Stanczak VJ, Benjamin SB (1988a) Refractory gastric ulcers and basal acid output (Abstr). Am J Gastroenterol 83:1031

Collen MJ, Ciarleglio CA, Stanczak VJ, Treem WR, Lewis JH (1988b) Basal gastric acid secretion in children with atypical epigastric pain. Am J Gastroenterol 83:923–926

Collen MJ, Stanczak VJ, Ciarleglio CA (1988c). Maximal acid output in patients with idiopathic gastric acid hypersecretion (Abstr). Gastroenterology 94:73

Collen MJ, Gallagher JE, Demissie E, Lewis JH (1989a). *Campylobacter pylori* in duodenal ulcer patients with idiopathic gastric acid hypersecretion (Abstr). Am J Gastroenterol 84:156

Collen MJ, LaMont B, Benjamin SB, Berlin RG (1989b) Inhibition of gastric acid secretion: no correlation between ranitidine and omeprazole (Abstr). Gastroenterology 96:94

Collen MJ, Lewis JH, Deschner WK, Ansher AF, Zurlo JJ, Benjamin SB, Frank MM (1989c) Abdominal pain in hereditary angioedema: the role of acid hypersecretion. Am J Gastroenterol 84:873–877

Collen MJ, Stanczak VJ, Ciarleglio CA (1989d). Refractory duodenal ulcers (nonhealing duodenal ulcers with standard doses of antisecretory medication). Dig Dis Sci 34:233–237

Collen MJ, Lewis JH, Benjamin SB (1990) Gastric acid hypersecretion in gastroesophageal reflux disease. Gastroenterology 98:654–661

Collen MJ, Kalloo AN, Lewis JH (1991). Bleeding duodenal ulcers: significant association with gastric acid hypersecretion. Dig Dis Sci (in press)

Feldman M (1979) Comparison of acid secretion rates measured by gastric aspiration and by in vivo intragastric titration in healthy human subjects. Gastroenterology 76:954–957

Feldman M, Richardson CT, Fordtran JS (1980) Effect of sham feeding on gastric acid secretion in healthy subjects and duodenal ulcer patients: evidence for increased basal vagal tone in some ulcer patients. Gastroenterology 79:796–800

Fich A, Talley NJ, Shorter RG, Phillips SF (1989) *Campylobacter pylori* in Zollinger-Ellison syndrome and chronic duodenal ulcer (Abstr). Am J Gastroenterol 84:1159

Fordtran JS, Walsh JH (1973) Gastric acid secretion rate and buffer content of the stomach after eating. Results in normal subjects and in patients with duodenal ulcer. J Clin Invest 52:645–657

Frucht H, Howard JM, Slaff JI, Wank SA, McCarthy DM, Maton PN, Vinayek R, Gardner JD, Jensen RT (1989) Secretin and calcium provocative tests in the Zollinger-Ellison syndrome: prospective study. Ann Intern Med 111:713–722

Gustavsson S, Adami H-O, Loof L, Nyberg A, Nyren O (1983) Rapid healing of duodenal ulcers with omeprazole: double-blind dose-comparative trial. Lancet 2:124–125

Hetzel DJ, Dent J, Reed WD, Narielvala FM, Mackinnon M, McCarthy JH, Mitchell B, Veberidge BR, Laurence BH, Gibson GG, Grant AK, Shearman JC, Whitehead R, Buckle PJ (1988) Healing and relapse of severe peptic esophagitis after treatment with omeprzaole. Gastroenterology 95:903–912

Howard JM, Chremos AN, Collen MJ, McArthur KE, Cherner JA, Maton PN, Ciarleglio CA, Cornelius MJ, Gardner JD, Jensen RT (1985) Famotidine, a new, potent, long-acting histamine H_2-receptor antagonist: comparison with cimetidine and ranitidine in the treatment of Zollinger-Ellison syndrome. Gastroenterology 88:1026–1033

Howden CW, Jones DB, Peace KE, Burget DW, Hunt RH (1988) The treatment of gastric ulcer with antisecretory drugs: relationship of pharmacological effect to healing rates. Dig Dis Sci 33:619–624

Hunt RH, Howden CW, Jones DB, Burget DW, Kerr GD (1986) The correlation between acid suppression and peptic ulcer healing. Scand J Gastroenterol [Suppl 125] 21:22–29

Jensen RT, Gardner JD, Raufman J-P, Pandol SJ, Doppman JL, Collen MJ (1983) Zollinger-Ellison syndrome – current concepts and management. Ann Intern Med 98:59–75

Jensen RT, Doppman JL, Gardner JD (1986) Gastrinoma. In: Go VLW, et al. (eds) The exocrine pancreas: biology, pathobiology and diseases. Raven, New York, pp 727–744

Jones DB, Howden CW, Burget DW, Kerr GD, Hunt RH (1987) Acid suppression in duodenal ulcer: a meta-analysis to define optimal dosing with antisecretory drugs. Gut 28:1120–1127

Kirkpatrick PM, Hirschowitz BI (1980) Duodenal ulcer with unexplained marked basal gastric acid hypersecretion. Gastroenterology 79:4–10

Koelz HR, Birchler A, Bretholz, Bron B, Capitaine Y, Delmore G, Fehr HF, Fumagalli I, Gehrig J, Gonvers JJ, Halter F, Hammer B, Kayasseh L, Kobler E, Miller G, Munst G, Pelloni S, Realini S, Schmid P, Voirol M, Blum AL (1986) Healing and relapse of reflux esophagitis during treatment with ranitidine. Gastroenterology 91:1198–1205

Malagelada J-R, Longstreth GF, Summerskill WHJ, Go VLW (1976) Measurement of gastric functions during digestion of ordinary solid meals in man. Gastroenterology 70:203–210

Maton PN, Vinayek R, Frucht H, McArthur KA, Miller LS, Saeed ZA, Gardner JD, Jensen RT (1989) Long-term efficacy and safety of omeprazole in patients with Zollinger-Ellison syndrome: a prospective study. Gastroenterology 97:827–836

McCarthy DM (1982) Zollinger-Ellison syndrome. Annu Rev Med 33:197–215

Miller LS, Vinayek R, Frucht H, Gardner JD, Jensen RT, Maton PN (1990) Reflux esophagitis in patients with Zollinger-Ellison syndrome. Gastroenterology 98:341–346

Paull G, Yardley JH (1988) Gastric and esophageal *Campylobacter pylori* in patients with Barrett's esophagus. Gastroenterology 95:216–218

Raufman J-P, Collins SM, Korman LY, Pandol SJ, Collen MJ, Cornelius MJ, Feld MK, McCarthy DM, Gardner JD, Jensen RT (1983) Reliability of symptoms in assessing control of gastric acid secretion in patients with Zollinger-Ellison syndrome. Gastroenterology 84:108–113

Rauws EAJ, Wies L, Houthoff HJ, Zanen HC, Tytgat GNJ (1988) *Campylobacter pyloridis*-associated chronic active antral gastritis: a prospective study of its prevalance and the effects of antibacterial and antiulcer treatment. Gastroenterology 94:33–40

Sandmark S, Carlsson R, Fausa O, Lundell L (1988) Omeprazole or ranitidine in the treatment of reflux esophagitis: results of a double-blind, randomized, Scandinavian multicenter study. Scand J Gastroenterol 23:625–632

Schnell GA, Schubert TT (1989) Usefulness of culture, histology, and urease testing in the detection of *Campylobacter pylori*. Am J Gastroentol 84:133–137

Spindel E, Harty RF, Leibach JR, McGuigan JE (1986) Decision analysis in evaluation of hypergastrinemia. Am J Med 80:11–17

Vantrappen G, Rutgeerts L, Schurmans P, Coenegrachts JL (1988) Omeprazole (40 mg) is superior to ranitidine in short-term treatment of ulcerative reflux esophagitis. Dig Dis Sci 33:523–529

CHAPTER 13

Zollinger-Ellison Syndrome: Advances in Diagnosis and Management

L.S. MILLER, J.D. GARDNER, J. DOPPMAN, and R.T. JENSEN

A. Introduction

In 1955 ZOLLINGER and ELLISON described two patients with recurrent peptic ulceration, a marked increase in gastric acid secretion, and islet cell tumors. This triad of findings became known as the Zollinger-Ellison syndrome (ZES). ZOLLINGER and ELLISON (1955) suggested that this syndrome was caused by a circulating hormone released from the tumor, which also caused gastric acid hypersecretion. Subsequent studies showed large amounts of the hormone gastrin in the serum and in tumors of patients with ZES (GREGORY et al. 1969; MCGUIGAN and TRUDEAU 1969; STREMPLE and MEADE 1968). Because these tumors synthesize and release large amounts of gastrin they have been called gastrinomas.

B. Pathophysiology

The early clinical manifestations of ZES (peptic ulcers, diarrhea, esophageal disease) are secondary to hypersecretion of gastric acid, which is produced by the parietal cells of the stomach in response to excess amounts of circulating gastrin. Evidence for this includes marked increased acid production and therapeutic response to total gastrectomy and H_2 blockers (JENSEN et al. 1983b, 1986; ZOLLINGER et al. 1980; THOMPSON et al. 1975; BONFILS et al. 1981; ISENBERG et al. 1973). Patients late in the course of the disease, with metastatic gastrinoma or large primary gastrinomas, may develop symptoms due to effects of the tumor per se, such as pain or cachexia. The pathogenesis of the diarrhea in patients with ZES is due to a number of consequences of gastric acid hypersecretion, including small intestinal mucosal injury, inactivation of pancreatic lipase, and precipitation of bile acids (JENSEN et al. 1983b, 1986; MCGUIGAN 1978; ISENBERG et al. 1973).

The pathogenesis of the peptic ulcer disease and esophageal disease involves direct mucosal injury from the increased acid production. In addition to causing stimulation of secretion of hydrogen ions from gastric parietal cells, gastrin also produces trophic changes in the gastric mucosa (JOHNSON 1987; DEMBINSKI and JOHNSON 1979). One consequence of this trophic action is that gastrin causes an increase in the number of gastric parietal cells and thereby increases the maximal gastric acid secretory capacity (NEUBURGER et al. 1972; SUM and PEREY 1969).

In the circulation gastrin is found to exist in three different molecular sizes: 34 amino acids ("big gastrin" or G34), 17 amino acids ("little gastrin" or G17), and 13 amino acids ("mini gastrin" or G13). Each form can exist in two different states, sulfated or nonsulfated. The predominant form of gastrin in gastrinomas is heptadecapeptide gastrin (G17), whereas the major form of circulating gastrin in patients with gastrinoma is the larger form G34 (GREGORY et al. 1969; YALOW and BERSON 1970; REHFELD et al. 1974). Most circulating gastrin in normal subjects in the fasting state is also G34, whereas antral gastrin in both normal subjects and patients with ZES is predominantly G17 (approximately 90%–95%). There is more variability in the proportion of G17 to G34 in gastrinoma tissue than in antral mucosa, and, on the average, 60%–90% of gastrin in gastrinomas is G17 (CREUTZFELD et al. 1975; DOCKRAY et al. 1975; REHFELD et al. 1973; WALSH and GROSSMAN 1975). Gastrin release from a gastrinoma is not influenced by the physiological stimulation which normally causes gastrin release from the gastric antrum. However, gastrin release can be affected by a number of different stimuli. Secretin and increased serum calcium cause increased serum gastrin levels in patients with gastrinoma (DEVENEY et al. 1977; LAMERS and VAN TONGEREN 1979).

C. Clinical Features

It is estimated that ZES occurs in one patient per 100000 population in Denmark (STADIL and STAGE 1979), approximately 0.1% of patients with duodenal ulcer disease in the United States (GROSSMAN 1981), and 0.5 patients per year per million population in Ireland (BUCHANAN et al. 1986).

The clinical features of ZES reported in several studies are summarized in Table 1. ZES is slightly more common in males (60%) than in females (40%); the mean age of patients is 45–50 years and approximately 25% have multiple endocrine neoplasia, type I (MEN-I). Abdominal pain remains the most common initial symptom, with 90%–95% of patients developing peptic ulcer disease at some time during the course of the disease. The abdominal pain cannot be distinguished from that which occurs in patients with idiopathic peptic esophagitis or peptic ulcer disease. In recent studies, diarrhea and esophageal disease are being reported more frequently as initial manifestations of the disease (JENSEN et al. 1983b, 1986).

Changes in presenting symptoms are reflected by changes in radiological and endoscopic findings. In early studies up to 93% of patients had a peptic ulcer, and in 36% of patients the ulcers were multiple or in unusual locations (ELLISON and WILSON 1964). Although atypical ulcers, when present, strongly suggest the diagnosis, today most patients with ZES have typical duodenal ulcers, and 18%–25% of patients have no ulcer at the time of diagnosis (JENSEN et al. 1983). The changes in presenting symptoms and severity of

Table 1. Clinical features of patients with ZES

	Ellison and Wilson (1964)	Regan and Mialiage-Liadia (1978)	Mignon et al. (1986)	NIH (Jensen et al. 1986)
No. of patients	260	40	144	80
Multiple endocrine neoplasia, type I (%)	21	23	24	21
Mean duration of symptoms before diagnosis (years)	ND (53% = 1–4) (27% = >4)	6.5	ND	3.8
First symptoms (%)				
Abdominal pain	93	98	26	43
Pain and diarrhea	30	28	49	29
Diarrhea only	7	2	15	35
Dysphagia/pyrosis	0	0	ND	13
Mean age at onset	ND	50.5	47	45
Sex (% male)	60	60	68	64

ND, no data.

peptic disease suggest that patients with ZES are being diagnosed earlier. Nevertheless, in almost all series there is still a delay of 3–6 years between the onset of symptoms and the diagnosis (JENSEN et al. 1983, 1986).

In two studies (RICHTER et al. 1981; MILLER et al. 1990) esophageal involvement, symptoms, or endoscopic signs are demonstrated to be a more common manifestation of ZES than previously suspected. In one study the investigators found that 61% of patients with ZES had one or more manifestations of esophageal disease, an incidence much higher than previously reported in other large series (MILLER et al. 1990).

The findings of gastric rugal hypertrophy, multiple ulcers, or ulceration of the distal duodenum and jejunum, although nonspecific, should warrant an investigation for ZES (ISENBERG et al. 1973; JENSEN et al. 1983b). Evidence of MEN-I is found in 15%–26% of patients with ZES (ELLISON and WILSON 1964; BONFILS and BADER 1970; CAMERSON and HOFFMAN 1974; REGAN and MALAGELADA 1978; STAGE and STADIL 1979; JENSEN et al. 1983, 1986). MEN-I is characterized by tumors or hyperplasia of multiple endocrine organs, with hypercalcemia due to hyperparathyroidism being the most common abnormality (EBERLE and GRUN 1981). Functioning islet cell adenomas of the pancreas are the second most frequent abnormality, but the frequency of gastrin-producing adenomas is not well documented, although estimates range from 11% to 55% (EBERLE and GRUN 1981). Kindreds with MEN-I should be screened for ZES with serum gastrin determinations. Conversely, patients with ZES syndrome should be screened for MEN-I by measuring serum calcium concentrations and serum parathyroid hormone concentrations.

Although ZOLLINGER and ELLISON (1955) defined the syndrome named after them as a triad of "primary peptic ulceration in unusual locations," "gastric hypersecretion of gigantic proportion," and the "identification of nonspecific islet cell tumor of the pancreas," none of these three criteria is currently required for a diagnosis of this syndrome (WOLFE and JENSEN 1987). The major factor responsible for this change in diagnostic criteria of ZES is the development and availability of gastrin radioimmunoassays. In patients with ZES, serum gastrin is almost always elevated; however, patients with unequivocal ZES may rarely have gastrin levels in the normal range (20–100 pg/ml) (JENSEN et al. 1983b; WOLFE et al. 1985; THOMPSON et al. 1975). In addition, values may fluctuate from day to day (JENSEN et al. 1983; THOMPSON et al. 1975; MCGUIGAN and TRUDEAU 1969); therefore, serum gastrin levels should be obtained on different days.

Disorders that raise serum gastrin levels but do not increase gastric acid hypersecretion (pernicious anemia, chronic gastritis, gastric cancer, vagotomy, pheochromocytoma; see Table 2) need to be excluded by the use of gastric acid analysis.

The most generally used gastric secretory criterion for diagnosing ZES is a basal acid output (BAO) that exceeds 15 mEq/h in patients without previous acid-reducing operations (JENSEN et al. 1983b, 1986; AOYAGI and

Table 2. Conditions associated with hypergastrinemia

Normal or decreased gastric acid	Increased gastric acid
Pernicious anemia	ZES
	Retained gastric antrum
Chronic gastritis	Gastric outlet obstruction
Gastric cancer	Renal failure
Vagotomy	Antral G cell hyperfunction
Pheochromocytoma	Antral G cell hyperplasia
	Short bowel syndrome

SUMMERSKILL 1966). Maximal acid output is not a useful criterion for diagnosing ZES, because mean values frequently overlap with those of duodenal ulcer patients (JENSEN et al. 1983b, 1986; AOYAGI and SUMMERSKILL 1966; KAYE et al. 1970).

Patients with ZES as well as patients with other islet cell tumors may develop clinical manifestations of excess release of additional peptide hormones, or a secondary symptomatic islet cell tumor (BARDRAM and STAGE 1985; DAWSON et al. 1983; WYNICK et al. 1988). In a recent study 62% of patients with ZES had an elevated serum concentration of another peptide [usually pancreatic polypeptide (PP), motilin, neurotensin, or gastrin-releasing peptide (GRP) (CHIANG et al. 1990)]; however, in all cases elevations of these peptides were not associated with clinically relevant manifestations. In a prospective study only 2% of patients with ZES followed for a median time of 11 years after onset of the disease developed a symptomatic secondary peptide tumor (CHIANG et al. 1990). Furthermore, in immunocytochemical studies of gastrinomas, elevated levels of PP, glucagon, somatostatin, or adrenocorticotropic hormone (ACTH)/corticotropin-like intermediate lobe peptide (CLIP) have been reported in 10%–50% (JENSEN et al. 1986).

Increased serum ACTH levels with associated Cushing's syndrome have been noted in 8% of 75 patients with ZES (MATON et al. 1986). Three of the 59 patients (5%) with sporadic gastrinoma had Cushing's syndrome, with severe symptoms produced by ACTH secretion by the islet cell tumor. Each patient had metastatic gastrinoma, which responded poorly to chemotherapy, and each died within 3 years of the diagnosis. Three of 16 MEN-I patients (19%) with ZES had Cushing's syndrome consequent upon pituitary release of ACTH and, in general, their symptoms were mild. Gastrinomas in these patients were not metastatic and prognosis was excellent.

D. Provocative Tests

Many patients evaluated for ZES will have marginal elevations in gastrin levels and basal gastric acid values in ranges that overlap with other conditions (WALSH and GROSSMAN 1975; STAGE and STADIL 1979; ISENBERG et al.

1973; THOMPSON et al. 1975; AOYAGI and SUMMERSKILL 1966; KAYE 1970; BARON 1979; STRAUSS and YALOW 1975; MCGUIGAN and WOLFE 1980), including retained gastric antrum, gastric outlet obstruction, renal failure, antral G cell hyperfunction, antral G cell hyperplasia, and short bowel syndrome. Thus, various provocative tests have been developed to attempt to distinguish these conditions from ZES.

The intravenous secretin test is the most reliable and the easiest to perform. In patients with ZES, intravenous secretin causes a marked increase in serum gastrin, whereas in patients without ZES, secretin causes no change, a small increase, or a decrease in serum gastrin levels (ISENBERG et al. 1972; WALSH and GROSSMAN 1975; STAGE and STADIL 1979; BARON 1979; STRAUSS and YALOW 1975; MCGUIGAN and WOLFE 1980; LAMERS and VAN TONGEREN 1979; DEVENEY et al. 1977; FRUCHT et al. 1989a). The test is currently done by administering 2 clinical units/kg body weight of secretin (Kabi) by intravenous bolus and measuring serum gastrin levels 10 min and 1 min before, and 2, 5, 10, and 20 min after administration (SLAFF et al. 1986; MCGUIGAN and WOLFE 1980). More than 90% of patients with ZES will show a rise in serum gastrin levels, which is usually greatest at 2–5 min after administration (FRUCHT et al. 1989a; SLAFF et al. 1986) (Fig. 1). An absolute increase of 200 pg/ml in serum gastrin level is generally regarded as diagnostic and is the recommended criterion for diagnosis (SLAFF et al. 1986; MCGUIGAN and WOLFE 1980). Although false-positive responses have been reported in patients with achlorhydria (FELDMAN et al. 1987), these patients can be easily excluded from having ZES by measuring gastric pH or output, and thus do not require a secretin test.

The calcium infusion test involves administering calcium, 5 mg/kg body weight per hour for 3 h, usually as calcium gluconate, and measuring serum calcium and serum gastrin levels (WALSH and GROSSMAN 1975; MCGUIGAN 1978; STAGE and STADIL 1979; THOMPSON et al. 1975; STRAUSS and YALOW 1975; MCGUIGAN and WOLFE 1980; LAMERS and VAN TONGEREN 1979; DEVENEY 1977; FRUCHT et al. 1989a). In patients with ZES there is an increase of serum gastrin levels of >395 pg/ml (Fig. 1). This test has generally been replaced by the secretin test because of adverse reactions to calcium infusion and occasional false-negatives and false-positives (MCGUIGAN and WOLFE 1980; JENSEN et al. 1983b, 1986; FRUCHT et al. 1989a).

The gastrin response to a standard meal is helpful in differentiating ZES from antral G cell hyperfunction and hyperplasia (WOLFE and JENSEN 1987). One meal commonly used includes one slice of bread, 200 ml milk, 50 g cheese, and one boiled egg, corresponding to 30 g protein, 20 g fat, and 25 g carbohydrate (LAMERS et al. 1977). Blood samples are drawn for determination of serum gastrin at 1 min before and at 15, 30, 45, 60, 90, 120, and 150 min after the start of the meal (Fig. 1). Patients with ZES usually have less than a 100% increase in postprandial serum gastrin levels (MCGUIGAN 1978; STAGE and STADIL 1979; BARON 1979; DEVENEY et al. 1977; STRAUSS and YALOW 1975; MCGUIGAN and WOLFE 1980; LAMERS and VAN TONGEREN

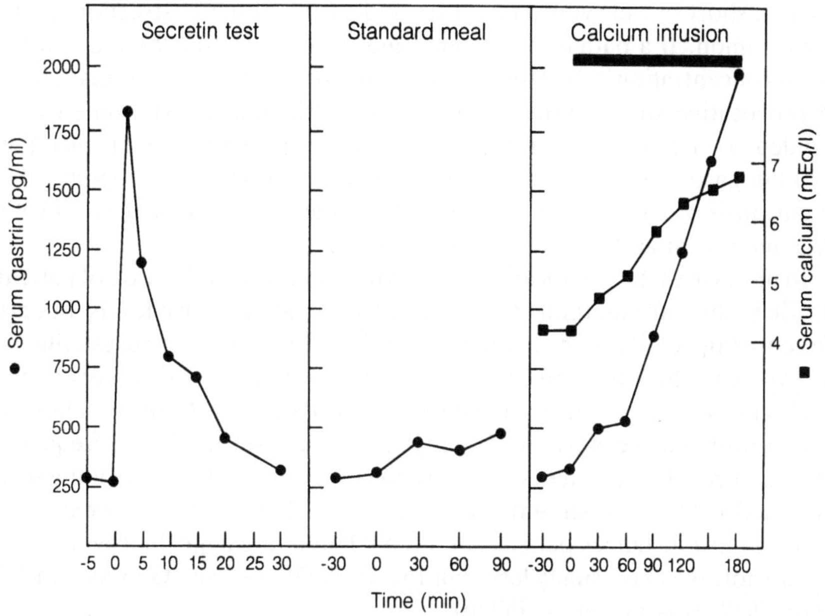

Fig. 1. Serum gastrin responses to different provocative tests in a patient with gastrinoma. Serum gastrin concentration was measured before and after an intravenous bolus injection of secretin (2 clinical units/kg of GIH secretin) (*left*), a standard meal consisting of 30 g protein, 20 g fat, and 25 g carbohydrate (*middle*), and an intravenous calcium infusion (5 mg calcium/kg body weight per hour for 3 h) (*right*). Serum calcium prior to and during the calcium infusion is shown in the *right panel*. (JENSEN et al. 1983b)

1979), but exaggerated responses have occasionally been reported (THOMPSON et al. 1975; DEVENEY et al. 1977; CREUTZFELDT et al. 1975; FRUCHT et al. 1989b). Patients with the syndromes of antral G cell hyperfunction and hyperplasia characteristically have a marked postprandial increase in serum gastrin (greater than 100%) (FRIESEN and TOMITA 1981; TAYLOR et al. 1981; WALSH and GROSSMAN 1975; GANGULI et al. 1974; LAMERS et al. 1978; BARON 1979).

Figure 1 summarizes the typical gastrin responses to various provocative tests in a patient with gastrinoma. No studies have evaluated whether H_2 receptor antagonists, with or without anticholinergic agents, change the pattern of response to any provocative tests.

E. Differential Diagnosis of Disorders with Increased Basal Acid Output and Increased Fasting Gastrin Concentration

Of the seven conditions listed in Table 2, in which gastric acid hypersecretion is secondary to hypergastrinemia (ZES, retained gastric antrum, gastric outlet obstruction, renal failure, antral G cell hyperplasia, antral G cell hyperfunction, short bowel syndrome), ZES and gastric outlet obstruction are the most common. If a patient has an elevated BAO (>15 mEq/h) and a fasting gastrin concentration >1000 pg/ml, the diagnosis of ZES can be made without provocative studies provided retained gastric antrum syndrome can be excluded by a history (WOLFE and JENSEN 1987). If there is an increased BAO but gastrin levels are only marginally elevated (100–1000 pg/ml), then the diagnosis of ZES must be excluded from the other causes of an elevated BAO and serum gastrin level listed in Table 2.

In most cases the provocative tests allow not only identification of patients with ZES who have marginally elevated gastric acid or gastrin levels, but also differentiation of ZES from other conditions that cause hypergastrinemia and hyperchlorhydria (JENSEN et al. 1986). The patient with massive small intestinal resection can be excluded by history. Patients with renal failure are rarely a problem, because even though serum gastrin levels are frequently elevated in renal insufficiency, there is no correlation between serum gastrin values and BAO (WALSH and GROSSMAN 1975; BARON 1979; KORMAN et al. 1972). In most instances patients with renal failure are hypochlorhydric; or if they are not, BAO is usually less than 15 mEq/h (WALSH and GROSSMAN 1975; BARON 1979; KORMAN et al. 1972b).

Retained gastric antrum is a rare condition that occurs in patients who have undergone partial gastric resection with a Billroth II gastroenterostomy in which part of the antrum is left attached to the excluded proximal duodenal stump (VAN HEEDEN et al. 1971). The normal inhibitory effect of gastric acid on release of gastrin does not occur because the antrum is excluded from the gastric acid stream; thus, these patients present with a syndrome that clinically resembles ZES. This syndrome should be suspected in any patient who has had a Billroth II type operation and presents with recurrent peptic ulcer. These patients can be distinguished from patients with ZES by the secretin test. Patients with retained gastric antrum do not show a rise in serum gastrin levels in response to injection of secretin, in contrast to patients with ZES, who show a marked increase in serum gastrin values (WALSH and GROSSMAN 1975; BARON 1979; KORMAN et al. 1972b).

Chronic gastric outlet obstruction can be difficult to distinguish from ZES because outlet obstruction can be caused by ZES or it can be secondary to other causes of duodenal obstruction. At present, provocative tests have not been adequately evaluated in patients with gastric outlet obstruction. If impaired emptying is shown or suspected, both serum gastrin and gastric acid output should be evaluated after prolonged suction with a nasogastric tube (JENSEN et al. 1983b, 1986).

The syndrome of antral G cell hyperplasia is characterized by elevated fasting gastrin levels, marked postprandial increases in serum gastrin (greater than 100% increase), no evidence of pancreatic tumor, increased numbers of antral G cells, and a decreased fasting serum gastrin after resection of the gastric antrum. Antral G cell hyperplasia can mimic ZES by presenting with basal hypergastrinemia, peptic ulcer, and hyperchlorhydria. Currently the

Table 3. Antisecretory agents used to treat ZES

Class of antisecretory agent	Drugs	Comment (potency, duration of action, safety, efficacy)
A. H_2 receptor antagonists	Cimetidine Ranitidine Famotidine	1. Famotidine = 10 times more potent than ranitidine and 30 times more than cimetidine (HOWARD et al. 1985) 2. Duration of action: famotidine = 1/3 longer than cimetidine or ranitidine (HOWARD et al. 1985) 3. Median doses required in ZES: famotidine – 0.25 g/day, ranitidine – 1.2 g/day, cimetidine – 3.6 g/day (WOLFE and JENSEN 1987) 4. Each safe at high doses but cimetidine causes antiandrogen side-effects in > 50% males at high doses (JENSEN et al. 1983b) 5. Cimetidine may cause clinically significant drug interactions with warfarin anticoagulants, phenytoin, lidocaine, and theophylline (BRODGEN et al. 1978)
B. H^+,K^+-ATPase	Omeprazole	1. Duration of action > 3 days (MCARTHUR et al. 1985) 2. Most patients require once or twice daily dosing with median dose = 80 mg (LLOYD-DAVIS et al. 1988; MATON et al. 1989; MCARTHUR et al. 1985) 3. Safe and effective in patients with ZES for up to 4 years, but with high doses causes ECL cell hyperplasia and carcinoid tumors in rats (MATON et al. 1988; LLOYD-DAVIS et al. 1988; EKMAN et al. 1985)
C. Prostaglandins	16,16-Dimethyl PGE Misoprostol Enprostil	1. Minimal experience in gastric hypersecretory states (IPPOLITI et al. 1981) 2. Causes diarrhea with higher doses and this may limit utility (JENSEN et al. 1986, 1988).
D. Anticholinergic agents	Nonselective (probanthine, isopropamide) Selective (pirenzepine)	1. Causes only 25%–30% reduction in acid secretion when used alone (MCCARTHY et al. 1982) 2. Potentiates the action of H_2 blockers (MCCARTHY et al. 1982; RICHARDSON et al. 1976) 3. High doses required frequently, with frequent anticholinergic side-effects which limit widespread use (MCCARTHY et al. 1983)
E. Gastrin receptor antagonists	Proglumide	1. Not used because of low potency

Table 3 (continued)

Class of antisecretory agent	Drugs	Comment (potency, duration of action, safety, efficacy)
F. Somatostatin	Somatostatin SMS 201–995	1. Inhibits gastrin-stimulated gastric secretion and gastrin secretion 2. Should not be used as primary antisecretory agent but may have antitumor effects or decrease tumor-induced effects on gastric mucosa (JENSEN et al. 1988; MATON et al. 1988; ELLISON et al. 1986a, b; VINIK et al. 1988; BONFILS et al. 1986; RUSZNIEWSKI et al. 1988)

syndrome can best be distinguished from ZES by the secretin test and by the serum gastrin response to a standard meal. Patients with antral G cell hyperplasia show a marked postprandial rise in gastrin levels (>100%) (GANGULI et al. 1974; FRIESEN and TOMITA 1981). During the secretin test, serum gastrin concentration has been reported to fall (WALSH and GROSSMAN 1975) or show only a small increase (FRIESEN and TOMITA 1981), in contrast to a marked increase seen in patients with ZES.

Antral G cell hyperfunction is a recently described syndrome characterized by basal acid hypersecretion, elevated fasting serum gastrin levels, an enhanced postprandial gastrin response to a meal, normal numbers of antral G cells, and, in some patients, association with hyperpepsinogenemia I and autosomal dominant inheritance (LAMERS et al. 1978; TAYLOR et al. 1981). These patients can be distinguished from patients with ZES by measuring the change in serum gastrin levels during secretin testing and after a standard meal. With secretin testing, patients with antral G cell hyperplasia show either a decrease in serum gastrin or only a slight increase (LAMERS et al. 1978, TAYLOR et al. 1981) and, with a standard meal, a marked increase in serum gastrin (greater than 100%) in contrast to no change or only a small increase in patients with ZES (LAMERS et al. 1978; TAYLOR et al. 1981).

F. Medical Therapy

H_2 receptor antagonists (cimetidine, ranitidine, famotidine) alone or in combination with anticholinergic agents (probanthine, isopropamide) and more recently the substituted benzimidazoles (omeprazole), which function as H^+,K^+-ATPase inhibitors, have been used successfully in the long-term treatment of gastric hypersecretion in ZES (JENSEN et al. 1990). Experience with the various antisecretory drugs in the treatment of gastric acid hypersecretory states, primarily ZES, is summarized in Table 3.

In general, with any of these agents, treatment is only effective if a reliable criterion of acid secretory control is used while the patient is taking medication (JENSEN et al. 1983b, 1986; WOLFE and JENSEN 1987; MATON et al.

1989c). If enough antisecretory drug is used to decrease gastric acid secretion to <10 mEq/h for the hour prior to the next dose of medication in patients without previous gastric surgery and to <5 mEq/h in patients with previous acid-reducing procedures, peptic ulcers will heal and complications of peptic ulcer disease will be prevented (JENSEN et al. 1983b; RAUFMAN et al. 1983; MCARTHUR et al. 1985; MCCARTHY et al. 1977). A recent study of esophageal disease complicating ZES shows that most patients with esophageal disease will also have resolution of symptoms and endoscopic signs of disease when the gastric acid secretion is lowered to <10 mEq/h but 23% will require the gastric acid to be reduced to <1 mEq/h before symptoms and signs resolve (MILLER et al. 1988). Another recent study (MATON et al. 1988a) demonstrates that the ≤10 mEq/h criterion is not adequate for patients with anastomotic ulcers and previous Billroth II gastroenterostomies. In these patients peptic ulcers will only heal if acid output is reduced to ≤5 mEq/h 1 h prior to the next dose of medication, and some refractory patients require reduction of gastric acid output to even lower values for ulcer healing to occur (MATON et al. 1988).

Relief of symptoms does not adequately reflect the effectiveness of antisecretory therapy and cannot be used as a reliable criterion for adjusting medication dosages (RAUFMAN et al. 1983; JENSEN et al. 1984). JENSEN et al. (1984) analyzed a number of different series and concluded that the principal factors contributing to the failure of antisecretory medication to control acid hypersecretion in ZES were the use of inadequate doses of antisecretory medication and the failure to use reliable criteria for assessing the ability of these agents to suppress acid output adequately.

The amount of antisecretory medication varies widely from patient to patient and increases slowly with time; thus, the optimal dose of medication must be determined for each patient initially and periodically reevaluated (JENSEN et al. 1983b, 1986; WOLFE and JENSEN 1987). Most patients require at least one increase in dose of medication per year while on H_2 blockers.

Long-term studies (JENSEN 1984; VINAYEK et al. 1986) have demonstrated that patients with ZES generally require higher doses of antisecretory medication than are usually recommended for common peptic ulcer disease. The dose required for a given patient with ZES on one H_2 blocker correlates closely with the required doses of other H_2 blockers. Therefore, a patient requiring a high dose of cimetidine will require a proportionally high dose of ranitidine or famotidine (HOWARD et al. 1985; VINAYEK et al. 1986). The required dose of omeprazole is also proportional to the required dose of H_2 receptor antagonist (MCARTHUR et al. 1985; MATON et al. 1988c).

I. H_2 Receptor Antagonists

1. General

The introduction of H_2 receptor antagonists has markedly changed the therapy for ZES. Instead of routine total gastrectomy, gastric acid hyper-

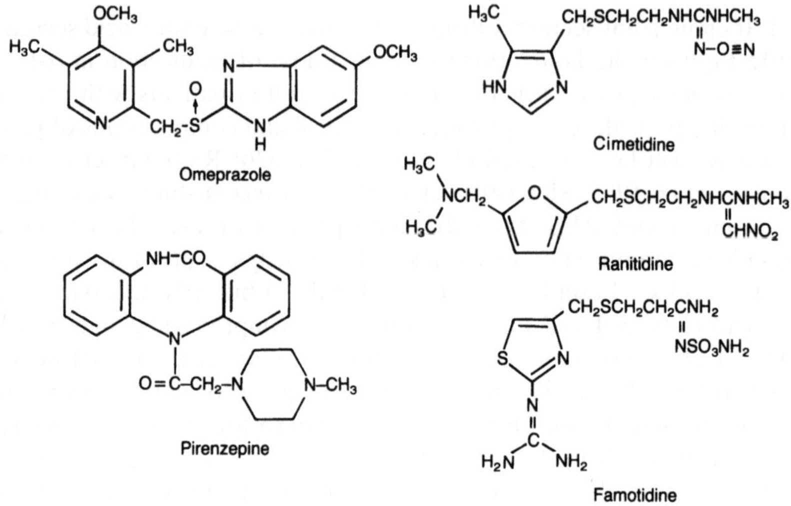

Fig. 2. Chemical structures of the H_2 receptor antagonists cimetidine, ranitidine, and famotidine, of the substituted benzimidazole omeprazole, and of the anticholinergic agent pirenzepine

secretion can now be successfully treated in almost all patients using an H_2 receptor antagonist alone or in combination with an anticholinergic agent (McCARTHY et al. 1977; BONFILS et al. 1977; McCARTHY 1978, 1980; JENSEN 1984; MATON et al. 1989c; JENSEN et al. 1990).

The chemical structures of the three currently available H_2 receptor antagonists used in ZES are shown in Fig. 2. Cimetidine, the first H_2 receptor antagonist to be introduced into general clinical use, contains an imidazole ring like histamine, but possesses a bulkier side chain, an ethyl guanidine side group (BRODGEN et al. 1978). However, the imidazole ring is not essential for interaction with the H_2 receptor. Ranitidine contains a furan ring with ethyl ethenediamine side group and famotidine contains a thiazole ring with a propionamidine side group (BRODGEN et al. 1978, 1982; CAMPOLI-RICHARDS and CLISSOLD 1986).

The H_2 blockers are reversible, competitive antagonists of the action of histamine on H_2 receptors. They are highly selective in their action and at the doses used clinically are virtually without effect on H_1 receptors (BRODGEN et al. 1978, 1982).

The most prominent pharmacological effect of the H_2 receptor blockers is their ability to inhibit histamine-stimulated gastric acid secretion in a competitive manner. The H_2 blockers also inhibit gastric secretion elicited by muscarinic agonists or by gastrin (BRODGEN et al. 1978, 1982). The mechanism of this latter effect is unclear. H_2 blockers do not interact with muscarinic cholinergic receptors or gastrin receptors (SOLL and BERGLINDH 1987). Possible explanations include: (a) histamine is the common mediator of the action of gastrin or muscarinic cholinergic agents, or (b) gastrin has very little stimulatory action when present alone, but its effect is markedly potentiated in the presence of histamine (BLACK and SHANKLEY 1978; SOLL and BERGLINDH 1987). Thus, by inhibiting the action of histamine, the ability of gastrin to stimulate acid secretion is inhibited.

2. Absorption and Excretion of H_2 Receptor Antagonists

In patients without ZES, cimetidine is well absorbed in the small intestine and reaches peak blood levels in 45–90 min, with a 2-h half-life. About 50% of the oral dose is excreted unchanged by the kidneys with the remainder being excreted after metabolism into a sulfoxide (BRODGEN et al. 1978).

Ranitidine is also rapidly and completely absorbed by orally. About 50% of a ranitidine dose is eliminated by hepatic metabolism (BRODGEN et al. 1982).

Famotidine is incompletely absorbed, with 37% reported to be bioavailable after absorption by the oral route (CAMPOLI-RICHARDS and CLISSOLD 1986). Mean urinary recovery was 25%–30% of orally administered and 65%–80% of intravenously administered dose. However, the degree of metabolism may vary widely (CAMPOLI-RICHARDS and CLISSOLD 1986). In patients with ZES, serum concentration of H_2 receptor antagonists correlated closely ($r = 0.95$) with changes in gastric acid hypersecretion (MCARTHUR et al. 1987).

3. Studies in Patients with Zollinger-Ellison Syndrome

The pharmacokinetics of the H_2 receptor antagonists differ in ZES patients when compared to normal or control individuals. A number of studies demonstrate that most patients with ZES require doses of cimetidine larger than the doses used to treat patients with duodenal ulcer (JENSEN 1984), and also require correspondingly large doses of ranitidine (COLLEN et al. 1984) or famotidine (HOWARD et al. 1985). Relative resistance to one H_2 receptor antagonist indicates relative resistance to other H_2 receptor antagonists (HOWARD et al. 1985; JENSEN et al. 1986). The reasons that ZES patients require such large doses of H_2 receptor antagonists are probably multiple. A number of possible explanations have been suggested including decreased absorption, increased metabolism, tachyphylaxis due to the high BAO, and parietal cell resistance (JENSEN 1984). Parietal cell resistance is defined as a higher than normal serum H_2 blocker concentration (IC_{50}) required to inhibit acid secretion (JENSEN 1984). One study reported three patients with ZES (ZIEMNIAK et al. 1983) and another study one patient with ZES (ANDERSEN et al. 1985) with parietal cell resistance to cimetidine. In a study of nine patients with ZES (MCARTHUR et al. 1987) it was estimated that one-third of patients with ZES may have parietal cell resistance. In this study the blood concentration of cimetidine required to produce a 50% inhibition of gastric acid secretion (EC_{50}) was calculated for each ZES patient and compared with

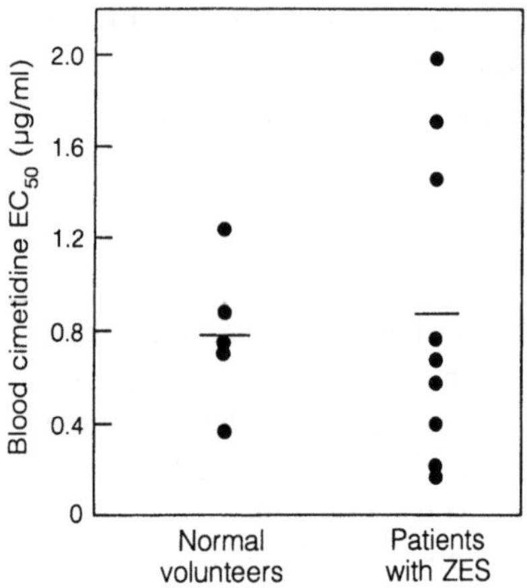

Fig. 3. Blood cimetidine concentrations that produced 50% inhibition (EC_{50}) of pentagastrin-stimulated gastric acid secretion in five normal volunteers or basal gastric acid secretion in nine patients with ZES. Mean EC_{50} for each group is indicated by a *horizontal line*. (MCARTHUR et al. 1987)

the blood cimetidine EC_{50} for normal volunteers (Fig. 3). There was no significant difference between the mean EC_{50} concentration of the two groups (normal volunteers 0.79 ± 0.32 µg/ml; patients with ZES 0.89 ± 0.67 µg/ml). However, three patients with ZES had EC_{50} concentrations > 2SD above the mean EC_{50} concentration for the normal volunteers, indicating possible parietal cell resistance (MCARTHUR et al. 1987) (Fig. 3). Similarly detailed studies have not been done with ranitidine or famotidine. However, a single patient with ZES requiring a high dose of ranitidine demonstrated that a serum ranitidine concentration of 1 µg/ml was required for half-maximal inhibition while in normal subjects only 0.2 µg/ml is required (JENSEN et al. 1984).

Decreased bioavailability of H_2 receptor antagonists was first demonstrated in two patients (ZIEMNIAK et al. 1983). In a systematic study of nine patients with ZES (MCARTHUR et al. 1987) the bioavailability of cimetidine was measured by comparing the area under the blood cimetidine curve (AUC) after an oral dose of cimetidine in patients with ZES with the AUC in normal controls (Fig. 4). These investigators found that the renal clearance of cimetidine in normal volunteers and patients with ZES was similar and that decreased total 24-h absorption of cimetidine was an uncommon cause for the increased dose requirement of the drug in patients with ZES (MCARTHUR et al. 1987). Only one of the nine patients had a decreased total bioavailability (MCARTHUR et al. 1987). However, peak serum cimetidine concentrations were markedly decreased in ZES patients when compared to peak concentrations in normal volunteers (Fig. 4). This indicates delayed absorption of oral cimetidine in 40% of patients with ZES. The mechanism of this delayed absorption is unknown. Therefore, 60% of patients with ZES had either a delayed or decreased bioavailability, which was not due to the fact that gastric acid hypersecretion was not controlled since in all patients acid secretion had been decreased to ≤10 mEq/h prior to the study (MCARTHUR et al. 1987).

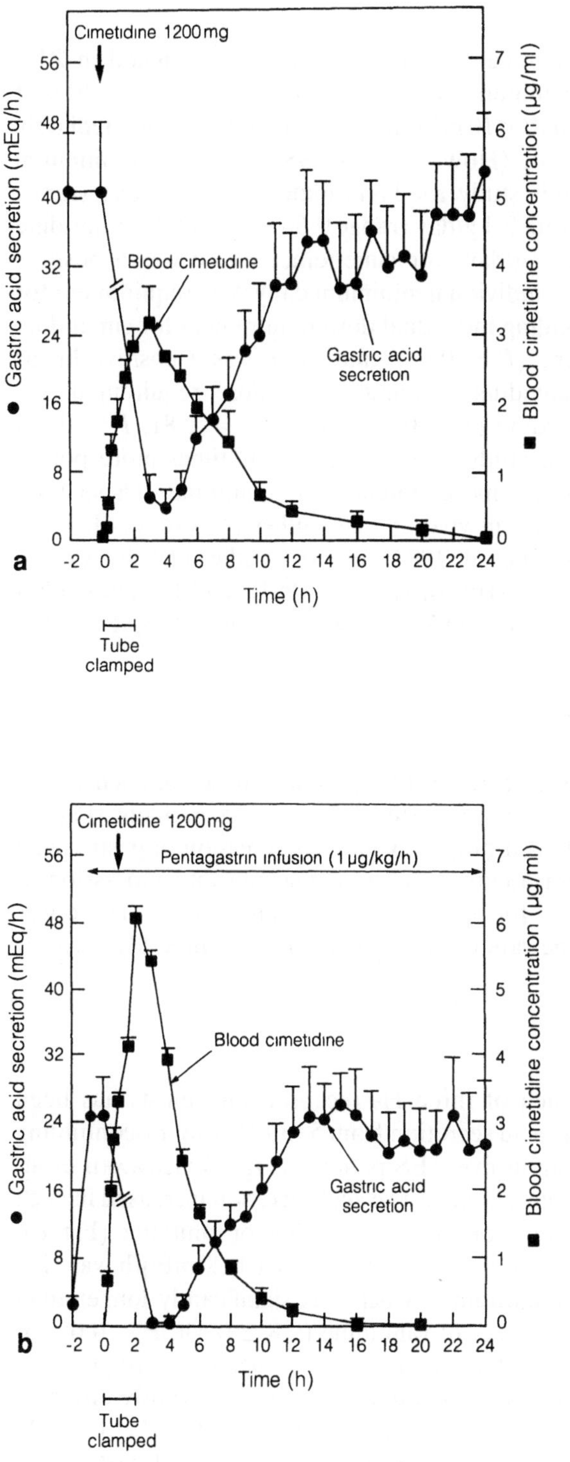

Fig. 4a, b. Comparison of the effect of a single oral dose of cimetidine (1200 mg) on basal gastric acid secretion in nine patients with ZES (**a**) and normal volunteers (**b**). Results given are the means. *Vertical bars* represent 1 SE. BAO was measured hourly for 2 h before cimetidine administration. The nasogastric tube was clamped for 2 h to allow for gastric emptying; then acid secretion was measured hourly for 24 h. Blood cimetidine concentrations were determined at the indicated times. Pentagastrin was given by continuous infusion at 1 µg/kg per hour to normal volunteers to maintain stimulated acid secretion. (McArthur et al. 1987)

4. Potency

Equipotent doses of each H_2 receptor antagonist were determined in ZES patients by establishing the minimum dose of each drug (given every 6 h) that reduced gastric acid secretion to <10 mEq/h during the last hour immediately preceding the next dose of drug (HOWARD et al. 1985). The mean minimum daily dose requirement in this study for famotidine was 0.24 g/day (range 0.08–0.48 g/day) compared with 2.1 g/day (range 0.6–3.6 g/day) for ranitidine and 7.8 g/day (range 1.2–13.2 g/day) for cimetidine. There was a positive linear correlation between the individual minimum daily dose requirement for famotidine and the corresponding individual dose requirement for cimetidine ($P < 0.05$) and for ranitidine ($P < 0.01$), and there was a positive linear correlation between the individual minimum daily dose requirement for ranitidine and that for cimetidine ($y = 0.34 + 0.25x$; $r = 0.81$; $P = 0.02$) (HOWARD et al. 1985). In this study, famotidine was 32 times more potent than cimetidine and nine times more potent than ranitidine. These findings are consistent with previous in vivo animal studies (TAKAGI et al. 1982; TAKEDA et al. 1983; PENDLETON et al. 1983), in vitro studies (TOMIOKA et al. 1982; PENDLETON et al. 1983; GAJTKOWSKI et al. 1983), and human studies (MIWA et al. 1982; SMITH et al. 1983; DAMMANN et al. 1983; CAMPOLI-RICHARDS et al. 1986).

5. Onset of Action

The time course for the onset of action of equipotent doses of each of the three H_2 receptor antagonists was reported in four ZES patients (Fig. 5) (HOWARD et al. 1985). With each drug maximum suppression of gastric acid secretion occurred 3–4 h after administration, and significant suppression of gastric acid secretion persisted for up to 7 h after administration. There was no significant difference in the rate of onset of action with three H_2 receptor antagonists.

6. Duration of Action

The duration of action of each of three H_2 receptor antagonists has been reported by measuring gastric acid secretion from 5 to 12 h after discontinuing equipotent doses of each drug in five ZES patients (Fig. 6) (HOWARD et al. 1985). After discontinuing famotidine, gastric acid secretion increased in each patient more slowly than after discontinuing cimetidine or ranitidine (Fig. 6). The mean time required for gastric acid secretion to reach 20 mEq/h was 12.2 ± 0.9 h after discontinuing famotidine, which was significantly longer than after discontinuing equipotent doses of ranitidine (9.8 ± 0.5 h, $P < 0.05$) or cimetidine (9.3 ± 0.6 h, $P < 0.001$). In contrast, the mean time required to reach 20 mEq/h after discontinuing cimetidine was not significantly different from the mean time after discontinuing ranitidine (9.8 vs 9.3 h, $P > 0.3$). At 12 h after discontinuing equipotent doses of drugs, inhibition of gastric acid

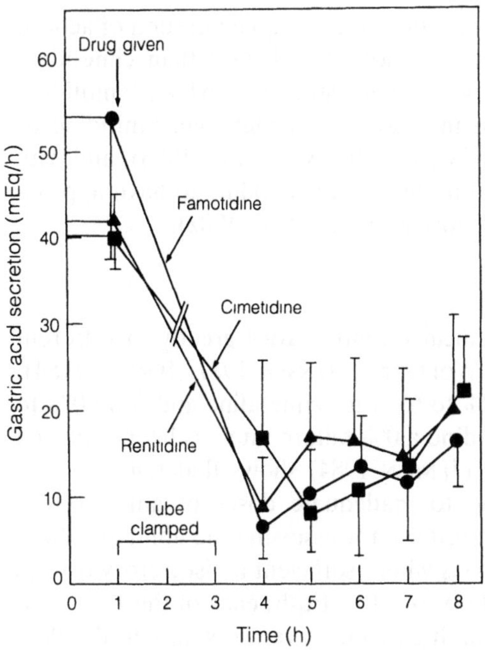

Fig. 5. Time course for the onset of action of single equipotent doses of famotidine, ranitidine, and cimetidine in four patients. The dose of each drug was one-quarter of the minimum daily dose of that drug. *Vertical bars* represent 1 SEM. The initial gastric acid secretion (time 0–1 h) before the time drugs were administered was 43 ± 6 mEq/h for ranitidine, 40 ± 7 mEq/h for cimetidine, and 53 ± 32 mEq/h for famotidine, values that were not statistically significantly different ($P > 0.01$). (HOWARD et al. 1985)

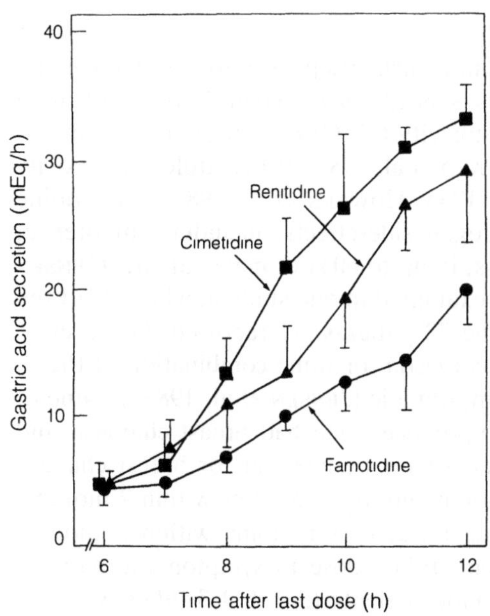

Fig. 6. Duration of action of equipotent doses of famotidine, ranitidine, and cimetidine in five patients. After discontinuing equipotent dose schedules of each drug, gastric acid secretion was measured from the beginning of the 6th hour to the end of the 12th hour after the last dose. The dose schedule of each drug was one-quarter of the minimum daily requirement of that drug given over 6 h. *Vertical bars* represent 1 SEM. (HOWARD et al. 1985)

secretion by famotidine was 58% ± 9% of the basal gastric acid secretory rate, which was significantly greater than the 27% ± 9% inhibition caused by cimetidine ($P < 0.01$) and the 38% ± 12% inhibition caused by ranitidine ($P < 0.005$) (HOWARD et al. 1985). From these results it was concluded that equipotent doses of cimetidine or ranitidine have an equal duration of action, whereas famotidine has a duration of action 30% longer than cimetidine or ranitidine. These results agree closely with studies in which famotidine was shown to inhibit acid secretion in dogs 30% longer than ranitidine or cimetidine (PENDLETON et al. 1983; CAMPOLI-RICHARDS et al. 1986), and with other studies which demonstrated ranitidine and cimetidine to have approximately equal durations of action (BRODGEN et al. 1978, 1982).

7. Failure

The number of patients failing medical therapy varies greatly in different series (JENSEN et al. 1983b, 1986; WOLFE and JENSEN 1987; JENSEN 1984); reported failure rates range from 0% to 65% for cimetidine and from 0% to 40% for ranitidine, while for famotidine a 0% failure rate has been reported (Table 4). Analysis of these series (JENSEN 1984) shows that failure of H_2 receptor antagonists is usually due to inadequate doses of antisecretory medication or failure to use reliable criteria for assessing the ability of these drugs to suppress acid output. In series where sufficient antisecretory drug is given to decrease gastric acid secretion to <10 mEq/h, each of the H_2 receptor antagonists has been shown to be highly effective (HOWARD et al. 1985; WOLFE and JENSEN 1987).

8. Safety

The long-term use of H_2 receptor antagonists has proven to be effective and safe (WOLFE and JENSEN 1987; JENSEN et al. 1986). High doses of all three drugs cause no dose-related hepatotoxicity (MCCARTHY et al. 1977; COLLEN et al. 1984; JENSEN et al. 1984; HOWARD et al. 1985) or hematological toxicity (JENSEN et al. 1984; COLLEN et al. 1984; HOWARD et al. 1985). Cimetidine at high doses does cause antiandrogen side-effects, including impotence, gynecomastia, and breast tenderness, in up to 60% of male patients (JENSEN et al. 1983a). The side-effects were examined in one study in which 20 of the 22 patients studied had ZES. Of the 22 patients, 11 reported the onset of impotence, breast tenderness, gynecomastia, or some combination of these, whereas the remaining 11 were asymptomatic (JENSEN et al. 1983a). Nine of the 11 symptomatic patients had impotence, nine had breast changes, and seven had both. The times of onset for impotence and for breast changes were similar, with seven of nine patients noting symptoms within 2 months, and all symptomatic patients noting onset of symptoms within 5 months of initiating the drug. The mean cimetidine dose in symptomatic patients (5.3 ± 3.6 g/day) and in asymptomatic patients (3.0 ± 1.3 g/day) was not statistically significantly different (JENSEN et al. 1983a). Nine of 11 patients with cimetidine-induced side-effects were treated with ranitidine with discontinuation of cimetidine. In the other two patients, cimetidine was discontinued in one after gastrinoma resection, and the dose of cimetidine was lowered in the other. Within 10 weeks of these changes symptoms of impotence resolved in all patients. Breast tenderness resolved in all patients within 8 weeks and gynecomastia improved in all patients, but three of five patients continued to have minimal gynecomastia at 3, 4, and 7 months. Long-term treatment with cimetidine in females, or with ranitidine or famotidine in patients of either sex, has been demonstrated to be safe (JENSEN et al. 1986; WOLFE and JENSEN 1987).

Cimetidine, apparently through an inhibitory effect on the mixed function oxidase system, has been reported to reduce the hepatic metabolism of warfarin-type anticoagulants, phenytoin, propranolol, chlordiazepoxide, diazepam, lidocaine, theophylline, and metronidazole, thereby delaying elimination and increasing blood levels of these drugs (BRODGEN et al. 1978, 1982). Dosage of these drugs may require adjustment when starting or stopping cimetidine since clinically significant effects have been reported with warfarin anticoagulants, phenytoin, lidocaine, and theophylline. Systematic studies of the effect of cimetidine on drug metabolism have not been carried out in patients with ZES. There is little or no effect of ranitidine or famotidine on drugs metabolized by the mixed function oxidase system (BRODGEN et al. 1982; CAMPOLI-RICHARDS et al. 1986).

Patients taking cimetidine have also been shown to have altered immunoregulation (WATSON et al. 1983), which may have an impact on rejection of kidney transplants and skin reactivity.

Central nervous system symptoms, including confusion, somnolence, and dizziness, have been reported with cimetidine. Altered mental status has been noted particularly in the elderly, in the ICU setting, and when compounded by renal or hepatic dysfunction (CERRA et al. 1986). Similar side-effects have been reported with ranitidine (BRODGEN et al. 1982).

Unusual reactions reported with both cimetidine and ranitidine include bone marrow depression, anaphylactoid reactions, interstitial nephritis, and rare cases of hepatitis, all which appear reversible (BRODGEN et al. 1978, 1982). These reactions have not been reported in patients with ZES treated with high doses of either drug, suggesting that the reactions are not dose related (JENSEN et al. 1984).

9. Use

To reduce gastric acid secretion to a safe level (<10 mEq/h for the hour prior to the next dose of H_2 receptor antagonist in patients without previous gastric surgery and <5 mEq/h in patients with previous gastric surgery or in some patients with esophageal disease), patients with ZES usually require more than twice the usual dose of H_2 receptor antagonist recommended for idiopathic peptic ulcer disease. In recent studies at the National Institutes of Health, the median doses were 3.6 g/day (range 1.2–12.6) for cimetidine, 1.2 g/day for ranitidine (range 0.45–6), and 0.25 g/day for famotidine (range 0.05–0.8) (WOLFE and JENSEN 1987; HOWARD et al. 1985; VINAYEK et al. 1986; JENSEN et al. 1984). As discussed in Sect. F.I.3, at present it is not clear why patients with ZES require more than the usual dose of H_2 antagonist to inhibit acid output adequately. Some patients have been shown to have a decreased sensitivity of the acid secretory process to antisecretory drugs or impaired absorption, but in 25% of patients no alteration in drug pharmacokinetics is found (McARTHUR et al. 1987; ZIEMNIAK et al. 1983). At present in females data suggest cimetidine, ranitidine, or famotidine are equally efficacious if sufficient doses are used (VINAYEK et al. 1986; HOWARD et al. 1985), and any of these three drugs can be used safely and effectively. In males, because of the antiandrogen side-effects of cimetidine, either ranitidine or famotidine is preferred. In a recent study famotidine was shown, because of its increased potency and 30% longer duration of action, to be preferable in patients who require use of anticholinergic agents with a H_2 receptor antagonist or who require cimetidine or ranitidine every 4 or 6h. In 30% of these patients famotidine will control acid hypersecretion without an anticholinergic agent, which frequently has bothersome side-effects. Furthermore, a number of the patients requiring cimetidine or ranitidine every 4 or 6h will require famotidine only every 6–8h (VINAYEK et al. 1986).

10. Use of Parenteral H_2 Receptor Antagonists

The importance of establishing effective criteria for controlling gastric hypersecretion for times when oral antisecretory agents cannot be used and when parenteral antisecretory agents are needed is underscored by the fact that almost all patients with ZES require parenteral antisecretory medication to control gastric acid hypersecretion at some time during the course of their disease. Parenteral antisecretory drugs are frequently required in patients with ZES presenting with nausea, vomiting, or severe diarrhea, in patients with metastatic disease receiving chemotherapy who have nausea and vomiting, and in patients with ZES undergoing surgery. Results of a study evaluating the continuous parenteral administration of H_2 receptor antagonists in 46 patients with ZES were reported by SAEED et al. (1989). In all patients it was possible to decrease gastric acid secretion to <10mEq/h with i.v. cimetidine infusion using a stepwise method of titration. For all 46 patients the mean minimum (±SEM) infusion dose of i.v. cimetidine required to achieve this level of control was 2.9 (±0.3) mg/kg per hour (median 2.5; range 0.5–7.0). Twenty-six (57%) of the 46 patients required 1.1–3.0mg/kg per hour of i.v. cimetidine by infusion to reduce gastric acid secretion to <10mEq/h. Five patients (11%) required <1mg/kg per hour, 12 patients (26%) required 3.1–5.0mg/kg per hour, and three patients (6%) required >5mg/kg per hour. Thirty-four patients who underwent surgery were treated with continuous i.v. cimetidine for a mean of 12 days (range 1–83 days). One-half of the patients did not require dose adjustment, whereas the remainder required an average of two dose adjustments, usually in the first 3 postoperative days. No patient developed any complication attributable to gastric acid hypersecretion in the postoperative period and there was no detectable neurological, hematological, or hepatic toxicity (SAEED et al. 1989). The minimum

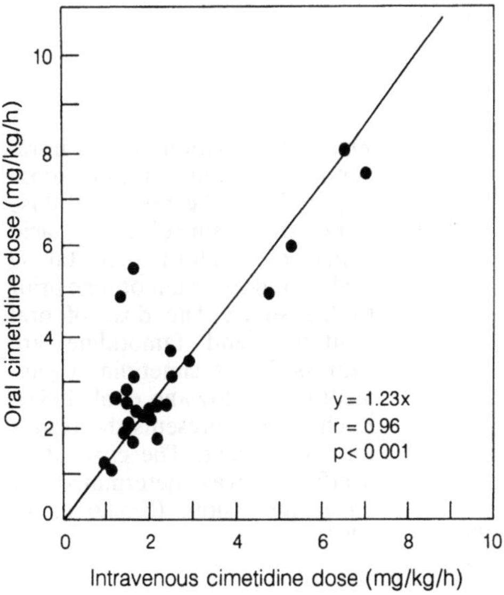

Fig. 7. Correlation of the intravenous cimetidine infusion dose required and the prior oral cimetidine dose required to control gastric acid hypersecretion for patients taking oral cimetidine prior to the study. Each *point* represents the results for one patient. The correlation coefficient was determined by linear regression. (SAEED et al. 1989)

i.v. cimetidine dose given to suppress gastric acid output to <10 mEq/h did not correlate with basal or maximal acid output or fasting gastrin concentration, but correlated closely with either the prior oral dose of cimetidine (Fig. 7) ($r = 0.96$, $P < 0.001$) or the prior oral dose of ranitidine or famotidine ($r = 0.95$, $P < 0.001$) (Fig. 8) (SAEED et al. 1989). A similar study has demonstrated that the continuous administration of intravenous ranitidine was also effective and without side-effects in controlling gastric acid hypersecretion in patients with ZES during surgery and in the postoperative period (FRAKER et al. 1988).

II. Omeprazole

1. General

Omeprazole, a substituted benzimidazole (Fig. 2), is a potent, long-acting inhibitor of gastric acid secretion in animals and man (LARSSON et al. 1983; OLBE et al. 1982). Omeprazole acts by inhibiting H^+,K^+-adenosine triphosphatase, which is responsible for hydrogen secretion by the gastric parietal cell (FELLENIUS et al. 1981).

2. Absorption, Metabolism, and Excretion

Omeprazole, which is a weak base, is absorbed from the small intestine at an alkaline pH. In the parietal cell the drug is trapped in the secretory canaliculus where the pH is acidic (SACHS 1984). The acid environment of the parietal cell causes formation of a sulfoxide metabolite of omeprazole that binds irreversibly to and inactivates H^+,K^+-ATPase and thus inhibits gastric acid secretion (FELLENIUS et al. 1981).

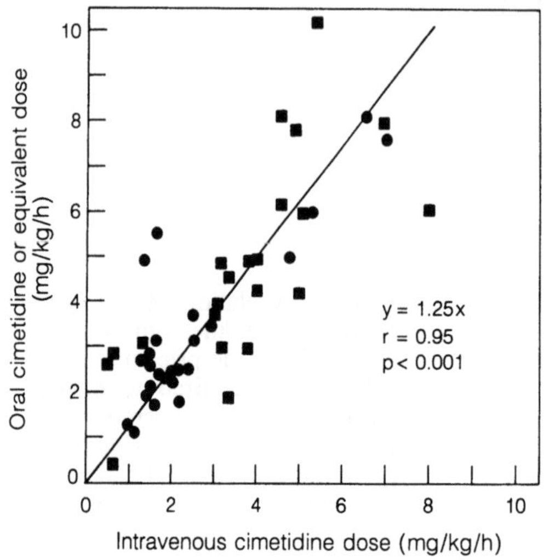

Fig. 8. Correlation of the intravenous cimetidine infusion dose required and the prior oral dose required to control gastric acid hypersecretion for patients taking oral ranitidine or famotidine prior to the study. The dose of oral ranitidine and famotidine are expressed as a cimetidine equivalent dose (HOWARD et al. 1985). Each *point* represents the results for one patient. The correlation coefficient was determined by linear regression. (SAEED et al. 1989)

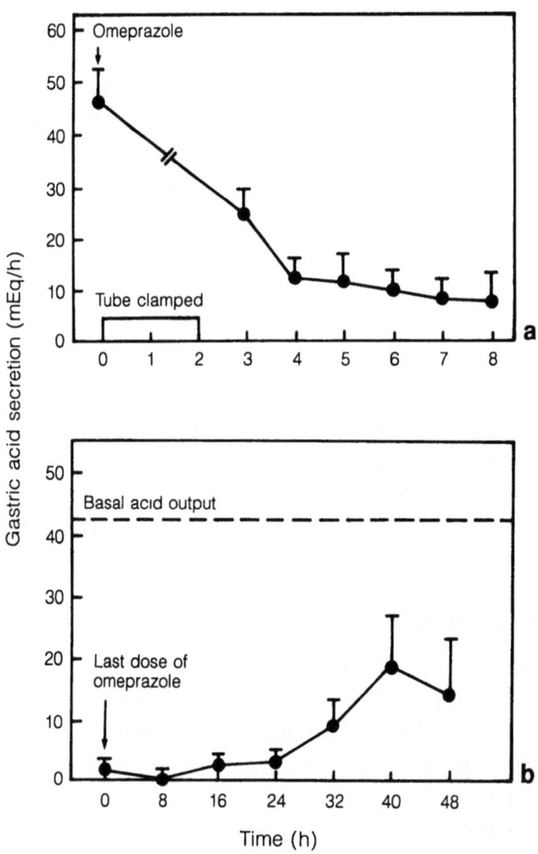

Fig. 9. a The effect of a single dose of omeprazole (60 mg) on gastric acid secretion in nine patients with ZES. Results given are means from the nine subjects. *Vertical bars* represent 1 SE (MCARTHUR et al. 1985) **b** Inhibition of gastric acid secretion after discontinuing omeprazole (mean dose, 56 mg) in five patients. BAO is the gastric acid secretion in milliequivalents per hour (mEq/h) measured after discontinuing all antisecretory medications as determined at the beginning of the study. Results given are the means from the five subjects. *Vertical bars* represent 1 SE. (MCARTHUR et al. 1985)

Because the active form of omeprazole is acid labile, the drug must be administered as a buffered suspension or in enteric-coated granules that dissolve at an alkaline pH. Absorption of omeprazole from enteric-coated granules peaks 3–4 h after administration (PRICHARD et al. 1985; CLISSOLD and CAMPOLI-RICHARDS 1986, 1988); however, plasma concentrations of omeprazole do not correlate with inhibition of gastric acid secretion (PRICHARD et al. 1988; CLISSOLD and CAMPOLI-RICHARDS 1986, 1988). Thus, although omeprazole disappears from the plasma 8–11 h after a single dose of the drug, inhibition of acid secretion lasts for up to 3 days (PRICHARD et al. 1988; CLISSOLD and CAMPOLI-RICHARDS 1986, 1988). Bioavailability of omeprazole increases with repeated doses (PRICHARD et al. 1988; CLISSOLD and CAMPOLI-RICHARDS 1986, 1988), possibly because absorption of the drug improves as gastric pH increases and less omeprazole is inactivated in the gastrointestinal tract.

3. Onset of Action

The time course for the onset of action of omeprazole has been studied by measuring gastric acid secretion after a single oral dose of omeprazole (60 mg) in nine patients with ZES (MCARTHUR et al. 1985). Basal gastric acid secretion was inhibited by 50% at 3 h, by 78% at 4 h, and by 86% at 8 h (Fig. 9a). In another study the maximum inhibition of gastric acid secretion occurred 6 h after a single dose of omeprazole (80 mg) in five patients with ZES (LAMERS et al. 1984). In the 2nd hour after ingestion of the drug, gastric acid secretion was inhibited by 98% ± 2%. Five patients were achlorhydric, while one patient having the lowest plasma omeprazole concentration had a 90% inhibition of gastric acid. At 24 h after ingestion of the drug, gastric acid was inhibited by 83% ± 6% (with a range of 56%–100%). At that time omeprazole was undetectable in plasma from four patients, while the omeprazole concentrations were very low in two other patients. Clinical symptoms, including diarrhea in five, gastric discomfort in two, and heartburn in two, were completely abolished for at least 48 h (LAMERS et al. 1984). No side-effects or laboratory abnormalities were induced by the drug. These studies demonstrate that even though there is marked gastric acid hypersecretion in patients with ZES and acid inactivates omeprazole, the omeprazole capsules have a time course of onset of action that is not different from that of H_2 receptor antagonists.

4. Duration of Action

When omeprazole therapy was discontinued in ZES patients on maintenance therapy, inhibition of gastric acid secretion persisted for up to 48 h (Fig. 9b) (MCARTHUR et al. 1985). Basal gastric acid secretion was inhibited by >80% during the first 24 h after omeprazole therapy and by >50% during the 24th–48th hour after omeprazole therapy. These results agree closely with recent studies in patients with peptic ulcer disease in which omeprazole was demonstrated to inhibit acid secretion, without a return to normal acid secretion, for 4 days after stopping the drug (CLISSOLD and CAMPOLI-RICHARDS 1986).

5. Potency

To establish the maintenance dose of omeprazole (the minimum dose required to reduce gastric acid secretion to <10 mEq/h for the last hour before the next dose) in 11 ZES patients omeprazole was given once in the morning every 24 h starting with 60 mg as the first dose (MCARTHUR et al. 1985). Gastric acid secretion was measured during the last 2 h before the next dose of medication. The drug dose was adjusted up or down based on the measured gastric acid secretion. If the patient required >200 mg omeprazole/day the dose was divided every 12 h. The minimum dose requirement of omeprazole was then compared to the minimum dose of H_2 receptor antagonist which these patients had previously required. The five patients taking cimetidine prior to the study required a mean cimetidine dose of 1650 mg every 6 h to control acid secretion (mean total daily requirement of 6.6 g). The six patients taking ranitidine prior to the study required a mean ranitidine dose of 1100 mg taken at 4- to 8-h intervals to control acid secretion (mean total daily requirement 5.2 g). Three patients also required an anticholinergic drug in addition to an H_2 receptor antagonist to control gastric acid secretion. The average total daily dose requirement for all patients taking omeprazole was 70 mg (range 20–160 mg). A positive correlation was found when the maintenance dose of omeprazole was plotted against the maintenance dose of cimetidine ($r = 0.936$, $P < 0.05$) and ranitidine ($r = 0.913$, $P < 0.05$). Similar results are reported in a large series involving 40 patients with ZES in which the dose of omeprazole was shown to correlate with the previous H_2 receptor antagonist dose ($r = 0.89$), BAO ($r = 0.43$, $P < 0.01$), and maximal acid output ($r = 0.39$, $P < 0.02$), but not with serum gastrin concentration ($r = -0.32$) (MATON et al. 1989b).

6. Failure

A failure rate from 0% to 7.5% is seen in various studies of omeprazole in hypersecretory states (Table 4). However, as with the reported failures of H_2 receptor antagonists, it is likely that this failure rate is due to inadequate doses of omeprazole (JENSEN et al. 1984).

7. Use

The first report on the effect of omeprazole on acid-peptic disease in a patient with refractory ulcers was published in 1982 (BLANCHI et al. 1982). Since then a number of small series of patients refractory to H_2 receptor antagonists but responsive to the use of omeprazole have been reported (OBERG and LINDSTROM 1983; LAMERS et al. 1984; DELCHIER et al. 1986; VEZZADINI et al. 1984; CLISSOLD and CAMPOLI-RICHARDS 1986, 1988). As well as for the treat-

Table 4. Results of long-term medical therapy of gastric hypersecretion in patients with ZES

Principal antisecretory drug	No. of patients	Percent failure	Duration of treatment (months)	Reference
Cimetidine	5	40	60%>6	CREUTZFELD (1977)
	13	61	–	BONFILS et al. (1979)
	14	0	11	STADIL and STAGE (1979)
	17	65	6/17 (mean 51)	DEVENEY et al. (1983)
Cimetidine[a]	61	8	12	McCARTHY (1978)
	20	50	33	STABILE et al. (1983)
	18	6	29	MALAGELADA et al. (1983)
	36	11	60%>24	JENSEN et al. (1983b)
Ranitidine	15	40	40%>18	MIGNON et al. (1982)
Ranitidine[a]	19	0	14	JENSEN et al. (1984)
Famotidine[a]	32	0	10	HOWARD et al. (1985) VINAYEK et al. (1986)
Omeprazole	7	0	14	LAMERS et al. (1984)
	11	0	6	McARTHUR et al. (1985)
	11	2	15	DELCHIER et al. (1986)
	31	3	8 days to 18 months	HIRSCHOWITZ et al. (1987)
	40	0	29	MATON et al. (1989)
	80	7.5	19	LLOYD-DAVIS et al. (1988)
	8	0	12	CADIOT et al. (1988)

[a] With anticholinergic agents.

ment of refractory ulcers, omeprazole has been used in a number of studies in patients with ZES which are summarized in Table 4. It is apparent that omeprazole controlled acid secretion in almost all patients. Two studies assessing the effect of long-term omeprazole therapy in ZES patients has been reported (LLOYD-DAVIES et al. 1988; MATON et al. 1989) and there are preliminary reports of three other studies (CADIOT et al. 1988; HIRSCHOWITZ et al. 1987; LAMERS et al. 1984). The published study is an international study evaluating the long-term use of omeprazole (LLOYD-DAVIES et al. 1988) in 80 patients with ZES from 39 centers. Acid secretion and laboratory variables were checked regularly and endoscopic examinations made at intervals. Dosage was adjusted primarily on the basis of BAO, but also if symptoms occurred. The starting dose was generally 60 mg daily and the median dose was 60–70 mg daily over the study period. There was no evidence of tachyphylaxis. More than 90% of the patients were successfully controlled on total daily doses of 120 mg or less; one-third of patients required divided doses. There were no obvious drug-related effects on laboratory variables, including fasting serum gastrin, and there were very few adverse events.

A recent long-term study on the use of omeprazole in ZES (MATON et al. 1989b) reported that doses of omeprazole required were greater than doses found to be effective in idiopathic duodenal ulcer disease (BARDHAN et al.

1986; CLASSEN et al. 1985; LAURITSEN et al. 1985) and reflux esophagitis (HAVELUND et al. 1988; KLINKENBERG-KNOL et al. 1987; DAMMANN et al. 1986). These findings are similar to findings reported with the use of H_2 receptor antagonists (MCCARTHY et al. 1977; MALAGELADA et al. 1983; COLLEN et al. 1984; RICHARDSON et al. 1985; BONFILS et al. 1981; VINAYEK et al. 1986). In 31 of the 40 patients in the study of MATON et al. (1989), acid was reduced to <10 mEq/h in the last hour before the next dose of drug by <120 mg dose of omeprazole once per day. The other nine patients required 60 mg omeprazole twice a day. It is somewhat surprising that division of the 120 mg dose into two equal 60 mg doses markedly increased the efficacy of the drug, in view of the fact that the duration of action has been reported to be in excess of 24 h in patients with ZES (MCARTHUR et al. 1985; LAMERS et al. 1984). The mean daily dose required to control acid secretion was 82.5 ± 31.4 mg/day (mean ± 1 SD) (median 100, range 20–120) (MATON et al. 1989b). Increases in the dose of omeprazole were required in nine patients (23%). This is in marked contrast to the use of H_2 receptor antagonists in ZES patients, who require an average of one increase in dose per year (COLLEN et al. 1984; RICHARDSON et al. 1985; LLOYD-DAVIES et al. 1988). Omeprazole was found to prevent mucosal disease in all patients, including 17 patients in whom H_2 receptor antagonist had produced only partial resolution despite acid output being <10 mEq/h (MATON et al. 1989b). MATON et al. (1989b) concluded that because of its potency, long duration of action, and lack of side-effects or toxicity, omeprazole is now the drug of first choice in patients with ZES.

The results of a multicenter U.S. study of omeprazole treatment of ZES have been reported in abstract form (HIRSCHOWITZ et al. 1987). In this study, 31 ZES patients were treated from 8 days to 18 months, the omeprazole dose was started at 60 mg/day, and the dose was adjusted after subsequent gastric analysis to keep the BAO < 10 mEq/h. The median effective dose of 60 mg/day reduced the BAO by an average of 83%. All patients were symptomatic before omeprazole, and all had endoscopic abnormalities, including an unexpectedly high (46%) incidence of esophagitis. Of the 18 patients endoscoped after 6 weeks to 6 months of treatment, seven were normal, four still had ulcers, four had erosions, and three had esophagitis, but with few symptoms. After treatment, heartburn, present at the start in 56% of patients, was totally relieved in all. Abdominal pain and diarrhea were relieved in 88% and 86%, respectively. No significant laboratory abnormalities occurred.

In a recent long-term study of the effect of omeprazole, seven ZES patients were continuously treated with omeprazole once or twice daily for 8–19 months (LAMERS et al. 1984). Treatment was started with 60 mg omeprazole. Six of these seven patients had symptoms that were resistant to high doses of H_2 receptor antagonists, and the seventh could not take high doses of cimetidine because of a possible drug-related increase in serum creatinine concentration. The inhibition of acid secretion, measured 24 h after daily ingestion of 60 mg of the drug, was measured on day 1, and the degree of inhibition did not change during the 1st month of treatment. Symptoms improved within 1–2 weeks, and peptic ulcers or esophagitis were healed in patients at endoscopy after 1 month of treatment. Omeprazole was effective for periods ranging from 8 to 19 months. In four patients the dose of omeprazole was decreased to 30 or 40 mg and in three patients a dose increase was required to keep the gastric acid secretion $\leq$10 mEq/h 24 h after the dose. No side-effects or adverse changes in laboratory values were observed in any of the patients.

8. Safety

An initial study in volunteers suggested that omeprazole might have some liver toxicity in some patients but subsequent studies have failed to show this (Howden et al. 1984; Clissold and Campoli-Richards 1986, 1988). Gastric carcinoids were observed in rats receiving long-term treatment with omeprazole (Ekman et al. 1985). The pathogenesis is thought to be drug-induced achlorhydria causing hypergastrinemia (Havu 1986; Larson et al. 1986). Others argue that omeprazole itself may be tumor promoting (Wormsley 1984). However, no gastric carcinoids have been detected in clinical studies of patients with ZES treated with omeprazole for up to 48 months (Lloyd-Davies et al. 1988; Maton et al. 1988), and in a recent study of 40 ZES patients on long-term omeprazole treatment (Maton et al. 1988), and a recent international study (Lloyd-Davies et al. 1988), omeprazole was not associated with significant side-effects, or with any evidence of hematological or biochemical toxicity. In patients with ZES long-term treatment with omeprazole did not change serum gastrin concentration in one study (Maton et al. 1988) whereas it caused elevations in some patients in another study (Cadiot et al. 1988). Altered metabolism of diazepam, phenytoin, and 7-hydroxycoumadin has been found with omeprazole, suggesting interactions with the hepatic cytochrome P_{450} (Gugler and Jensen 1985; Henry et al. 1984; Clissold and Campoli-Richards 1986, 1988), but the importance of drug interactions with omeprazole remains to be defined.

III. Anticholinergic Agents

Both classical anticholinergic agents such as probanthine (propantheline) or isopropamide, and selective M_1 muscarinic cholinergic receptor antagonists such as pirenzepine, have been used in patients with ZES. In general, anticholinergic agents only decrease basal acid output by 25%–30% when used alone (McCarthy and Hyman 1982). However, the combination of an H_2 receptor antagonist and an anticholinergic drug has been shown to be more effective than an H_2 receptor antagonist alone in patients with ZES (Richardson and Walsh 1976; McCarthy and Hyman 1982). Ranitidine plus pirenzepine or other anticholinergic agents, and famotidine plus probanthine or isopropamide have been used in combination in treating some patients with ZES (Collen et al. 1982).

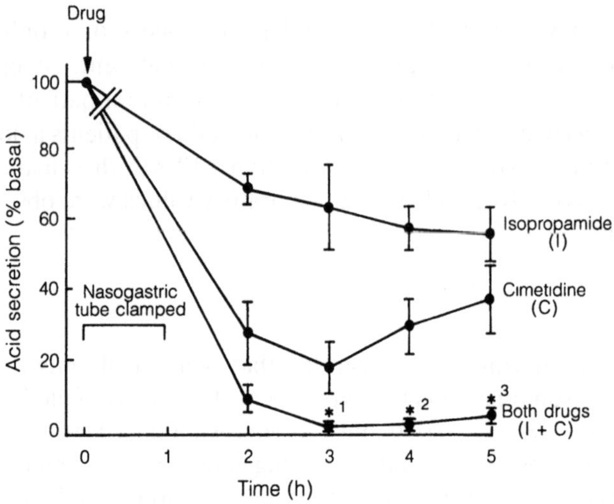

Fig. 10. Time courses of the effect of drugs on acid output, expressed as percentages of the mean BAO of the individual cases. *Vertical bars* represent ± SE of the mean acid output of the six patients at each hour. The significance of between-drug differences at each point in time was assessed by Student's *t*-test for paired data. Doses of cimetidine required to show the effect varied, but were 600 mg in four cases and 300 mg in two cases. The dose of isopropamide was 20 mg in all cases. For isopropamide + cimetidine ($I + C$) versus cimetidine (C), $*^1 = P < 0.025$; $*^2 = P < 0.005$; $*^3 = P < 0.01$. (McCARTHY and HYMAN 1982)

The effect of isopropamide on the response to oral cimetidine in six ZES patients has been reported (McCARTHY and HYMAN 1982). All patients were relatively resistant to cimetidine as judged by the persistence of hypersecretion of acid or epigastric pain following a 300 mg dose of cimetidine in four patients and a 450 mg dose in two patients. In five of six cases combination therapy caused a statistically significantly greater suppression of acid secretion than either drug alone. The time courses of the responses in the group as a whole to the doses of drugs are indicated in Fig. 10. It can be seen that the effect of isopropamide is gradual in onset and maintained to the end of the test period. By contrast, the peak effect of cimetidine is seen 3 h after ingestion of the drug. The response to the combination of drugs is significantly greater than that to either drug alone, with $P < 0.001$ (hour 6) when compared to cimetidine, and $P < 0.0001$ for hours 4, 5, and 6 when compared to isopropamide. The authors also found that the combination of cimetidine plus isopropamide was statistically significantly more effective in suppressing acid secretion than the next highest tested dose of cimetidine alone in four of the six patients tested (McCARTHY and HYMAN 1982).

The ability of pirenzepine, a selective M_1 muscarinic cholinergic antagonist (Fig. 2), to control gastric acid secretion in five patients with ZES who were being treated with cimetidine plus isopropamide or probanthine but who developed severe anticholinergic side-effects has been reported (COLLEN et al. 1982). With cimetidine alone (1.8–7.2 mg/day), gastric acid secretion was reduced to a mean value of 16 ± 6 mEq/h 1 h prior to the next dose of medication, whereas with the same dose of cimetidine plus pirenzepine (75–125 mg/day) gastric acid secretion was 5 ± 3 mEq/h. No patient developed adverse side-effects with pirenzepine, and each patient was treated with cimetidine plus pirenzepine for 2–5 months with no evidence of toxicity or side-effects. In another study, five ZES patients were studied using a combination of cimetidine and pirenzepine (72 mg/day) after failing therapy with the same dose of cimetidine (2.4–3.2 g/day) alone (MIGNON et al. 1980). In four cases i.v. cimetidine and i.v. pirenzepine were administered together as a treatment and were successful in three of the cases as judged by the disappearance of clinical symptoms and the healing of gastroduodenal and jejunal mucosal ulceration within 14 days or less. The efficacy of the treatment was judged by continuous or repeated aspiration of the gastric contents and by measurement of the daily fecal output over two consecutive 24-h periods. In three cases it was apparent that the combination of the two drugs (oral cimetidine 2.4 g plus pirenzepine 1 mg/kg) caused anacidity in a significantly greater number of acid specimens than was the case during treatment with cimetidine alone (i.e., 2.4 g). In one patient the duration and efficacy of pirenzepine alone in suppressing gastric secretion was studied on three separate days. Studies were begun 3 h after stopping an i.v. infusion of cimetidine and after determining the 1-h secretory output. Pirenzepine was given intramuscularly in a dose of 0.5 mg/kg. The mean output of acid was 79 mEq/h before pirenzepine, 17.5 mEq/h at 2 h after injection, and 32 mEq/h at 9 h after injection.

Until the development of the H^+,K^+-ATPase inhibitor omeprazole, or more powerful H_2 receptor antagonists such as famotidine, anticholinergic agents were frequently added to H_2 receptor antagonists (JENSEN et al. 1986); JENSEN and GARDNER 1986). However, with the classical anticholinergic agents side-effects such as dry mouth and difficulty with vision occurred in a significant number of patients. Therefore, these agents were not well tolerated. The selective antagonist, pirenzepine, causes fewer side-effects, but too few patients have been treated to assess the true frequency of side-effects.

IV. Prostaglandins

Only one published study has examined the effect of prostaglandin on patients with ZES (IPPOLITI et al. 1981). Oral 16, 16-dimethyl prostaglandin E_2 (PGE_2) was given in a dose of 1 µg/kg to six unoperated ZES patients. IPPOLITI et al. (1981) found that oral dimethyl PGE_2 significantly inhibited basal gastric acid secretion for 3 h ($P < 0.001$). Two hours after giving 0.15 M NaCl to these patients mean gastric acid secretion was 53.3 ± 12.5 mEq/2 h (range 29–101 mEq/2 h); during the 2 h after 1 µg/kg dimethyl PGE_2 acid secretion was 8.2 ± 1.5 mEq/2 h, and basal hypergastrinemia in these patients was not altered.

The most common side-effect of misoprostol is diarrhea, which occurs in from 4%–15% of patients treated in various series. When misoprostol is used in conventional doses diarrhea is reported to be transient and to stop despite continued administration (EULER 1987). Prostaglandins are rarely used in hypersecretory states because the high doses required cause frequent side-effects, including diarrhea, limiting its utility (JENSEN et al. 1986).

V. Somatostatin or SMS 201-995

Somatostatin is a naturally occurring cyclic peptide containing 14 amino acids that inhibits the release of numerous peptide hormones and has many effects on gastrointestinal function (ADRIAN et al. 1981). One of these effects is the inhibition of pentagastrin-stimulated gastric secretion and inhibition of gastrin secretion. Because of these effects the use of native somatostatin and a long-acting somatostatin analogue (SMS 201-995) has been proposed in the symptomatic treatment of ZES. Native somatostatin has a very short half-life (2–3 min) (KUTZ et al. 1986), making it impractical to use long-term. In contrast, the new synthetic analogue SMS 201-995, a cyclic octapeptide (D-Phe-Cys-Phe-D-Trp-Cys-Thr-Cys-Throl) has a duration of action of 90 min (PLESS et al. 1986) and can be used intermittently by subcutaneous injection.

Native somatostatin infusions in eight patients with ZES resulted in short-term reductions in serum gastrin levels (40% ± 7%) and acid output (ARNOLD et al. 1975). In another report a patient with ZES experienced rebound acid secretion following infusion of native somatostatin, but it was not clear if the patient's serum gastrin concentration was reduced (BONFILS et al. 1982). A case report described a patient with ZES who received SMS 201-995 with a decrease in serum gastrin concentrations and improvement in symptoms. However, when SMS 201-995 treatment was discontinued after 3 months the patient had a rebound in symptoms and serum gastrin levels (BUCK et al. 1987). ELLISON et al. (1986a) studied ten patients with gastrinoma in order to define the duration of action and the variability of inhibition in serum gastrin caused by SMS 201-995 and also to determine the effect on stimulated serum gastrin secretion. They reported a significant reduction in serum gastrin levels beginning 1 h and persisting for 16 h after a single subcutaneous injection of SMS 201-995. Maximum inhibition of gastrin occurred 6 h after administration of the drug (a mean of 25% of basal levels, with a range of 11%–37%). Gastrin levels were noted to begin to increase after 6 h, returning to baseline levels by 18 h. No rebound or overshoot above baseline in serum gastrin was noted for the 18 h of the study (ELLISON et al. 1986a,b).

In a second series of experiments the effect of subcutaneous administration of SMS 201-995 (1 µg/kg) on secretin-stimulated gastrin secretion (three patients) and calcium-stimulated gastrin secretion (three patients) was studied (ELLISON et al. 1986). During the 1st hour after the administration of secretin without pretreatment with SMS 201-995, the integrated change in gastrin was 36.8 ± 11 mg·60 min/ml. Following pretreatment with SMS 201-995, the mean integrated change in gastrin levels was -1.1 ± 0.76 hg·60 min/ml. In the control group, the expected stimulation occurred, with a peak level of stimulation observed between 2 and 5 min. Following administration of SMS 201-995, no stimulation was observed. During the 1st hour following the administration of calcium without pretreatment with SMS 201-995, the mean integrated change in gastrin was 129 ± 30 hg ·60 min/ml, compared with -29 ± 28 hg·60 min/ml following SMS 201-995 pretreatment ($P < 0.05$). As occurred after secretin stimulation, there was no delayed calcium stimulation of gastrin secretion during the 12 h following administration of SMS 201-995. At present somatostatin therapy for relief of symptoms due to acid hypersecretion in ZES is not recommended since much more efficacious therapy such as the potent H_2 receptor antagonists or omeprazole is available (JENSEN 1988).

VI. Gastrin Receptor Antagonists

The gastrin receptor antagonist proglumide has not been successful at controlling gastric acid hypersecretion in patients with ZES. In a preliminary study at NIH even very high doses of proglumide (1.4 g bolus and 1.0 g/h) in five patients with ZES failed to change the BAO (COLLINS, unpublished data).

G. Surgical Therapy

The ideal treatment of ZES is surgical excision of the gastrinoma. In early studies surgical cure was only possible in 5% of patients (JENSEN et al. 1984; WOLFE and JENSEN 1987; THOMPSON et al. 1975; DEVENEY et al. 1978). Recent studies suggest a higher cure rate, averaging approximately 20% (see Table 5). A number of recent developments may lead to surgical cure rates even higher than 20% in the future. These include first, the development of effective antisecretory agents, which allow patients to undergo extensive preoperative investigational studies and allow surgeons to perform elective operations directed at gastrinoma localization and removal without the emphasis on performing surgery to control gastric acid hypersecretion. Second, preoperative localization allows the identification of metastatic liver disease in more than 90% of patients with metastatic hepatic gastrinoma, obviating unnecessary attempts at curative surgery (JENSEN et al. 1986; WOLFE and JENSEN 1987; WANK et al. 1987; MATON et al. 1987). Third, clinical distinction between patients with and without MEN-I allows identification of groups with different potential for cure. Fourth, in patients with nonmetastatic, sporadic gastrinoma, the cure rate may be much higher in those patients with extrapancreatic gastrinoma (up to 66%) than in those with pancreatic gastrinoma (THOMPSON et al. 1983; MATON et al. 1986; DEVENEY et al. 1983; MALAGELADA et al. 1983; HOFMANN et al. 1973; WOLFE et al. 1982). For the

Table 5. Results of attempts at complete surgical resection of gastrinoma

No. of patients operated[a]	% with normal serum gastrin postop.	Reference
25	4	STAGE and STADIL (1979)
42	5	ZOLLINGER et al. (1980)
32	6	BONFILS et al. (1981)
23	39	FRIESEN (1982)
18	22	WOLFE et al. (1982)
26	12	THOMPSON et al. (1983)
52	12	DEVENEY et al. (1983)
44	16	MALAGELADA et al. (1983)
45	11	STABILE et al. (1984)
22	18	RICHARDSON et al. (1985)
29	43 (postop.) 30 (6 mo–4 yr)	NORTON et al. (1986c)
20	25	VOGEL et al. (1987)

[a] No. of patients includes the total of patients reported to have undergone exploratory laparotomy in each series.

above reasons the current recommendation is for all patients with sporadic gastrinoma, i.e., ZES that is not associated with MEN-I and no serious contraindications to surgery, to undergo tumor localization studies. If no metastases are found, the patient should undergo surgical exploration.

The single most important factor in achieving a good surgical result is the expertise of the surgeon (JENSEN et al. 1986; WOLFE and JENSEN 1987). At surgery either a long midline or a bilateral subcostal incision is used. The liver, small intestine, pancreas, stomach, duodenum, mesenteric and retroperitoneal regions in the upper abdomen, and the pelvis, particularly the ovaries in a female, are carefully explored and palpated. The pancreas should be examined visually and by careful palpation. The pancreatic head should be inspected after an extended Kocher maneuver (NORTON et al. 1986c). The pancreatic body and tail are inspected by opening the lesser sac along the avascular plane of the transverse colon and the inferior border of the pancreas is dissected free so that the body and tail can be palpated between two fingers. The entire duodenum should be carefully palpated and any suspicious nodule is better exposed by opening the duodenum. Any suspicious pancreatic, stomach, duodenal, bowel, or peripancreatic nodule or lymph node should be removed for pathological examination. The same extensive search should be made regardless of the preoperative localization information. Furthermore, even if one gastrinoma is found the extensive search should still be completed because gastrinomas are frequently multiple or metastatic. If a gastrinoma is found as a solitary lesion in the liver, it should be removed, provided the resection can be performed safely. If a gastrinoma is found in the pancreatic head it should be enucleated (NORTON et al. 1986; WOLFE and JENSEN 1987). If an unresectable gastrinoma is found in the pancreatic head area, a pancreaticoduodenectomy is not indicated. No studies have demonstrated an increased survival overall in patients with ZES after pancreaticoduodenectomy. Because of the marked morbidity and mortality associated with this operation (up to 37% in one study) (ROCHE et al. 1982) and the excellent long-term prognosis of these patients, it has not been established that the adverse consequences of the performance of a pancreaticoduodenectomy might not outweigh the adverse consequences of an unresected solitary gastrinoma. If no gastrinoma is found at surgery, as occurs in 30% of cases overall but was the case in up to 60% of patients in one series (RICHARDSON et al. 1985), a blind distal pancreatectomy should not be performed, since 65%–90% of gastrinomas are now found in the pancreatic head or duodenum (gastrinoma triangle) (STABILE et al. 1984; NORTON et al. 1986c) and since such an approach has not improved cure rates (WOLFE and JENSEN 1987). If no tumor is found at laparotomy, or if the gastrinoma is unresectable or metastatic to the liver and the patient had a high antisecretory drug requirement prior to surgery (>4.8 g/day cimetidine), a highly selective vagotomy may be considered.

At present the role of surgery in the treatment of patients with ZES with MEN-I is unclear (JENSEN et al. 1986; NORTON 1984). Because of the low possibility of cure, because recent studies suggest that gastrinomas in familial cases are less malignant, and because these patients almost always have multiple small gastrinomas (THOMPSON et al. 1984), some groups recommend no exploratory laparotomy (STABILE et al. 1984; MALAGELADA et al. 1978) or recommend a laparotomy only if a localized lesion is predicted by a localized gastrin gradient from selective venous sampling for gastrin (THOMPSON et al. 1981) or if the fasting serum pancreatic polypeptide concentration is more than three times normal (FRIESEN et al. 1983). It is not established that familial gastrinoma has a less malignant course (JENSEN et al. 1983b). Also, too few patients have had exploratory laparotomies after measurement of pancreatic polypeptide concentrations or gastrin sampling studies to assess adequately their potiential usefulness. Because many of these patients' parents died of metastatic gastrinoma and many of the patients present at relatively young ages with a large tumor, for a particular kindred a surgical approach similar to the one used in patients with sporadic disease may be warranted (WOLFE and JENSEN 1987). Therefore, at present, we currently recommend that all patients with ZES and MEN-I undergo extensive tumor localization studies, but that only those patients with unequivocally positive imaging studies undergo surgical exploration. This approach is predicated on the fact that without total pancreaticoduodenectomy these patients cannot be cured, and that the imaging studies detect most large tumors (>3 cm) (MATON et al. 1987; WANK et al. 1987) which may metastasize if left untreated.

The effect of parathyroidectomy in patients with hyperparathyroidism, ZES, and MEN-I was studied prospectively (NORTON et al. 1987). This group

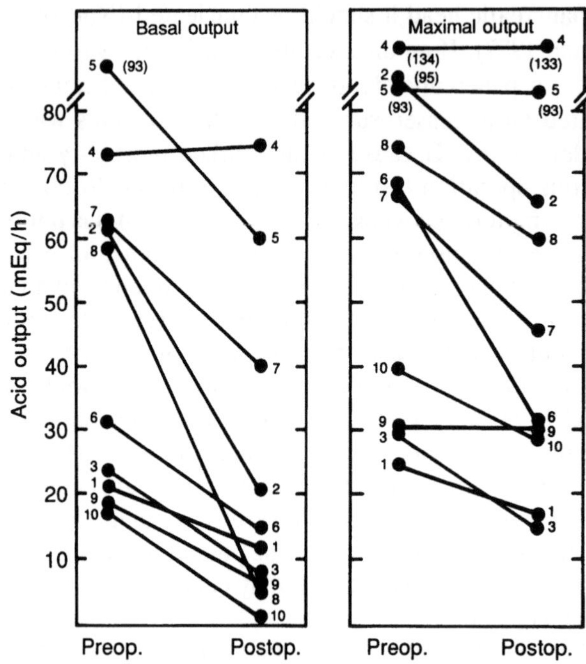

Fig. 11. The basal acid output (*left*) and maximal acid output (*right*) are shown before and after parathyroidectomy for ten patients with hyperparathyroidism, ZES, and MEN-I. Basal gastric hypersecretion was defined as greater than 15 mEq/h in patients without previous gastric surgery (patients 1–2, 4–10) or greater than 5 mEq/h in patients with previous gastric surgery (patient 3). Except for patient 4, all patients were normocalcemic after surgery. *Numbers* refer to individual patients. (NORTON et al. 1987)

found that all patients who were normocalcemic postoperatively (90%) had a decline in BAO, 80% had a decline in maximal acid output, 80% had a decrease in fasting serum gastrin, and 33% had a negative secretin test (Fig. 11). Antisecretory medication could be reduced because patients had an increased sensitivity to H_2 receptor antagonists and a lower BAO (Fig. 12) (NORTON et al. 1987).

H. Tumor Localization

Precise localization of the gastrinoma has become an increasingly important factor in evaluating patients with ZES. With the increased ability to control gastric acid hypersecretion long-term, the growth and possible metastatic spread of the gastrinoma has become a major determinant of long-term survival (ZOLLINGER and ELLISON 1955; JENSEN et al. 1986; ZOLLINGER et al. 1976; FOX et al. 1974).

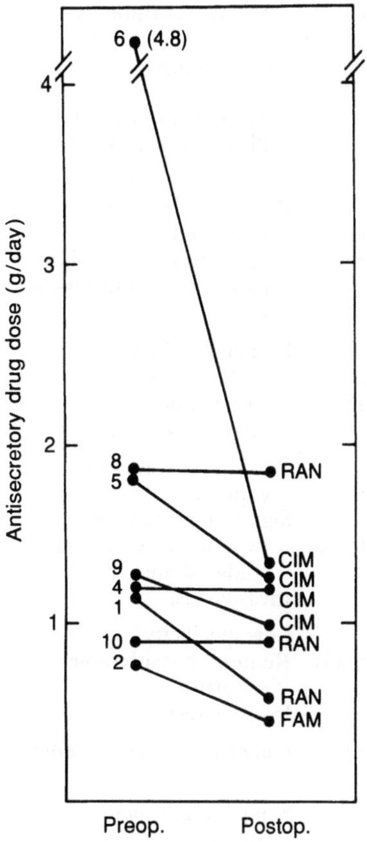

Fig. 12. The antisecretory drug dose before and after parathyroidectomy for eight patients with hyperparathyroidism, ZES, and MEN-I. *RAN*, ranitidine; *CIM*, cimetidine; *FAM*, famotidine. (NORTON et al. 1987)

Careful imaging studies may assist the surgeon in localizing the tumor. A number of different techniques, including abdominal ultrasound (HANCKE 1979; SHAWKER et al. 1982; NORTON et al. 1986c), CT scanning (THOMPSON et al. 1983; DAMGAARD-PETERSEN et al. 1979; DUNNICK et al. 1980; STARK et al. 1984; KRUDY et al. 1984; WANK et al. 1987), selective abdominal angiography (BURCHARTH et al. 1979; ROCHE et al. 1982; MATON et al. 1987; KRUDY et al. 1984; RUSZNEWSKI et al. 1986), selective venous sampling for gastrin from portal venous tributaries (ROCHE et al. 1982; BURCHARTH et al. 1979; GLOWNIAK et al. 1982; CHERNER et al. 1986), venous sampling after arterial secretion injection (IMAMURA et al. 1988), MRI scanning (ANDERSSON et al. 1987; SAEED et al. 1988a; STARK et al. 1983), and intraoperative ultrasonography (SIGEL et al. 1982; CHARBONEAU et al. 1983; CROMACK et al. 1987; NORTON et al. 1988a,b), have all been reported to be helpful in localizing gastrinomas (Tables 6–8).

In general abdominal ultrasound has a low sensitivity, with studies demonstrating a sensitivity of 14% and a specificity of 100% for hepatic metas-

Table 6. Advantages and disadvantages of tests used in localizing gastrinomas

Modality	Advantages	Disadvantages
1. Upper gastrointestinal endoscopy or radiology	Widely available	Almost never localizes duodenal gastrinoma
2. Ultrasound	Widely available Localizes large tumors No radiation exposure	Rarely localizes small primary tumors Frequently does not show gastrinoma metastatic to liver
3. Computed tomography with oral and intravenous contrast (CT)	Widely available Localizes most hepatic gastrinomas and many primaries	Frequently does not localize primary gastrinoma Radiation exposure
4. Selective abdominal angiography	Localizes primary gastrinoma and liver metastases not identified by other tests	Requires considerable expertise Significant radiation exposure if sequential studies done Invasive test
5. Selective portal venous sampling for gastrin (PVS)	Localizes area where functional gastrinoma is present	Low specificity Requires considerable expertise Invasive test
6. Arterial secretin with venous sampling	Less expertise required than with PVS	Only a few patients studied
7. Intraoperative ultrasound	Direct confirmation to surgeon May identify malignant tumors	Not generally available Equipment expensive Requires considerable expertise Limited data
8. Magnetic resonance imaging (MRI)	No radiation exposure	Limited experience Low sensitivity and specificity Current MRI scanners have long scanning time
9. Intraoperative endoscopy	Allows transillumination of the duodenum Detects high frequency of duodenal gastrinoma	Limited data

tases and a sensitivity of 21%–28% and a specificity of 92%–93% for primary gastrinoma (NORTON et al. 1986; HANCKE 1979; SHAWKER et al. 1982). CT scanning performed with intravenous contrast in recent studies had a sensitivity of 35%–72% and a specificity of 98%–100% for primary gastrinomas (Fig. 13) (NORTON et al. 1986; WOLFE and JENSEN 1987; STARK et al. 1984; DUNNICK et al. 1980; KRUDY et al. 1984; WANK et al. 1987; RUSZNIEWSKI et al. 1986). Selective abdominal angiography was originally reported to give high

Table 7. Ability of various imaging tests to detect primary gastrinoma found at surgery

	Sensitivity Mean (range) (%)	Specificity Mean (range) (%)
Ultrasound	23 (21–28)	92
CT scan	50 (35–59)	90 (83–100)
Angiography	68 (35–68)	95
PVS	73	33
IOUS	83	Not evaluated
MRI	21	33

Sensitivity = true-positives/(true-positives + false-negatives); specificity = true-negatives/(true-negatives + false-positives); CT scan = computed tomography with contrast (oral and intravenous); angiography = selective abdominal angiography; PVS = portal venous sampling for gastrin; IOUS = intraoperative ultrasound; MRI = magnetic resonance imaging.

Table 8. Ability of various imaging modalities to detect metastatic gastrinoma to the liver found at surgery

	Sensitivity Mean (range) (%)	Specificity Mean (range) (%)
Ultrasound	14	100
CT scan	54 (35–72)	99 (98–100)
Angiography	62 (33–86)	98
PVS	Not evaluated	Not evaluated
IOUS	Not evaluated	Not evaluated
MRI	67	Not evaluated

Sensitivity = true-positives/(true-positives + false-negatives); specificity = true-negatives/(true-negatives + false-positives); CT scan = computed tomography with contrast (oral and intravenous); angiography = selective abdominal angiography; PVS = portal venous sampling for gastrin; IOUS = intraoperative ultrasound; MRI = magnetic resonance imaging.

false-positive and false-negative rates (Thompson et al. 1983; Roche et al. 1982). However, in recent studies selective angiography has been shown to have a high sensitivity and specificity (Fig. 13). Recently angiography was found to have a sensitivity of 33%–86% and specificity of 96%–100% for hepatic metastases and a sensitivity of 35%–68% and specificity of 84%–94% for primary gastrinoma (Norton et al. 1986; Wolfe and Jensen 1987; Ruszniewski et al. 1986; Maton et al. 1987). In a recent comparative study of CT and angiography, angiography identified 17% more hepatic metastases (Maton et al. 1987). Angiography identified 13% more primary gastrinomas than CT, and combination of the techniques identified the same number as did angiography alone. The specificity of CT was 98% and the specificity of angiography was 100% (Maton et al. 1987). CT scanning should be the initial imaging procedure done because of its general availability, ease of perform-

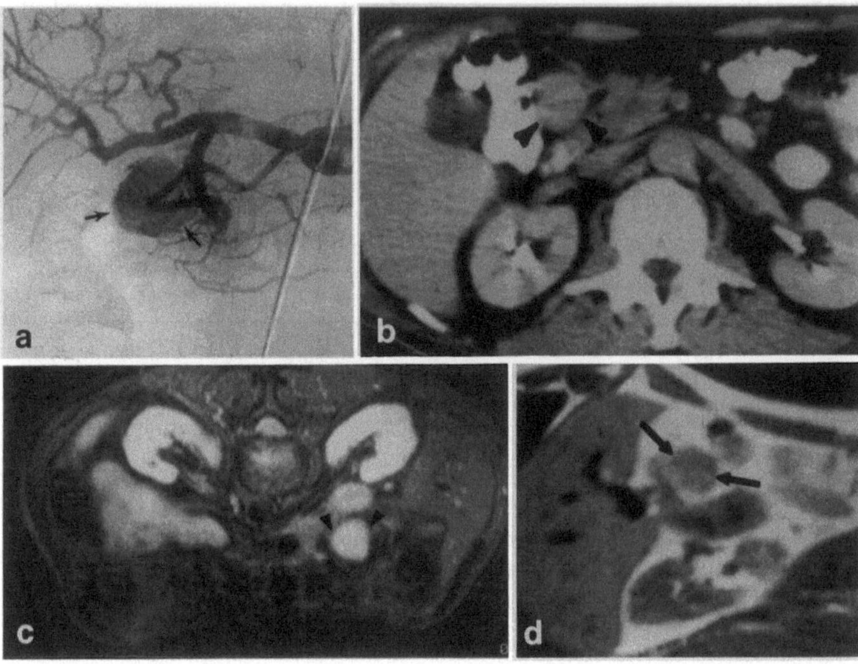

Fig. 13. a–d. Localization of gastrinoma by angiography, CT scanning, and MRI in a single patient with ZES. **a** shows results of selective abdominal angiogram with a selective injection into the gastroduodenal artery demonstrating a 3 cm gastrinoma (*arrows*). **b** is a CT scan demonstrating a 2-cm gastrinoma medial to the hepatic flexures (*arrows*). **c** a stir-weighed MRI scan (transverse section) and **d** is a T1-weighed image (sagittal panel). *Arrows* in the *right-hand panels* indicate the gastrinoma

ance, sensitivity, and specificity (WANK et al. 1987). If the localization and extent of tumor are still in question, selective angiography should be performed (MATON et al. 1987).

Recently four new techniques, selective venous sampling for gastrin from portal venous tributaries, (Fig. 14), venous sampling after intra-arterial secretin, MRI scanning (Fig. 13), and intraoperative ultrasonography, have been reported to be useful in localizing gastrinomas. Whereas initial studies suggested selective venous sampling for gastrin would be very helpful (BURCHARTH et al. 1979; ROCHE et al. 1982; GLOWNIAK et al. 1982), a recent prospective study (CHERNER et al. 1986) demonstrated that a combination of selective venous sampling and imaging yielded only marginally better results than imaging alone in identifying gastrinomas preoperatively, that were subsequently found at surgery. Therefore, selective venous sampling for gastrin, although occasionally helpful, should not be used routinely (CHERNER et al. 1986; WOLFE and JENSEN 1987). Venous sampling after intra-arterial secretin has been reported to localize gastrinomas (IMAMURA et al. 1988) but experience to date is too limited to assess this technique (Table 6).

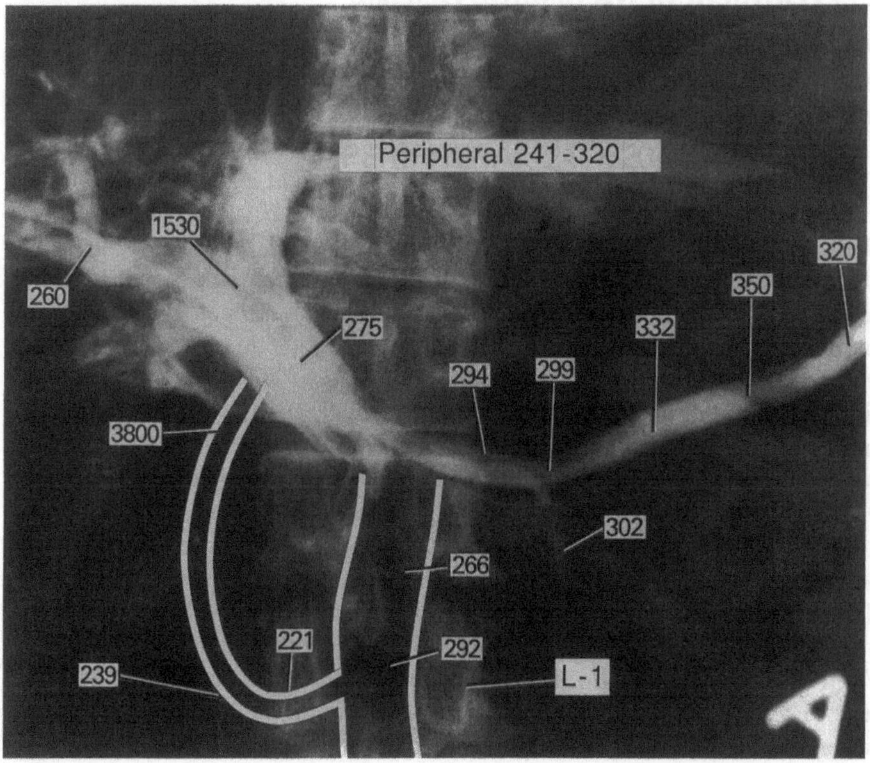

Fig. 14. Portal venous sampling for gastrin in a patient with ZES. Values shown are serum gastrin concentrations in pg/ml in the location from which the sample was taken. *Peripheral* indicates the simultaneous peripheral venous value. This patient had a gastrin concentration of 3800 pg/ml in the superior pancreaticoduodenal vein with an average peripheral gastrin concentration of 275 pg/ml, giving a localized gastrin gradient of 1307%. At surgery a localized gastrinoma was removed from the pancreatic head in the area suggested by the localization

Intraoperative ultrasonography has been reported to be helpful in localizing gastrinomas at surgery (Sigel et al. 1982; Charboneau et al. 1983; Cromack et al. 1987; Norton et al. 1988). In one recent report, this procedure led to a change in operative management in 10% of all ZES cases operated on, either by localizing additional gastrinomas or by determining that a gastrinoma was malignant (Norton et al. 1988). Although the equipment is expensive and requires considerable experience, these results suggest that intraoperative ultrasonography will play an increasing role in the future (see Table 6).

In the past MRI scanning (Fig. 13) was found to be useful for imaging islet tumors (Stark et al. 1983; Andersson et al. 1987); however, in a recent prospective study involving 24 patients with ZES, it was found to be less sensitive than CT scanning or angiography (Frucht et al. 1987; Saeed et al. 1988a) (Table 6).

J. Treatment of Metastatic Disease

With the ability to control gastric acid hypersecretion, increasing numbers of patients will develop metastatic disease. Therefore, there is an increasing need for effective treatment of disseminated disease. Chemotherapy, hepatic embolization (MATON et al. 1983; CARRASCO et al. 1983), systemic removal of all resectable tumor (ZOLLINGER et al. 1980; NORTON et al. 1986b), hormonal therapy with a somatostatin analogue such as SMS 201-995 (MATON et al. 1988), and treatment with interferon (ERICKSON et al. 1986) have all been advocated (Table 9). The current role of all of these therapies remains uncertain and awaits further trials. Chemotherapy using streptozotocin alone or in combination with 5-fluorouracil, or 5-fluorouracil plus doxorubicin has been reported to be effective at reducing tumor size in 20%–63% of patients with islet cell tumors. In one study (MOERTEL et al. 1980) the combination of streptozotocin plus 5-fluorouracil was more effective than streptozotocin alone. Dacarbazine and doxorubicin have given poor response rates alone (9%–20%) and chlorozotocin has given approximately the same response rate (i.e., 50%) as streptozotocin alone. Almost all large studies investigating the effects of chemotherapeutic agents on islet cell tumors have combined all islet cell tumors together (i.e., generally insulinomas, gastrinomas, nonfunctioning islet cell tumors, and pancreatic polypeptide releasing tumors). Whether these results can be extrapolated to metastatic gastrinoma is unclear. Two studies have demonstrated no difference in response rates of various islet cell tumors to streptozotocin (MOERTEL et al. 1980; BUCHANAN et al. 1986b); however, these were small studies comparing different types of islet cell tumor. When results are combined from a number of small series, streptozotocin alone appears to cause an objective response in 50% of patients with metastatic gastrinoma (Table 9). Streptozotocin combined with 5-fluorouracil or 5-fluorouracil plus doxorubicin causes an objective response

Table 9. Drug therapy for gastrinomas

	No. of patients	Objective responses	Reference
STZ	24	12 (50%)	JENSEN et al. (1983b) MOERTEL et al. (1980) BRODER and CARTER (1973)
DTIC	5	0 (0%)	NIH (1987)
STZ + 5-FU	3	1 (33%)	MOERTEL et al. (1980)
	10	8 (80%)	MIGNON et al. (1986)
	5	1 (20%)	ZOLLINGER et al. (1976)
STZ + 5-FU STZ	28 17	(42%)	BONFILS et al. (1986a)
STZ + 5-FU + DOX	10	4 (40%)	VON SCHRENCK et al. (1988)
SMS 201-995	4	3 (75%)	MATON et al. (1989)
Interferon	4	2 (50%)	ERICKSON et al. (1986)

Abbreviations: STZ, streptozotocin; DOX, doxorubicin; 5-FU, 5-fluorouracil; DTIC, dacarbazine; interferon, human leukocyte interferon.

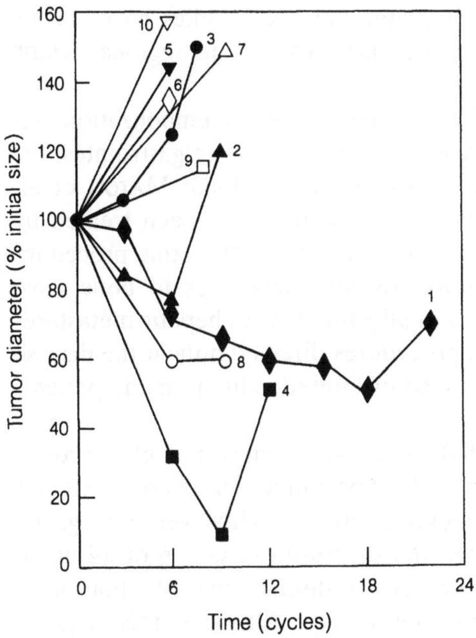

Fig. 15. Effect of chemotherapy on tumor diameter evaluated by CT scan. The largest diameter of the most clearly measurable tumor lesion was measured before chemotherapy and at each of the indicated times after starting chemotherapy. Tumor diameter at times after starting chemotherapy was expressed as the percentage of the tumor diameter before chemotherapy. The *numbers* refer to individual patients. (von Schrenck et al. 1988)

in 20%–80% of patients with metastatic gastrinoma (Table 9). For all islet cell tumors the combination of streptozotocin plus 5-fluorouracil gave a response rate of 63%, which was significantly better than the 40% response rate with streptozotocin alone (Moertel et al. 1980). Whether similar results would be obtained with gastrinoma alone is unknow. Furthermore, in a recent prospective study of ten patients with metastatic gastrinoma to the liver that increased in size over a 6-month period prior to entry to the study, chemotherapy with streptozotocin, 5-fluorouracil, and doxorubicin resulted in a 40% response rate (≥25% decrease in tumor size with no new lesions) (von Schrenck et al. 1988). Responses occurred at 3.7 ± 0.7 months and lasted 9.7 ± 2.8 cycles. No complete responses occurred and survival was not significantly different in responders and nonresponders (Fig. 15) (von Schrenck et al. 1988). Therefore, the precise role and efficacy of chemotherapy in patients with metastatic gastrinoma have not been established. Also not established is when chemotherapy should be considered in a given patient with metastatic disease. Some patients have been followed for 20 years with stable metastatic disease (Zollinger et al. 1976) whereas most die within 5 years with the mean survival being 3–5 years (Zollinger et al. 1980; Bonfils et al. 1981; Thompson et al. 1983; Deveney et al. 1978; Norton et al. 1986b). Of the two groups with considerable experience treating metastatic gastrinoma, one group proposes that patients be treated with chemotherapy when they become symptomatic (Moertel et al. 1980). However, if gastric acid hypersecretion is controlled adequately, symptoms due to the tumor only arise very late in the course of the disease. The other group (Jensen et al. 1983b, 1986) proposes that after the initial evaluation patients be reassessed in 3–6 months and that those patients with increasing hepatic metastases should be treated with chemotherapy. No studies have recommended chemotherapy in patients with metastases only to regional lymph nodes.

For tumors metastatic to the liver, hepatic arterial embolization has been recommended in patients with gastrinoma and other gastrointestinal endocrine tumors (carcinoids, etc.) (CARRASCO et al. 1983; MATON et al. 1983). However, only small numbers of gastrinomas have been treated by this technique and it is not possible to determine whether this procedure affects long-term survival. Furthermore, distant metastases to bone have been reported recently to occur in 12% of all patients with hepatic metastases (BARTON et al. 1986), suggesting that procedures directed only at the disease in the liver, such as embolization, may be of limited value in many patients with extensive disease.

The data of ZOLLINGER et al. (1980) suggest that removal of all resectable tumor or "debulking surgery" prolongs life expectancy. There are no studies that have systemically evaluated debulking surgery. However, one group (NORTON et al. 1986) recently reported the successful resection of all metastatic disease in 4 of 20 patients with extensive disease, two of whom have maintained normal gastrin levels postoperatively. Although this requires systematic evaluation before it can be routinely recommended, these results raise the possibility that a small percentage of patients with extensive disease can be identified in whom removal of all resectable tumor may provide prolonged benefit.

Hormonal therapy with the long-acting somatostatin analogue, SMS 201-995, has been shown to be effective in controlling the symptoms due to a number of different islet cell or carcinoid-like tumors, including VIPomas, glucagonomas, GRFomas, insulinomas, gastrinomas, and carcinoids (MATON et al. 1989) (Table 9). SMS 201-995 has been reported to decrease the size of metastases or growth of islet cell tumors in animals (REUBI 1985) and humans (KVOLS et al. 1987). Studies have reported a decrease in hepatic metastases in two patients with gastrinoma (SHEPARD and SENATOR 1986; BONFILS et al. 1986b, MATON et al. 1988); however, another recent study of nine patients with metastatic gastrinoma treated with SMS 201-995 for 1–11 months reported no effect (KVOLS et al. 1987). Therefore, at present, until controlled trials are done, treatment with SMS 201-995 cannot be recommended for routine use in patients with metastatic gastrinoma.

A recent study has demonstrated that human leukocyte interferon (ERICKSON et al. 1986) may be helpful in patients with metastatic islet cell tumors, including gastrinoma (Table 9). In this study 17 of 22 patients, most of whom had previously failed chemotherapy, demonstrated an objective response (defined as a decrease of more than 50% in tumor size or in tumor markers) with interferon treatment. Two of four patients with metastatic gastrinoma responded (Table 9). However, because of the small numbers of cases and limited follow-up, it is unclear whether interferon will provide long-term benefit for patients with metastatic gastrinoma.

References

Adrian TE, Barnes AJ, Long RG, O'Shaughessy DJ, Brown MR, Rivier J, Vale W, Blackburn AM, Bloom SR (1981) The effect of somatostatin analogs on secretion of growth, pancreatic and gastrointestinal hormones in man. J Clin Endocrinol Metab 53:675–681

Andersen BN, Larsen NE, Rune SJ, Worning H (1985) Development of cimetidine resistance in Zollinger-Ellison syndrome. Gut 26:1263–1265

Andersson T, Eriksson B, Hemmingsson A, et al. (1987) Angiography, computed tomography, magnetic resonance imaging and ultrasonography in detection of liver metastasis from endocrine gastrointestinal tumors. Acta Radiol 28:535–539

Aoyagi T, Summerskill WHJ (1966) Gastric secretion with ulcerogenic islet cell tumor: importance of basal acid output. Arch Intern Med 117:667–672

Arnold R, Kobberling J, Track NS, Creutzfeldt W (1975) Lowering of basal and stimulated serum immunoreactive gastrin and gastric secretion in patients with Zollinger-Ellison syndrome by somatostatin (Abstr). Acta Endocrinol [Suppl] (Copenh) 193:75

Bardman KD, Bianchi Porro G, Bose K, Daly K, Hinchliffe RFC (1986) Comparison of two different doses of omeprazole versus ranitidine treatment of duodenal ulcers. J Clin Gastroenterol 8:403–413

Bardram L, Stage JG (1985) Frequency of endocrine disorders in patients with the Zollinger-Ellison syndrome. Scand J Gastroenterol 20:233–238

Baron JH (1979) Clinical tests of gastric secretion – history, methodology and interpretation, Oxford University Press New York, pp 123–136

Barton JC, Hirschowitz BI, Maton PN, Jensen RT (1986) Bone metastases in malignant gastrinoma. Gastroenterology 91:1179–1185

Black JW, Shankley NP (1987) How does gastrin act to stimulate oxyntic cell secretion. Trends Pharm Sci 8:486–490

Blanchi A, Delchier JC, Soule JC, Payen D, Bader JP (1982) Control of acute Zollinger-Ellison syndrome with intravenous omeprazole. Lancet 2:1223–1224

Bonfils S, Bader J-P (1970) The diagnosis of Zollinger-Ellison syndrome with special reference to the multiple endocrine adenomas. 2:332–355

Bonfils S, Mignon M, Jian R, Lkoeti G (1977) Biological studies during long-term cimetidine administration in Zollinger-Ellison syndrome. In: Burland WL, Simkins MA (eds) Cimetidine: Proceedings of the Second International Symposium on Histamine H_2-receptor Antagonists. Excerpta Medica, Amsterdam, pp 311–321

Bonfils S, Mignon M, Grutton J (1979) Cimetidine treatment of acute and chronic Zollinger-Ellison syndrome. World J Surg 3:597–604

Bonfils S, Landor JH, Mignon M, Hervoir P (1981) Results of surgical management in 92 consecutive patients with Zollinger-Ellison syndrome. Ann Surg 194:692–697

Bonfils C, Chevalier T, Rene E, Rigaud D, Accary JP (1982) Interest of a somatostatin inhibition test in hormone secreting tumors (Abstr). Hepatogastroenterology 29:87

Bonfils S, Ruszniewski P, Hannar S, Laucournet H (1986a) Chemotherapy of hepatic motastases (HM) in Zollinger-Elligon syndrome (ZES). Report of a multicenteric analysis (Abstr). Dig Dis Sci 31:WS51

Bonfils S, Ruszniewski P, Laucouret H, Costil V, Rene W, Mignon M (1986b) Long-term management of Zollinger-Ellison syndrome with SMS 201-995, a long acting somatostatin analogue (Abstr). Can J Physiol Pharmacol 63

Broder LE, Carter SK (1973) Pancreatic islet cell carcinoma. Ann Intern Med 79:108–117

Brodgen RN, Heel TC, Speight TM, Avery GS (1978) Cimetidine: a review of its pharmacological and therapeutic efficacy in peptic ulcer disease. Drugs 15:93–131

Brodgen RN, Carmine AA, Heel RC, Speight TM, Avery GS (1982) Ranitidine: a review of its pharmacology and therapeutic use in peptic ulcer disease and other allied diseases. Drugs 24:267–303

Buchanan KD, Johnston CF, O'Hare MMT, Ardill JES, Shaw C, Collins JSA, Watson P, Atkinson AB, Hadden DR, Kennedy TL, Sloan JM (1986a) Neuroendocrine tumors: a European view. Am J Med [Suppl 6B] 81:14–23

Buchanan KD, O'Hare MMT, Russel CJF, Kennedy TL, Hadden DR (1986b) Factors involved in the responsiveness of gastrointestinal apudomas to streptozotocin. Dig Dis Sci 31:511S

Buck M, Kvols L, O'Dorisio T (1987) Rebound hypergastrinemia after cessation of a somatostatin analogue (SMS 201–995) in malignant gastrinoma. Am J Med 82:92–95

Burcharth F, Stage JG, Stadil F, Jensen LI, Fischermann K (1979) Localization of gastrinoma by transhepatic portal catheterization and gastrin assay. Gastroenterology 77:444–450

Cadiot G, Lehy T, Mignon M, Ruszniewski P, Elauaer-Blanc L, Bonfils S, Lewin M (1988) Comparative behavior of gastric endocrine cells and serum gastrin levels in Zollinger-Ellison patients during long term treatment with omeprazole or H_2 receptor antagonists (Abstr). Gastroenerology 94:A56

Cameron AJ, Hoffman HN (1974) Zollinger-Ellison syndrome. Clinical features and long term follow-up. Mayo Clin Proc 49:44–51

Campoli-Richards DM, Clissold SP (1986) Famotidine: pharmacodynamics and pharmacokinetic properties and a preliminary review of its therapuetic use in peptic ulcer disease and Zollinger Ellison syndrome. Drugs 32:197–221

Carrasco CH, Chuang VP, Wallace S (1983) Apudoma metastatic to the liver: treatment by hepatic artery embolization. Radiology 149:79–83

Cerra FB, Schentag JJ, McMillen M, Karwande SV, Fitzgerald GC, Leising M (1986) Mental status, the intensive care unit and cimetidine. Ann Surg 191:565–570

Charboneau WJ, James EM, van Heerden JA, et al. (1983) Intraoperative realtime ultrasonographic localization of pancreatic insulinomas. J Ultrasound Med 2: 251–255

Cherner JA, Doppman JL, Norton JA, Miller DL, Krudy AG, Raufman JP, Collen MJ, Maton PN, Gardner JD, Jensen RT (1986) Prospective assessment of selective venous sampling for gastrin to localize gastrinomas. Ann Intern Med 105:841–847

Chiang H-CV, O'Dorisio TM, Maton P, Gardner JD, Jensen RT (1990) Multiple hormonal elevation in patients with Zollinger-Ellison syndrome: Prospective study of clinical significance and of development of a second symptomatic pancreatic endocrine tumor syndrome. Gastroenterology 99:1565–1575

Classen M, Dammann HG, Domschke W, Hengels. KJ, Hutteman W, Londong W, Rehner M, Simon B, Witzel L, Berger UJ (1985) Kurzzeittherapie des Ulcus duodeni mit Omeprazol und Ranitidin. Dsct Med Wochenschr 110:210–215

Clissold SP, Campoli-Richards DM (1986) Omeprazole. Drugs 32:15–47

Clissold SP, Campoli-Richards DM (1988) Omeprazole: an updated review. Drugs 34:1–41

Collen MJ, Pandol SJ, Raufman JP, Allende HD, Gardner JD, Jensen RT (1982) Beneficial effects of pirenzepine, a selective anticholinergic agent in patients with Zollinger-Ellison syndrome. Gastroenterology 82:1035

Collen MJ, Howard JM, McArthur KE, Raufman JP, Cornelius AJ, Ciarleglio CA, Gardner JD, Jensen RT (1984) Comparison of ranitidine and cimetidine in the treatment of gastric hypersecretion. Ann Intern Med 100:52–58

Creutzfeldt W (1977) Discussion. In: Creutzfeldt W. (ed) Cimetidine. Excerpta Medica, Amsterdam, P 149

Creutzfeldt W, Arnold R, Creutzfeldt C, Track NS (1975) Pathomorphological, biochemical, and diagnostic aspects of gastrinomas (Zollinger-Ellison syndrome). Hum Pathol 6:47–76

Cromack DT, Norton JA, Sigel B, Shawker TH, Sigel B, Doppman JL, Maton PN, Jensen RT (1987) The use of high-resolution intraoperative ultrasound to localize gastrinomas: an initial report of a prospective study. World J Surg 11:648–653

Damgaard-Petersen K, Stage JG (1979) CT scanning in patients with Zollinger-Ellison syndrome and carcinoid syndrome. Scand J Gastroenterol 53:117–122
Dammann H-G, Muller P, Simon B (1983) 24 Hour intragastric acidity and single night-time dose of three H_2-blockers. Lancet 2:1078
Dammann H-G, Blum AL, Lux G, Rehner M, Riecken EO, Schiessel R, Wienbeck M, Witzel L, Berger J (1986) Differences in healing tendency of reflux esophagitis with omeprazole and ranitidine. Results of an Austrian-German-Swiss multicenter trial. Dtsch Med Wochenschr 6(111):123–128, 144
Dawson J, Bloom SR, Cockel RA (1983) Unique apudoma producing the glucagonoma and gastrinoma syndromes. Postgrad Med J 59:315–316
Delchier JC, Soule JC, Mignon M, Goldfam D, Cortot A, Bonfils SJ (1986) Effectiveness of omeprazole in seven patients with Zollinger-Ellison syndrome resistant to histamine H_2-receptor antagonists. Dig Dis Sci 31:693–699
Dembinski AB, Johnson LR (1979) Growth of pancreas and gastrointestinal mucosa in antrectomized and gastrin-treated rats. Endocrinology 105:769–773
Deveney CW, Deveney KS, Jaffe BM, Jones RS, Way LW (1977) Use of calcium and secretin in the diagnosis of gastrinoma (Zollinger-Ellison syndrome). Ann Intern Med 87:680–686
Deveney CW, Deveney KS, Way LW (1978) The Zollinger-Ellison syndrome – 23 years later. Ann Surg 188:384–393
Deveney CW, Deveney KS, Stark D, Moss A, Stein S, Way LW (1983) Resection of gastrinomas. Ann Surg 198:546–553
Dockray GJ, Walsh JH, Passaro E Jr (1975) Relative abundance of big and little gastrins in the tumors and blood of patients with Zollinger-Ellison syndrome. Gut 16:353–358
Dunnick NR, Doppman JL, Mills SR, Mills SR, McCarthy DM (1980) Computed tomographic detection of nonbeta pancreatic islet cell tumors. Radiology 135: 117–120
Eberle F, Grun R (1981) Multiple endocrine neoplasia, type I (MEN I). Ergeb Inn Med Kinderheilkd 46:75–150
Ekman L, Hansson E, Havu N, Carlsson E, Lundberg C (1985) Toxicological studies on omeprazole. Scand J Gastroenterol [Suppl] 108:53–69
Ellison EC, O'Dorisio TM, Sparks J, Mekjian HS, Fromkes JJ, Wottering EA, Carey LL (1986a) Observations on the effect of somatostatin analogue in the Zollinger-Ellison syndrome: implications for treatment of apudomas. Surgery 100:437–444
Ellison EC, Grower WR, Elkhammas E, Woltering EA, Sparks J, O'Dorision TM, Fabri PJ (1986b) Characterization of the in vivo and in vitro inhibition of gastrin secretion from gastrinoma by a somatostatin analogue (SMS 201–995). Am J Med [Suppl 6B] 81:56–64
Ellison EH, Wilson SD (1964) The Zollinger-Ellison syndrome: re-appraisal and evaluation of 260 registered cases. Ann Surg 160:512–530
Erickson B, Oberg K, Alm G, Karlsson A, Lundqvist G, Andersson T, Wilander E, Wide L (1986) Treatment of malignant endocrine pancreatic tumors with human leucocyte interferon. Lancet 2:1307–1309
Euler A (1987) Prostaglandins-gastrointestinal, therapeutic clinical experiences. In: Szabo S, Mozsik G (eds) New pharmacology of ulcer disease. Elsevier, Amsterdam, pp 329–337
Feldman M, Schiller LR, Walsh JH, Fordtran JS, Richardson CT (1987) Positive intravenous secretin test in patients with achlorhydria-related hypergastrinemia. Gastroenterology 93:59–62
Fellenius E, Berglindh T, Sachs G, Olbe L, Elander B, Sjostrand SE, Bjorn W (1981) Substituted benzimidazoles inhibit gastric acid secretion by blocking (H^+-K^+) ATPase. Nature 290:159–161
Fox PS, Hofmann JW, Wilson SD, DeCosse JJ (1974) Surgical management of the Zollinger-Ellison syndrome. Surg Clin North Am 54:395–407

Fraker D, Norton J, Saeed Z, Maton PN, Gardner JD, Jensen RT (1988) A prospective study of pre- and post-operative control of acid hypersecretion in patients with Zollinger-Ellison syndrome. Surgery 104:1054–1063
Friesen SR (1982) Treatment of the Zollinger-Ellison syndrome. Am J Surg 143: 331–338
Friesen SR, Tomita T (1981) Pseudo-Zollinger-Ellison syndrome: hypergastrinemia, hyperchlorhydria without tumor. Ann Surg 194:481–493
Friesen SR, Tomita T, Kimmel JR (1983) Pancreatic polypeptide update: its role in detection of the trait for multiple endocrine adenopathy syndrome, type 1 and pancreatic polypeptide-secreting tumors. Surgery 94:1028–1037
Frucht H, Doppman JL, Maton PN Norton JA, Wank SA, Vinayek R, Gardner JD, Jensen RT (1987) Prospective study of the ability of magnetic resonance imaging to localize gastrinomas (Abstr). Gastroenterology 92:1397
Frucht H, Howard JM, Laff JIS, McCarthy DM, Maton PN, Wank SA, Vinayek R, Gardner JD, Jensen RT (1989a) Secretin and calcium provocative tests in the Zollinger-Ellison syndrome: A prospective study. Ann Int Med 111:713–722
Frucht H, Howard JM, Stook HA, McCarthy DM, Maton PN, Goodsen JD, Jensen RT (1989b) Prospective study of meal provocative gastrin testing in patients with Zollinger-Ellison syndrome. Am J Med 87:524–536
Gajtkowski GA, Norris DB, Rising TJ, Wood TP (1983) Specific binding of ^{3}H-tiotidine to histamine H_2-receptors in guinea pig cerebral cortex. Nature 304: 65–67
Ganguli PC, Polak JM, Pearse AGE, Elder JB, Hegarty M (1974) Antral-gastrin cell hyperplasia in peptic-ulcer disease. Lancet 1:83–86
Glowniak JV, Shapiro B, Vinnik AI Glaser B, Thompson NM, Cho KT (1982) Percutaneous transhepatic venous sampling of gastrin. N Engl J Med 307: 293–297
Gregory RA, Grossman MI, Tracy HJ, Agarwal KL (1969) Amino acid constitution of two gastrins isolated from Zollinger-Ellison tumor tissue. Gut 10:603–608
Grossman MI (1981) Peptic ulcer. Yearbook Medical Publishers, Chicago, pp 141–151
Gugler R, Jensen JC (1985) Omeprazole inhibits oxidative drug metabolism. Gastroenterology 89:1235–1241
Hancke S (1979) Localization of hormone-producing gastrointestinal tumors by ultrasonic scanning. Scand J Gastroenterol 53:115–116
Havelund T, Laursen LS, Skoubo-Kristensen E, Andersen BN, Pedersen SA, Jensen KB, Fenger C, Hanberg-Sorensen F, Lauritsen K (1988) Omeprazole and ranitidine in treatment of reflux esophagitis. Br Med J 296:89–92
Havu N (1984) Enterochromaffin-like cell carcinoids of gastric mucosa in rats after life-long inhibition of gastrin secretion. Digestion [Suppl 1] 35:42–55
Henry DA, Somerville KW, Kitchingman G, Langman MJS (1984) Omeprazole: effects on oxidative drug metabolism. Br J Clin Pharmacol 18:195–200
Hirschowitz BI, Peren J, Raufman JP, Lamont B, Berman R, Humphries T (1987) A multicenter US study of omeprazole treatment of Zollinger-Ellison syndrome (Abstr). Gastroenterology 94:A188
Hofmann JW, Fox PS, Wilson SD (1973) Duodenal wall tumors and the Zollinger-Ellison syndrome. Arch Surg 107:334–339
Howard J, Chremos AN, Collen MJ, McArthur KE, Cherner JA, Maton PN, Ciarleglio CA, Cornelius MJ, Gardner JD, Jensen RT (1985) Famotidine: a new, potent, long-acting histamine H_2-receptor antagonist: comparison with cimetidine and ranitidine in the treatment of Zollinger-Ellison syndrome (ZES). Gastroenterology 88:1026–1033
Howden CW, Reid JL, Forrest JSH (1984) Effect of omeprazole on gastric acid secretion in human volunteers. Gut 25:707–710
Imamura M, Minematsu S, Hattori Y, Shimada Y, Tobe T (1988) Localization of gut hormone producing tumors by selective arterial injection of various hormones (Abstr). Biomed Res [Suppl] 9:29

Ippoliti AF, Isenberg JI, Hagie L (1981) Effect of oral and intravenous 16, 16-dimethyl prostaglandin E_2 in duodenal ulcer and Zollinger-Ellison syndrome patients. Gastroenterology 80:55–59

Isenberg JI, Walsh JH, Passaro EJ (1972) Unusual effect of secretin on serum gastrin, serum calcium, and gastric acid secretion in a patient with suspected Zollinger-Ellison syndrome. Gastroenterology 62:626–631

Isenberg JI, Walsh JH, Grossman MI (1973) Zollinger-Ellison syndrome. Gastroenterology 65:140–165

Jensen RT (1984) Basis for failure of cimetidine in patients with Zollinger-Ellison syndrome. Dig Dis Sci 39:353–358

Jensen RT (1988) Gastric hypersecretory states. Regul Peptide Newslett 1(2):3–6

Jensen RT, Gardner JD (1986) Gastrinoma. In: Bayless TM (ed) Current therapy in gastroenterology and liver disease. Decker, Philadelphia, pp 77–80

Jensen RT, Maton PN (1990) Zollinger-Ellison syndrome. In: Gustavsson S, Kumar D, Groham DY (eds) The Sarrah Churchill Livingstone Press, London, (in press)

Jensen RT, Collen MJ, Allende HD, Raufman, Bissonette BM, Duncan WC, Durgin PL, Gillin JC, Gardner JD (1983a) Cimetidine induced impotence and breast changes in patients with gastric hypersecretory states. N Engl J Med 308:883–887

Jensen RT, Gardner JD, Raufman J-P, Pandol SJ, Doppman JL, Collen MJ (1983b) Zollinger-Ellison syndrome, NIH combined clinical staff conference. Ann Intern Med 98:59–75

Jensen RT, Collen MJ, McArthur KE, Howard JM, Maton PN, Cherner JA, Gardner JD (1984) Comparison of the effectiveness of ranitidine and cimetidine in inhibiting acid secretion in patients with gastric hypersecretory states. Am J Med 77:90–105

Jensen RT, Doppman JL, Gardner JD (1986) Gastrinoma. In: Go VLW, et al. (eds) The exocrine pancreas: biology, pathobiology and diseases. Raven, New York, pp 727–744

Johnson LR (1987) Regulation of mucosal growth. In: Johnson Le (ed) Physiology of the GI tract. Raven, New York, pp 301–334

Kaye MD, Rhodes J, Beck P (1970) Gastric secretion in duodenal ulcer, with particular reference to the diagnosis of Zollinger-Ellison syndrome. Gastroenterology 58:476–481

Klinkenberg-Knol EC, Jansen JBMJ, Festen HPM, Meuwissen SGM, Lamers CBHW (1987) Double-blind multicentre comparison of omeprazole and ranitidine in the treatment of reflux oesophagitis. Lancet 2:349–351

Konturek SJ, Tasler J, Cieszkowski M, Coy DH, Schally AV (1976) Effect of growth hormone release-inhibiting hormone on gastric secretion, mucosal blood flow, and serum gastrin. Gastroenterology 70:737–741

Korman MG, Laver MC, Hansky J (1972a) Hypergastrinemia in chronic renal failure. Br Med J 1:209–210

Korman MG, Scott DF, Hansky J, Wilson H (1972b) Hypergastrinemia due to excluded gastric antrum: a proposed method for differentiation from Zollinger-Ellison syndrome. Aust N Z J Med 3:266–271

Krudy AG, Doppman JL, Jensen RT, et al. (1984) Localization of islet cell tumors by dynamic CT. A JR 143:585

Kutz K, Nuesch E, Rosenthaler J (1986) Pharmacokinetics of SMS-201-995 in healthy subjects. Scand J Gastroenteorl [Suppl 119] 21:65–72

Kvols LK, Buck M, Moertel CG, Schutt AJ, Rubin J, O'Connell J, Hahn RG (1987) Treatment of metastatic islet cell carcinoma with somatostatin analogue (SMS-201-995). Ann Intern Med 107:162–168

Lamers CBH, van Tongeren JHM (1977) Comparative study of the value of calcium, secretin, and meal stimulated increase in serum gastrin in the diagnosis of the Zollinger-Ellison syndrome. Gut 18:128–134

Lamers CBH, Ruland CM, Joosten HJM, Verkooyen HCM, Tongeren JHM, Rehfeld JF (1978) Hypergastrinemia of antral origin in duodenal ulcer. Dig Dis Sci 23:998–1002

Lamers CBH, Lind T, Moberg S, Jansen JBMJ, Olbe L (1984) Omeprazole in Zollinger-Ellison syndrome. Effects of a single dose and long-term treatment in patients resistant to histamine H_2-receptor antagonists. N Engl J Med 310: 758–761

Larsson H, Carlsson E, Junggren U, Oble L, Sjostrand SE, Skanberg I, Sundell G (1983) Inhibition of gastric acid secretion by omeprazole in the dog and rat. Gastroenterology 85:900–907

Larsson H, Carlsson E, Mattsson H (1986) Plasma gastrin and gastric enterochromaffin cell activation and proliferation – studies with omeprazole and ranitidine in intact and antrectamized rats. Gastroenterology 90:319–99

Lauritsen K, Rune SJ, Bytzer P, Kelbaek H (1985) Effect of omeprazole and cimetidine on duodenal ulcer. N Engl J Med 312:958–961

Levine RA, Kohen KR, Schwartzek EH, Ramsay CE (1982) Prostaglandin E_2-histamine interactions on cAMP, cGMP and acid production in isolated fundic glands. Am J Physiol 242:G21–G29

Lloyd-Davies KA, Rutgersson, Solvell L (1988) Omeprazole in the treatment of Zollinger-Ellison syndrome: a 4 year international study. Aliment Pharmacol Ther 2:13–37

Malagelada JR, Edis AJ, Adson MA, von Heenden JA, Go VLW (1983) Medical and surgical options in the management of patients with gastrinoma. Gastroenterology 84:1524–1532

Maton PN, Camilleri M, Griffin G, Allison DJ, Hodgson HJF, Chadwick VS (1983) Role of hepatic arterial embolization in the carcinoid syndrome. Br Med J 287:932–935

Maton PN, Gardner JD, Jensen RT (1986) Cushing's syndrome in patients with the Zollinger-Ellison syndrome. N Engl J Med 315:1–5

Maton PN, Miller DL, Doppman JL, Collen MJ, Norton JA, Vinayek R, Slaff JI, Wank SA, Gardner JS, Jensen RT (1987) Role of selective angiography in the management of Zollinger-Ellison syndrome. Gastroenterology 92:913–919

Maton PN, Frucht H, Vinayek R, Wank SA, Gardner JD, Jensen RT (1988a) Medical management of patients with Zollinger-Ellison syndrome who have had previous gastric surgery: a prospective study. Gastroenterology 94:294–299

Maton PN, Gardner JD, Jensen RT (1989a) The use of the long-acting analogue SMS 201-995 in patients with pancreatic islet cell tumors. Dig Dis Sci 34:28–375

Maton PN, Vinayek R, Frucht H, McArthur KA, Miller LS, Saeed ZA, Gardner JD, Jensen RT (1989b) Long term efficiency and safety of omeprazole in patients with Zollinger-Ellison syndrome: A Prospective study. Gastroenterology 97: 827–836

Maton PN, Gardner UD, Jensen RT (1989c) Recent advances in the management of gastrin and hypersecretion in patients with Zollinger-Ellison syndrome. Med Clin North Am 18:847–863

Maton PN; Lack EE, Collen MJ, Cornelius MJ, David E, Gardner JD, Jensen RT (1990) Effect of Zollinger-Ellison syndrome and omeprazole therapry on gastric endocrine cells. Gastroenterology 99:943–950

McArthur KE, Collen MJ, Maton PN, Cherner, JA, Howard JM, Ciarleglio CA, Cornelius MJ, Jensen RT, Gardner JD (1985) Omeprazole: effective, convenient therapy for Zollinger-Ellison syndrome. Gastroenterology 88:939–944

McArthur KE, Raufman JP, Seaman JJ, Ziemniak JA, Collen MJ, Gardner JD, Jensen RT (1987) Cimetidine pharmacodynamics in patients with Zollinger-Ellison syndrome. Gastroenterology 93:69–76

McCarthy DM (1978) Report on the United States experience with cimetidine in the Zollinger-Ellison syndrome and other hypersecretory states. Gastroenterology 74:453–458

McCarthy DM (1980) The place of surgery in the Zollinger-Ellison syndrome. N Engl J Med 302:1844–1847

McCarthy DM, Hyman PE (1982) Effect of isopropamide on response to oral cimetidine in patients with Zollinger-Ellison syndrome. Dig Dis Sci 27:353–359

McCarthy DM, Olinger EJ, May RJ, Long BW, Gardner JD (1977) H_2-histamine receptor blocking agents in the Zollinger-Ellison syndrome. Ann Intern Med 87:668–675

McGuigan JE (1978) The Zollinger-Ellison syndrome. In: Sleisinger MH, Fordtran JS, (eds) Gastrointestinal disease. Saunders, Philadelphia, pp 860–875

McGuigan JE, Trudeau WL (1969) Immunochemical measurement of elevated levels of gastrin in the serum of patients with pancreatic tumors of the Zollinger-Ellison variety. N Engl J Med 278:1308–1313

McGuigan JE, Wolfe MM (1980) Secretin injection test in the diagnosis of gastrinoma. Gastroenterology 79:1324–1331

Mignon M, Vallot T, Galmiche JP, Dupas JL, Bonfils S (1980) Interest of a combined antisecretory treatment, cimetidine and pirenzepine, in the management of severe forms of Zollinger-Ellison syndrome. Digestion 20:56–61

Mignon M, Vallot T, Hervoir P, Benfredj P, Bonfils (1982) Ranitidine versus cimetidine in the management of Zollinger-Ellison syndrome. In: Riley AJ Salmon PR (eds) Ranitidine, Excerpta Medica, Amsterdam, pp 169–177

Mignon M, Ruszniewski R, Haffar S, Rigaud D, Rene E, Bonfils S (1986) Current approach to the management of tumoral process in patients with gastrinoma. World J Surg 10:702–709

Miller LS, Frucht H, Saeed ZA, Stark H, Jensen RT, Maton PN (1990) Reflux esophagitis in patients with Zollinger-Ellison syndrome (ZES) (Abstr). Gastroenterology 98:341–346

Miwa M, Senoue I, Nomiyami T, Suzuki S, Harasawa S, Tani N, Miwa T (1982) The newest H_2-receptor antagonist, YM-11170. Scand J Gastroenterol [Suppl 78] 17:107

Moertel CG, Hanley JA, Johnson LA (1980) Streptozotocin alone compared with streptozotocin plus fluorouracil in the treatment of advanced islet-cell carcinoma. N Engl J Med 303:1189–1192

Neuburger PH, Lewin M, Bonfils S (1972) Parietal and chief cell populations in four cases of the Zollinger-Ellison syndrome. Gastroenterology 63:937–944

Norton JA (1984) Invited commentary. World J Surg 8:575

Norton JA, Sugarbaker PH, Doppman JL, Wesley RN, Maton PN, Gardner JD, Jensen RT (1986b) Aggressive resection of metastatic disease in selected patients with malignant gastrinoma. Ann Surg 203:352–359

Norton JA, Cromack DT, Shawker TH, Doppman JL, Comi R, Gorden P, Maton, Gardner JD, Jensen RT (1986c) Intraoperative ultrasonographic localization of islet cell tumors: a prospective comparison to palpation. Ann Surg 207:160–168

Norton JA, Cornelius MJ, Doppman JL, Maton PN, Gardner JD, Jensen RT (1987) Effect of parathyroidectomy in patients with hyperparathyroidism and Zollinger-Ellison syndrome and multiple endocrine neoplasia type I: a prospective study. Surgery 102:958–966

Norton JA, Doppman JL, Collen MJ, Harmon JW, Maton PN, Gardner JD, Jensen RT (1988) Prospective study of gastrinoma localization and resection in patients with Zollinger-Ellison syndrome. Ann Surg 204:468–479

Oberg K, Lindstrom H (1983) Reduction of gastric hypersecretion in Zollinger-Ellison syndrome with omeprazole. Lancet 1:66–67

Olbe L, Haglund U, Leth R, Tore L, Cederberg C, Ekenved G, Elander B, Fellenius E, Lundborg P, Wallmark B (1982) Effects of substituted benzimidazole (H 149/94) on gastric acid secretion in humans. Gastroenterology 83:193–198

Pendleton RG, Torchiana ML, Chung C, Cook P, Wiese S, Clineschmidt BV (1983) Studies on MK-208 (YM-11170), a new, slowly dissociable H_2-receptor antagonist. Arch Int Pharmacodyn Ther 266:4–16

Pless J, Bauer W, Briner U, Doepfner D, Marbach P, Maurer R, Fletcher TJ, Reubi J-C, Vonderscher J (1986) Chemistry and pharmacology of SMS-201-995, a long acting octapeptide analogue of somatostatin. Scand J Gastroenterol [Suppl 119] 21:54–64
Prichard PJ, Yeomas ND, Mihaley GW, Jones DB, Buckle PJ, Smallwood RA, Louis WJ (1985) Omeprazole: a study of its inhibition of gastrin pH and oral pharmacokinetics after morning or evening dosage. Gastroenterology 88:64–69
Raufman JP, Collins SM, Korman LY, Collen MJ, Pandol SJ, Cornelius MJ, Feld ME, McCarthy DM, Gardner JD, Jensen RT (1983) Reliability of symptoms in assessing control gastric acid secretion in patients with Zollinger-Ellison syndrome. Gastroenterology 84:108–113
Regan PT, Malagelada JR (1978) A reappraisal of clinical, roentgenographic, and endoscopic features of the Zollinger-Ellison syndrome. Mayo Clin Proc 53: 19–23
Rehfeld JF, Stadil F (1973) Gel filtration studies an immunoreactive gastrin serum from Zollinger-Ellison patients. Gut 14:369–373
Rehfeld JF, Stadil F, Vikelsoe J (1974) Immunoreactive gastric components in human serum. Gut 15:102
Reubi JC (1985) Somatostatin analogues inhibits chondrosarcoma and insulinoma tumor growth. Acta Endocrinol (Copenh) 109:108–112
Richardson CT, Walsh JH (1976) The value of histamine H_2-receptor antagonists in the management of patients with Zollinger-Ellison syndrome. N Engl Med 294:133–135
Richardson CT, Peters MN, Feldman M, McClelland RN, Walsh JH, Cooper KH, Willeford G, Dukerman RM, Fordtran JS (1985) Treatment of Zollinger-Ellison syndrome with exploratory laparotomy, proximal gastric vagotomy, and H_2-receptor antagonists: a prospective study. Gastroenterology 89:357–367
Richter JE, Pandol SJ, Castell SO, McCarthy DM (1981) Gastroesophageal reflux disease in the Zollinger-Ellison syndrome. Ann Intern Med 95:37–43
Roche A, Raisonnier A, Gillon-Savouret MC (1982) Pancreatic venous sampling and arteriography in localizing insulinomas and gastrinomas: procedure and results in 55 cases. Radiology 145:621–627
Ruszniewski P, Mignon M, Rene E, Bonfils S (1986) Localization of tumoral process in Zollinger-Ellison syndrome (ZES). A retrospective study in 76 patients (Abstr). Gastroenterology 90:1610
Ruszniewski P, Laucournet H, Elouaer-Blanc L, Mignon M, Bonfils A (1988) Long-acting somatostatin (SMS-201-995) in the management of Zollinger-Ellison syndrome: evidence for sustained efficacy. Pancreas 3:145–152
Sachs G (1984) Pump blockers and ulcers disease. N Engl J Med 310:785–786
Saeed ZA, Doppman JL, Norton J, Maton PN, Gardner JD, Jensen RT (1988a) Gastrinoma localization in Zollinger-Ellison syndrome. Intern Med Specialist 9:79–99
Saeed ZA, Frank W, Frucht H, Frank Wo, Young MD, Maton PN, Gardner JD, Jensen RT (1989) Parenteral antisecretory drug therapy in patients with Zollinger-Ellison syndrome (ZES) (Abstr). Gastroenterology 96:1393–1402
Shawker TH, Doppman JL, Dunnick NR, et al. (1982) Ultrasound investigation of pancreatic islet cell tumors. J Ultrasound Med 1:193–200
Shepherd JJ, Senator GB (1986) Regression of liver metastases in patients with gastrin secreting tumor treated with SMS 201-995. Lancet 2:274
Sigel B, Colho JCU, Nyhus, LM, Velasco JM, Donahue PE, Wood DX, Spigus DS (1982) Detection of pancreatic tumors by ultrasound during surgery. Arch Radiol 117:1058–1061
Slaff JI, Howard JM, Maton PN, Vinayek R, Wank SA, McCarthy DM, Gardner JD, Jensen RT (1986) Prospective assessment of provocative gastrin tests in 81 consecutive patients with Zollinger-Ellison syndrome (ZES) (Abstr). Gastroenterology 90:1637

Smith JL, Gamal M, Chremos AN, Graham DY (1983) Effect of an H_2-receptor antagonist, MK-208, on gastric parietal and nonparietal secretion (Abstr). Gastroenterology 84:1314
Soll AH, Berglindh T (1987) Physiology of gastric glands and parietal cells: receptors and effectors regulating function. In: Johnson LR (ed) Physiology of the gastrointestinal tract, 2nd edn. Raven, New York, pp 883–909
Stabile BE, Ippoliti AF, Walsh JH, Passaro E Jr (1983) Failure of histamine H_2-receptor antagonist therapy in Zollinger-Ellison syndrome. Am J Surg 145:17–23
Stabile BE, Morrow DJ, Passaro E Jr (1984) The gastrinoma triangle. Operative implications. Am J Surg 147:25–32
Stadil F, Stage JG (1979) The Zollinger-Ellison syndrome, Clin Endocrinol Metab 9:433–446
Stage JG, Stadil R (1979) The clinical diagnosis of the Zollinger-Ellison syndrome. Scand J Gastroenterol [Suppl 53] 14:79–91
Stark DD, Moss AA, Goldberg HI, Deveney W, Way L (1983) Computed tomography and nuclear magnetic resonance imaging of pancreatic islet cell tumors. Surgery 94:1024–1027
Stark DP, Moss AA, Goldberg HI, Deveney W, Way L (1984) CT of pancreatic islet cell tumors. Radiology 150:491–495
Strauss E, Yalow RS (1975) Differential diagnosis of hypergastrinemia. In: Thompson JC (ed) Gastrointestinal hormones. University of Texas Press, Austin, pp 99–113
Stremple JF, Meade FCC (1968) Production of antibodies to synthetic human gastrin I and radioimmunoassay of gastrin in the serum of patients with Zollinger-Ellison syndrome. Surgery 64:165–174
Sum P, Perey BJ (1969) Parietal cell mass on a patient with Zollinger-Ellison syndrome. Can J Surg 12:285–288
Takagi T, Takeda M, Maeno H (1982) Effect of a new potent H_2-blocker, 3-[[[2-[(diaminomethylene) amino]-4-thiazolyl]methyl]-thio] N^2-sulfamoylpropionamidine (YM-11170), on gastric secretion, ulcer formation and weight of male accessory sex organs in rats. Arzneimitdelforschung 32:734–737
Takeda M, Takagi T, Maeno H (1983) Kinetics of antisecretory action of a new H_2-antagonist, YM-11170, in conscious dogs. Eur J Pharmacol 91:371–379
Taylor IL, Calam J, Rotter JI, Vaillant C, Samloff IM, Cook A, Simkin E, Dockray GJ (1981) Family studies of hypergastrinemic hyperpepsinogenemic I duodenal ulcer. Ann Intern Med 95:421–425
Thompson JC, Reeder DD, Villar HV, Fender HR (1975) Natural history and experience with diagnosis and treatment of the Zollinger-Ellison syndrome. Surg Gynecol Obstet 140:721–739
Thompson JC, Lewis BG, Wiener I, Townsend CM (1983) The role of surgery in the Zollinger-Ellison syndrome. Ann Surg 197:594–607
Thompson NW (1983) Surgical consideration in the MEN-I syndrome. In: Johnston IDA, Johnston NW (eds) Endocrine surgery. Butterworth, London, pp 144–163
Thompson NW, Lloyd RU, Nishiyama RH, et al. (1984) MEN-I pancreas: a histological and immunohistochemical study. World J Surg 8:561–568
Tomioka K, Yamada T, Tachikawa S (1983) Effects of famotidine (YM-11170), an H_2-receptor antagonist, on in vivo immediate and delayed type hypersensitivity reactions and antibody formation. Drug Exp Clin Res 9:881–889
Tsai St, Lewis EM, Vinik AI (1985) Long-acting somatostatin analog for patients with gastrinoma syndrome (Abstr). Clin Res 33:876A
Van Heerden JA, Bernatz PE, Rovelstad RA (1971) The retained gastric antrum – clinical considerations, Mayo Clin Proc 46:25–27
Vezzadini P, Tomassett P, Toni R, Bonora G, Labo G (1984) Omeprazole in the medical treatment of Zollinger-Ellison syndrome. Curr Ther Res 35:772–776
Vinayek R, Howard JM, Maton PN, Wank SA, Slaff SE, Gardner JD (1986) Famotidine in the therapy of gastric hypersecretory states. Am J Med [Suppl 4B] 81:49–59

Vinik A, Tsai S-T, Moattari AR, Cheung P (1988) Somatostatin analogue in patients with gastrinomas. Surgery 104:834–842
Vogel SB, Wolfe MM, McGuigan JE, Hawkins IF, Howard RJ, Woodward ER (1987) Localization and resection of gastrinomas in Zollinger-Ellison syndrome. Ann Surg 205:550–558
Von Schrenck T, Howard JM, Doppman JL, Norton JA, Smith F, Maton PN, Vinayek R, Frucht H, Wank AS, Gardner JD, Jensen RT (1988) Prospective study of chemotherapy in patients with metastatic gastrinoma. Gastroenterology 94:1326–1334
Walsh JH, Grossman MI (1975) Gastrin. N Engl J Med 292:1324–1334, 1377–1384
Wank SA, Doppman JL, Miller DL, Collen MJ, Maton PN, Vinayek R, Slaff JI, Norton JA, Gardner JD, Jensen RT (1987) Prospective study of the ability of computerized axial tomography to localize gastrinomas in patients with Zollinger-Ellison syndrome. Gastroenterology 92:905–912
Watson AJS, Dalbow MH, Stachura I, Fragola JA, Rubin MF, Watson RM, Bourke E (1983) Immunologic studies in cimetidine induced nephropathy and polymyositis. N Engl J Med 308(3):142
Wolfe MM, Jensen RT (1987) Zollinger-Ellison syndrome. N Engl J Med 317: 1200–1219
Wolfe MM, Alexander RW, McGuigon JE (1982) Extrapancreatic, extraintestinal gastrinoma. N Engl J Med 306:1533–1536
Wolfe MM, Jain PK, Edgerton JR (1985) Zollinger-Ellison syndrome associated with persistently normal fasting serum gastrin concentrations. Ann Intern Med 103: 215–217
Wormsley KG (1984) Assessing the safety of drugs for the long-term treatment of peptic ulcers. Gut 25:1416–1423
Wynick D, Williams SJ, Bloom SR (1988) Symptomatic secondary hormone syndromes in patients with established pancreatic endocrine tumors. N Engl J Med 319:608–614
Yalow RS, Berson SA (1970) Size and charge distinctions between endogenous human plasma gastrin in peripheral blood and heptadecapeptide gastrins. Gastroenterology 58:609
Ziemniak JA, Madura M, Adamonis AJ, Olinger EJ, Dreyer M, Schentag JJ (1983) Failure of cimetidine in Zollinger-Ellison syndrome. Dig Dis Sci 28:976–980
Zollinger RM, Ellison EH (1955) Primary peptic ulcerations of the jejunum associated with islet cell tumors of the pancreas. Ann Surg 142:709–723
Zollinger RM, Martin EW, Carey LC, Sparks J, Mintar JP (1976) Observations on the postoperative tumor growth behavior of certain islet cell tumors. Ann Surg 184:525–530
Zollinger RM, Ellison EC, Fabri PJ, Johnson J, Sparks J, Carey LC (1980) Primary peptic ulceration of the jejunum associated with islet cell tumors: twenty-five year appraisal. Ann Surg 192:422–430

CHAPTER 14

The Pathophysiology and Treatment of Gastroesophageal Reflux Disease

S.B. BENJAMIN

A. Introduction

Symptoms attributable to reflux of gastric contents from the stomach into the esophagus are recognized by almost all individuals as something that they "think" they have experienced at one time or another. These symptoms are the subject of jokes and are perceived by most as an annoyance, not a disease or even a potentially serious problem. When closely examined, however, our understanding of gastroesophageal reflux, from its etiology to the degree of injury that it may produce, has increased to the point where we now recognize that a variety of serious medical problems may occur secondary to this phenomenon. Even with this understanding our knowledge is at best limited and undergoing extremely rapid change as this whole concept is subjected to very careful examination and clinical investigation. This chapter will review our present understanding of why reflux of material from the stomach into the esophagus occurs, discuss what factors are responsible for the variability in response to this noxious material, consider whether the esophagus is the only site of injury, review the material supporting the claim that the consequences of gastroesophageal reflux are more widespread and potentially clinically significant than has heretofore been recognized, and finally, on this basis, consider how we can effectively treat individuals with this problem, either medically or surgically. However, prior to the examination of the data, agreement is required regarding appropriate nosology in respect of gastroesophageal reflux.

B. The Nosology of Reflux

As in other areas of science, it is a requirement of the scientific method that, when individuals use terms, these terms have the same meaning to everyone. The implementation of a meaningful nosology that is able to change as our understanding of this problem increases is imperative. This is best accomplished by recognizing the wide range and variability of gastroesophageal reflux. Reflux that occurs as a normal event in the postprandial period as the stomach empties itself of gas, representing swallowed ambient air, is best referred to as *physiologic reflux*. This is reflected in 24-h pH monitoring as the small amount of acid exposure seen in the upright position, almost all in the postprandial period (DEMEESTER et al. 1976; FINK and MCCULLUM 1984). The remaining categories in this terminology reflect the presence or absence of symptoms and/or end-organ injury as a result of gastroesophageal reflux (BENJAMIN 1986). Patients may have *symptomatic reflux*, that is, symptoms of heartburn or pain associated with reflux of gastric contents, but there may or may not be evidence of any end-organ injury. These symptoms may occur in any period, representing either physiologic or pathologic reflux, but for reasons as yet unknown they do not have to result in evidence of tissue injury; in fact, in many situations there is an inverse correlation between symptoms and the degree of mucosal injury in the esophagus (DEMEESTER et al. 1976). The final major category in this classification is *gastroesophageal reflux disease*. These patients have evidence of "disease" related to the reflux of gastric contents into the esophagus, more proximal hypopharyngeal areas, and mouth or lungs. It is critical to recognize that symptoms need not be present in such individuals, i.e., silent reflux of gastric contents can produce significant injury without the recognition by the patient that it has occurred or it may trigger, via neural pathways, bronchospasm, tachyarrhythmias, or angina. The best example of this phenomenon of "silent reflux" is Barrett's esophagus, in which up to a third of patients do not have symptoms yet have obvious evidence on 24-h pH monitoring of pathologic degrees of gastroesophageal reflux (IASCONE et al. 1983).

These three "sets" of patients cover the entire range of reflux, from that occurring as a part of normal digestion to occult aspiration with unexplained lung disease (Fig. 1). It is important to recognize that regardless of whether patterns of gastroesophageal reflux, as measured by 24-h pH monitoring, show acid or alkaline reflux or supine or upright reflux, it is possible to measure and quantify the reflux and determine whether the amount or pattern is pathologic or falls within an acceptable range; however, only when we recognize the variety of outcomes in this very common event can we further our understanding of its great variability of expression. Further confounding our ability to understand reflux is the observation that a "nonpathologic" amount of gastroesophageal reflux may trigger reflex events such as bronchospasm.

C. Why Do Humans Reflux?

Fundamental to our understanding and the eventual treatment of this condition is an elucidation of the events that lead to gastroesophageal reflux as a pathologic event, since we recognize that some degree of reflux is physiologic, occurring as a normal part of digestion. Gastroesophageal reflux should be considered a syndrome since a variety of conditions may lead to the same end result, that is, an abnormal amount of gastric contents and/or prolonged exposure of tissues proximal to the stomach (i.e., esophagus, hypopharynx, mouth, or lungs) to these gastric contents (Fig. 2). The major potential causes

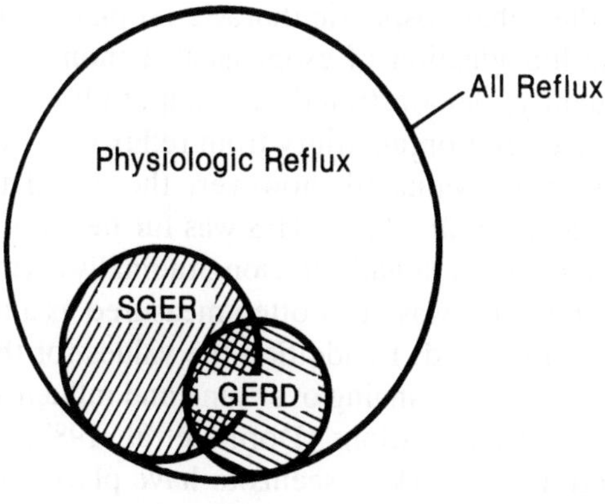

Fig. 1. The "sets" of gastroesophageal reflux. *SGER*, symptomatic gastroesophageal reflux; *GERD*, gastroesophageal reflux disease. (BENJAMIN 1986)

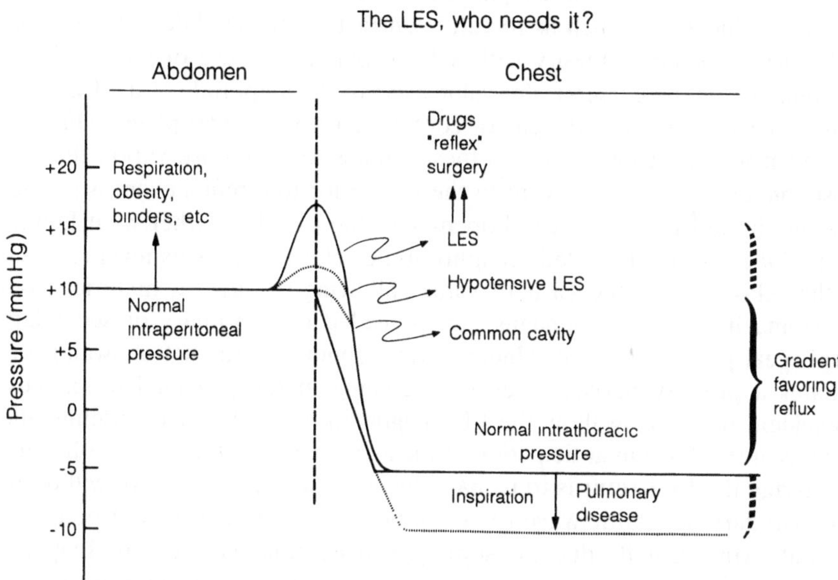

Fig. 2. Factors involved in gastroesophageal reflux. A variety of factors are simultaneously operative and their summation will determine the degree of reflux

of reflux are the incompetence of the lower esophageal sphincter (LES), the "aggressiveness" of the material refluxed, and abnormal function of the stomach (DODDS et al. 1982; LILLEMOE et al. 1982; MCCALLUM et al. 1984).

Our understanding of the role of the LES has increased dramatically over the last 10 years. Teleologically this high pressure zone exists as a barrier preventing the movement of gastric contents in the high pressure abdominal environment into the subatmospheric thoracic esophagus. Original observations following the introduction of esophageal manometry, and repeatedly confirmed subsequently, demonstrated that amplitudes of the LES did correlate with evidence of end-organ injury from reflux (e.g., esophagitis) when a group of patients was evaluated; however, the correlation in individual patients was poor (KATZ et al. 1986). This was further confused by the characteristics of this sphincter, a radially and longitudinally asymmetric sphincter, whose value on manometry was most often measured as a mean value of the four different values recorded. In addition the values for this sphincter have been shown to be dynamic, changing over time and influenced by events such as eating and a host of medications (DODDS et al. 1982). The very elegant work of DODDS and his co-workers seems to have placed most, if not all, of these variables in order. The LES is a dynamic muscular sphincter which maintains a high pressure barrier preventing the movement of gastric contents, as had been hypothesized. If this high pressure zone falls to levels below those of intraabdominal pressure then gastric contents can move or be "forced" into the thoracic esophagus. In situations where intraabdominal pressure is increased, such as forceful contraction of the abdominal muscles (a belch), exogenous obesity with a large pannus, or use of tight – fitting abdominal binders (corsets), this value exceeds the amplitude of the LES, the sphincter is forced open, and gastric contents pass into the esophagus (Fig. 2).

What was most interesting in these studies was the observation that the most common antecedent event in the LES prior to a reflux event is neither low amplitude LES nor forceful opening of the LES but rather what DODDS et al. (1982) originally called "inappropriate relaxation." This term referred to the relaxation of the LES to values allowing passage of material from the stomach into the esophagus, *not* preceded by a primary or secondary esophageal peristaltic wave. Under normal conditions the act of swallowing initiates a primary peristaltic event beginning in the proximal esophagus. Coincident with the swallow the LES begins to relax to gastric baseline and remains at this level in anticipation of the arriving peristaltic wave. Following its passage the LES returns to its basal levels. This same sequence will occur if a secondary peristaltic wave (by definition a peristaltic wave not preceded by swallowing, usually due to esophageal distention) is initiated. Inappropriate relaxation was not preceded by either of these events and was initially thought to be pathologic. Current opinion suggests that these relaxations are similar to the ruminant reflex that is well described in herbivores, and they are currently referred to as "LES transients" (as suggested by DENT et al. 1983). The majority of reflux events in a group of patients with esophagitis were preceded by this heretofore unrecognized behavior of the human LES. How this event is triggered and whether it represents the initial cause of pathologic reflux or is a secondary phenomenon due to preceding injury remains to be elucidated. Information derived from a wide array of surgical research may provide some information salient to this discussion and will be discussed below; however, concepts of how the sphincter functions and how it can be modified are still changing. Thus the sphincter is being considered not only in terms of absolute pressure; rather its length and the environment in which it is located (intrathoracic vs intraabdominal) are also receiving attention (BONAVIANA et al. 1986). Furthermore, measurements of the force exerted by this sphincter have now been obtained and may be a more accurate predictor of sphincter competence (BOMBECK et al. 1987).

It seems appropriate to consider gastroesophageal reflux as a syndrome in which essentially all the etiologies are abnormalities of gastric function. Most authors would agree that the lower "esophageal" sphincter is really located on the gastric side of the gastroesophageal junction, and primarily represented in oblique gastric musculature (CASTELL 1975). In addition several other abnormalities of gastric physiology may play a role in causing or aggravating gastroesophageal reflux. Although disagreement exists, it would appear that abnormalities of gastric emptying may play a role in some patients with reflux (MCCALLUM et al. 1984). Notwithstanding the problems with methodology that plague gastric emptying studies, there are data to support the concept that disordered motility may lead to the movement of material into the esophagus in a subset of patients with gastroesophageal reflux. In addition, patients with significant increases in gastric acid production (either Zollinger-Ellison syndrome or idiopathic gastric acid hypersecretion) appear to be at increased risk for esophageal mucosal injury, presumably due to the dramatic increase in hydrogen ion concentration and the increased volume of gastric juice found in such individuals (RICHTER et al. 1981; COLLEN et al. 1990). Gastric volume is another factor that is often given too little attention in understanding gastroesophageal reflux and especially in treating it. There is a clear relationship between gastric volume and the likelihood of reflux, and it becomes necessary to reduce intragastric volume dramatically when one attempts to treat reflux (COLLEN et al. 1990).

Although arbitrary separation of patient groups is likely to prove inaccurate, since more than one event may be found in many individuals, it is important to understand clearly the major variables playing a role. Not only does this further our understanding of this complex condition, but in individual patient situations it may be critical to proper diagnosis and management. For example, it is appropriate to consider evaluation for gastric acid hypersecretion, either idiopathic gastric acid hypersecretion or Zollinger-Ellison syndrome, in patients poorly responsive to standard therapy for gastroesophageal reflux with esophagitis, and to exclude mechanical pyloric outlet obstruction in patients with delayed gastric emptying prior to the use of prokinetic agents.

D. Variability of Tissue Response to Reflux

An often ignored but extremely important aspect of gastroesophageal reflux is the variability of the material refluxed and the sensitivity of the tissue exposed (HARMON et al. 1981; ORLANDO 1985). Only in recent years have we made significant advances in understanding these variables. Gastric juice is a complex and dynamic solution reflecting changing concentrations of acid, pepsin, bile acids, pancreatic enzymes, peptide hormones, and a practically undefinable variety of ingested exogenous compounds ranging from tobacco products to the complex materials found in alcoholic products. Because we can simply and reproducibly measure acid, we have focused much of our attention on hydrogen ion concentration. Data collected from animal experimentation suggest that the concentrations of acid that are recorded as "abnormal" during pH monitoring ($pH < 4$) are not in themselves injurious to the esophagus and that concentrations of acid reflected by a pH less than or equal to 1 are necessary to induce injury by themselves (HARMON et al. 1981). It has been shown for a variety of experimental systems that the addition of a small amount of pepsin to acid in concentrations insufficient to cause injury will produce significant damage. It is likely that under most circumstances it is not acid alone that produces injury in the esophagus, but this may not be the case if acid is introduced to other organ systems, particularly the lungs (MORAN 1955). Given the dynamic nature of gastric contents and the wide variety of things the omnivore that is *Homo sapiens* adds to this mixture, we are unlikely to quantify or standardize gastric contents. It is critical, however, that we recognize the complexity of this material.

The other side of this equation is the ability of tissues to protect themselves from the presence of gastric contents. Obviously the stomach has the ability to protect itself from this most noxious of environments, and under certain circumstances the esophagus may show surprisingly little damage despite exposure comparable to that of a patient with severe esophagitis. As we are rediscovering in other areas of the upper gastrointestinal tract, there is a balance between those factors likely to cause damage (aggressive factors) and those working to protect the tissue from injury (defensive factors). ORLANDO and co-workers have shown us that the esophageal mucosa has the ability to withstand the onslaught of acid for considerable periods of time (ORLANDO 1985). Prolonged exposure, increased hydrogen ion concentration, and the presence of pepsin are all factors contributing to the inability of this mucosa to withstand gastric juice exposure.

Additional variables may be present that affect this side of the equation, i.e., the defense. Esophageal sensitivity involving mechanisms as yet to be elucidated, salivary flow, a level of consciousness allowing nocturnal response to refluxed acid (alcoholic intoxication or sedative-hypnotic drugs, for example, prevent recognition of reflux due to diminished level of consciousness), and factors such as epidermal growth factor found in salivary secretions (in which there is newly rekindled interest) all potentially have a significant role in enabling the mucosa of the upper gastrointestinal tract to resist injury.

The increased risk of upper gastrointestinal injury and poor response to therapy in cigarette smokers may be due to the effect of cigarette smoke in reducing salivary bicarbonate flow and/or the secretion of growth factors (HELM et al. 1987; ORR et al. 1981; SKOV OLSEN et al. 1984). It is obvious that the defensive side of upper gastrointestinal tract diseases has taken a back seat to our interest in the aggressive factors, and particularly acid, primarily since we have been able to treat this parameter effectively, but a clear understanding of all the parameters that may play a role in the pathogenesis of tissue injury will only add to both our understanding and our ability to provide such individuals with better treatment.

E. Sequelae of Gastroesophageal Reflux

Given the large number of variables operative in both the pathogenesis of gastroesophageal reflux and the tissue responsiveness to the materials refluxed, it should not be a surprise to anyone that the clinical response to reflux can be quite variable. We have traditionally assumed that almost all of the significant pathology encountered will be found in the esophagus. However, as will be discussed in detail later in this chapter, the esophageal manifestations of gastroesophageal reflux may be only the tip of the iceberg as far as the clinical consequences of reflux are concerned.

The effects of acid on the esophagus are those that we would expect when a tissue not adapted to its presence finds itself exposed to significant concentrations of hydrogen ion and pepsin. The development of esophagitis, peptic stricture, or Barrett's esophagus is accepted as a potential response to pathologic amounts of refluxed gastric material (URSCHEL and PAULSON 1967; OGOREK and FISHER 1989; EASTWOOD 1983). It has been clearly demonstrated that patients with these abnormalities have a dramatic increase in exposure to gastric contents as reflected by monitoring acid reflux. Nevertheless, the exact pathogenesis of peptic strictures remains to be clearly elucidated. Specifically there is little information to suggest that the deeper layers of the esophageal wall are affected, even in the presence of active esophagitis. How a mucosal event, esophagitis, translates into a peptic stricture is unclear. The data, however, are overwhelmingly in support of this concept.

Much of the interest that relates to the response of the esophagus to gastroesophageal reflux is centered on Barrett's esophagus. For some time there was considerable discussion about the exact relationship of gastroesophageal reflux to Barrett's esophagus and whether or not this was an acquired or a congenital lesion (EASTWOOD and BONNICE 1985). The weight of the evidence currently supports the concept that Barrett's esophagus develops as a sequela to longstanding gastroesophageal reflux. How and why it develops in a small subset of patients with reflux is unknown, although a variety of mechanisms have been suggested (EASTWOOD and BONNICE 1985).

Consideration must be given to a variety of other potential outcomes of gastroesophageal reflux. Irritation without tissue injury has certainly been recognized; such irritation results in chest pain syndromes and conceivably may be the trigger for a variety of effects distant to the esophagus, including reflex bronchospasm and reflex myocardial ischemia (cf. Sect. F).

F. Extraesophageal Manifestations of Reflux

In recent years, interest has been rekindled in evaluating the potential relationship between gastroesophageal reflux and disease states that occur outside of the esophagus (Benjamin 1986). Physicians have for the most part adopted a parochial attitude toward this potential association, assuming that only the esophagus is at risk from the movement of gastric contents from the stomach. Nevertheless, for many years individual physicians have speculated that a wide array of problems – from recurrent pneumonia due to aspiration of gastric contents to recurrent sore throat, early enamel loss, and even "reflux dyspareunia" – may be due to pathologic gastroesophageal reflux (Table 1) (Belcher 1949; Kennedy 1962; Mansfield and Stien 1978; Nelson 1984; Kirk 1986; Goldman and Bennett 1988). Slowly objective data have accumulated in support of this view. The exact extent of the problem and the variety of clinical syndromes that can be causally linked to gastroesophageal reflux remain to be clarified. We are clearly at a point where our suspicions have been heightened and technology is being developed that will hopefully resolve some of these interesting and important questions (Benjamin 1986).

It has long been appreciated that the aspiration of gastric contents can result in aspiration pneumonia or pulmonary abscess as a direct consequence of the noxious effects of gastric contents (Belcher 1949; Kennedy 1962). Many authors have speculated over the years that occult aspiration might be responsible for some of the pulmonary complications that were previously thought to be "idiopathic." It is possible that chronic cough is related to irritation of the "tussive center" in the esophagus. Using the limited resources available it was hypothesized that idiopathic pulmonary fibrosis without autoimmune markers might be related to occult aspiration of gastric contents (Mays et al. 1976). This hypothesis was supported by experimental data in animals and the occasional patient known to have massive aspiration with the subsequent development of restrictive pulmonary disease (Moran 1955). Further information on the potential relationship between gastroesophageal reflux and pulmonary disease came with the demonstration that irritation of the distal esophagus could result in obstructive physiology as measured by pulmonary function testing (Mansfield and Stien 1978).

The development of more sophisticated methodology and equipment has added to our understanding of the potential relationship between esophageal irritation and asthma (Mausfield et al. 1981; Boyle et al. 1985; Spaulding et al. 1982; Wilson et al. 1985; Andersen et al. 1986). From the available data it is clear that in a percentage of asthmatic patients, esophageal irritation in the absence of aspiration produces airway obstruction, with symptoms of wheezing and/or cough, almost certainly by neurally mediated signals. The

Table 1. Extraesophageal manifestations of gastroesophageal reflux

Pulmonary	
	Aspiration pneumonia
	Cough
	Asthma
	Chronic intestinal lung disease[a]
Cardiac	
	Tachyarrhythmias
	Angina[a]
Head and neck manifestations	
	Vocal cord granuloma
	Recurrent sore throat
	Eustachian tube dysfunction
	Enamel loss

[a] Possible manifestations of gastroesophageal reflux.

more sophisticated the test, the smaller the changes that can be appreciated. Additional information supporting this concept is empiric, arising from the use of H_2 receptor antagonist therapy in patients with asthma (GOODALL et al. 1981; HARPER et al. 1987). From these studies it became clear that the use of these medications helped some but not all patients with asthma (Fig. 3). In the absence of bronchial H_2 receptors the presumption is that by decreasing the aggressiveness of the gastric contents less esophageal irritation was induced, leading to clinical improvement.

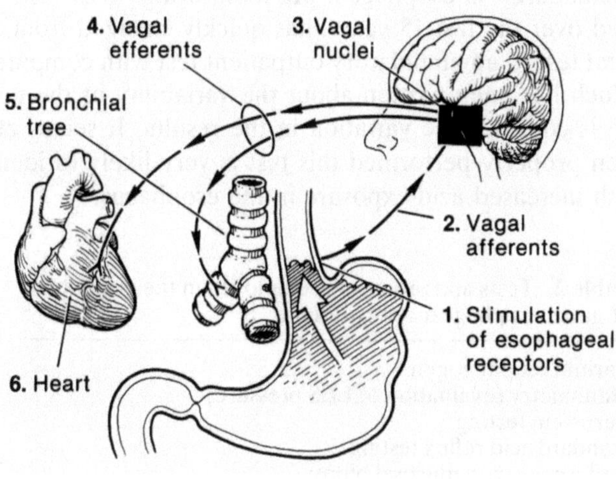

Fig. 3. Potential relationship between gastroesophageal reflux and reflex events triggered in the lungs and/or heart (BENJAMIN 1986)

Given the weight of this circumstantial evidence, what remains is to determine in individual disease states whether there is direct aspiration or a triggered "reflex" event. In diseases like progressive systemic sclerosis where severe pulmonary fibrosis and esophageal disease go hand in hand there is increasing reason to believe that reflux and aspiration may in fact be the cause of the lung disease (JOHNSON et al. 1989). Clarification of the extent to which such problems exist awaits the general introduction of technology which will allow documentation of reflux with aspiration.

G. Testing in Gastroesophageal Reflux

Despite the weight of evidence that supports the association of reflux and a wide array of complications, a variety of problems are encountered when dealing with individual patients with symptoms suggestive of reflux – problems related to the use of tests to confirm the association between reflux and a set of symptoms. The variety of tests that can be used is a testimony to the difficulty clinicians have in confirming that association (Table 2).

Our desire to test for reflux has several aspects, ranging from the confirmation of a clinical suspicion to the development of a clinical research protocol where the association between a given condition and reflux is being evaluated. In many common clinical conditions where end-organ injury is detected there is little reason to use sophisticated testing since the association between reflux and the injury is well established (e.g., esophagitis); however, a knowledge of the tests that are available is mandatory in the setting of clinical research (e.g., regarding the association between reflux and lung disease).

Of the many tests that can be performed the test that has assumed the role of "gold standard" is esophageal pH monitoring. This test, which has been developed over the last 15 years, has quickly changed from a cumbersome in-hospital test to an ambulatory outpatient test with computer-assisted evaluation. Much has been written about the variability of the test and the fact that there is considerable variation in the results. It seems clear, however, that when properly performed this test is very likely to identify those individuals with increased acid exposure in the esophagus.

Table 2. Tests and procedures employed in the evaluation of gastroesophageal reflux disease

Barium esophagogram
Manometry (evaluation of LES pressure)
Bernstein testing
Standard acid reflux testing
Endoscopy with mucosal biopsy
pH monitoring
Radionuclide scintiscanning

A review of all of the tests that have been or can be used to evaluate gastroesophageal reflux or its consequences is beyond the scope of this chapter, but these tests can be generally divided into those that document the presence of reflux and those that are principally used to evaluate the consequences of reflux, i.e., end-organ injury. Barium studies have been evaluated as a means of both showing that reflux occurs and evaluating for possible end-organ injury. Although much has been written about how to use barium studies in reflux, we are often left having to state that spontaneous reflux during a barium study correlates quite well with reflux but is not sensitive (OTT et al. 1981). Scintigraphy has been used to define reflux, but because of the rapid egress of material from the stomach its principal, albeit limited, use has been in the exclusion of aspiration as a consequence of reflux (JOHNSON et al. 1989; FISHER et al. 1976; JONA et al. 1981). Clearly none of these modalities compare favorably to pH monitoring (DEMEESTER et al. 1976; RICHTER et al. 1987; WERNER et al. 1988).

Compared with barium studies, endoscopy is a more sensitive and specific way to exclude esophageal injury as a result of gastroesophageal reflux. The additional information that can be obtained from biopsy of the esophageal mucosa only adds to the mandate to use endoscopy when questions about possible esophageal injury are raised (JOHNSON et al. 1978). The use of real-time videoendoscopy or even digital imaging technology in clinical trials in patients with esophagitis may add considerably to our ability to quantify the response of the esophagus to therapy.

H. Treatment of Gastroesophageal Reflux

The frequency with which gastroesophageal reflux is found in the population is reflected in the enormous literature that has developed regarding the treatment of this condition. As with other acid-peptic disorders, much of this literature is an outgrowth of the introduction of the H_2 blockers and other recent additions to our medical armamentarium (APRILL et al. 1979; BENNETT et al. 1983). In reviewing this extensive literature several things become immediately apparent: (a) gastroesophageal reflux is a *chronic* condition, which relapses rapidly, even if effectively treated medically; (b) gastroesophageal reflux and peptic esophagitis *had* been extremely difficult to treat and/or heal; (c) a clear understanding of the pathophysiology was not reflected in the design or evaluation of many of these studies.

These facts are all very closely interconnected and have been brought to the fore by the recent introduction of omeprazole (KLINKENBERG-KNOL et al. 1987). Since the introduction of omeprazole multiple trials have been undertaken in the medical treatment of gastroesophageal reflux, and using this drug a remarkable improvement in our ability to treat and heal patients with peptic esophagitis secondary to gastroesophageal reflux has become apparent. Why should this disorder, which had been so frustrating to treat with "standard medical therapy," be so responsive to this new class of agents? The answer lies in the pathophysiology of gastroesophageal reflux and the pharmacologic effects of the drugs employed!

Our current understanding of gastroesophageal reflux and peptic esophagitis is that it is contact time with the esophagus that is crucial to the initiation and perpetuation of injury, whether this be reflected in an increased number of reflux episodes or prolonged duration of a smaller number of episodes. We also realize that in patients with an incompetent antireflux barrier, the crucial factor that relates to reflux is gastric volume (COLLEN et al. 1990). In order to decrease reflux to levels allowing remission of symptoms and a signifigant decrease in tissue exposure, intragastric volume must be *dramatically* decreased. In trials using H_2 blockers in "standard" doses, this is essentially never accomplished, but in trials with omeprazole it is almost always achieved. Decreases in intragastric volume similar to those seen with omeprazole can be achieved with H_2 blockers (COLLEN et al. 1990). It becomes very clear that the problem has never been the disease but our understanding or lack of understanding about why this condition was often "refractory" to treatment. We can accomplish the same end-result with H_2 blockers as is achieved with omeprazole if attention is paid to individualizing treatment so that acid production and therefore intragastric volume are reduced to levels where reflux is significantly reduced (COLLEN et al. 1990).

Confirmation of this concept is readily provided when patients who have been treated with omeprazole are followed after discontinuation of the drug. Rapid relapse to pretreatment levels occurs, just as had been seen with H_2 blockers (BENNETT et al. 1983). Gastroesophageal reflux is a chronic disease and in cases where significant end-organ injury is apparent this must be kept in mind; the patient is likely to require lifelong treatment, or consideration for surgical therapy.

J. Surgery in Gastroesophageal Reflux

The chronic nature of gastroesophageal reflux and our inability to treat it effectively, especially in the pre-H_2 blocker era, led to the development of a variety of surgical interventions to correct the problem. The history of surgery as a treatment for gastroesophageal reflux is unique in that a series of empiric operations evolved and a host of speculations were forwarded to explain their effectiveness (SEIWERT et al. 1974; DEMEESTER 1985; DEMEESTER et al. 1979). In retrospect these operative manipulations have added considerably to our understanding of what is necessary to prevent reflux. Most of the procedures accomplish one or more of these effects:

1. Placing the LES on "stretch"
2. Preventing "distraction" of the cardia (preventing widening of the cardia leading to LES opening)
3. Placing the LES in the intraabdominal enrvironment where it functions more effectively

It would appear that these operations have the combined effect of enhancing the effectiveness of the LES and preventing "mechanical failure" (BOMBECK et al. 1987; SEIWERT et al. 1974; DEMEESTER 1985). The consequences that the procedures have in common are: preventing reflux and increasing the "resting tone" of the LES.

Although the evaluation of antireflux surgery was based on logic and not an understanding of the pathophysiology of reflux, future research is likely to show that a combination of the effects of surgery is responsible for its effectiveness. In addition to increasing LES resting tone, "wrapping" of the cardia may be responsible for preventing the initiation of LES transients if this is finally found to be controlled by distention of the cardia. Although new strategies are being developed for the surgical treatment of gastroesophageal reflux, the increasing effectiveness of medical therapy had led to a marked decline in the frequency with which such surgery is being performed. However, given the chronic nature of this process and the expense of medical therapy, surgery may become increasing popular in the approaching era of cost-effective health care delivery.

K. Management in Real Life

Practicing physicians of almost every type are likely to see patients with complaints related to gastroesophageal reflux in their practice. Multiple algorithms have been developed to allow the physician to work through the complex series of potential events that may transpire. Certainly the initial complaint of heartburn should lead to an attempt to exclude any associated symptom that would mandate urgent workup, e.g., dysphagia, associated pulmonary complaints, and weight loss. If these are not present then a therapeutic trial of antacids or H_2 blockers in conjunction with dietary restrictions and life-style modification is appropriate, with clearly outlined follow-up instructions. Failure to respond to these measures should prompt evaluation, which can involve either double-contrast upper gastrointestinal series or preferably endoscopy.

In the absence of any significant pathology, therapy can be pursued by increasing the dose of H_2 blocker. The presence of severe esophagitis or Barrett's esophagus would prompt gastric acid analysis. The measurement of gastric acid over time is the most predictable way to assure that individualized and effective therapy is being delivered. Increasing the dose of medication to levels sufficient to reduce acid exposure to less than 5% in 24 h and gastric volumes to well below 10% of normal will assure effective therapy (COLLEN et al. 1990). Remember that this is what is happening to patients being treated with omeprazole; the very same thing can be accomplished with H_2 blockers but it requires individual dosing.

Consideration at some time must be given to the possibility of antireflux surgery, especially if the patient has pulmonary symptoms related to reflux.

Although this is difficult to prove at the present time it should be suspected in all patients and attempts made to confirm the association. In the near future omeprazole or other new potassium-hydrogen ATPase inhibitors will likely serve the function of providing the "therapeutic trial" that confirms or denies the association between reflux and other disorders. Remembering that it may be a long time before omeprazole is recommended for indefinite use, patients who respond would be considered potential surgery candidates, although we should expect that most patients or physicians would not opt for this.

L. Summary

Just as in other areas of acid-peptic disease, our concepts regarding gastroesophageal reflux have changed dramatically in the last several years. In all areas of this very common disorder we now have a better understanding of the pathophysiology and possible therapies. Many of our difficulties in understanding and treating gastroesophageal reflux stem from the parochial attitude taken to this disease. Our failure to understand why standard doses of H_2 blockers, which very effectively healed duodenal ulcers, would not heal esophagitis, and our current inability to elucidate the scope of extraesophageal manifestations of gastroesophageal reflux, stand out as two of the major results of that attitude.

We are now entering an era in which we can effectively treat essentially all patients with gastroesphageal reflux, at least in the short term, and one in which the technology exists to document the relationships between reflux and other potential manifestations outside the esophagus. Using the information we have gained is mandatory as we approach both our patients and our research.

References

Andersen LI, Schmidt A, Bundgaard A (1986) Pulmonary function and acid application in the esophagus. Chest 90:358–363

Aprill N, Echrich J, Wang C, Clementschitsch P, DeMeester JR, Winans C (1979) Quantitative reduction of gastroesophageal acid reflux by cimetidine. Gastroenterology 76:1092

Belcher JR (1949) The pulmonary complications of dysphagia. Thorax 4:44–56

Benjamin SB (1986) Extraesophageal complications of gastroesophageal reflux. J Clin Gastroenterol [Suppl 1] 8:68–71

Bennett JR, Buckton G, Morten HD (1983) Cimetidine in gastroesophageal reflux. Digestion 26:166–172

Bombeck CT, Vaz O, DeSalvo J, Donahue PE, Hyhus LM (1987) Computerized axial manometry of the esophagus. Ann Surg 206:465–472

Bonaviana L, Evander A, Demeester TR et al. (1986) Length of the distal esophageal sphincter and competence of the cardia. Am J Surg 151:25–34

Boyle JT, Tuchman DN, Altschuler SM, Noxon TE, Pack AI, Cohen S (1985) Mechanisms for the association of gastroesophageal reflux and bronchospasm. Am Rev Resp Dis 131:516–520

Castell DO (1975) The lower esophageal sphincter: physiologic and clinical aspects. Am J Med 83:390–401

Collen MJ, Lewis JH, Benjamin SB (1990) Gastric acid hypersecretion in refractory gastroesophageal reflux. Gastroenterology 98:654-661
DeMeester TR (1985) Surgical management of gastroesophageal reflux. In: Castell DO, Wu WC, Ott DJ (eds) Gastroesophageal reflux disease: pathogenesis, diagnosis, therapy. Futura, Mount Kisco, pp 243–280
DeMeester TR, Johnson LF, Joseph GJ, Toscano MS, Hall AW, Skinner DB (1976) Patterns of gastroesophageal reflux in health and disease. Ann Surg 184:459–470
DeMeester TR, Wemly JA, Bryant GH, Little AG, Skinner OB (1979) Clinical and in vitro analysis of determinants of gastroesophageal competence. A study of the principles of antireflux surgery. Am J Surg 137:39–46
Dent J, Dodds WJ, Sekiguchi T, Hogan WJ, Arndorfer RC (1983) Interdigestive phasic contractions of the human lower esophageal sphincter. Gastroenterology 84:453–460
Dodds WJ, Dent J, Hogan WJ, Helm JF, Hauser R, Patel GK, Egide MS (1982) Mechanism of gastroesophageal reflux in patients with reflux esophagitis. N Engl J Med 307:1547–1552
Eastwood GL (1983) Esophagitis and its consequences. In: Castell DO, Johnson LF (eds) Esophageal function in health and disease. Elsevier, New York, pp 176–186
Eastwood GL, Bonnice CA (1985) Barrett's esophagus – a special problem. In: Castell DO, Wu W, Oh DJ (eds) Gastroesophageal reflux disease. Futura, Mount Kisco, pp 801–320
Fink SM, McCullum RW (1984) The role of prolonged esophageal pH monitoring in the diagnosis of gastroesophageal reflux. JAMA 252:1160–1164
Fisher RS, Malmud LS, Roberts GS, Lobis IF (1976) Gastroesophageal (GE) scintiscanning to detect and quantitate GI reflux. Gastroenterology 70:301–308
Goldman J, Bennett TR (1988) Gastroesophageal reflux and respiratory disorders in adults. Lancet 2:493–494
Goodall RJR, Earis JE, Cooper DM, Bernstein A, Temple JG (1981) Relationship between asthma and gastro-oesophageal reflux. Thorax 36:116–121
Harmon JW, Johnson LF, Maydonovitch CL (1981) Effects of acid and bile salts on the rabbit esophageal mucosa. Dig Dis Sci 26:6572
Harper PC, Bergner A, Kaye MD (1987) Antireflux treatment for asthma. Improvement in patients with associated gastroesophageal reflux. Arch Intern Med 147:56–60
Helm JF, Dodds WJ, Hogan WJ (1987) Salivary response to esophageal acid in normal subjects and patients with reflux esophagitis. Gastroenterology 93:1393–1397
Iascone C, DeMeester TR, Little AG, Skinner DB (1983) Barrett's esophagus. Functional assessment, proposed pathogenesis, and surgical therapy. Arch Surg 118:543–549
Johnson DA, Orane WE, Curran J, Cattau EL, Ciarleglio C, Khan A, Cottingham J, Benjamin SB (1989) Pulmonary disease in progressive systemic sclerosis – a complication of gastroesophageal reflux and occult aspiration? Arch Intern Med 149:589–593
Johnson LF, De Meester TR, Haggitt RC (1978) Esophageal epithelial response to gastroesophageal reflux: a quantitative study. Am J Dig Dis 23:198–509
Jona JZ, Sty JR, Glicklich M (1981) Simplified radiostope technique for assessing gastroesophageal reflux in children. J Pediatr Surg 16:114–117
Katz PO, Knuff TE, Benjamin SB, Castell DO (1986) Abnormal esophageal motility in reflux esophagitis: cause or effect? Am J Gastroenterol 81:744–746
Kennedy JH (1962) "Silent" gastroesophageal reflux: an important but little known cause of pulmonary complications. Dis Chest 42:42–45
Kirk AJB (1986) Reflux dyspareunia. Thorax 41:215–221
Klinkenberg-Knol EC, Jansen JMBJ, Festen HPM, Meuwissey SGU, Lancers CBHE (1987) Double-blind multicenter comparison of omeprazole and ranitidine in the treatment of reflux esophagitis. Lancet 1:349–351
Lillemoe KD, Johnson LF, Harmond JW (1982) Role of the components of the gastroduodenal contents in experimental acid esophagitis. Surgery 92:276–284

Mansfield LE, Stien MR (1978) Gastroesophageal reflux and asthma: a possible reflex mechanism. Ann Allergy 41:224–226
Mansfield LE, Hameister HH, Spaulding HS, Smith NJ, Glab N (1981) The role of the vagus nerve in airway narrowing caused by intraesophageal hydrochloric acid provocation and esophageal distention. Ann Allergy 47:431–434
Mays EE, Dubois JJ, Hamilton GB (1976) Pulmonary fibrosis associated with tracheobronchial asthma. Chest 69:512–515
McCallum RW, Fink SM, Winnan GR, Avella J, Callachan C (1984) Metoclopramide in gastroesophageal reflux disease: rationale for its use and results of a double-blind trial. Am J Gastroenterology 79:165–172
Moran TJ (1955) Experimental aspiration pneumonia. Arch Pathol 60:122–129
Nelson HS (1984) Gastroesophageal reflux and pulmonary disease. J Allergy Clin Immunol 73:547–556
Ogorek CP, Fisher RS (1989) Detection and treatment of gastroesophageal reflux disease. Gastroenterol Clin North Am 18:293–323
Orlando RC (1985) Esophageal epithelial resistance. In: Castell DO, Wu WC, Ott DJ (eds) Gastroesophageal reflux disease. Futura, Mount Kisco, pp 55–80
Orr WC, Robinson MG, Johnson LF (1981) Acid clearance during sleep in the pathogenesis of reflux esophagitis. Dig Dis Sci 26:423–427
Ott DJ, Wu WC, Gelfand DW (1981) Reflux esophagitis revisited: prospective analysis of radiologic accuracy. Gastrointest Radiol 6:1–7
Richter JE, Paneol SJ, Castell DO, McCarthy DM (1981) Gastroesophageal reflux disease in the Zollinger-Ellison Syndrome. Ann Intern Med 95:37–43
Richter JE, Wu WC, Johns DN, Blackwell JN, Nelson JL, Castell JA, Castell DO (1987) Esophageal manometry in 95 health adult volunteers. Dig Dis Sci 32: 583–592
Seiwert R, Jennewein HM, Waldeck F (1974) Mechanism of action of fundoplication. Proceedings of the fourth international symposium on gastrointestinal mobility. Mitchell, Van Couver, pp 143–15
Skov Olsen PSS, Kirkegaard P, Nexo E (1984) Role of submandibular saliva and epidermal growth factor in gastric cytoprotection. Gastroenterology 87:103–108
Spaulding HS, Mansfield LE, Stein MR, Sellner JC, Gremillion DE (1982) Further investigation of the association between gastroesophageal reflux and bronchoconstriction. J Allergy Clin Immunol 69:516–521
Urschel HC Jr, Paulson DL (1967) Gastroesophageal reflux and hiatal hernia: complications and therapy. J Thorac Cardiovasc Surg 53:2132
Werner GJ, Mongan TM, Cooper JB, Wu WC, Castell DO, Sinclair JW, Richter JC (1988) Ambulatory 24 hr pH monitoring: reproducibility and variability of pH parameters. Dig Dis Sci 33:1127–1133
Wilson NM, Charette L, Thomson NH, Silverman M (1985) Gastro-oesophageal reflux and childhood asthma: the acid test. Thorax 40:592–597

CHAPTER 15

Endoscopy in the Evaluation and Treatment of Acid-Peptic Disease

P.N. YAKSHE and E.L. CATTAU

A. Introduction

Endoscopy has revolutionized the clinical approach to gastrointestinal disease. The authors assume the reader is familiar with the fundamental design and operation of modern gastrointestinal endoscopes. The advent of specialized probes, catheters, and endoscopes has transformed this diagnostic instrument into a versatile therapeutic tool. Wire snares enable the removal of polyps, needles permit the injection of chemical agents used for sclerosis, several probes deliver electrical energy for cauterization or cutting, and optical fibers transmit laser light for hemostasis and the palliative ablation of tumors. Although in some areas the implementation of new technology has preceded documentation of clinical efficacy, it is this unique ability of gastrointestinal endoscopy to concomitantly make a diagnosis, obtain tissue for histologic confirmation, and provide treatment that has revolutionized our approach to acid-peptide disease. In this chapter, detailed attention is given to the indications for endoscopy, the value of information obtained by endoscopy, and the basic principles and clinical efficacy of therapeutic devices used in complicated acid-peptic disease.

B. Accuracy

Many comparative studies have shown that endoscopy has greater diagnostic accuracy than radiology ("accuracy" is defined as the sum of the true-positives and true-negatives divided by the total number of observations). The accuracy of esophagogastroduodenoscopy (EGD) ranges from 90% to 97% compared with 70% to 88% for the double contrast barium meal (DCBM) (BROWN et al. 1978; WILJASALO et al. 1980; KIIL and ANDERSON 1980; DOOLEY et al. 1984). Regarding peptic ulcer disease, two comparative studies are noteworthy. The first involved a prospective evaluation of 50 patients with chronic duodenal ulcer disease, in which elective surgery served as the final arbiter for the presence of disease. The diagnostic accuracy of EGD was 90% compared to 82% for DCBM (BROWN et al. 1978). In the other study, the presence of a gastroduodenal ulcer or malignancy was assessed in 173 dyspeptic patients. The final diagnosis was arrived at by specific criteria. EGD had a diagnostic accuracy of 97% compared to 88% for DCBM

(KIIL and ANDERSON 1980). The combination of increased accuracy and ability to obtain tissue for analysis has made endoscopy the preferred diagnostic approach in the evaluation of peptic ulcer disease (ASGE 1988b).

In certain circumstances, radiology is preferred over endoscopy. When symptoms are suggestive of a disorder of transit, as in dysphagia or persistent vomiting, an initial barium meal may provide more useful information about esophageal and gastric function or the severity and extent of a mechanical obstruction (COTTON and SHORVON 1984; COLIN-JONES 1986). When there is known or suspected perforation of a viscus, endoscopy is contraindicated and x-rays of the chest and abdomen and Gastrografin meals are indispensable (ASGE 1988b; Health and Public Policy Committee 1987). Therefore, the physician must choose the diagnostic procedure which is best suited to answer the clinical question.

C. Safety

Upper endoscopy carries a small risk to the patient. The most common complications are cardiopulmonary (0.08%), perforation (0.04%), and bleeding (0.03%) (SILVIS et al. 1976; COLIN-JONES et al. 1978; SHAHMIR and SCHUMAN 1980). The overall mortality resulting from these complications is about 0.01%–0.02% (DEKKER and TYTGAT 1977; COLIN-JONES et al. 1978; COLIN-JONES 1986). Endoscopic complications are more likely to occur during urgent evaluations of seriously ill patients; here the mortality approaches 0.15% (GILBERT et al. 1981a).

The possibility of infection has two considerations. First, transient bacteremia may occur during instrumentation of the gastrointestinal tract; therefore, antibiotic prophylaxis is recommended for patients with a prior history of endocarditis or a prosthetic heart valve (FLEISCHER 1989). Second, to minimize the potential for endoscopic transmission of infectious agents such as viral hepatitis (VENNES 1981; BIRNIE et al. 1983) or the human immunodeficiency virus, established procedures for cleansing and disinfection should be followed (ASGE 1988c; British Society of Gastroenterology 1988).

D. Uncomplicated Acid-Peptic Disease

I. Endoscopy as the Initial Diagnostic Modality

When confronted with suspected acid peptic disease, a clinical appraisal of the patient's signs and symptoms will determine the need for a diagnostic test. For example, in a patient whose only complaint is dyspepsia, it is reasonable to initiate a 6- to 8-week therapeutic trial of antiulcer therapy combined with the discontinuation of offending agents such as alcohol, cigarettes, and ulcerogenic medication. This approach to uncomplicated dyspepsia will target two groups of people in whom endoscopy is indicated as the initial diagnostic test: (a) those patients who do not respond to therapy after a week to 10 days and (b) those patients who have residual symptoms at the end of the therapeutic trial. While this management strategy is not intended for patients at increased risk for cancer, it will obviate diagnostic tests in the majority of patients with isolated dyspepsia, conserve resources, and utilize the procedure with the highest diagnostic accuracy in those who ultimately require evaluation. Conversely, if more serious disease is suggested by the presence of anorexia, early satiety, persistent vomiting, weight loss, signs of bleeding, evidence of obstruction, or systemic illness, then the patient should undergo an immediate diagnostic evaluation (Health and Public Policy Committee 1985; 1987; ASGE 1988b). Endoscopy should be the initial diagnostic procedure in all of these patients except for those with bowel obstruction or perforation. Earlier diagnostic evaluation is also indicated during the therapeutic trial if the patient with isolated dyspepsia develops an exacerbation of symptoms, complications of peptic disease, or signs of a severe systemic illness.

II. Endoscopy Following a Radiologic Procedure

In a patient who has already had upper gastrointestinal x-rays, the need for subsequent endoscopic evaluation depends on an assessment of the prior radiologic findings and the relevance of the additional information to the patient's clinical management.

1. Negative Upper Gastrointestinal Series

A patient with a negative upper gastrointestinal series and persistent dyspepsia despite medical therapy deserves further evaluation by endoscopy. For gastroduodenal ulcers, the negative predictive value of a DCBM (the chance of a patient having no ulcer when the test is negative) ranges from 43% to 91% and is inferior to that of endoscopy (BROWN et al. 1978; KIIL and ANDERSON 1980). Although the diagnosis of superficial mucosal lesions is most commonly missed by radiology (WILJASALO et al. 1980), the superior sensitivity and specificity of endoscopy remain significant even if these lesions are excluded from the analysis (DOOLEY et al. 1984). Consequently, endoscopic evaluation can increase the percentage of correct diagnoses over that made with DCBM by almost 20% (DOOLEY et al. 1984).

2. Gastric Ulcer

If additional endoscopic information will be used in the patient's management, all gastric ulcers meeting radiologic criteria for "malignant" or "indeterminant" should be promptly evaluated by gastroscopy with brushing and biopsy to obtain a pretreatment tissue diagnosis (WEINSTEIN 1977; ASGE 1988b; Health and Public Policy Committee 1987).

The need for endoscopic evaluation of a radiologically "benign" gastric ulcer is less clear. Some authors believe that a gastric ulcer, clearly demonstrated as benign on a DCBM study, can be followed radiologically to complete healing (WEINSTEIN 1977; THOMPSON et al. 1983; GELFAND et al. 1984). The arguments against this approach are compelling. During the life cycle of early gastric cancer, approximately 70% of malignant ulcers may undergo partial or complete mucosal repair (SAKITA et al. 1971). Despite radiologic appearance, roughly 3%–7% of gastric ulcers initially classified as benign turn out to be gastric carcinoma (GRAHAM et al. 1982; RICHARDSON 1983). Furthermore, endoscopic visualization alone cannot reliably discriminate a benign from a malignant gastric ulcer (DEKKER and TYTGAT 1977; WITZEL et al. 1976; GRAHAM et al. 1982; SANCHO-POCH et al. 1978; FARINI et al. 1983; PODOLSKY et al. 1988). Based on these considerations, the authors advocate endoscopic biopsy and cytology of all "benign" gastric ulcers.

3. Duodenal Ulcer

Endoscopy may be required when a prior radiologic procedure demonstrates duodenal disease. If the upper gastrointestinal x-rays are equivocal (duodenal deformity, spasm, or thickened folds), the greater sensitivity of endoscopy can establish a diagnosis. If the x-rays clearly demonstrate a duodenal ulcer but the patient fails to respond to an appropriate course of medical therapy, endoscopy may detect the presence of another condition such as esophagitis, gastric ulcer, or neoplasm which may alter the patient's management. There is currently no role for biopsy in duodenal ulcer disease (ASGE 1988b). Ongoing research into the relationship between *Helicobacter pylori* and duodenal ulcer disease may alter this approach in the future.

III. Biopsy and Cytology

Biopsy technique is critical for successful differentiation of benign and malignant gastric ulcers. The importance of biopsy site was demonstrated in an in vitro study of 20 freshly resected specimens of ulcerated gastric carcinoma (HATFIELD et al. 1975). The sensitivity of detecting cancerous tissue was highest when biopsies were obtained from the rim (80%) and the center (75%) of the ulcer. When these biopsy sites were combined, the yield increased to 95%. Equally important is the total number of biopsies taken (KASUGAI 1968; DEKKER and TYTGAT 1977; SANCHO-POCH et al. 1978; GRAHAM et al. 1982). Although the recommended number varies, at least eight biopsies are required (when biopsy is used alone) to achieve a 99% probability of sampling malignant tissue (SANCHO-POCH et al. 1978).

The value of adding brush cytology to biopsy is controversial. While its specificity is usually comparable to that of biopsy, in some studies cytology tends to have a higher rate of false-positive diagnoses (WITZEL et al. 1976; KIIL et al. 1979; QIZILBASH et al. 1980; COOK et al. 1988) and may be more sensitive in diagnosing tumors of the cardia and malignant stenotic lesions (WITZEL et al. 1976). In published series, the combined sensitivity of biopsy and cytology in detecting gastroesophageal malignancy ranges from 91% to 96%. Using both techniques, it seems reasonable to obtain at least six biopsy specimens: one from each quadrant of the rim, one from the ulcer base, and one or more from where the endoscopist suspects malignancy.

While the negative predictive value of combined biopsy and cytology is high, it is important to recognize that these techniques cannot always detect malignancy when it is present. Submucosally infiltrating and necrotic ulcerating tumors may be missed by both techniques. Therefore, negative results should not override one's clinical impression when deciding on surgical intervention.

IV. Disease Follow-up

Gastric ulcers warrant follow-up. Gastric malignancy has eluded detection with a benign radiographic appearance (GROSSMAN 1971; WELCH and BURKE 1969) and negative endoscopic biopsies (FARINI et al. 1983; PODOLSKY et al. 1988). Since the time required for healing of a gastric ulcer is related to its size (GROSSMAN 1971), follow-up should be performed approximately 8–12 weeks from the initial procedure (ASGE 1988b). Provided endoscopy with biopsy is performed at initial diagnosis, follow-up can be done by either radiology or endoscopy.

Because the risk of malignancy is so low, endoscopy is not indicated in the routine clinical follow-up of uncomplicated duodenal ulcer disease.

E. Gastrointestinal Bleeding from Acid-Peptic Disease

I. Guidelines for Intervention

Endoscopy has assumed a key role in the diagnosis of upper gastrointestinal hemorrhage. It has superior accuracy compared to radiology (DRONFIELD et al. 1982; MORRIS et al. 1975; ALLAN and DYKES 1974) and it can determine which of several potential sites is responsible for the bleeding (PALMER 1969; COTTON et al. 1973; GILBERT et al. 1981b). Should additional diagnostic or therapeutic procedures be required, it does not interfere with interventional radiology.

The timing of endoscopy is associated with the likelihood of identifying the bleeding site. Urgent endoscopy should be performed in all patients with clinical evidence of active persistent bleeding, ideally as soon as the patient's hemodynamic status can be stabilized and generally within 12 h of admission (ASGE 1988c). As the interval between admission and endoscopy increases, the number of actively bleeding lesions identified decreases significantly (GILBERT et al. 1981) and the chance of not identifying the bleeding site increases. In two studies (COTTON et al. 1973; ALLEN et al. 1973), the bleeding site was found in 79% and 90% of patients endoscoped within 48 h of admission, compared to 5% and 33% of those endoscoped beyond 48 h. In hemodynamically stable patients with evidence of acute self-limited blood loss, elective endoscopy is most accurate in determining the site of bleeding when it is performed within the first 24 h (GILBERT et al. 1981b; COTTON et al. 1973).

Historically, advances in diagnostic endoscopy have exceeded our ability to manage upper gastrointestinal hemorrhage. Numerous studies showed that although routine early endoscopy resulted in an increased diagnostic accuracy, this was not associated with an improvement in transfusion requirements, length of hospital stay, or patient survival (PETERSON et al. 1981; GRAHAM 1980; EASTWOOD 1977; DRONFIELD et al. 1982). There are two explanations for these observations. First, the studies looked at gastrointestinal bleeding from a variety of causes for which specific tailored therapy was not available. To paraphrase COTTON (1977), if more accurate diagnosis does not lead to better outcome, surely the management must be wrong. Second, the studies evaluated consecutive series of patients. Since the majority of gastrointestinal hemorrhage tends to be self-limited, a much larger number of patients would be required to show a small benefit. Consequently, endoscopists have attempted to identify features of gastrointestinal lesions having prognostic significance toward patient outcome. Conceptually, if one can identify subgroups of patients at increased risk for persistent or recurrent bleeding, then therapeutic intervention may demonstrate a reduction in morbidity and mortality.

II. Stigmata of Bleeding

FOSTER et al. (1978) were among the first to establish criteria for accepting a lesion as the source of hemorrhage and to show the prognostic value of endoscopic findings. These criteria were termed "stigmata" of bleeding and included: (a) fresh blood coming from the lesion, (b) fresh or altered blood clot or black slough adherent to the lesion, and (c) a vessel protruding from the base or margin of an ulcer. Of 60 ulcer patients with stigmata, 25 (42%) had further hemorrhage and roughly 53% required surgery. In contrast, only 1 of 29 (3%) ulcer patients without stigmata had further hemorrhage and required surgery. These criteria identified those ulcers that definitely bled, were associated with a 50% risk of rebleeding, and were found to be superior to any other single factor or combination of factors in predicting rebleeding and the need for emergency surgery.

Subsequent authors reached contradictory conclusions about the relative value of endoscopic stigmata in predicting patient outcome. For instance, the prognostic value of the visible vessel has been corroborated by GRIFFITHS et al. (1979) and STOREY et al. (1981) but refuted by WARA (1985) and CHANG-CHIEN et al. (1988). The importance of other stigmata of bleeding in predicting outcome is also unclear. In an attempt to clarify this issue, we reviewed the English literature for endoscopic findings in patients with upper gastrointestinal bleeding. Articles that failed to define criteria for stigmata of bleeding were excluded from further analysis. Even among papers that defined their terms, there was great variability in the meaning of "stigmata" of recent hemorrhage, in the subgrouping of stigmata, and in the definitions used for recurrent hemorrhage, emergency surgery, and even mortality. Therefore, for the purposes of comparison, we defined the following endoscopic categories:

1. Clean ulcer; an ulcer with a clean base, having neither evidence of stigmata of recent hemorrhage nor active bleeding as defined in the other categories.
2. Flat spot or stain; evidence of focal red, blue, brown, or black spots or stains that are flush with the surface of the ulcer base.
3. Old clot or black slough; black-colored slough or blood clot adherent to the ulcer base (presumably indicating an older organized clot).
4. Fresh red clot; a relatively large, fresh, adherent red blood clot.
5. Active oozing; continuous nonspurting bleeding from the base or margin of the ulcer.
6. Visible vessel; a relatively small, pigmented object definitely protruding above the surface of the ulcer. Included in this category are terms such as pulsating pseudoaneurysm, sentinel clot, pigmented protuberance, protruding spot or vessel, and yellow-white rod sticking out of the ulcer base.
7. Spurting arterial bleed; active bleeding that has a pulsatile character.

The endoscopic findings in the literature were collated into these categories along with information about persistent or recurrent bleeding. If two or more endoscopic findings were identified within the same ulcer base, the ulcer was placed in the category with the higher number. Because there is no consensus in the literature on criteria for rebleeding, and for the sake of simplifying the comparison, we took the position that any evidence of further bleeding (persistent or recurrent) is clinically relevant to the patient's management (since it would, at the very least, prolong the patient's hospitalization). Since emergent surgery and mortality data were not available in all of the studies, they were not included in our evaluation. The results are illustrated in Fig. 1.

When the literature on stigmata of bleeding is sorted in this manner, some general observations can be made. First, there is a spectrum of endoscopic findings having prognostic value. As one might predict, peptic ulcers with evidence of a spurting arterial bleed carry the worst prognosis for further hemorrhage (77%), while ulcers with a clean base are very unlikely to bleed again (2%). Between these extremes, there is an increased risk of rebleeding with visible vessels (48%), followed by active oozing (34%) and fresh clot (28%), while old clot (8%) and focal flat spot or stain (3%) have a minimally

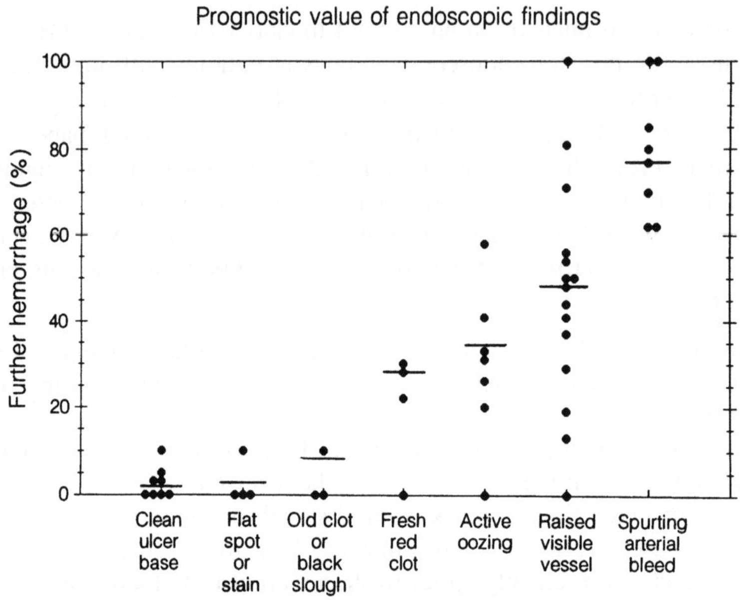

Fig. 1. Risk of further hemorrhage (defined as persistent bleeding or rebleeding) from a gastroduodenal ulcer based on endoscopic appearance

increased risk of rebleeding. Interestingly, when studies that either combine fresh and old blood clot together or do not differentiate between them are summed, averaged, and compared with Fig. 1, the percentage having further bleeding (17%) falls in between the rates for fresh and old clot alone. There did not appear to be a prognostic advantage to flat spots or stains or old clot as suggested by some (Bornman et al. 1985).

An important observation is that endoscopic findings alone are an unreliable predictor of further hemorrhage. Note that while the average rebleeding risk for a "visible vessel" is 48%, the individual studies range from 0% to 100%. This variation may be explained by differences in selection criteria between studies. Wara (1985) and Krejs et al. (1987) found further bleeding in only 19% and 13% of patients with visible vessels respectively; however, they excluded patients who were hemodynamically unstable. This would tend to support the contention by Bornman et al. (1985) that the combination of shock and important endoscopic findings is a better predictor of patient outcome than either factor alone. In addition, heterogeneity within the term "visible vessel" may be another reason for the variable outcome. As currently used, this term includes a variety of endoscopic descriptions, within which there are probably subgroups having differing natural histories. The variables of color, size, and duration of time between the bleeding episode and endoscopic description are likely to be important in this regard. For example, red visible vessels may be more ominous than black or white ones. Additional studies are needed to elucidate these points.

Another controversial issue is whether one should dislodge an adherent clot to determine whether a visible vessel lurks in the ulcer base below. In one study, 11 patients with adherent clot rebled; at least nine were found to have a visible vessel at the time of surgery (BORNMAN et al. 1985). We advocate meticulous endoscopic inspection of the ulcer base in all patients. Irrigation of the lesion with water has been shown to be safe and effective and should be routinely performed. Since approximately 70% of patients with fresh clot stop bleeding spontaneously, removal of adherent clot by other mechanical means does not seem warranted unless additional factors such as active oozing beneath the clot or a clinical setting of recurrent hemorrhage are present. Clearly, one should be prepared for the possibility of active hemorrhage, be experienced in therapeutic endoscopy, and have prompt surgical backup before attempting such measures.

III. Endoscopic Hemostasis

Endoscopy now has the potential to treat actively bleeding ulcers and reduce the incidence of rebleeding. While a variety of techniques have demonstrated efficacy in animal models and shown promise in uncontrolled clinical trials, the following section focuses primarily on those tested in prospectively controlled clinical trials. The modalities are introduced with a brief discussion of the underlying principles important to successful and safe clinical application and are summarized with a comment on their merits and limitations.

1. Electrocoagulation

Electrocoagulation uses high frequency electrical currents to achieve tissue coagulation. When an electric current greater than 100,000 cycles per second is applied to living tissue, resistance to the flow of current (tissue impedance) produces intense heat without causing muscle contraction or nerve stimulation (CURTISS 1973). The desired histologic effect of thermal energy is coagulation, which corresponds with the biochemical denaturation of proteins (SIGEL and DUNN 1965).

Coagulation is confined to the treatment site by one of two methods. In monopolar electrocoagulation, a small active electrode is placed into contact with the target tissue and the electric current passes through the patient to a large dispersal pad applied to the skin. Because the current density (amperes/mm^2) is highest where the small electrode comes into contact with the tissue, coagulation is restricted to that area. In contrast, bipolar electrocoagulation has both electrodes at the tip of the probe. Therefore, the current of electricity spans only the tissue in close proximity to the contact points and does not travel through the patient (PAPP 1982). The main difference between the two methods is that monopolar electrocoagulation produces a greater depth of injury (MOORE et al. 1978; PROTELL et al. 1981).

The use of electrocoagulation for the treatment of gastrointestinal bleeding is linked to experiments by SIGEL and co-workers (SIGEL and DUNN 1965;

SIGEL and HATKE 1967). These authors described the closure of blood vessels by two mechanisms: (a) obliterative coagulation, where current is applied to the general area around a blood vessel, resulting in shrinkage of the vessel wall and closure of its lumen via intraluminal thrombosis and contracting coagulated tissue, and (b) coaptive coagulation, in which the vessel's walls are mechanically opposed and sealed or "welded" together. The former technique is best suited for small vessels, whereas the latter is usually required for vessels larger than 1 mm in diameter. Some principles of coaptive coagulation warrant emphasis. The strength of the coaptive bond is directly related to the pressure exerted on the blood vessel. Maximal bond strength is also related to the level of energy input (and degree of tissue heating). Whereas suboptimal energy input produces a weak bond, an excessive amount damages surrounding tissue, destroys connective tissue fibers (which give strength to the bond), and creates an amorphous coagulum that may separate from normal tissue. Ideally, coaptive coagulation should preserve the stromal connective tissue fibers and allow a reparative process to occur without inciting an inflammatory response (SIGEL and HATKE 1967).

a) Monopolar Electrocoagulation

Three prospective, randomized, controlled studies have evaluated monopolar electrocoagulation in the treatment of gastrointestinal bleeding (Fig. 2). PAPP (1982), one of the first investigators to recognize the importance of the visible

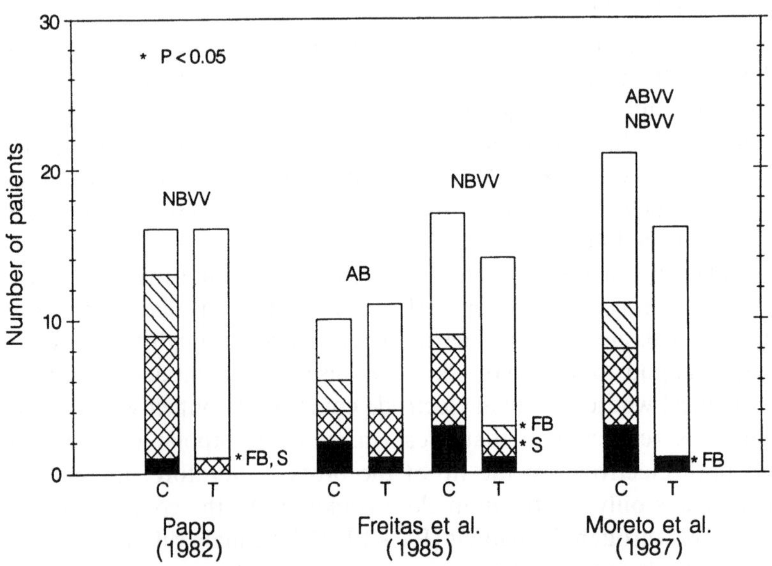

Fig. 2. Prospective, controlled clinical trials of monopolar electrocoagulation. *C*, control group; *T*, treatment group; *AB*, active bleeding; *ABVV* and *NBVV*, actively bleeding or nonbleeding visible vessel; \\\\ or *FB*, further bleeding; crosshatched area, both further bleeding and surgery; *blackened area*, mortality

ulcer vessel, found that only 1 of 16 (6%) patients treated with monopolar electrocoagulation rebled compared to 13 of 16 (81%) in the control group ($P < 0.05$). This study demonstrated a reduction in the average hospital stay and total costs to the patient. MORETO et al. (1987) also found monopolar electrocoagulation effective in reducing further hemorrhage in patients with active bleeding and nonbleeding visible vessels. FREITAS et al. (1985) found that patients with visible vessels treated with a modified liquid monopolar electrode had a statistically significant reduction in the rate of recurrent hemorrhage and surgery.

Despite its demonstrated efficacy, technical considerations have dampened enthusiasm for monopolar electrocoagulation. The probe's design and energy distribution usually require an en face approach to the lesion for successful therapy. Compared with other contact probes, direct contact with the visible vessel carries a higher risk of precipitating active hemorrhage and the greater depth of tissue injury may be associated with an increased risk of perforation. Finally, tissue adherence to the probe's tip may require repeated cleaning which prolongs endoscopy time.

b) Bipolar Electrocoagulation

Six prospective, randomized, controlled clinical trials of the BICAP system (acronym for bipolar circumactive probe) in gastrointestinal bleeding have yielded varying results (Fig. 3). Two early studies did not show bipolar electrocoagulation to be effective. KERNOHAN et al. (1984) evaluated patients with peptic ulcer disease bearing stigmata of recent hemorrhage (defined as a vessel or spot, bleeding or nonbleeding). Eleven of 17 patients (65%) in the treatment group and 7 of 22 patients (32%) in the control group had recurrent hemorrhage. GOUDIE et al. (1984) studied patients with solitary peptic ulcers bearing stigmata of recent hemorrhage (not defined). Rebleeding occurred in 7 of 21 patients (33%) in the treatment group compared to 5 of 25 patients (20%) in the control group and no difference was found in the rate of surgical intervention, mean transfusion requirements, or length of hospital stay.

In contrast, four subsequent studies showed bipolar electrocoagulation to be effective in the management of bleeding peptic ulcers. O'BRIEN et al. (1986) identified peptic ulcer disease with active bleeding or signs of recent hemorrhage (defined as a visible vessel or adherent clot) in 204 patients with upper gastrointestinal bleeding. Recurrent hemorrhage occurred in 17 of 101 patients randomized to the treatment group compared to 34 of 103 controls. Patients with visible vessels, especially those who were actively bleeding at the time of treatment, received the greatest benefit from bipolar electrocoagulation. BICAP therapy was found to be advantageous despite an older treatment group with a lower mean hemoglobin concentration and a higher proportion of hemodynamically compromised patients. Although the rate of surgery and bleeding-associated mortality were lower in the treated group, these did not reach statistical significance. Favorable results were also re-

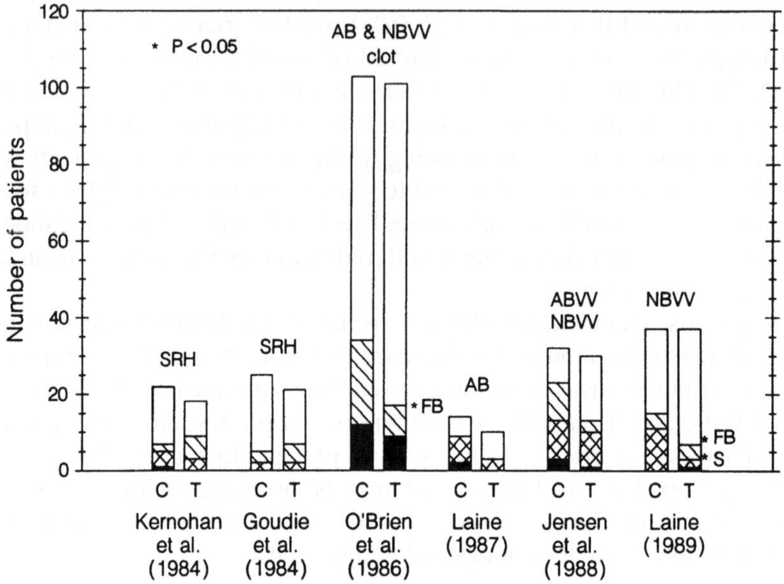

Fig. 3. Prospective, controlled clinical trials of bipolar electrocoagulation. *C*, control group; *T*, treatment group; *SRH*, stigmata of recent hemorrhage; *AB*, active bleeding; *ABVV* and *NBVV*, actively bleeding or nonbleeding visible vessel; \\\\ or *FB*, further bleeding; *crosshatched area*, both further bleeding and surgery; *blackened area*, mortality

ported by Laine (1987). Peptic ulcer disease accounted for active gastrointestinal bleeding (defined as a continuous flow of blood for 5 min) in 24 patients; 10 patients were randomized to the treatment group and 14 to the control group. Persistent or recurrent hemorrhage occurred in 30% of the treatment group compared with about 64% of controls. While only trends were seen in the reduction of surgery and mortality, statistical significance was achieved in the amount of blood transfused, the length of hospital stay, and a reduction in cost to the patient. Jensen et al. (1988) found bipolar electrocoagulation effective in achieving hemostasis in active hemorrhage and noted a nonsignificant trend in the reduction of recurrent hemorrhage and surgery. In a separate report, Laine (1989) also found bipolar electrocoagulation effective in nonbleeding visible vessels. Of 37 sham-treated control patients, 15 (41%) had recurrent hemorrhage compared to 7 of 38 (18%) treated patients. There was a statistically significant reduction in the rate of emergency surgery, length of hospital stay, and hospital costs.

How can one account for the discrepancies between these studies? The relatively small size of the negative studies may be an important factor. First, there is a learning curve associated with any new technique; hence inexperience with application of the probe may have obscured the benefit in the smaller studies (O'Brien et al. 1986). It is interesting to note that 50% of the patients in the study by Kernohan et al. (1984) were reported to have suboptimal treatment. Second, the small numbers of patients in the negative studies increase the chance of a type II error (failure to show a difference when one exists). Differences in entry criteria, treatment endpoints, and energy delivery may also explain the discrepant results. For example, Laine's study on active bleeding had a definite endpoint for successful electrocoagulation: hemostasis. O'BRIEN et al. (1986) also noted that patients with actively bleeding visible vessels received the greatest benefit. In contrast, the study by GOUDIE et al. (1984) apparently excluded patients with active bleeding and studied only patients with "stigmata of recent hemorrhage." These authors had to rely on charring of the ulcer base as a treatment endpoint. How much energy should one deliver to a nonbleeding lesion? Three studies provide sufficient information for comparison. The median application time of 44 and 41 s at a power setting of 5 reported by LAINE (1987, 1989) is nearly twice the energy delivered in the negative study by GOUDIE et al. (1984), who reported a median application time of 17 s at a power setting of 7. Recent experimental data suggest more effective hemostasis may be achieved by prolonged use of bipolar electrocoagulation (HARRISON and MORRIS 1989). Finally, the use of the 7-French probe in the earlier studies may have put the investigators at a disadvantage. Animal studies show that the larger size probe is more effective in treating larger arteries (MORRIS et al. 1985).

Bipolar electrocoagulation has the advantage of being relatively inexpensive and safe in experienced hands; in addition the BICAP system is readily portable. The probe's central channel is connected to a peristaltic water pump and is convenient for removing blood and debris from the ulcer bed. Since it can be applied in a tangential fashion, more ulcers are accessible to endoscopic treatment. The probe's flexible shaft, however, is suboptimal for successful coaptation in some situations. Coagulated tissue also tends to adhere to the probe, which may precipitate bleeding or require periodic removal and cleaning of the probe.

2. Photocoagulation

In gastrointestinal endoscopy, LASER (an acronym for light amplification by the stimulated emission of radiation) is a powerful beam of monochromatic light that is primarily used as a noncontact thermal device. Laser light is transmitted to the mucosa through the endoscope via an optical fiber. When laser light hits living tissue, four physical effects may occur: reflection, scattering, transmission, and absorption (BOWN et al. 1979). The histologic changes induced by laser are the result of absorption; chromophores within the tissue absorb the light and convert it into thermal energy. The resulting tissue effect varies depending on the total energy received (FLEISCHER 1984). It is the coagulative effect of laser energy that has been used to achieve hemostasis in gastrointestinal bleeding.

Two types of laser have been used for endoscopic therapy. The argon ion laser produces visible light with a wavelength in the blue–green region of the spectrum (~500 nm) and the neodymium: yttrium aluminum garnet (Nd:YAG) laser emits an invisible beam in the near-infrared region of the spectrum (1064 nm). Because the wavelength of the argon laser is absorbed by hemoglobin, technical problems are encountered when blood or bloodclot overlies an ulcer. Conversely, the greater power of the Nd:YAG laser can easily cause full thickness tissue damage and increases the risk of perforation.

a) Argon Laser

Prospective, randomized controlled clinical trials with the argon laser have yielded varying results (Fig. 4). VALLON et al. (1981) found that patients with actively bleeding ulcers seemed to benefit from laser therapy, but this did not reach statistical significance unless two patients were excluded from the analysis because of technical difficulties. SWAIN et al. (1981), in an excellent study, evaluated 76 patients with peptic ulcer disease bearing stigmata of bleeding (well-defined subgroups). Among the 52 patients with visible vessels, further hemorrhage was seen in 8 of 24 (33%) laser-treated compared to 17 of 28 (61%) control patients. The study also showed a significant reduction in mortality; none of the laser-treated patients died compared to seven deaths in the control group. All of the deaths occurred in patients who rebled and all but one followed emergency surgery. In a small trial of patients with arterial bleeding or nonbleeding visible vessels, JENSEN et al. (1984) found

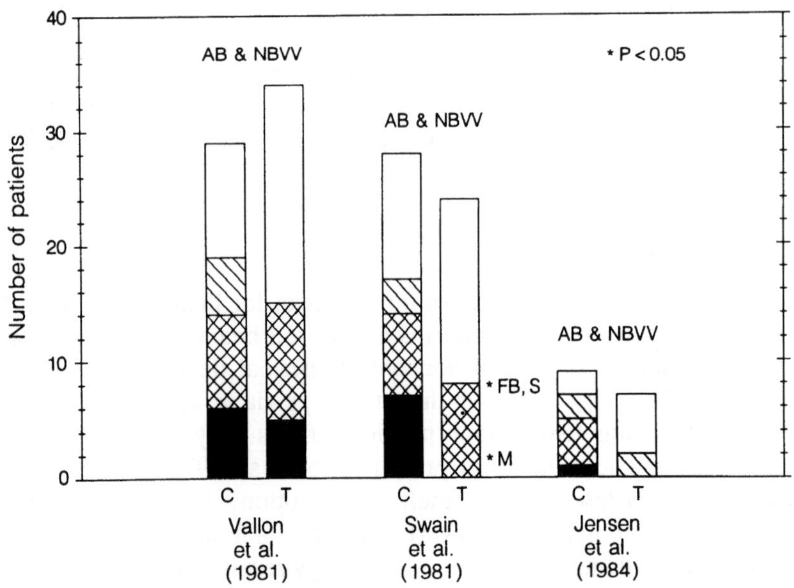

Fig. 4. Prospective, controlled clinical trials of argon laser photocoagulation. *C*, control group; *T*, treatment group; *AB* and *NBVV*, actively bleeding or nonbleeding visible vessel; \\\\ or *FB*, further bleeding; *crosshatched area*, both further bleeding and surgery; *blackened area* or *M*, mortality

that laser-treated patients fared better than control patients regarding mean units of blood transfused, further bleeding, emergency surgery, and death. On balance, argon laser therapy appears to confer a benefit on selected groups of patients with visible vessels or active bleeding from peptic ulcer disease. Because of the advantages of the Nd:YAG laser, few people are currently using argon laser for photocoagulation of bleeding peptic ulcers.

b) Nd:YAG Laser

Discrepant results were also obtained among seven prospective randomized controlled studies evaluating the Nd:YAG laser (Fig. 5). Two studies showed no benefit. IHRE et al. (1981) studied 135 consecutive patients with massive gastrointestinal bleeding and found no differences in mortality, blood transfusions, or length of hospital stay between laser-treated and control groups. However, the results were weakened by poor study design. First, the treatment group was too diverse (including everything from esophageal varices to duodenitis). Second, insufficient information was provided about specific subgroups. Active bleeding from peptic ulcer disease was seen in 12 of 36 (33%) patients in the treatment group and 6 of 31 (19%) controls, but no information regarding stigmata of recent bleeding was given in the remaining patients and one cannot decipher which subgroups had recurrent hemorrhage. Third, laser therapy was performed at a maximum power output of

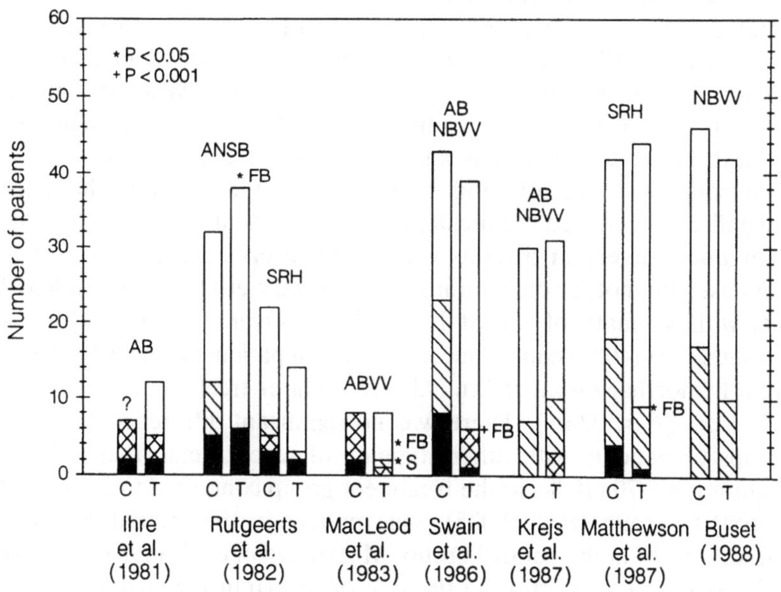

Fig. 5. Prospective, controlled clinical trials of Nd:YAG laser photocoagulation. *C*, control group; *T*, treatment group; *SRH*, stigmata of recent hemorrhage; *AB*, active bleeding; *ABVV* and *NBVV*, actively bleeding or nonbleeding visible vessel; \\\\ or *FB*, further bleeding; *crosshatched area*, both further bleeding and surgery

50 W, which is low compared with animal experiments (JOHNSTON et al. 1980) and other clinical studies reviewed in this section. Finally, only 15 out of 66 patients in the treatment group actually received laser therapy; 12 of these had bleeding from peptic ulcer disease and the other three from esophageal varices. It is noteworthy, however, that initial hemostasis was obtained in 14, recurrent hemorrhage occurred in 50%, and an exacerbation of bleeding was encountered in one. KREJS et al. (1987) randomized 174 peptic ulcer patients with either active bleeding or stigmata of recent hemorrhage. In comparison to the control group, laser therapy was of no benefit in terms of the need for blood transfusions, the rate of rebleeding, the length of stay in the intensive care unit or hospital, or the mortality. However, this study has received strong criticism. Compared to most trials, the rebleeding rate in the control group was very low, probably because the sickest patients were excluded from the study; 21% of the patients initially evaluated for acute gastrointestinal bleeding were considered too unstable to be moved to the laser room. In addition, the treatments were performed by fellows (HEIER et al. 1988).

In contrast, four studies demonstrated a significant benefit and a fifth showed a nonsignificant trend toward benefit in Nd:YAG laser-treated patients. RUTGEERTS et al. (1982) demonstrated laser photocoagulation was significantly better in achieving hemostasis than conservative management in patients with active nonspurting bleeding. Reductions were noted in the rate of rebleeding and surgery, but only the subgroup of patients with active hemorrhage from peptic ulcers reached statistical significance. The authors were not permitted to randomize patients with a spurting arterial bleed because the hospital's ethics committee felt the risk of eventual operation was greater than the risk of endoscopy and laser therapy. When this group of patients was treated in an uncontrolled fashion, hemostasis was achieved in 87% and the need for operation was reduced to 61% compared to 95% in historical controls. MACLEOD et al. (1983) showed that Nd:YAG laser treatment significantly reduced the incidence of further hemorrhage and the need for emergency surgery in patients with active arterial bleeding from peptic ulcer disease. In another outstanding study, SWAIN et al. (1986) studied 138 patients with stigmata of recent hemorrhage. Overall, 7/70 (10%) laser-treated and 27/68 (40%) control ulcers rebled. In patients with visible vessels, recurrent hemorrhage occurred in 6/39 (15%) laser-treated and 23/43 (53%) control ulcers ($P < 0.001$). There was no significant difference detected in the groups of patients with other stigmata of recent hemorrhage. Surgery was required in 7/70 (10%) in the treatment group compared to 24/68 (35%) in the control group ($P < 0.005$). One patient in the treated group died compared to eight in the control group. MATTHEWSON et al. (1987) also documented a significant reduction in the rate of recurrent hemorrhage in laser-treated patients as compared to controls. Finally, BUSET et al. (1988) showed a small reduction in the rate of recurrent hemorrhage in laser-treated patients, but this was not statistically significant.

Although laser therapy has been shown to benefit selected patients with bleeding from peptic ulcer disease, there are many reasons why it is not the best method of endoscopic therapy. Compared to other treatment modalities described in this chapter, laser equipment costs more, portability remains suboptimal, and the technical skills necessary for successful therapy tend to be more difficult to master. Repeat laser therapy for recurrent hemorrhage is relatively contraindicated due to the frequency of transmural damage and increased risk of perforation. In summary, the merits of laser photocoagulation therapy are outweighed by the disadvantages of this modality and it will probably assume a limited role in the treatment of gastrointestinal bleeding from peptic ulcer disease.

3. Heater Probe

The heater probe is another system using thermal energy to achieve hemostasis. Heat is generated at the probe's tip as electric current flows through a resistance coil and is transmitted by diffusion to tissue in contact with the probe (Protell et al. 1978). In experimental studies, the heater probe is comparable to BICAP in that it causes significantly less transmural tissue damage than other treatment modalities (Johnston et al. 1987) and is superior to BICAP with regard to maximum arterial bond strength and avoidance of tissue adherence.

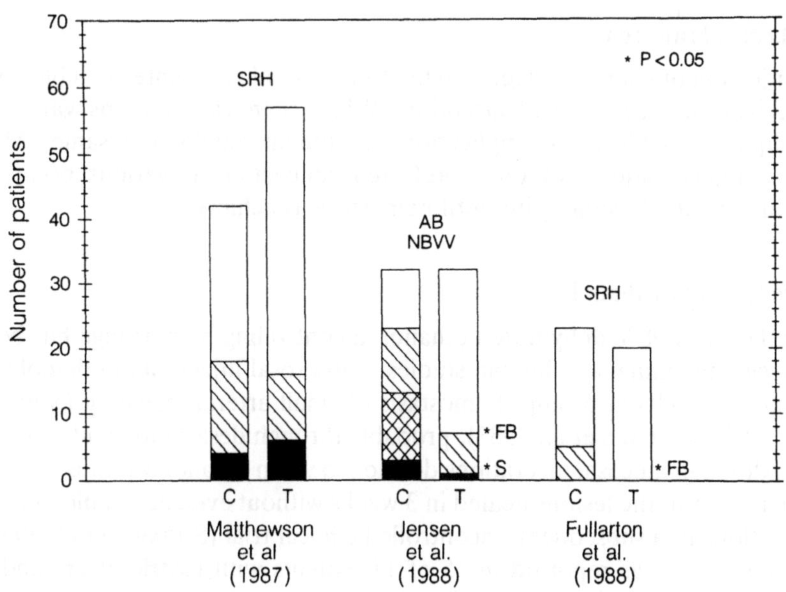

Fig. 6. Prospective, controlled clinical trials of heater probe. *C*, control group; *T*, treatment group; *AB* and *NBVV*, actively bleeding or nonbleeding visible vessel; \\\\ or *FB*, Further bleeding; *crosshatched area*, both further bleeding and surgery; *blackened area* or *M*, mortality

Prospectively controlled trials have shown encouraging results (Fig. 6). MATTHEWSON et al. (1987) showed a trend in benefit from the heater probe; 28% of 57 treated patients had recurrent hemorrhage compared to 42% of 42 controls ($P > 0.05$). JENSEN et al. (1988) demonstrated that the heater probe was 93% effective in stopping active bleeding from peptic ulcers. Among patients with either active hemorrhage or nonbleeding visible vessels, statistically significant reductions were noted in the rates of recurrent hemorrhage (72% in controls vs 22% in treated patients) and in the need for surgery (41% in controls vs 3% in treated patients). FULLARTON et al. (1988) also found the heater probe to be effective in patients with active bleeding or major stigmata of recent hemorrhage; none of the 20 treated patients rebled compared to 5 of 23 (22%) sham-treated controls ($P < 0.05$).

The heater probe has many desirable features. It has demonstrated efficacy that is equal or superior to other modalities. Its greater probe stiffness allows for a higher appositional force during coaptive coagulation (JOHNSTON et al. 1985), and energy delivery per pulse and resultant tissue coagulation are reproducible despite changes in application force and angulation (SWAIN et al. 1984). Design modifications also allow irrigation of the visual field while tamponade is being applied to the bleeding lesion. In contrast to laser, it is relatively inexpensive and can easily be taken to the patient's bedside. While additional prospective studies are needed, the heater probe is one of the most promising therapeutic devices currently available.

4. Chemical Injection

The injection of sclerosing agents in the treatment of gastrointestinal bleeding is receiving a great deal of attention. While chemical solutions vary, the techniques of endoscopic application are fundamentally the same. Most authors inject aliquots of their preferred concoction at various points in proximity to the bleeding site until hemostasis is achieved.

a) Dehydrated Ethanol

The efficacy of 98% dehydrated ethanol in controlling hemorrhage has been chronicled in animal and human studies. Subserosal injection of ethanol in a dog model results in prompt hemostasis of small arterial bleeding (SUGAWA et al. 1984; RANDALL et al. 1987), probably through desiccation and coagulation. Although mucosal ulcerations developed when ethanol was injected into normal mucosa, the lesions healed in 3 weeks without evidence of bleeding or perforation. In a subsequent uncontrolled clinical trial (SUGAWA et al. 1986), clinical success was reported in 15 of 17 patients with gastric ulcers and in 10 of 11 patients with duodenal ulcers. In two patients who underwent operation shortly after successful hemostasis, the ulcers reportedly showed no additional tissue damage induced by ethanol injection except for thrombosis of the vessel and nondescript "perivascular changes."

b) Epinephrine and Hypertonic Saline

Another promising chemical agent is epinephrine, with or without associated vehicles or sclerosants. Conceptually, a mixture of epinephrine and hypertonic saline promotes hemostasis through the physiologic effects of epinephrine coupled with the physicochemical properties of hypertonic saline: epinephrine promotes vasoconstriction and activation of platelets, while hypertonic saline provides local tamponade and fibrinoid degeneration of the vascular wall.

In an uncontrolled clinical trial (HIRAO et al. 1985), prompt hemostasis was achieved in 98% of 114 patients with bleeding from a gastric ulcer. Complete cessation of hemorrhage was maintained for at least a week in 95%, rebleeding occurred within a week in 4%, and initial hemostasis could not be achieved in two cases (2%). In 15 duodenal ulcers, sustained and temporary hemostasis was achieved in 80% and 13% respectively. To combat recurrent hemorrhage, the authors adopted a treatment regimen whereby injections were repeated at 24 and 48 h. Compared to historical controls, this regimen reduced the rate of emergency operation from 22% (15/69) to 0.8% (1/128).

c) Epinephrine and Polidocanol

The combination of epinephrine and polidocanol (a sclerosing agent) has been shown to be effective in the immediate control of severe gastrointestinal bleeding. In an uncontrolled study, 21 patients with gastric ulcers and 16 patients with duodenal ulcers were among 56 patients treated for massive bleeding. Endoscopic injection of 5–10 cc epinephrine (1:10,000) followed by 3–5 cc 1% polidocanol achieved hemostasis in 90% of 29 patients with spurting hemorrhage and in all of the remaining patients with active oozing. Rebleeding occurred in 17% and 29% respectively. Another prospective series demonstrated definitive hemostasis in 98% of 50 actively bleeding lesions. Twenty-eight of these were from peptic ulcer disease (SOEHENDRA et al. 1985).

In a prospective randomized controlled trial of patients with peptic ulcer disease and signs of recent hemorrhage (Fig. 7), PANES et al. (1987) found that endoscopic injection of epinephrine (1:10,000) followed by 1% polidocanol significantly reduced the rate of major rebleeding and emergency surgery. The number of units transfused and the duration of hospital stay were also significantly reduced in the treatment group. There was no significant difference in the number of minor rebleeds or deaths during the study. Treatment groups fared significantly better whether the ulcer showed an actively bleeding visible vessel, nonbleeding vessel, oozing, or clot.

d) Epinephrine

Epinephrine alone (1:10,000) has also been shown to be an effective hemostatic agent. In an uncontrolled study of actively bleeding peptic ulcers,

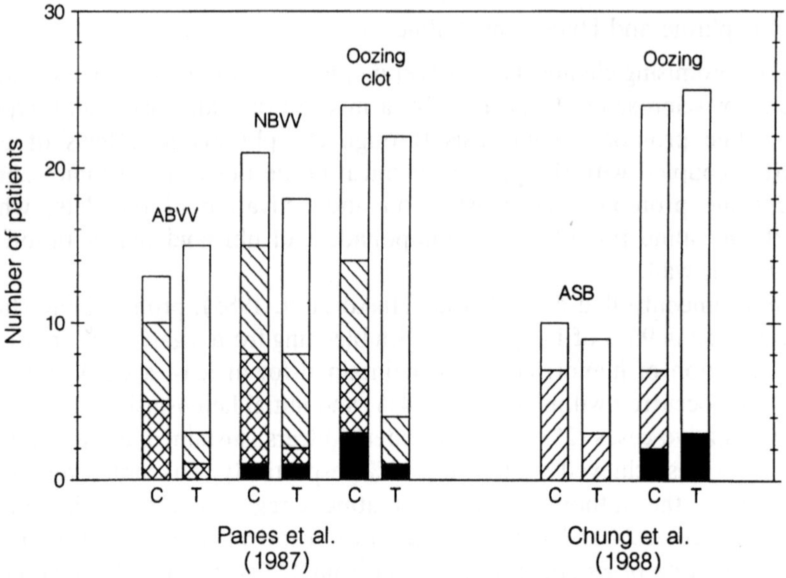

Fig. 7. Prospective, controlled clinical trials of injection therapy. *C*, control group; *T*, treatment group; *ABVV* and *NBVV*, actively bleeding or nonbleeding visible vessel; \\\\, further bleeding; ////, required surgery; *crosshatched area*, both further bleeding and surgery; *blackened area*, mortality ASB; arterial bleed

initial and definitive hemostasis was achieved in 37 (100%) and 34 (92%) patients respectively (Leung and Chung 1987). Five patients rebled within 4 days after therapy; one stopped spontaneously, one responded to retreatment, and three required emergent surgery. Endoscopic follow-up showed that injected ulcers healed at the same rate as noninjected ulcers.

In a subsequent prospective controlled trial (Fig. 7), 68 patients with actively bleeding ulcers were randomized to receive endoscopic injection of epinephrine or no endoscopic treatment (Chung et al. 1988). Emergency operations were performed only if patients met previously established criteria. While initial hemostasis was achieved in all 34 patients in the treatment group, two had recurrent hemorrhage within 24 h and required surgery. Follow-up endoscopy at 24 h in the remaining 32 patients revealed six ulcers were bleeding again, but hemostasis was restored by repeat injections in all patients. Three of the six patients found to be rebleeding required surgery within 48 h of the initial injection. Consequently, five patients in the treatment group and 14 patients in the control group required emergent surgery ($P < 0.05$). Both the median number of units of blood transfused (3 vs 5) and the median stay in the hospital (6 vs 8 days) were statistically lower in the treatment group. No complications were observed with the injection of epinephrine, and the rate of healing of ulcers at 6 weeks was about 80% in both groups.

Injection therapy of bleeding peptic ulcers has distinct advantages over other treatment options. It is readily available, inexpensive, portable, and relatively easy to learn.

5. Comparison of Hemostatic Modalities

Several studies compare therapeutic modalities in the management of gastrointestinal bleeding. Among the thermal devices, BICAP and Nd:YAG laser therapy were found to have equal efficacy (RUTGEERTS et al. 1987a; GOFF 1986). Although retrospective comparisons favor heater probe over Nd:YAG laser therapy on the basis of ease of use, efficacy, and cost (JOHNSTON et al. 1985; ENGEL and GOLDMAN 1986), a prospective randomized comparison found a nonsignificant trend favoring Nd:YAG laser therapy over heater probe based on reductions in rebleeding rate and mortality (MATTHEWSON et al. 1987). Both heater probe and BICAP were found to stop active ulcer bleeding; however, only heater probe had a significant reduction in the rate of recurrent hemorrhage and need for ulcer surgery (JENSEN et al. 1988).

Other studies have compared injection therapy to thermal devices. RUTGEERTS et al. (1987b) found epinephrine followed by polidocanol to be significantly better than either epinephrine alone or epinephrine followed by Nd:YAG laser therapy in achieving hemostasis. WOODS et al. (1988), LAINE (1989), and WARING et al. (1989) concluded that BICAP and ethanol injection were of equal efficacy and safety. The heater probe had better initial and ultimate hemostasis in comparison to ethanol (LIN et al. 1988) and was similar to epinephrine alone (CHUNG et al. 1988).

CHIOZZINI et al. (1989) found ethanol and epinephrine equally effective in controlling gastroduodenal bleeding.

F. Gastric Outlet Obstruction

Therapeutic endoscopy has entered another surgical domain: strictures of the gastrointestinal tract. The logic is the same; one hopes to achieve an acceptable result using an endoscopic approach and avoid the potential morbidity, mortality, and postoperative sequelae associated with surgery.

The management of gastric outlet obstruction due to acid-peptic disease depends on the severity and duration of disease. Local edema and spasm from acute ulceration are more likely to respond to conventional medical management (NPO, nasogastric suction, and antiulcer therapy) than is cicatricial scarring from chronic disease. In a retrospective review, an operation was ultimately required in 64% of patients with acute disease and 98% of patients with chronic disease. Vagotomy and either pyloroplasty or antrectomy were performed with almost equal frequency. Nearly 10% of the patients had postoperative complications and 24% had postoperative sequelae including small bowel obstruction and dumping syndrome (WEILAND et al. 1982). To avoid the sequelae of drainage procedures, some surgeons have successfully used highly selective vagotomy with digital dilation of the stenotic pylorus (JOHNSTON et al. 1973). The logical extension of this approach is the combination of transluminal endoscopic dilation of the pylorus and H_2 blocker therapy (GRAHAM 1987).

Endoscopic dilatation of pyloric stenosis has progressed from the use of the endoscope itself to the use of sophisticated balloon-tipped catheters. Synthetic polymers used in the construction of low compliance balloons allow radial distribution of high pressures without a significant change in the maximum balloon diameter. The deflated balloon is endoscopically positioned within the narrowed pylorus and a hydrostatic force is applied to dilate the stenosis. Initial reports by BENJAMIN et al. (1982, 1984) and SOLT et al. (1984) demonstrated the feasibility of this technique, usually in patients considered high risk for surgery. LINDOR et al. (1985) reported their experience with balloon dilatation in 111 patients with upper digestive tract strictures. Although the procedure was technically successful in about 87% of patients with pyloric stenosis, only 67% reported symptomatic improvement. The duration of the improvement was a median of 12 months and nearly one-third required retreatment. Despite the lack of controlled data, a national survey (KOZAREK 1986) demonstrates that hydrostatic balloon dilatation of digestive tract strictures is being widely used. In 207 patients treated with balloon dilatation of pyloric stenosis, technical success was achieved in 76%. Immediate symptomatic relief was noted in 67% and objective improvement in 54%; however, these percentages decreased to 56% and 37% at 3 months, respectively. Symptomatic relief was associated with balloon size: immediate symptomatic improvement was noted in 39% when a balloon less than 20 French had been used, compared to 82% with a balloon greater than 52 French. One perforation was reported, for a complication rate of 0.5%.

The role of endoscopic management of pyloric stenosis is uncertain. It is clear that the procedure is technically feasible, relatively safe, and results in symptomatic improvement in approximately two-thirds of patients. In comparison with strictures elsewhere in the digestive tract, endoscopic balloon dilatation of a narrowed pylorus is technically more difficult to perform and fraught with the problem of restenosis. Although there are no prospectively controlled trials, at least one author recommends an initial attempt at endoscopic balloon dilation in all patients with nonmalignant gastric outlet obstruction (SHAPIRO 1987).

G. Summary

Gastrointestinal endoscopy is the preferred diagnostic and therapeutic approach in the management of peptic ulcer disease. In uncomplicated dyspepsia, endoscopic evaluation should be carried out in select groups of patients who fail empiric medical therapy. Patients with complicated acid-peptic disease should undergo prompt diagnostic evaluation. Endoscopy should play a major role in orchestrating the management of upper gastrointestinal bleeding. The prognostic information obtained by meticulous inspection of the ulcer base, in conjunction with clinical parameters, should guide medical management and the utilization of hospital resources more effectively. Given the potential to reduce the risk of recurrent hemorrhage, emergency surgery, and even mortality, gastrointestinal endoscopists should be able to identify and differentiate stigmata of hemorrhage, be trained in the techniques of endoscopic hemostasis, and have an understanding of which groups of patients require this intervention. Even in exsanguinating hemorrhage requiring surgical intervention, endoscopic localization of the bleeding site can provide important information relevant to surgical management. Further increases in knowledge and advances in therapeutic endoscopy should provide a better understanding of which subgroups of patients are at increased risk for poor outcome, which patients will benefit most from therapeutic intervention, and which of the therapeutic options are both practical and efficacious. Endoscopic balloon dilatation of pyloric stenosis is still at an embryonic stage and its role needs to be elucidated by prospectively controlled trials.

References

Allan R, Dykes P (1974) A comparison of routine and selective endoscopy in the management of acute gastrointestinal hemorrhage. Gastrointest Endosc 20: 154–155

Allen HM, Block MA, Schuman BM (1973) Gastroduodenal endoscopy: management of acute upper gastrointestinal hemorrhage. Arch Surg 106:450–455

ASGE (1988a) The role of endoscopy in the management of upper gastrointestinal hemorrhage. Gastrointest Endosc 34:4S–5S

ASGE (1988b) The role of endoscopy in the management of the patient with peptic ulcer disease. Gastrointest Endosc 34:21S–22S

ASGE (1988c) Infection control during gastrointestinal endoscopy. Gastrointest Endosc 34:37S–40S

Beckly DE, Casebow MP (1986) Prediction of rebleeding from peptic ulcer experience with an endoscopic Doppler device. Gut 27(1):96–99

Benjamin SB, Cattau EL, Glass RL (1982) Balloon dilation of the pylorus: therapy for gastric outlet obstruction. Gastrointest Endosc 28:253–254

Benjamin SB, Glass RL, Cattau EL, Miller WB (1984) Preliminary experience with balloon dilation of the pylorus. Gastrointest Endosc 30:93–95

Birnie GG, Quigley EM, Clements GB, Follett GAC, Watkinson G (1983) Endoscopic transmission of hepatitis B virus. Gut 24:171–174

Bornman PC, Theodorou NA, Shuttleworth RD, Essel HP, Marks IN (1985) Importance of hypovolaemic shock and endoscopic signs in predicting recurrent haemorrhage from peptic ulceration: a prospective evaluation. Br Med J [Clin Res] 291(6490):245–247

Bown SG, Salman PR, Kelly DF, Calder BM, Pearson H, Weaver BMQ, Read AE (1979) Argon laser photocoagulation in the dog gut. Gut 20:680–687

Brearly S, Morris DL, Hawker PC, Dykes PW, Keighley MR (1985) Prediction of mortality at endoscopy in bleeding peptic ulcer disease. Endoscopy 17(5): 173–174

British Society of Gastroenterology (1988) Cleaning and disinfection of equipment for gastrointestinal flexible endoscopy: interim recommendations of a working party of the British Society of Gastroenterology. Gut 29:1134–1151

Brown P, Salmon PR, Burwood RJ, Know AJ, Clendinnen BG, Read AE (1978) The endoscopic radiologic and surgical findings in chronic duodenal ulceration. Scand J Gastroenterol 13:551–560

Buset M, Des Marez B, Vandermeeven A, Baize M, Cremer M (1988) Laser therapy for non bleeding visible vessels in peptic ulcer hemorrhage: a prospective randomized study. Gastrointest Endosc 34:173–174

Chang-Chien CS, Wu CS, Chen PC, Lin DY, Chu CM, Fang KM, Sheen IS, Liaw YF (1988) Different implications of stigmata of recent hemorrhage in gastric and duodenal ulcers. Dig Dis Sci 33(4):400–404

Chiozzini G, Bortoluzzi F, Pallini P, Betetto G, Costantini R, Costa F, Vitalba A, Saggioro A (1989) Controlled trial of absolute ethanol vs. epinephrine as injection agent in gastroduodenal bleeding. Gastroenterology 96(II) Suppl A-86

Chung SC, Leung JW, Steele RJ, Crofts TJ, Li AK (1988) Endoscopic injection of adrenaline for actively bleeding ulcers: a randomized trial. Br Med J [Clin Res] 296(6637):1631–1633

Colin-Jones DG (1986) Endoscopy or radiology for upper gastrointestinal symptoms? Lancet 1:1022–1023

Colin-Jones DG, Cockel R, Schiller KFR (1978) Current endoscopic practice in the United Kingdom. Clin Gastroenterol 4:775–786

Cook IJ, de Carle DJ, Haneman B, Hunt DR, Talley NA, Miller D (1988) Acta Cytol 32:461–464

Cotton PB (1977) Endoscopy versus radiology in acute upper gastrointestinal tract bleeding. Lancet 1:1367

Cotton PB, Shorvon PJ (1984) Analysis of endoscopy and radiography in the diagnosis, followup and treatment of peptic ulcer disease. Clin Gastroenterol 13:383–403

Cotton PB, Rosenberg MT, Waldram RPL, Axon ATR (1973) Early endoscopy of oesophagus, stomach and duodenal bulb in patients with hematemesis and melaena. Br Med J 2:505–509

Curtiss LE (1973) High frequency currents in endoscopy: a review of principles and precautions. Gastrointest Endosc 20:9–12

Dekker W, Tytgat GN (1977) Diagnostic accuracy of fiberendoscopy in the detection of upper intestinal malignancy: a follow-up analysis. Gastroenterology 73: 710–714

Dixon JA, Berenson MM, McCloskey DW (1979) Neodymium-YAG laser treatment of experimental canine gastric bleeding. Gastroenterology 77:647–651

Dooley CP, Larson AW, Stace NH, Renner IG, Valenzuela JE, Eliasoph J, Colletti PM, Halls JM, Weiner JM (1984) Double-contrast barium meal and upper gastrointestinal endoscopy. Ann Intern Med 101:538–545

Dronfield MW, Langman MJS, Atkinson M, Balfour TW, Bell GD, Vellacott KD, Amar SS, Knapp DR (1982) Outcome of endoscopy and barium radiography for acute upper gastrointestinal bleeding: controlled trial in 1037 patients. Br Med J 284:545–548

Eastwood GL (1977) Does early endoscopy benefit the patient with active upper gastrointestinal bleeding? Gastroenterology 72:737–739

Engel JJ, Goldman J (1986) Neodymium YAG laser and heater probe in the treatment of acute gastrointestinal bleeding (Abstr). Gastrointest Endosc 32:174

Farini R, Farinati F, Cardin F, DiMano F, Vianello F, Paguini C Arslan, Naccarato R (1983) Evidence of gastric carcinoma during follow-up of apparently benign gastric ulcer. Gut 24:A486

Fleischer D (1984) Endoscopic laser therapy for gastrointestinal disease. Arch Intern Med 144:1225–1230

Fleischer D (1989) Recommendations for antibiotic prophylaxis before endoscopy. Am J Gastroenterol 84:1489–1491

Foster DN, Miloszewski KTA, Losowsky MS (1978) Stigmata of recent hemorrhage in diagnosis and prognosis of upper gastrointestinal bleeding. Br Med J 1:1173–1177

Freitas D, Donato A, Monteiro JG (1985) Controlled trial of liquid monopolar electrocoagulation in bleeding peptic ulcers. Am J Gastroenterol 80:853–857

Fullarton GM, Birnie GG, MacDonald A, Murray WR (1988) Controlled study of heater probe (HP) in bleeding peptic ulcers. Gut 29:A701

Gelfand DW, Ott DJ, Munitz AH, Chen YM (1984) Radiology and endoscopy. a radiologic viewpoint. Ann Intern Med 101:550–552

Gilbert DA, Silverstein FE, Tedesco FJ, and 277 members of the ASGE (1981a) National ASGE survey on upper gastrointestinal bleeding, complications of endoscopy. Dig Dis Sci 26:555–595

Gilbert DA, Silverstein FE, Tedesco FJ, Buenger NK, Persing J (1981b) The National ASGE survey on upper gastrointestinal bleeding. Gastrointest Endosc 27:94–102

Goff JS (1986) Bipolar electrocoagulation versus Nd-YAG laser photocoagulation for upper gastrointestinal bleeding lesions. Dig Dis Sci 31:906–910

Goudie BM, Mitchell KG, Birnie GG, Mackay C (1984) Controlled trial of endoscopic bipolar electrocoagulation in the treatment of bleeding peptic ulcers (Abstr). Gut 25:1185

Graham DY (1980) Limited value of early endoscopy in the management of acute upper gastrointestinal bleeding: prospective controlled trial. Am J Surg 140: 284-290

Graham DY (1987) Endoscopic therapy of pyloric stenosis. ASGE course syllabus, 20–29

Graham DY, Schwartz JT, Cain GD, Gyorkey F (1982) Prospective evaluation of biopsy number in the diagnosis of esophageal and gastric carcinoma. Gastroenterology 82:228–231

Griffiths WJ, Neuman DA, Welsh JD (1979) The visible vessel as an indicator of uncontrolled or recurrent gastrointestinal hemorrhage. N Engl J Med 300: 1411–1413

Grossman M (1971) Resumé and comment. Gastroenterology 61:635–638

Harrison JD, Morris DL (1989) Does bipolar electrocoagulation time affect vessel weld strength? Gastroenterology 96:A199

Hatfield ARW, Slavin G, Segal AW, Levi AJ (1975) Importance of the site of endoscopic gastric biopsy in ulcerating lesions of the stomach. Gut 16:884–886

Health and Public Policy Committee, American College of Physicians (1985) Endoscopy in the evaluation of dyspepsia. Ann Intern Med 102:266–269

Health and Public Policy Committee, American College of Physicians (1987) Clinical competence in diagnostic esophagogastroduodenoscopy. Ann Intern Med 107: 937–939

Heier SK, Lebovics E, Rosenthal WS (1988) Endoscopic coagulation for gastrointestinal bleeding (Letter). N Engl J Med 318:185

Hirao M, Kobayashi T, Masuda K, Yamaguchi S, Noda K, Matsuura K, Naka H, Kawauchi H, Namiki M (1985) Endoscopic local injection of hypertonic saline-epinephrine solution to arrest hemorrhage from the upper gastrointestinal tract. Gastrointest Endosc 31(5):313–317

Ihre T, Johansson C, Seligson U, Torngren S (1981) Endoscopic YAG-laser treatment in massive upper gastrointestinal bleeding: report of a controlled randomized study. Scand J Gastroenterol 16(5):633–640

Jensen DM, Machicado GA, Tapia JI, Elashoff J (1984) Controlled trial of endoscopic argon laser for severe ulcer hemorrhage. Gastroenterology 86:1125

Jensen DM, Machicado GA, Kovacs TOG, van Deventer G, Randall GM, Reedy T, Silpa M, Sue M (1988) Controlled, randomized study of heater probe and BICAP for hemostasis of severe ulcer bleeding. Gastroenterology 94:A208

Johnston D, Lyndon PJ, Smith RB, Humphrey CS (1973) Highly selective vagotomy without a drainage procedure in the treatment of haemorrhage, perforation and pyloric stenosis due to peptic ulcer. Br J Surg 60:790–797

Johnston JH, Jensen DM, Mautner W (1979) Comparison of laser photocoagulation and electrocoagulation in endoscopic treatment of UGI bleeding. Gastroenterology 76:1162
Johnston JH, Jensen DM, Mautner W, Elashoff J (1980) YAG laser treatment of experimental bleeding canine gastric ulcers. Gastroenterology 79(6):1252–1261
Johnston JH, Rawson S, Namihira Y (1985) Experimental comparison of heater probe and BICAP for endoscopic control of gastrointestinal bleeding. Gastrointest Endosc 31:155–156
Johnston JH, Jensen DM, Auth DG (1987) Experimental comparison of endoscopic yttrium-aluminum-garnet laser, electrosurgery, and heater probe for canine gut arterial coagulation. Importance of compression and avoidance of erosion. Gastroenterology 92:1101–1108
Kasugai T (1968) Gastric lavage cytology and biopsy for early gastric cancer under direct vision by the fibergastroscope. Gastrointest Endosc 14:205–208
Kernohan RM, Anderson JR, McKelvey ST, Kennedy TL (1984) A controlled trial of bipolar electrocoagulation in patients with upper gastrointestinal bleeding. Br J Surg 71:889–891
Kiil J, Anderson D (1980) x-ray examination and/or endoscopy in the diagnosis of gastroduodenal ulcer and cancer. Scand J Gastroenterol 15:39–43
Kiil J, Anderson D, Myhre Jensen O (1979) Biopsy and brush cytology in the diagnosis of gastric cancer. Scand J Gastroenterol 14:189–191
Kozarek RA (1986) Hydrostatic balloon dilation of gastrointestinal stenoses: a national survey. Gastrointest Endosc 32:15–19
Krejs GJ, Little KH, Westergaard H, Hamilton JK, Spady DK, Polter DE (1987) Laser photocoagulation for the treatment of acute peptic-ulcer bleeding. A randomized controlled clinical trial. N Engl J Med 316:1618–1621
Laine L (1987) Multiple electrocoagulation in the treatment of active upper gastrointestinal tract hemorrhage: a prospective controlled trial. N Engl J Med 316: 1613–1617
Laine L (1989) Multiple electrocoagulation in the treatment of peptic ulcers with nonbleeding visible vessels. Ann Intern Med 110:510–514
Leung JW, Chung SC (1987) Endoscopic injection of adrenalin in bleeding peptic ulcers. Gastrointest Endosc 33:73–75
Lin HJ, Yang TT, Shou DL, Kwok HL, Lee FY, Ching YL, Chen HL (1988) A prospectively randomized trial of heat probe thermocoagulation versus pure alcohol injection in nonvariceal peptic ulcer hemorrhage. Am J Gastroenterol 83:283–286
Lindor KD, Oh BJ, Hughes RW (1985) Balloon dilation of upper digestive tract strictures. Gastroenterology 89:545–548
MacLeod IA, Mills PR, MacKenzie JF, Joffe SN, Russell RI, Carter DC (1983) Neodymium yttrium aluminum garnet laser photocoagulation for major haemorrhage from peptic ulcers and single vessels; a single blind controlled study. Br Med J [Clin Res] 286:345–348
Matthewson K, Swash CP, Bland M, Kirkham JS, Boun SG, Northfield TC (1987) Randomized comparison of Nd:YAG laser heater probe and no endoscopic therapy for bleeding peptic ulcer. Gastroenterology 92:1522
Moore JP, Silvis SE, Vennes JA (1978) Evaluation of bipolar electrocoagulation in canine stomachs. Gastrointest Endosc 24:148–151
Moreto M, Zaballa M, Ibanez S, Setien F, Figa M (1987) Efficacy of monopolar electrocoagulation in the treatment of bleeding gastric ulcer: a controlled trial. Endoscopy 19:54–56
Morris DL, Brearley S, Thompson H, Keighley MRB (1985) A comparison of the efficacy of gastric wall injury with 3.2 and 2.3 mm bipolar probes in canine arterial hemorrhage. Gastrointest Endosc 31:361–363
Morris DW, Levine GM, Soloway RD, Miller TM, Marin GA (1975) Prospective, randomized study of diagnosis and outcome in acute upper gastrointestinal

bleeding: endoscopy versus conventional radiography. Dig Dis Sci 20:1103–1109

Nudel J, Guavena J, Mitman PJ, Grant D, Ceccetti C, Falkenstein DB, Zimmon BS (1977) Endoscopic diagnosis of active bleeding: a prognostic sign in upper gastrointestinal hemorrhage. Gastrointest Endosc 23:237

O'Brien JD, Day SJ, Burnham WR (1986) Controlled trial of small bipolar probe in bleeding peptic ulcers. Lancet 1(8479):464–467

Palmer ED (1969) The vigorous diagnostic approach to upper-gastrointestinal hemorrhage. JAMA 207:1477–1480

Panes J, Viver J, Forne M, Garcia-Olivares E, Marco C, Garau J (1987) Controlled trial of endoscopic sclerosis in bleeding peptic ulcers. Lancet 2:1292–1294

Papp JP (1982) Endoscopic electrocoagulation in the management of upper gastrointestinal tract bleeding. Surg Clin North Am 62:797–806

Peterson WL, Barnett CC, Smith HT, Allen MH, Corbett DB (1981) Routine early endoscopy in upper gastrointestinal tract bleeding. N Engl J Med 304:925–929

Podolsky I, Storms PR, Richardson CT, Peterson WL, Fordtran JS (1988) Gastric adenocarcinoma masquerading endoscopically as a benign gastric ulcer. Dig Dis Sci 33:1057–1063

Protell RL, Rubin CE, Auth DG, Silverstein FE, Terou F, Dennis M, Piercey JRA (1978) The heater probe: a new endoscopic method for stopping massive gastrointestinal bleeding. Gastroenterology 74:257–262

Protell RL, Gilbert DA, Silverstein FE, Jensen DM, Hulett FM, Auth DC (1981) Computer assisted electrocoagulation: bipolar vs. monopolar in the treatment of experimental canine gastric ulcer bleeding. Gastroenterology 80:451–455

Qizilbash AH, Castelli M, Kowalski MA, Churly A (1980) Endoscopic brush cytology and biopsy in the diagnosis of cancer in the upper gastrointestinal tract. Acta Cytol 24:313–318

Randall GM, Jensen DM, Hirabayashi K, Machicado GA (1987) Controlled trial of sclerosing agents for hemostasis of canine gut arteries. Gastrointest Endosc 33:182

Richardson CT (1983) Gastric ulcer. In: Sleisenger MH, Fordtran JS (eds) Gastrointestinal disease. Saunders, Philadelphia, p 676

Rutgeerts P, Vantrappen G, Broeckaert L, Janssens J, Coremans G, Geboes K, Schurmans P (1982) Controlled trial of YAG laser treatment of upper digestive hemorrhage. Gastroenterology 83:410–416

Rutgeerts P, Vantrappen G, van Hootegem P, Broeckaert L, Janssens J, Coremans G, Geboes K (1987a) Neodymium-YAG laser photocoagulation versus multipolar electrocoagulation for the treatment of severely bleeding ulcers; a randomized comparison. Gastrointest Endosc 33(3):199–202

Rutgeerts P, Broeckaert L, Coremans G, Janssens J, van Isveldt J, Vantrappen G (1987b) Randomized comparison of three hemostasis modalities for severely bleeding peptic ulcers. Gastrointest Endosc 33:182

Sakita T, Oguro Y, Takasu S, Fukutomi H, Miwa T, Yoshimori M (1971) Observations on the healing of ulcerations in early gastric cancer. Gastroenterology 60:835–844

Sancho-Poch FJ, Balanzo J, Ocana J, Presa E, Sala-Caldera E, Cusso X, Valardell F (1978) An evaluation of gastric biopsy in the diagnosis of gastric cancer. Gastrointest Endosc 24:281–282

Shahmir M, Schuman BM (1980) Complications of fiberoptic endoscopy. Gastrointest Endosc 26:86–91

Shapiro M (1987) Gastric outlet obstruction: endoscopic vs surgical management. ASGE course notes:120–128

Sigel B, Dunn MR (1965) The mechanism of blood vessel closure by high frequency electrocoagulation. Surg Gynecol Obstet 121:823–831

Sigel B, Hatke FL (1967) Physical factors in electrocoagulation of blood vessels. Arch Surg 95:54–58

Silverstein FE, Protell RL, Gilbert DA, Gulacsik C, Auth DC, Dennis MB, Rubin CE (1979) Argon vs. neodymium YAG laser photocoagulation of experimental canine gastric ulcers. Gastroenterology 77:491–496

Silvis SE, Nebel O, Rogers G, Sugawa C, Mandelstam P (1976) Endoscopic complications: results of the 1974 American Society for Gastrointestinal Endoscopy Survey. JAMA 235:928–930

Soehendra N, Grimm H, Stenzel M (1985) Injection of nonvariceal bleeding lesions of the upper gastrointestinal tract. Endoscopy 17:129–132

Solt J, Rauth J, Papp Z, Bohensky G (1984) Balloon catheter dilation of gastric outlet stenosis. Gastrointest Endosc 30:359–361

Storey DW, Bown SE, Swain CP, Salmon PR, Kirkham JS, Northfield TC (1981) Endoscopic prediction of recurrent bleeding in peptic ulcers. N Engl J Med 305:915–916

Sugawa C, Ikeda T, Fujita Y, Walt AJ (1984) Endoscopic hemostasis of gastrointestinal hemorrhage by local injection of 98% ethanol: an experimental study. Gastrointest Endosc 30:155

Sugawa C, Fujita V, Ikeda T, Walt AJ (1986) Endoscopic hemostasis of bleeding in the upper gastrointestinal tract by local injection of ninety-eight percent ethanol. Surg Gynecol Obstet 162:159–163

Swain CP, Bown SG, Storey DW, Kirkam JS, Northfield TC, Salmon PR (1981) Controlled trial of argon laser photocoagulation in bleeding peptic ulcers. Lancet 2:1313–1316

Swain CP, Mills TN, Shemesh E, Dark JM, Lewin MR, Clifton JS, Northfield TC, Cotton PB, Salmon PR (1984) Which electrode? A comparison of four endoscopic methods of electrocoagulation in experimental bleeding ulcers. Gut 25: 1424–1431

Swain CP, Kirkham JS, Salmon PR, Bown SG, Northfield TC (1986) Controlled trial of Nd-YAG laser photocoagulation in bleeding peptic ulcers. Lancet 1:1113–1117

Thompson G, Somers S, Stevenson GW (1983) Benign gastric ulcer: a reliable radiologic diagnosis? AJR 141:331–333

Vallon AG, Cotton PB, Laurence BH, Armengol Miro JR, Salord Oses JC (1981) Randomized trial of endoscopic argon laser photocoagulation in bleeding peptic ulcers. Gut 22:228–233

Vennes JA (1981) Infectious complications of gastrointestinal endoscopy, Dig Dis Sci 26:605–645

Wara P (1985) Endoscopic prediction of major rebleeding: a prospective study of stigmata of hemorrhage in bleeding ulcer. Gastroenterology 88:1209–1214

Waring JP, Sanowski RA, Woods CA, Sawyer RL, Foutch PG (1989) BICAP vs injection sclerotherapy for bleeding ulcers: a randomized, controlled study. Am J Gastroenterol 84:1172

Weiland D, Dunn DH, Humphrey EW, Schwartz ML (1982) Gastric outlet obstruction in peptic ulcer disease: an indication for surgery. Am J Surg 143:90–93

Weinstein WM (1977) Gastroscopy for gastric ulcer. Gastroenterology 73:1160–1162

Welch CE, Burke JF (1969) Gastric ulcer reappraisal. Surgery 65:708–715

Wiljasalo M, Tallroth K, Korhola O, Ihamaki T (1980) A comparison of double contrast barium meal and endoscopy. Diagn Imaging 49:1–5

Witzel L, Halter F, Gretillat PA, Scheurer U, Keller M (1976) Evaluation of specific value of endoscopic biopsies and brush cytology for malignancies of the esophagus and stomach. Gut 17:375–377

Woods A, Sanowski RA, Waring JP, Foutch PG (1988) Endoscopic therapy for gastric and duodenal ulcer bleeding, a comparison of BICAP coagulation versus ethanol sclerotherapy. Gastrointest Endosc 34:209

CHAPTER 16

Videoendoscopy and Digital Imaging

A.M. ROSEN and D.E. FLEISCHER

> I had opportunities for the examination of the interior of the stomach, and its secretions, which has never before been so fully offered to any one. This most important organ, its secretions and its operations, have been submitted to my observation in a very extraordinary manner . . .
>
> WILLIAM BEAUMONT, *Experiments and Observations on the Gastric Juice and the Physiology of Digestion* (1833)

A. Introduction

Ever since he had the extraordinary opportunity to view – through a trauma-induced gastrocutaneous fistula – the gastric lining of his patient Alexis St. Martin, Dr. William Beaumont has been admired by all who seek better ways to view the interior of the gastrointestinal tract. It was not until 1958 that the modern age of gastrointestinal endoscopy began with the introduction by Hirschowitz (HIRSCHOWITZ et al. 1958) of a prototype fiberoptic gastroscope. Previously, Schindler had developed first the rigid, and then the semiflexible gastroscope, the latter using a series of lenses and prisms. With the development of coherent, insulated optical glass fibers, however, the path was cleared for construction of a fully flexible endoscope.

During the 1960s and 1970s, technical developments fostered the remarkable growth and acceptance of gastrointestinal endoscopy. As optical glass fibers became smaller and fiber bundles more flexible, endoscopic images improved. In fact, modern fibers, at a diameter of 8–10 μm each, approach the smallest width that can adequately transmit light (WILLIAMS 1989). What was lacking, however, was a convenient system for providing high quality hard copies of endoscopic images. In 1983, the introduction of electronic (or video) endoscopy solved this problem and constituted the most significant advance in gastrointestinal endoscopy since the first use of the optical fiber bundle.

The revolutionary advance at the heart of electronic endoscopy was the charge-coupled device (or CCD). Developed in 1969 at Bell Laboratories by Willard S. Boyle and George E. Smith and patented in 1974, its initial use was in astronomy, and its first medical endoscopic application was reported in 1984.

The rudiments of digital imaging and analysis can be found in agricultural studies conducted in the 1960s. Digital image processing, applied to multispectral data collected from aircraft flying over an agricultural field in Indiana in 1966, was able to distinguish wheat from oats. In the 1970s, several studies of vegetation were developed which employed digital pattern recognition and manual interpretation of infrared and aerial photographs. This early work led to an appreciation of the different kinds of information that could be provided by different wavelengths of light (Committee on Planetary Biology 1986). Further sophistication and miniaturization of digital imagery techniques and hardware ultimately led to vastly improved endoscopic image production and storage.

In this review, we will discuss how CCDs and videoendoscopes work, the practical advantages they offer in documentation and teaching, the unique applications of digital technology to gastrointestinal endoscopy, and speculations regarding what effects this technology may have on the future of diagnosis and treatment of gastrointestinal disease.

B. Charge-Coupled Devices and Videoendoscopy – How They Work

I. Background

The term "pixel" has been used commonly – but ambiguously – in the literature of videoendoscopy and digital imaging. It has been used to refer both to a picture element (the smallest discernible portion of a picture) and to an individual sensing element of an imaging device. KNYRIM et al. (1989a) have articulated an important distinction between the terms "sensing elements," referring to a sensor device, and "picture elements," referring to an image. In the present discussion, "pixel" is employed only when context clearly indicates whether the reference is to a sensor device or an image.

The number of sensing elements in a fiberscope is limited to the number of fiberoptic bundles in the instrument, usually 30000–40000. The key to appreciating the advantages and potential of videoendoscopy is to understand the design and function of the CCD, which permits more reliable and reproducible image transfer than fiberbundles and which can accommodate over 100000 sensing elements.

II. CCD Function

A CCD, also known as a "chip," is a small silicon wafer incorporating diodes, capacitors, and resistors (DEMLING and HAGEL 1985) which converts incident light into electrical signals. The physicochemical basis for this function is the inherent property of some forms of silicon to generate an electric current when struck by light. When light strikes the silicon device, the silicon's electrical resistance decreases, thereby generating carriers of current, i.e., electrons or positively charged electron holes (temporary absences of electrons within the silicon substrate). One photon (a unit of light) yields one electron and one electron hole. As the intensity of incident light increases, more charge and more current are generated (SIVAK 1988a). The emitted energies that are sensed by the CCD are ultimately transformed by computer into an image (BENJAMIN 1989).

A CCD comprises a grid-like array of discrete photosensitive elements known as potential wells, each approximately 10 μm in width. The chip itself is approximately 4 × 4 mm in size. In aggregrate, the wells constitute an electrical representation of the image focused on the silicon chip by a lens, as each well functions independently to generate electrons in proportion to the number of incident photons (SIVAK 1988a). The charges generated by the potential wells must be transferred in an organized, interpretable fashion. This is achieved by arranging the wells in rows called channels. Electrons are confined to the channels by barriers known as channel stops. Electrodes, also known as gates, are oriented perpendicular to the channels. The channel stops and gates, then, divide the chip into pixels. Voltage changes applied to the gates serve to sequentially march the packets of electrical charge, accumulated within each pixel, to the edge of the silicon wafer. The charge-coupled device derives its name from this process of charge coupling wherein the directed movement of electrical charges is effected by the rapidly sequenced on/off switching of applied current.

At the chip's edge, an isolating region, known as a transfer gate, receives each row of charges. Then, charges move into an output shift register, which operates the same way as the imaging section of the wafer, moving pixels, except that the rows of charges are arranged end-to-end and moved to an amplifier where each pixel's charge is measured (SIVAK 1986, 1988a).

III. Image Transfer

At this point, to continue the trafficking of electrical information, the videoendoscopy system must overcome a fundamental problem of the CCD: its inability to simultaneously store and move electrical charges. Three methods have been developed to overcome this problem.

Frame transfer employs two adjacent CCDs, one for imaging and charge collection, the other for image storage and transfer. The frame transfer device, although easier to construct, is relatively bulky and therefore not ideal for endoscopic use.

The *interline transfer method* has lines on the chip alternating between rows of imaging pixels (wells) and shift registers. Once collected, charges are transferred (gated) to the shift register. While the imaging pixels collect more charges, the shift register "reads" those previously collected. Interline transfer chips are smaller than the frame transfer type, but are complex and difficult to build. Their sensitivity is reduced because those portions of the CCD devoted to the transport process must be shielded from light (CLASSEN et al. 1987).

The *cycling or sequential method* (which also has important applications to color generation, as will be described below) employs a smaller chip whose entire surface area is used for photon collection and is quite suitable for endoscopic use. Use of this one CCD for both photogeneration and transfer of charges requires that the photogeneration process be temporarily and repeatedly suspended by interrupting illumination of the imaged object while the charges are read (SIVAK 1988a).

IV. Microprocessor Function

The required components of a videoendoscopy system include a videoendoscope, a videomicroprocessor, and a television (TV) monitor. The videoendoscope contains, except for the imaging fiberoptic bundle, all components of a conventional endoscope, including a fiberoptic bundle to provide light. Most systems also incorporate a keyboard used to annotate the monitored and recorded image with patient identification, date, procedure name, and anatomical location. Additional hardware and software can be used to edit and further label stored images. The CCD itself is an analog device, i.e., it collects and stores variable quantities (photons, charges). The microprocessor converts the analog signals to computer-usable signals, discrete numerical values in binary (digital) code. These digitized data can be presented and manipulated in many ways. They are required for the sequential method of image production and for displaying single images (freeze-frame) and permit retention of images in computer memory, the exact reproduction of images, and telephone transmission. The microprocessor ultimately converts the digitized signal back to analog for synthesis of the image seen on the TV monitor. The process whereby the microprocessor "transcribes" the initial analog signal to a digital code and then retranscribes it back to analog is somewhat analogous to the transcription sequence of DNA's conversion to RNA (by RNA polymerase) and RNA's reconversion (by reverse transcriptase "processor") back to DNA. Facsimile machines work similarly, converting an analog image to a digital signal for telephone transmission, then reconverting the signal to analog for image reproduction.

Another function of the processor is to adjust the intensity of illumination at the endoscope tip to compensate for variation in reflected light (SIVAK 1988b). CCDs are very sensitive to light. Potential wells have a finite capacity for photons which, when exceeded, causes photons to spill over into adjacent pixels, causing a distortion called "blooming." This constant, nearly instantaneous readjustment of illumination, therefore, is required to maintain an interpretable image.

V. Color

1. Background

An appreciation of some concepts of color and its interpretation aids the understanding of videoendoscopic methods of color reproduction. The color of an object is based on the way it reflects light. Pure white light comprises all colors (wavelengths) in the electromagnetic spectrum. The perceived color of an object depends on the illuminating light (Sivak 1988a). The human eye has three different types of receptors (or, more precisely, retinal cones) for the red, green, and blue (RGB) regions of the visible light spectrum (visible light: 400–700 nm wavelength) (Knyrim et al. 1989a).

With fiberscopes, the eye is the principal color sensor; the fiberbundles carry the image to the eye. Electronic endoscopes do not "see" color; rather, they synthesize it. The principal sensor is the CCD and the eye sees only the image as synthesized by the processor (Knyrim et al. 1989a).

Color can be expressed in terms of its saturation, hue, and brightness. "Saturation" refers to the amount of white in the color that "dilutes" its effect. "Hue" differentiates shades of color and "brightness" represents luminosity (Knyrim et al. 1989a).

2. Videoendoscopic Color Reproduction

All CCDs are fundamentally arrays of black-and-white photo cells, and are, therefore, "color blind" (Williams 1989). The potential wells of a CCD measure light intensity (photons), not color per se.

There are two basic systems used to transmit color in videoendoscopy: the *mosaic filter* (or color chip) and the *sequential* (monochrome, rotating color wheel). A color chip is so called because it is covered with a mosaic transparent to the three primary colors (RGB) or the complementary counterparts (cyan, magenta, and yellow). Every third pixel, therefore, receives a different color illumination. A specific color is associated with each pixel and all colors are transmitted simultaneously (Classen et al. 1987) as a composite signal.

A color television picture is composed of parallel lines on a cathode ray tube. The picture is produced by three signals produced by three electron guns within the picture tube, one each for red, green, and blue. Each color beam activates a separate set of phosphor dots (Sivak 1988b). A television monitor has approximately half a million pixels on its entire screen. The image from an endoscope, electronic or fiberoptic, occupies only part of the screen.

As described above, then, one approach to videoendoscopic color transmission is to use a CCD with three sets of color pixels. However, the assignment of pixels to specific colors is done, at least theoretically, at the expense of resolving power, because only a fraction of the total number of sensing elements is sensitive to each color (Knyrim et al. 1989a).

The sequential (color wheel) method is used more commonly and employs all pixels for all colors using a strobed light, sequentially illuminating the object of interest with the three primary colors through the light bundles. A rapidly rotating color wheel, with filters for the three primary colors, releases short "bursts" of red, green, and blue light on the target (CLASSEN et al. 1987). The RGB beams of light hit the mucosa and are reflected from it, depending on the target's color content (KNYRIM et al. 1989a). The CCD measures the intensity of reflected light three times, once for each of the three colors. The light intensity pattern is recorded in separate digital memories, one for each color. The processor contains a timing circuit which switches signals from the chip's sensor during a red illumination period to the red image memory, working similarly for green and blue (CLASSEN et al. 1987). With each memory simultaneously supplying its separate signal to the appropriate electron gun, the processor composes an apparently real-time television image (SIVAK 1988b). The chip is read approximately 90 times a second; i.e., the three-color sequence occurs 30 times a second. At this speed of repetition, the separate colors are indistinguishable, and the television display appears as a single image, although the endoscope tip shows a strobe effect if viewed directly.

The rotating color wheel also interrupts object illumination and thereby allows photo-generated electrical charges to be shifted from the CCD to an output register, completing the sequence of photo-generation transfer as described previously in the discussion of image transfer mechanisms. Again, the sequential method allows for the use of a smaller and less complicated CCD. Technical analysis has shown that color reproduction generated by the rotating wheel approach is quite accurate, and that color chips, although they obviate strobed light, are not required for good color reproduction. Refinements of sequential-type videoendoscopy systems have decreased undesirable blurring and color fringes seen when the endoscope tip is moved fast, problems not seen at all with the color chip systems. However, for a given chip size, the color saturation is poorer with the color chips because each pixel "sees" only one color. To summarize, in the "color chip" system, potential wells are constantly illuminated by white light through an interposed color mosaic; in the sequential, all wells are intermittently illuminated by strobed red, green, and blue light. Regardless of chip type, though, all new videoendoscopes produce images whose quality equals or surpasses that of fiberscopes.

VI. Technical Evaluation

Performance of videoendoscopy can be evaluated by measuring technical characteristics such as focal range and resolution. Focal range is defined as the distance between the endoscope lens and the target at which the target remains in focus. The focal range of the endoscope is a function of both the lens that focuses the image on a CCD (or fiberbundle) and characteristics of the CCD itself. Most videoendoscopes presently used have a minimum focal distance of 4–5 mm, whereas fiberoptic endoscopes can focus at 3 mm.

Resolution is measured as the shortest distance (*d*) between two picture elements, a picture element being defined as the smallest discernible portion of a picture (i.e., a pixel). At distances greater than *d*, two adjacent points appear separate; at distances less than *d*, they appear fused (KNYRIM et al. 1989a). The greater the resolving power of a lens or CCD or system, the greater its ability to recognize separate picture elements as separate. KNYRIM et al. (1987b), who published the first technical evaluation of videoendoscopes, prefer to define resolution, as it relates to optoelectronic technology, as "the maximum number of pairs of black and white lines per mm which can be resolved."

Resolution is determined in part by the number of sensing pixels. Smaller size of potential wells permits greater number of sensors per unit area and, theoretically, more accurate reproduction. However, minimum pixel size is restricted by lens resolution and manufacturing capabilities. In addition to the number of sensors on a CCD, resolution also depends on the angle of view (determined by the objective lens) and the distance of the lens from the target. As the angle of view decreases, peak resolution improves, but the amount of the target remaining visible decreases. All endoscopic systems, fiberoptic and video, constitute a compromise between angle of view and peak resolution (KNYRIM et al. 1989a).

Sensing chips can have over 600 000 pixels. Most current videoendoscopes have 30 000–200 000. For optical reasons, not all of a CCD's sensor area can be illuminated by the lens at the scope tip. Therefore, in the critical evaluation and comparison of different endoscopes, what counts most is not the number of pixels on the chip, but rather the number of picture elements in the final image. These two values may differ significantly. Lenses are round; CCDs are square or rectangular. This difference of shape dictates which focal ranges and viewing angles are usable. Newer videoendoscopes with better lens–chip matching permit an increased number of sensing elements to be illuminated and therefore produce an image of a larger area with greater resolving power.

Adaptors have been developed to provide users of fiberoptic endoscopes with many of the advantages of direct videoendoscopy. In this "indirect videoendoscopy" system, a chip camera is attached to the eyepiece of the fiberscope, so the video image is picked up "second hand." There is, therefore, an inevitable loss of resolution and luminosity. Initially, the light (and image) crosses the fiberoptic interface at the scope tip, travels (losing intensity) "down the fiberoptic bundle, passes through the ocular lens (with an antireflective coating that causes a further decrease), and then strikes the receiving microchip camera surface" (SATAVA 1987). Once received, however, this attenuated image is processed exactly like that acquired in direct videoendoscopy.

VII. Clinical Use

In 1984, the first two reports of clinical use of videoendoscopes were published. SIVAK and FLEISCHER (1984a) described their experience with videocolonoscopy in 79 patients, and CLASSEN and PHILLIP (1984) reported results of 43 esophago-gastroduodenoscopies and eight colonoscopies. Both groups were favorably impressed by the ease of use and quality of image produced by the new "chip scopes." Since that time videoendoscopy has gained wide acceptance, both for its immediately obvious practical benefits, as documented in SCHAPIRO et al. (1987) series of 1200 cases, and for its possible research uses. These advantages and potential applications are discussed in the sections that follow.

C. Practical Benefits and Advantages of Videoendoscopy

I. Image Storage, Retrieval, and Transfer

The ability to make an enduring, high quality record of endoscopic images has been a major advance made possible by videoendoscopy and digital imaging. The major types of devices used for recording are videotape recorders, optical discs, and floppy discs. Most endoscopists record on videotape and usually use ¾″ tape for greater clarity (than ½″ tape).

Optical discs use laser technology to store electronic images and are also known as laser discs. Because the technology employed differs from that of the CCD, the quality of the recorded images, although excellent, does not equal that obtained when reproductions are reconstructed from digital code. Each image, when placed on the disc, is assigned a unique identification number and is unerasable. It can be stored and retrieved (by number) quite rapidly. Erasable optical discs are being developed.

The chief advantage of using an optical disc is its extraordinary capacity, as each disc, costing approximately $300, can store up to 40 000 frames. The recording machine itself costs approximately $25 000–$30 000. A small disadvantage is that the controls used to record images are separate from the endoscope.

Floppy discs store images as digital code, directly accepting RGB video input, and therefore can reproduce endoscopic pictures with unexcelled fidelity. However, so much code is required for each frame that each standard 5¼″disc can store only relatively few images. Even smaller discs are used with current recording systems and can store a maximum of only 25 frames. Hard discs also can be used for storage, but, again, capacity is limited. Controls for storing images are located on the control heads of many videoendoscopes and indirect video adaptors.

Endoscopic photography, prior to video, was poor. Instant photos were of low quality, and, without the freeze-frame function present in all video-systems, even good 35-mm slides and prints (which then required processing) were difficult to obtain, store, and retrieve. Television cameras attached to the endoscope headpiece ocular were very bulky, and the movies obtained were not nearly as good as those now obtained even with indirect video-endoscopy (SIVAK 1986). This greater ability to record endoscopic pictures is particularly welcome, as it has arisen in an era when documentation has become increasingly important in patient care, scientific research, and medically related litigation.

Currently available cameras and thermal printers turn out excellent reproductions. However, storage on optical and floppy disc provides benefits far beyond simply reproducing a good picture. Both systems are compatible with computer software database systems for reporting endoscopic procedures. To review a prior endoscopic examination, one can retrieve, with the appropriate software and a patient identification number, both the written report and all images stored in conjunction with the report (SIVAK 1986). Retrieval of an old image helps to objectify changes in a lesion over time, e.g., as a response to therapy.

It is possible to search a disc to collect all images for any diagnosis in a database. Digitized images can be transmitted over telephone lines or by satellite, and, because they are coded, the electronic images are not subject to the attenuation of transmitted light.

II. Teaching/Other

Implications for teaching and teamwork are obvious. With a real-time endoscopic image visible on television monitor, there is no limit to the number of people who can observe a procedure. No longer is an inconvenient fiberoptic extension "teaching head" or "lecture scope" necessary. Endoscopy assistants, rather than relying solely on instructions spoken by the endoscopist, can now participate with greater efficiency and coordination as they respond to visual cues to help obtain specimens or perform therapeutic procedures. To share an interesting case, whether for teaching or consultation, one can simply replay the videotape so that all who witness it can see the procedure as if they had performed it themselves.

Several practical benefits derive from videoendoscopy. As the instrument no longer must be held up to one eye, back/neck and eye strain are substantially diminished. They image, although not stereoscopic, is binocular, and there is some magnification provided by the television monitor. One can stand or sit, comfortably holding the endoscope's control head at waist level, making the procedure less tiring. There is greater freedom to turn or torque the instrument. With greater distance between the endoscopist and the patient, there is less risk to the operator of facial contamination with infectious or offensive fluids.

Because they can be recorded in their entirety, some procedures can be performed by nonphysicians and subsequently reviewed by physicians. The wisdom of having paraprofessionals perform endoscopy is not universally accepted, but Schroy et al. (1988) have reported a successful program where videoendoscopy was done for colorectal cancer screening by nurse practitioners with the recordings subsequently reviewed by physician endoscopists.

D. Special Applications

I. Measurement of Lesion Size

One of the most straightforward applications of digital imaging is in measurement of lesion size. Korman et al. (1988) reported a study of dogs with laser-induced gastric ulcers in which each lesion was measured using two to five images. A rectangular or circular reference probe of known area was placed in the plane of the lesion for each recorded image. The area of the probes, as determined by image analysis, was found to be quite accurate, and, as would be expected, the coefficient of variation was greatest for the smaller lesions. The authors found that quantitative analysis of ulcer area in a system which captured, digitized, stored, and retrieved images was reproducible and capable of detecting differences of 10%–20% in ulcer size. Using a similar method in humans, Nardi et al. (1988) also obtained favorable results in evaluating the reproducibility of measurements of area independent of shape. The relative ease of this approach can be appreciated especially when compared to cumbersome methods such as comparing endoscopic photographs of ulcers and mesh patterns of squares of known size (Okabe et al. 1986), or analyzing the parallax in dot patterns on a photograph of an ulcer illuminated by an argon laser projected through an optical grid (Yamaguchi et al. 1988).

II. Real-Time Image Analysis

Kurosaka et al. (1985) developed a real-time image analyzer using indirect videoendoscopy. Upper endoscopy was performed in humans with a system designed to highlight subtle changes of texture or color possibly indicating underlying pathology. The videomonitor was divided into a matrix and a computerized system was adjusted to recognize differences in luminance between neighboring blocks of the matrix. When a difference exceeded a selected value, an alarm bar signal appeared on the monitor at the site of the difference (or lesion). False alarms (due to technical reasons obvious to the investigators) occurred in 4% of 206 cases. The system was designed to eliminate human error due to inattention or fatigue and, indeed, was apparently sensitive to most lesions visible to the eye (the authors did not specify the rates of sensitivity or concordance) but did not identify more subtle lesions. Nevertheless, it does represent an example of an "intelligent endoscope," i.e., one that is capable of analysis.

III. Image Modification

Rey et al. (1988) developed a videoelectronic cmoputer classification of lesions of esophagitis by quantifying colorimetric modifications of esophageal mucosa. They manipulated a digitized image of distal esophagus, varying the intensity of individual RGB channels and analyzing each pixel with a scale of 256 gray steps. Variations of color intensity of esophageal mucosa were determined on a colorimetric scale. Microulcerations (appearing white endoscopically) were processed in an arbitrarily chosen color – blue – allowing the computer to read automatically the aggregate of microulcerations in the image. Classification was according to the surface area, in pixels, of each zone of different coloration. The computer picked out the totality of the points on the screen whose intensity equalled or exceeded a reference level. This system provided a reproducible, consistent, and unbiased determination of area of abnormality, rendering classification more objective, and serves as a good illustration of possible applications of image processing to videoendoscopy.

Sivak et al. (1987) tested a video image enhancement system (VIES) to determine whether computer images augmented visual diagnosis. The VIES functions were as follows: magnification, edge enhancement, signal selection (R, G, or B), image subselection (window), topographic images, contrast enhancement and reversal (i.e., negative image), and graphic display of reflected light intensity. Although it appeared subjectively that some of the VIES manipulations increased image detail and revealed additional features, objective analysis using an imaging chamber failed to demonstrate such advantages.

IV. Chromoscopy and Infrared Imaging

Taking advantage of CCDs' sensitivity to infrared light, Kohso et al. (1988) studied gąstric mucosal vasculature using intravenous indocyanine green (ICG) to enhance vessel contrast. The mucosa was viewed with a videoendoscope equipped with a modified infrared filter, with illumination supplied by an infrared ray from a laser diode. ICG injection was performed while the mucosa was in endoscopic view and revealed a fine vascular pattern. This study provides an example of combining chromoscopy (i.e., dye-enhanced endoscopy) and illumination by nonvisible wavelengths. It is not known how this compares to other methods used to enhance vascular structures (e.g., tinted glass filters (McWhorter et al. 1986).

V. Mucosal Hemodynamics

Many of the functions of videoendoscopy constitute improvements or refinements of techniques that are already achievable by fiberoptic imaging. A remarkable technique that is unique to videoendoscopy was developed by TSUJI et al. (1988), who, noting the difficulties of measuring gastric mucosal blood flow by the complicated techniques of reflectance spectrophotometry (LEUNG et al. 1987), H_2 gas clearance under endoscopy, and laser Doppler velocimetry, devised a method for real-time analysis of gastric mucosal hemodynamics using electronic endoscopic images and an image processing system. To investigate a rat model of hemorrhagic shock, the videoendoscope and processor were directly coupled to a microcomputer which algorithmically processed the ratio of red to green electric signals, yielding a calculated index. The index correlated strongly with the index of gastric mucosal hemoglobin concentration determined by reflectance spectrophotometry (a slow technique) and also the mucosal blood flow measured by hydrogen gas clearance (which required that an electrode be placed into or onto the mucosa). Contact techniques are problematic, as constant pressure is not only difficult to apply but also alters mucosal microcirculation. The chief advantages of the non-touch videoendoscope method, therefore, were its rapidity of measurement and its nonperturbation of what it was measuring. And, only by combining electronic endoscopy with digital imaging and processing, could such testing be accomplished.

A variation on TSUJI et al. theme was demonstrated by KASHIMURA et al. (1989), who, using a similar rat model, compared the speed of gastric mucosal blood flow as measured by laser velocimetry to that obtained by analyzing the RGB components of a videoendoscopic image. They found that the ratio of red to blue (R:B) values correlated strongly with blood flow speed, and that the endoscopic image could be manipulated with the R/B values to create a hemodynamic image displaying mucosal blood perfusion.

TSUJI et al. (1989) reported a modification of their previous technique to estimate hemoglobin oxygen saturation and hemoglobin concentration. They matched a videoendoscope to an infrared lighting system with rotating filters so that the mucosa was illuminated by lights of different infrared wavelengths. An image analyzer calculated, according to an algorithm, an index of hemoglobin saturation for each captured image. In this rat stomach model with ethanol-induced injury, mucosal lesions were seen to develop in areas where hemoglobin oxygen saturation decreased.

OBATA et al. (1989) studied video images of regenerating colonic mucosa in patients with ulcerative colitis. Images of mucosal blood vessels were processed from the gray level of the green color component. The number and pattern of vessels were quantified and compared over time. Some of the features so obtained correlated with the patients' clinical course.

TSUJII et al. (1989) used reflectance spectrophotometry and videoendoscopy to investigate colonic mucosal hemodynamics and tissue oxygenation in patients with ulcerative colitis. Calculated indices of mucosal blood volume and blood oxygenation were correlated with endoscopic and histological findings. In active disease, mucosal blood volume and blood oxygenation were significantly increased and decreased, respectively, compared to controls. The heterogeneous distribution of hemoglobin, seen especially at the margins of mucosal ulceration, was clearly shown in a computer-assisted color image of mucosal hemoglobin content.

VI. Videoenteroscopy

In the absence of fiberoptic imaging bundles, there is no constraint on an endoscope's insertion tube length. Dabezies et al. (1989) reported on examinations of six patients with a videoenteroscope, an instrument 400 cm long (43% longer than the fiberoptic enteroscope) used for viewing the jejunum and the ileum. A standard videoprocessor/light source was used. It is not clear that the additional length of the videoenteroscope (i.e., compared to the fiberoptic enteroscope) offered any advantage, as the ileum was reached in only half the patients; however, the same benefits of image recording and processing would have applied.

E. The Future

The advent of electronic imaging has vastly improved many of the technical aspects of performing gastrointestinal endoscopy, and of storing, retrieving, and even manipulating images. But the greatest potential benefit of this new technology will be its contribution to patient care, to improving endoscopic diagnosis and treatment. What are some of the ways in which this might occur?

With the exception of a few examples previously described, the only endoscopic information used currently is that which is visible to the human eye. Visible light, however, is only a small part of the electromagnetic spectrum which also includes ultraviolet and x-rays (shorter wavelengths) and infrared and radiowaves (longer wavelengths). The range of the CCD as a detector of electromagnetic radiation is much broader than that of the human eye or even photographic film. (An example: light from an Nd:YAG laser that is invisible to humans is detected by the CCD and has required that special coatings be applied to tips of videoendoscopes used for laser work to avoid overwhelming the detector.) Silicon and CCDs, which are not uniformly sensitive to all wavelengths of light, can be modified to detect specific ranges of wavelengths by applying special optical coatings or adding to the silicon small amounts of impurities, such as antimony, which "focuses" on far infrared. Several detectors of different infrared ranges can be sandwiched together, effectively providing several pixel arrays, each specific for certain wavelengths (Sivak 1988a).

Fiberscope light sources filter out most infrared light because the thermal component of infrared light can damage fibers. Videoscopes, unrestricted by this problem, could be applied, for example, to infrared reflectance spectroscopy. Human (and other) tissues, when stimulated with specific wavelengths, have characteristic reflectance spectra. Laser-induced fluorescent spectroscopy is under investigation as a tool for distinguishing normal and neoplastic human colonic mucosa (YAKSHE et al. 1989; PETRAS et al. 1989). CCDs might be ideally suited for spectroscopic imaging of the gastrointestinal tract.

Perhaps subtle mucosal changes could be made conspicuous by combining different specific wavelengths of illumination with different chromoscopic techniques using dyes injected intravenously or sprayed topically. SILVERSTEIN (1988) has speculated about other applications of digital technology, such as digital subtraction endoscopic angiography, in which dye-dependent detection of gastric mucosal vasculature, using wavelengths visible to the CCD but not the eye, might be enhanced by subtracting a control image of the mucosa obtained before the dye was injected.

If infrared spectral imaging analysis of reflectance, video image enhancement, and measurement of mucosal blood flow could be refined to identify – specifically and reproducibly – features such as textural and vascular change, there would be extraordinary potential for diagnosis of many lesions: dysplasia or carcinoma in Barrett's esophagus, gastritis or early gastric cancer, mucosal ischemia, dysplasia or carcinoma in ulcerative colitis, or early polyps. So-called intelligent endoscopes might be able to indicate what areas should be biopsied, especially when coupled with endoscopic ultrasound probes. Further, a sophisticated system incorporating image processing might automatically and selectively direct therapy, such as laser ablation of tumors, to areas it determines to be malignant or premalignant. The autofocusing of laser beams has already been proven in coronary angioplasty (BAILLIE 1989).

Simulation programs could be used for teaching endoscopy technique. As CCD architecture and lens–chip matching improve, it may become feasible to mount two chips on an endoscope tip to generate true three-dimensional images (BAILLIE et al. 1989). Higher definition television monitors (i.e., with more pixels) and CCDs with smaller sensing elements could combine to produce images of extraordinarily fine resolution.

References

Baillie J (1989) Computer simulation of endoscopy and the intelligent endoscope. ASGE Midyear Course Syllabus, Boston

Baillie J, Anderson NC, Cotton PB (1989) Three dimensional stereoscopic imaging of the gut: a new tool for endoscopic training by simulation (Abstr). Gastrointest Endosc 35:177

Benjamin SB (1989) The research applications of videoendoscopy. ASGE Midyear Course Syllabus, Boston

Benjamin SB, Fleischer DE (1988) Videoendoscopy – a fluke or the future? Contemp Gastroenterol 1:39–43

Classen M, Phillip J (1984) Electronic endoscopy of the gastrointestinal tract: initial experience with a new type of endoscope that has no fiberoptic bundle for imaging. Endoscopy 16:16–19

Classen M, Knyrim K, Seidlitz HK, Hagenmuller F (1987). Electronic endoscopy – the latest technology. Endoscopy 19:118–123

Committee on Planetary Biology (1986) Remote sensing of the biosphere. National Academy Press, Washington

Dabezies MA, Fisher RS, Krevsky B (1989) Preliminary experience with a video small bowel endoscope (Abstr). Gastrointest Endosc 35:179

DeDombal FT (1988) Endoscopists, computers and the man on the Micklefield train (Editorial). Endoscopy 20:66–69

Demling L, Hagel HJ (1985) Videoendoscopy, fundamentals and problems (Editorial). Endoscopy 17:167–169

DeReuck M, DeKoster E (1988) Comparing the diagnostic accuracy of live and recorded electronic videoendoscopy and fiberoptic endoscopy (Letter). Gastrointest Endosc 34:77

Graham DY, Smith JL, Schwartz JT (1986) Endoscopic television: traditional and video endoscopy (Editorial). Gastrointest Endosc 32:49–51

Hatada Y, Iwane S, Sano M, Munakata A, Yoshida Y (1989) Study of a new method to measure the size of lesions using electronic endoscope and image processor (Abstr). Gastrointest Endosc 35:180

Hirschowitz BI, Curtiss LE, Peters CW, Pollard HM (1958) Demonstration of a new gastroscope, the "fiberscope." Gastroenterology 35:50–53

Kashimura H, Nakahara A, Tsushima K, Hara K, Fukutomi H, Oosuga T (1989) Imaging of the gastric mucosal hemodynamics by digital processing of videoendoscopic view (Abstr). Gastroenterology 96:A250

Knyrim K, Seidlitz HK, Hagenmuller F, Classen M (1987a) Color performance of videoendoscopes: quantitative measurement of color reproduction. Endoscopy 19:233–236

Knyrim K, Seidlitz HK, Hagenmuller F, Classen M (1987b) Videoendoscopes in comparison with fiberscopes: quantitative measurement of optical resolution. Endoscopy 19:156–159

Knyrim K, Seidlitz H, Vakil N, Hagenmuller F, Classen M (1989a) Optical performance of electronic imaging systems for the colon. Gastroenterology 96:776–782

Knyrim K, Vakil N, Seidlitz H, Classen M (1989b) Resolution measurements with a new generation of electronic gastroscopes (Abstr). Gastroenterology 96:A261

Kohso H, Tatsumi Y, Fujino H, Kodama T (1989) Infrared electronic endoscope with rapid intravenous injection of indocyanine green (Abstr). Gastroenterology 96:A265

Korman LY, Nardi RV, Overholt BF (1988) Quantitative analysis of endoscopic images: ulcer area measurement using computer-based image morphometry (Abstr). Gastroenterology 94:A236

Kurosaka H, Oohara T, Andoh T (1985) Objective automatic evaluation of endoscopic images by a real time image analyzer. Gastrointest Endosc 31:395–396

Kuwayama H, Kohashi E, Ikeda Y, Furukawa M, Takeuchi K, Tashiro Y, Matano Y, Kurihara R (1987) Filing and transmittance of electronic endoscopy data (Abstr). Gastrointest Endosc 33:174

Leung FW (1988) Endoscopic measurement of human gastric mucosal blood flow by hydrogen gas clearance (Abstr). Gastrointest Endosc 34:206

Leung FW, Slodownik E, Jensen DM, van Deventer GM, Guth PH (1987) Gastroduodenal mucosal hemodynamics by endoscopic reflectance spectrophotometry. Gastrointest Endosc 33:284–288

Lux G, Knyrim K, Scheubel R, Classen M (1986) Electronic endoscopy – fibres or chips? Z Gastroenterol 24:337–343

Matek W, Lux G, Riemann JF, Demling L (1984) Initial experience with the new electronic endoscope. Endoscopy 16:20–21

McWhorter JH, Schneir E, Roe DC, Springer DL (1986) The use of glass filters to minimize the decrease in sensitivity while viewing through endoscopes (Letter). Gastrointest Endosc 32:306–307
Morrissey JF (1984) Thoughts on the Video Endoscope (TM) (Editorial). Gastrointest Endosc 30:43
Nardi, RV, Overholt BF, Benjamin S, Fleischer D, Zimmon D, Korman L (1988) Quantitative endoscopy: morphometric analysis of gastrointestinal lesions (Abstr). Gastroenterology 94:A321
Noble JA (1989) Computer applications in endoscopy. ASGE Midyear Course Syllabus, Boston
Obata A, Kitano A, Okawa K, Matsumoto T, Oshitani N, Kobayashi K (1989) Computer analysis of video-image of blood vessels in regenerating colonic mucosa (Abstr). Gastroenterology 96:A370
Okabe H, Ohida M, Okada N, Mitsuhashi T, Katsumata T, Saigengi K, Nakahashi K (1986) A new disk method for the endoscopic determination of gastric ulcer area. Gastrointest Endosc 32:20–24
Okano H, Kodama T, Takino T (1988) Development of an clinical experience with a new TV monitoring system in electronic endoscopy. Endoscopy 20:45–47
Overholt BF, Sudman T (1985) Endoscopic image reproduction: Computer digital system (Abstr). Am J Gastroenterol 80:868
Overholt BF, DeNovo EC, Nardi RV (1989) Kinetic analysis of ulcer re-epithelialization in a canine gastric ulcer healing model (Abstr). Gastrointest Endosc 35:156
Petras RE, Richards-Kortum R, Tong L, Fitzmaurice M, Feld M, Sivak M (1989) Fluorescence spectroscopy of colonic adenomas: implications for an endoscopic laser diagnostics system. Gastrointest Endosc 35:181
Petrini JL Jr (1987) Video endoscopy. In: Sivak MV Jr (ed) Gastroenterologic endoscopy. Saunders, Philadelphia, pp 253–269
Rey JF, Albuisson M, Greff M, Bidart JM, Mouget JM (1988) Electronic video-endoscopy: preliminary results of imaging modification. Endoscopy 20:8–10
Satava RM (1986) Comments on endoscopic TV editorial (Letter). Gastrointest Endosc 32:368–369
Satava RM (1987) A comparison of direct and indirect videoendoscopy. Gastrointest Endosc 33:69–72
Satava RM, Poe W, Joyce G (1988) Current generation videoendoscopes – a critical evaluation. Am Surg 54:73–77
Schapiro M, Auslander MO, Schapiro MB (1987) The electronic videoendoscope: clinical experience with 1200 diagnostic and therapeutic cases in the community hospital. Gastrointest Endosc 33:63–68
Schroy PC, Wiggins T, Winawer SJ, Diaz B, Lightdale CJ (1988) Videoendoscopy by nurse practitioners: a model for colorectal cancer screening. Gastrointest Endosc 34:390–394
Seidlitz H, Knyrim K, Vakil N, Classen M (1989) Mechanism of distorted perception in the red color range with electronic endoscopes (Abstr). Gastroenterology 96:A460
Silverstein FE (1988) The future of videoendoscopy (Editorial). Gastrointest Endosc 34:361–362
Sivak M, Skipper G, Turinic W, Petrini J (1987) Endoscopic image enhancement using a videoendoscope and computer (Abstr). Gastrointest Endosc 33:178
Sivak MV (1986) Video endoscopy. Clin Gastroenterol 15:207–234
Sivak MV Jr (1988a) Videoendoscopy. Digestive Disease Week Syllabus, Washington
Sivak MV (1988b) Videoendoscopy. In: Cotton PB, Tytgat GNJ, Williams CB (eds) Annual of gastrointestinal endoscopy 1988. Gower, London, pp 115–125
Sivak MV Jr (1989) Endoscopic documentation: overview. In: Cotton PB, Tytgat GNJ, Williams CB (eds) Annual of gastrointestinal endoscopy 1989. Current Science, London, pp 149–157
Sivak MV Jr, Fleischer DE (1984a) Colonoscopy with a Video Endoscope (TM): preliminary experience. Gastrointest Endosc 30:1–5

Sivak MV Jr, Fleischer DE (1984b) Reply to Dr. Morrissey's editorial on the Video Endoscope (TM) (Letter). Gastrointest Endosc 30:271

Tsuji S, Sato N, Kawano S, Kamada T (1988) Functional imaging for the analysis of the mucosal blood hemoglobin distribution using electronic endoscopy. Gastrointest Endosc 34:332–335

Tsuji S, Sato N, Kawano S, Hayashi N, Tsujii M, Kamada T (1989) Evaluation of oxygen metabolism in digestive organs using computer-assisted electronic endoscopy (Abstr). Gastroenterology 96:A517

Tsujii M, Ogihara T, Kawano S, Sato N, Kamada T (1989) Colonic mucosal hemodynamics in patients with ulcerative colitis (Abstr). Gastroenterology 96:A517

Williams CB (1989) Endoscopic instrumentation. In: Cotton PB, Tytgat GNJ, Williams CB (eds) Annual of gastrointestinal endoscopy 1989. Current Science, London, pp 143–148

Yakshe PN, Bonner RF, Patterson R, Leon MB, Fleischer DE (1989) Laser-induced fluorescence spectroscopy (LIFS): can it be used in the diagnosis and treatment of colonic malignancy? (Abstract). Am J Gastroenterol 84:1199

Yamaguchi M, Okazaki Y, Yanai H, Takemoto T (1988) Three dimensional determination of gastric ulcer size with laser endoscopy. Endoscopy 20:263–266

Subject Index

Handbook of Experimental Pharmacology

Volume 56
Cardiac Glycosides

Part 1: **Experimental Pharmacology**

Part 2: **Pharmacokinetics and Clinical Pharmacology**

Volume 57
Tissue Growth Factors

Volume 58
Cyclic Nucleotides

Part 1: **Biochemistry**

Part 2: **Physiology and Pharmacology**

Volume 59
Mediators and Drugs in Gastrointestinal Motility

Part 1: **Morphological Basis and Neurophysiological Control**

Part 2: **Endogenous and Exogenous Agents**

Volume 60
Pyretics and Antipyretics

Volume 61
Chemotherapy of Viral Infections

Volume 62
Aminoglycoside Antibiotics

Volume 63
Allergic Reactions to Drugs

Volume 64
Inhibition of Folate Metabolism in Chemotherapy

Volume 65
Teratogenesis and Reproductive Toxicology

Volume 66
Part 1: **Glucagon I**

Part 2: **Glucagon II**

Volume 67
Part 1: **Antibiotics Containing the Beta-Lactam Structure I**

Part 2: **Antibiotics Containing the Beta-Lactam Structure II**

Volume 68
Antimalarial Drugs

Part 1: **Biological Background, Experimental Methods and Drug Resistance**

Part 2: **Current Antimalarias and New Drug Developments**

Volume 69
Pharmacology of the Eye

Volume 70
Part 1: **Pharmacology of Intestinal Permeation I**

Part 2: **Pharmacology of Intestinal Permeation II**

Volume 71
Interferons and Their Applications

Volume 72
Antitumor Drug Resistance

Volume 73
Radiocontrast Agents

Volume 74
Antieliptic Drugs

Volume 75
Toxicology of Inhaled Materials

Volume 76
Clinical Pharmacology of Antiangial Drugs

Springer-Verlag
Berlin
Heidelberg
New York
London
Paris
Tokyo
Hong Kong
Barcelona
Budapest

Handbook of Experimental Pharmacology

Editorial Board: G. V. R. Born, P. Cuatrecasas, H. Herken

Volume 77
Chemotherapy of Gastrointestinal Helminths

Volume 78
The Tetracyclines

Volume 79
New Neuromuscular Blocking Agents

Volume 80
Cadmium

Volume 81
Local Anesthetics

Volume 82
Radioimmunoassay in Basic and Clinical Pharmacology

Volume 83
Calcium in Drug Actions

Volume 84
Antituberculosis Drugs

Volume 85
The Pharmacology of Lymphocytes

Volume 86
The Cholinergic Synapse

Volume 87
Part 1: **Pharmacology of the Skin I**
Part 2: **Pharmacology of the Skin II**

Volume 88
Drugs for the Treatment of Parkinson's Disease

Volume 89
Antiarrhythmic Drugs

Volume 90
Part 1: **Catecholamines I**
Part 2: **Catecholamines II**

Volume 91
Microbial Resistance to Drugs

Volume 92
Insulin

Volume 93
Pharmacology of Antihypertensive Therapeutics

Volume 94
Part 1: **Chemical Carcinogenesis and Mutagenesis I**
Part 2: **Chemical Carcinogenesis and Mutagenesis II**

Volume 95
Part 1: **Peptide Growth Factors and Their Receptors I**
Part 2: **Peptide Growth Factors and Their Receptors II**

Volume 96
Chemotherapy of Fungal Diseases

Volume 97
Histamine and Histamine Antagonists

Volume 98
Pharmacology of Asthma

Volume 99
Pharmacology of Peptic Ulcer Disease

Volume 100
Targeted Drug Delivery

Springer-Verlag
Berlin
Heidelberg
New York
London
Paris
Tokyo
Hong Kong
Barcelona
Budapest

MIX
Papier aus verantwortungsvollen Quellen
Paper from responsible sources
FSC® C105338

If you have any concerns about our products,
you can contact us on
ProductSafety@springernature.com

In case Publisher is established outside the EU,
the EU authorized representative is:
Springer Nature Customer Service Center GmbH
Europaplatz 3, 69115 Heidelberg, Germany

Printed by Libri Plureos GmbH
in Hamburg, Germany